HERPESVIRIDAE – A LOOK INTO THIS UNIQUE FAMILY OF VIRUSES

Edited by **George D. Magel** and **Stephen Tyring**

Herpesviridae – A Look into This Unique Family of Viruses
Edited by George D. Magel and Stephen Tyring

Published by InTech
Janeza Trdine 9, 51000 Rijeka, Croatia

Publishing Process Manager Ivona Lovric

Technical Editor Teodora Smiljanic

Cover Designer InTech Design Team

Additional hard copies can be obtained from orders@intechopen.com

Herpesviridae – A Look into This Unique Family of Viruses,
Edited by George D. Magel and Stephen Tyring
p. cm.
978-953-51-0186-4

For EU product safety concerns:
IN TECH d.o.o., Prolaz Marije Krucifikse Kozulić 3, 51000 Rijeka, Croatia,
info@intechopen.com or visit our website at intechopen.com.

Meet the editors

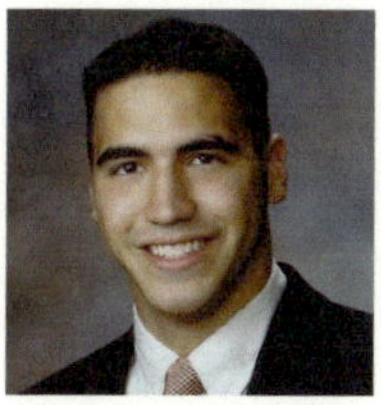

George D. Magel, M.D., is currently a clinical research fellow at the Indiana University School of Medicine Department of Dermatology in Indianapolis, Indiana, and will be completing his dermatology residency there in 2015. His work over the last two years includes several trials dealing with psoriasis, psoriatic arthritis, non-melanoma skin cancer, HPV infection, postherpetic neuralgia, HSV infection, herpes zoster infection, and eczema. His work has led to the approval of various medications, indicated for psoriasis, psoriatic arthritis, and HSV infections and the development of novel techniques to treat non-melanoma skin cancer. Over the last two years, he has published numerous peer-reviewed articles and book chapters in the field of dermatology and has presented his work at several meetings, including the Texas Dermatological Society Meeting and the American Academy of Dermatology Annual Meeting.

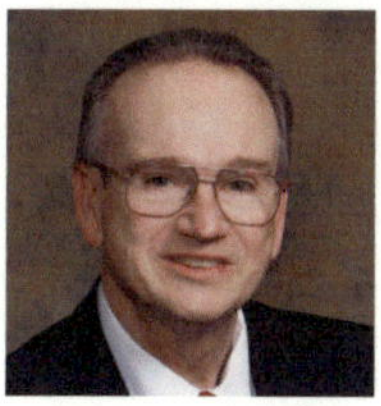

Dr Stephen Tyring is a Clinical Professor in the Departments of Dermatology, Microbiology/Molecular Genetics and Internal Medicine at the University of Texas Health Science Center at Houston. He is board certified by the American Academy of Dermatology (AAD), and is a member of the Infectious Disease Society of America, as well as the American Federation for Clinical Research. Dr Tyring sits on several editorial boards and serves as a reviewer for a number of journals. He is the author of over 600 journal articles and book chapters as well as eight books. Dr Tyring received his undergraduate degree from Indiana State University, his Master's Degree from Abilene Christian University, his medical degree from the University of Texas Medical Branch, his doctorate from Texas Tech University and his MBA from Rice University.

Contents

Preface

In order to fully understand the nature of viruses, it is important to look at them from both, their basic science and clinical, standpoints. Our goal with this book was to dissect Herpesviridae into its biological properties and clinical significance in order to provide a logical, as well as practical, approach to understanding and treating the various conditions caused by this unique family of viruses. In addition to their up-to-date and extensive text, each chapter is laced with a variety of diagrams, tables, charts, and images, aimed at helping us achieve our goal. We hope that this book will serve as a reference tool for clinicians of various specialties worldwide.

We want to thank the numerous authors from across the world who contributed to this book. *Herpesviridae - A Look Into This Unique Family of Viruses* is a collaboration of their experiences, expertise, and research. It truly was an honor and pleasure working with them.

George D. Magel, M.D.
Indiana University School of Medicine, Department of Dermatology,
Indianapolis, Indiana
USA

Stephen K. Tyring, M.D., Ph.D.
Department of Dermatology, University of Texas Health Science Center,
Houston, Texas,
USA

Part 1

Genome and Biological Properties

1

Interferon, the Cell Cycle and Herpesvirus

H. Costa, S. Correia, R. Nascimento and R.M.E. Parkhouse
Instituto Gulbenkian de Ciência
Portugal

1. Introduction

Herpesviruses are a large group of successful, and widely distributed, double-stranded DNA viruses of serious medical and veterinary importance. Although they infect many different animal species, they are host specific at the individual species level. On the other hand, they share a common life style, first with an acute infection in epithelial cells which is followed by the establishment of persistence in neurons (α-herpesvirus), monocytes (β-herpesvirus), or B lymphocytes (γ-herpesvirus). The varied pathology of these different groups of herpesvirus is typically associated with reactivation of a persistent infection and the subsequent production of virus. Thus, the immune system faces three distinct challenges: how to control the acute phase, the persistent virus, and the consequences of reactivation. For this reason, control of herpesvirus infection calls on the many functional arms of both the innate and adaptive immune systems, which in turn have exerted the selection pressure that has driven the evolution of many strategies of immune evasion. This chapter will focus on herpesviruses host evasion genes manipulating cell cycle progression and interferon.

All members of order *Herpesvirales* have a biphasic infection cycle consisting of replicative (lytic) and latent phases. During the lytic cycle and viral reactivation, most of the viral genes are expressed in a cascade manner and large numbers of infectious virus particles are released. Latency, on the other hand, is characterized by limited gene expression, lack of virion production and, in the case of γ-herpesviruses, is associated with immortalization and transformation of infected cells. Virus survival at each phase depends on evasion of the host immune response. Thus, the escape from immune detection in the early phases of infection may be almost as important as in the latent phase (Vider-Shalit *et al.*, 2007). The typical herpesvirus life cycle is a challenge for the development of a global antiviral therapy or protective vaccines. Although all herpesviruses present a similar lytic phase and are able to establish latency in a specific set of cells, the cell types in which they remain latent, and thus have evolved virus host cell evasion molecular mechanisms, differ widely from one virus to another (Pellet & Roizman, 2007). One promising approach is to explore new viral targets, particularly viral proteins involved in host immune evasion. An effective herpesvirus vaccine would therefore be a genetically targeted mutant with one or more non-immunogenic host evasion genes deleted, and with appropriate investigation of the pathogenesis to ensure safety.

Bioinformatic analysis of putative homologues showed that 39 conserved herpesvirus protein families and 20 single proteins had significant sequence similarity to human gene products, with 54% of them being involved in host-virus interaction, particularly control of apoptosis and immune response (Holzerlandt *et al.*, 2002). There are, however, evasion proteins encoded by genes without sequence homology to cellular genes. In these cases, the viral protein function can only be accessed by functional assays or sophisticated structural assays, such as x-ray crystallography (Cooray *et al.*, 2007). Virus proteins without sequence homology with cellular genes can still be functional homologues of cellular proteins. One interesting example is the HSV-1 US3, a viral protein kinase, that has no sequence homology to the cellular kinase Akt, yet it is able to phosphorylate tuberous sclerosis complex 2 (TSC2) on S939 and T1462, the same sites targeted by cellular Akt to inhibit TSC activity and activate mTORC1 in uninfected cells. This strategy allows the virus to bypass the strict limits normally imposed on the cellular Akt, promoting mTORC1 activation even when Akt activity is low or undetectable, as may be the case in non-proliferating cells (Chuluunbaatar *et al.*, 2010).

Virus host evasion strategies conserved in all herpesviruses are likely to manipulate conserved cellular pathways that are regulated by all herpesviruses. Others, on the other hand, may be restricted to one subfamily or species, with a function related to a more restricted specific aspect of the virus life cycle, particularly during latency. While the latter can be explored for the development of a specific herpesvirus therapy, functional studies of herpesvirus homologous protein families are advantageous for a global herpesvirus treatment.

Herpesviruses have evolved a wide repertoire of host evasion genes that impact on many components of the immune response, such as antigen presentation, autophagy, and apoptosis, which have been extensively reviewed and are not included in this chapter. Here, we focus on two virus proteins conserved in all herpesviruses, ORF36 and UL24. The first contains a conserved kinase domain with cellular homology, while UL24 is an unassigned gene with no cellular homolog. Their roles in manipulating interferon and the cell cycle have been the focus of our laboratory and will be described in detail.

2. The immune response to viruses

The immune system is an astoundingly resourceful defence system which has evolved to protect animals from external and internal threats, that is, invading pathogens and tissue damage, respectively. It is able to generate a number of different cells, secreted effector molecules and intracellular mechanisms that act independently and together. This wide variety of possible responses reflects the equally wide variety of extracellular and intracellular threats and life-styles. As a necessary correlate, the immune system must distinguish between pathogen molecules ("non self") and its own cells and proteins ("self"), and also select and apply the most "appropriate" immune effector mechanism.

Following the elimination of the pathogen, it is equally important to switch off the selected immune effector mechanisms. Failure at either the level of self-non-self discrimination, or appropriate regulation of immune responses, can lead to non-infectious diseases - for example, autoimmune and inflammatory diseases. As pathogens have evolved many mechanisms to manipulate the immune system, however, these provide "ready-made tools" for the development of novel therapeutic approaches; for example, viruses have evolved a variety of mechanisms to inhibit the inflammatory response.

The immune response against virus infections can be divided into innate and adaptive defence components. The innate immune response is the first line of defence as it is always present and rapidly activated in a normal host upon exposure to the invading virus. Many viral infections are resolved by the innate immune system before intervention by the

adaptive immune system, which is the second-line of defence to be mobilized. This adaptive response comprises the antibody response and the lymphocyte cell-mediated response, usually called humoral and cell-mediated immune responses, respectively (Flint, 2004). A successful immune response to an infection must be appropriately selected and regulated, as inefficient or inappropriate regulation can fail to eliminate the invader and/or cause disease. Viruses, in particular, have evolved multiple strategies to down-regulate, or terminate, immune responses, and thus provide enormous potential as source of strategies for immunomodulation, as indicated above.
This section will focus on virus manipulation of innate immunity, particularly the interferon system.

2.1 Innate immunity

Innate immunity is the most immediate line of response to pathogens, which needs to be potent and rapid, and functions to eliminate and prevent the spread of the pathogen prior to the subsequent action of the adaptive immune response. However, it must also be transient because its continued activity can damage the host. Importantly, innate immunity also shapes and regulates the subsequent adaptive immune response as a result of the combined influence of antigen presentation and the secreted cytokine/chemokine profile. Among these secreted effectors, interferon is absolutely essential for virus immunity.
Viruses are recognised as foreign, and thus potentially dangerous, by a limited number of germline-encoded host pattern-recognition receptors (PRRs), which recognize viral pathogen-associated molecular patterns (PAMPs). As PAMPS are highly conserved structures, the corresponding PRRs are also conserved. Of particular interest for virus infection is the TLR3 molecule that interacts with double-stranded RNA of viral origin. There is, in addition, TLR7/8 and TLR9 which also localise to endosomes and recognise viral DNA. Cells also recognise viruses in their cytoplasm through the retinoic acid-inducible gene I (RIG-I)-like helicases (RLHs), consisting of RIG-I and the melanoma differentiation-associated gene-5 (MDA5), that recognise viral RNA. Other sensors such as DAI or IFI16 detect viral DNA. These molecules initiate similar signalling transduction pathways which also results in the production of type I IFN and pro-inflammatory cytokines (Takeuchi & Akira, 2007). Pro-inflammatory cytokines can also be induced independently of IFN, by activation of the inflammasome which also has specific sensors localised both in endosomes and in the cytoplasm.

2.2 The interferon system

The interferons constitute three groups of cytokines (type I, II, and III) with overlapping, specific and redundant activities, and plays a major role in virus immunity. They are secreted by a variety of cell types as a result of disparate pathogen molecular signals, which in turn activate similarly overlapping, specific, and redundant intracellular signalling pathways. The complexity of the system has presumably evolved together with the co-evolution of virus mechanisms for its subversion. Thus, in order to discuss virus strategies for the manipulation of the interferon system, we must first describe its essentials in some detail.
Interferons control a variety of biological functions, including modulation of the immune system, regulation of apoptosis, inhibition of proliferation, induction of differentiation, and inhibition of angiogenesis. The importance of the interferon response against viral infections has been dramatised by demonstrating increased susceptibility to virus infection

of mice deficient for different components of the IFN system (Arnheiter *et al.*, 1996; Chee *et al.*, 2003; Haller *et al.*, 1981; Hefti *et al.*, 1999).

2.2.1 Induction of IFN expression

Four major families of PRRs with relevance for IFN have been identified: Toll-like receptors (TLRs), RIG-I-like receptors, NOD-like receptors, and C-type lectin receptors. Recently, several cytosolic nucleic acid sensors have also been found, such as DAI, AIM-2, RNA polymerase III and LRRFIP1. The PRRs detect pathogens invading from different routes through their differential localization in distinct subcellular compartments, such as the cell surface, endosome, and cytoplasm. Upon recognition of the pathogen, PRRs trigger major downstream signalling pathways, involving NF-κB, MAPK, and/or IRF3/7, to induce the production of inflammatory cytokines and/or type I interferons (IFNs), thereby leading to antimicrobial immune responses.

2.2.2 Transcriptional control of IFN expression

Although, as described above, there are different routes to initiate transcription of IFN type I, the downstream kinases and transcription factors are common to all. The induction of Type I IFN is primarily regulated at the level of transcription, with the IFN regulatory factors (IRFs) IRF-1, IRF-3, IRF-5 and IRF-7 and NF-κB having major roles (Barnes *et al.*, 2001; Watanabe *et al.*, 1991; Wathelet *et al.*, 1998).

Transcription of the IFN-β gene involves the formation of a large, multi-subunit complex called the "enhanceosome". It comprises the promoter-specific transcription factors, associated structural elements, and basal transcriptional machinery to enhance gene expression. The promoter enhancer region is composed of four positive regulatory regions (PRDI-IV) (Hiscott *et al.*, 2006). The PRDI and PRDIII sequences contain sites for binding of IRF-3 and IRF-7, the PRDII site binds NF-κB heterodimers, while PRDIV binds ATF-2 and c-Jun heterodimers. Upon binding to the promoter region by the different activated transcription factors, and the high-mobility group (HMG) chromatin-associated protein HMGI(Y), the complete transcriptional machinery of the enhanceosome is formed by the additional recruitment of CBP/p300 (Honda *et al.*, 2006).

The induction of IFN-α expression is less well understood. Its promoter region contains binding sites for IRFs but lacks binding sites for NF-κB. Although the identity of the IRF member that stimulates IFN-α is uncertain, there is some evidence that IRF-7 is required for induction; for example, in fibroblast cells there is no primary induction of IFN-α gene, as IRF-7 gene expression is dependent on feedback induction by IFN-β. On the other hand, with regards to plasmocytoid DCs, which constitutively express IRF-7 and induce the expression of massive amounts of IFN type I, the induction of IFN-α is not dependent on the primary induction of IFN-β and its feedback loop (Lin *et al.*, 2000; Marie *et al.*, 1998).

The induction of type II interferon secretion is restricted to a small group of cells, with NK cells and CD8 T cells being the main source of IFN-γ. However, other cell types, such as macrophages and DCs, have also been reported to produce type II IFN under specific conditions (Darwich *et al.*, 2009).

2.2.3 Signalling responses to IFN

As secreted factors, type I IFNs regulate a range of immune responses through binding to the type I IFN receptor, composed of two subunits, IFN-α receptor 1 (IFNAR1) and IFNAR2.

Upon interferon binding, the two subunits of the receptor associate and facilitate the activation of Tyk2 and Jak1. The phosphorylation of the IFNAR1 by Tyk2 creates a docking site for STAT2 and its subsequent phosphorylation by Tyk2, while Jak1 phosphorylates STAT1 (Colamonici *et al.*, 1994; Novick *et al.*, 1994; Shuai *et al.*, 1993). The activated STATs dissociate from the receptor forming a stable heterodimer and associate with p48 (also known as IRF-9), forming the ISGF3 multimeric complex that translocates to the nucleus and binds to IFN-stimulated response elements (ISRE) present in the promoter region of IFN-stimulated genes (ISGs) (Mogensen *et al.*, 1999; Stark *et al.*, 1998). Until recently, the assembly of the ISGF3 complex was thought to be in the nucleus. However it has been recently shown that it is IFNAR2 that forms a docking site for p48 which, together with STAT1 and STAT2, then becomes acetylated (Tang *et al.*, 2007). The transcriptional co-factor CREB-binding protein (CBP) is a mediator for these acetylation reactions, implying that acetylation plays a major role in the signal transduction pathway activated by the receptors (Tang *et al.*, 2007).

The Type II IFN receptor also consists of two subunits: the IFNGR1 that associates with Jak1, and the IFNGR2, which constitutively associates with Jak2. Binding of IFN-γ to the receptor leads to its dimerization, which brings Jak1 and Jak2 into close proximity, resulting in the activation of Jak2 and trans-phosphorylation of Jak1. Activated Jaks phosphorylate the C-terminus of IFNGR1 which creates a pair of binding sites for STAT1, which are then phosphorylated and dissociate from the receptor. The STAT1 homodimer translocates to the nucleus and binds to unique elements of IFN-γ stimulated genes, the gamma-activation sequence (GAS), and stimulates transcription. Of note is the fact that type I IFN stimulation is also able to form STAT1-homodimers and leads to the induction of genes containing GAS elements in their promoter region (Bach *et al.*, 1997; Stark *et al.*, 1998). The Jak-Stat pathway plays an important role in the response to IFN and in mounting an effective and rapid anti-viral response through the induction of ISGs. The subsequent decay of the response requires negative regulators of STAT signalling, which include cytoplasmic tyrosine phosphatases, nuclear and cytoplasmic regulators and truncated forms of STAT proteins.

2.2.4 IFN-induced antiviral state

One of the major functions of interferon is the induction of an anti-viral state in cells infected by viruses. The anti-viral state is characterized by the expression of genes that are induced by interferon in order to limit virus replication and subsequent spread to neighbouring cells. The interferon stimulated genes (ISGs) are crucial components of the interferon responses as they set up the antiviral, antiproliferative and immunoregulatory state in the host cells. The best-characterized IFN inducible components that have been already reviewed are the enzymes dsRNA-dependent protein kinase (PKR), 2′,5′-oligoadenylate synthetase (2′5′OAS), and Mx proteins (Garcia *et al.*, 2006; Haller *et al.*, 2007; Silverman, 2007). Other proteins that are induced and play important roles in the antiviral response are ISG15, ISG54 and ISG56, ISG20, PML, and TRIM.

2.3 Viral evasion of interferon responses

Whatever its lifestyle, a virus will always have appropriate and complementary strategies for evasion of host defences. The interferon system is a powerful and first line of defence against virus infections, and so it is not surprising that viruses have evolved multiple means of down-regulating IFN responses. These include inhibiting IFN production, inhibiting the

IFN-mediated signalling pathways, and blocking the action of IFN-induced enzymes with antiviral activity. Even within one of these strategies, viruses have evolved multiple molecular mechanisms to achieve the same result. During the past few years, much has been learned about the molecular mechanisms used by viruses to manipulate and escape the host interferon response. The exact strategy exploited by a virus will presumably depend on the biology of the host-virus interaction, and will be a major factor that will influence the pathogenesis of that virus infection (Randall & Goodbourn, 2008).

2.4 Herpesviruses evasion of the interferon system

As herpesviruses are known to trigger the induction of type I IFN during the primary infection of a cell (Ankel *et al.*, 1998; Boehme *et al.*, 2004; Mossman *et al.*, 2001), it is not surprising that an effective evasion of these initial type I IFN responses is essential for virus replication and establishment of latency.

The modulation of interferon responses by herpesviruses is already an extensive area of research, with several proteins already been described to inhibit IFN signalling, antagonizing IFN-initiated gene transcription, and target IRF-3 and IRF-7 activation. The multiplicity of these genes reflects the importance of diminishing IFN responses for virus survival. Understanding their strategies of evasion might lead to the development of new treatments or prevention strategies for diseases associated with these viruses.

The Kaposi's Sarcoma Herpesvirus (KSHV) is one of the examples of a herpesvirus modulating interferon responses. During primary infection, a decreased transcription of type I IFN genes and subsequent binding to the receptors has been demonstrated (Naranatt *et al.*, 2004). One of the candidate genes responsible for this evasion strategy is ORF45, which is a major component of the KSHV viral tegument, thus delivered into the host cells at the most early stages of infection (Zhu *et al.*, 2005; Zhu & Yuan, 2003). In addition, ORF45 has been found to inhibit the phosphorylation and nuclear translocation of IRF-7 (Zhu *et al.*, 2002). The combination of these two effects points to the ORF45 protein as a significant contributor in the antagonism of type I IFN in *de novo* KSHV infections.

During lytic reactivation, several KSHV proteins are also involved in evasion of IFN responses. The ORF10 (RIF) inhibitory function is not at the level of IFN induction but rather at the IFN signalling pathway, by forming complexes with several critical factors of the signalling pathway such as the type I IFN receptor subunits, the janus kinases and STAT2 (Bisson *et al.*, 2009). The multiple targeting of components of this signalling pathway ensures that the ISGF3 complex is not formed and does not translocate into the nucleus thus inhibiting the transcription of ISGs. The ORF50 protein functions as a transcription factor and is essential for KSHV reactivation from latency (Sun *et al.*, 1998). This viral protein targets IRF-7 for proteasomal degradation (Yu *et al.*, 2005), and more recently has been shown to mediate degradation of TRIF also by targeting it for proteasomal degradation (Ahmad *et al.*, 2011). The ORF K8 (K-bZIP) has been shown to inhibit IRF-3, but instead of direct interaction with the transcription factor, this viral protein binds efficiently to the PRDIII-I region of the IFN-β promoter, thus inhibiting the binding of the IRF-3-CBP/p300 complex (Lefort *et al.*, 2007). This strategy leads to inhibition of formation of a functional enhanceosome complex, thereby resulting in a defective transcription of IFN-β.

There are several IRF member homologues in KSHV. For example, the protein encoded by ORF K9 was described as the first viral member of the family, vIRF-1 (Moore *et al.*, 1996). The vIRF-1 protein interferes with the transactivation ability of both IRF-1 and IRF-3 by targeting a common transcriptional cofactor; CBP/p300 (Burysek *et al.*, 1999; Lin *et al.*, 2001). The vIRF2 is also an inhibitor of the expression of IFN inducible genes, which are regulated by IRF-1, IRF-3 and ISGF3, but not by IRF-7 (Fuld *et al.*, 2006). In addition, this viral protein also interacts with PKR and thereby prevents the antiviral effects mediated by PKR (Burysek & Pitha, 2001).

The KSHV has also evolved multiple strategies to avoid host immune responses during latency, including antagonizing type I IFN signaling pathways. Examples of these are the expression of latent proteins such as LANA, which inhibits function of IRF-3 (Cloutier & Flamand, 2010) and vIRF-3, which binds to IRF-7 (Joo *et al.*, 2007).

In the case of HCMV infection, the mechanisms for subversion of interferon have been extensively studied. However, only a small number of genes have been identified as being responsible for modulation of the interferon response. The immediate-early proteins of HCMV are the obvious candidates, as they are the first genes being expressed, and indeed, the IE72 protein has been shown to play a role in inhibiting the antiviral state by binding to promyelocytic leukemia (PML) protein and disrupting PML-associated nuclear bodies (NBs) leading to the displacement of PML-NB associated proteins such as PML, Sp100 and Daxx (Ahn *et al.*, 1998; Ahn & Hayward, 1997; Korioth *et al.*, 1996; Wilkinson *et al.*, 1998). In addition, IE72 also binds to Stat2, and to a lesser extent, to STAT1, thereby inhibiting the IFN signaling pathway (Huh *et al.*, 2008; Paulus *et al.*, 2006). The IE86 protein has been described as an inhibitor of IFN-β production by blocking NF-κB (Taylor & Bresnahan, 2005). On the other hand, UL83 has been also shown to inhibit IFN-β production, but in this case by inhibiting IRF-3 phosphorylation and translocation into the nucleus (Abate *et al.*, 2004). HCMV also encode two PKR antagonists, proteins IRS1 and TRS1 (Cassady, 2005; Hakki & Geballe, 2005). Recently, an HCMV protein without known function, ORF94, was identified as an inhibitor of OAS expression during infection, therefore limiting the induction of OAS-mediated antiviral response (Tan *et al.*, 2011).

In order to replicate and persist, the HSV-1 virus, like the above described herpesviruses, also elicits innate immune responses just after virus entry - for example, through activation of IRF-3 (Preston *et al.*, 2001). Such evasion strategies include the expression of genes that target the IRF-3 signaling pathway, thereby inhibiting the production of IFN type I, and interfering with the signaling through the receptors and inhibiting the anti-viral state. Examples of such early expressed HSV-1 evasion genes include ICP0 and ICP27 which already had a described function, but were subsequently found to also inhibit IRF-3 accumulation in the nucleus (Eidson *et al.*, 2002; Melroe *et al.*, 2004), and to inhibit STAT1 phosphorylation and its subsequent translocation to the nucleus (Johnson & Knipe, 2010; Johnson *et al.*, 2008), respectively. Another HSV-1 protein, ICP34.5, was identified as playing a role in the PKR signaling pathway due to its sequence homology with mouse MyD116 (He *et al.*, 1998; He *et al.*, 1997). More recently, ICP34.5 has been found to form a complex with TBK1, thereby disrupting the interaction between TBK1 and IRF-3 (Verpooten *et al.*, 2009). Finally, US11 and UL41 have been shown to: bind to PKR (Cassady *et al.*, 1998), to block the activation of OAS (Sanchez & Mohr, 2007); and to mediate the degradation of cellular proteins such as ISGs (Kwong & Frenkel, 1989; Matis & Kudelova, 2001; Paladino & Mossman, 2009).

2.5 The herpesviruses viral protein kinases family

All of the α-, β- and γ-herpesviruses genomes contain several genes that are conserved between families. One of these is the protein kinase family, which includes ORF36 from KSHV, UL13 from HSV, BGLF4 from Epstein-Barr virus, and UL97 from HCMV.

Conservation of these viral protein kinase domains among the herpesviruses suggests that they are indispensable for survival of herpesviruses. The HCMV UL97 protein was the first to be defined and described as a protein that phosphorylates the antiviral nucleoside analogue ganciclovir, and therefore, could be a useful tool in the understanding of the antiviral activity of new selective anti-HCMV compounds (Littler *et al.*, 1992). Subsequently, other groups demonstrated that UL97 is an auto-phosphorylating serine-threonine kinase (He *et al.*, 1997). Along with a conserved role, these individual kinases may have unique functions in the context of viral infection. For example, the inhibition of the activity of HCMV UL97 protein kinase by a number of compounds that exhibit a pronounced antiviral effect is not shared by other protein kinases, such as BGLF4, illustrating the fact that low homology between the members of this group complicates the design of compounds able to target all herpesviruses, and suggesting that structure-based inhibitor designed for each group of herpesviruses might be more effective. On the other hand, Cyclopropavir (CPV), with a mechanism of action similar to ganciclovir, is active against HCMV as well as both 28 variants of HHV 6 and KSHV (James *et al.*, 2011).

The kinase domain containing KSHV ORF36 homologue was tested, and indeed, not only displayed an intrinsic protein kinase activity but was also autophosphorylated on a serine residue (Park *et al.*, 2000). Several studies have demonstrated that these conserved herpesvirus protein kinases impact at multiple steps in the virus life cycle, such as regulation of viral and cellular genes, nuclear egress, virus maturation and replication, chromosome condensation, and tissue tropism (Asai *et al.*, 2007; Gershburg & Pagano, 2008; Hamza *et al.*, 2004; Izumiya *et al.*, 2007; Kawaguchi & Kato, 2003; Michel & Mertens, 2004).

The ORF36 proteins from KSHV, HSV (UL13), HCMV (UL97) and Epstein-Barr virus (BGLF4) localize predominantly in the nucleus of cells (Daikoku *et al.*, 1997; Marschall *et al.*, 2005; Park *et al.*, 2000), and are only expressed several hours post-infection, with an early-late kinetics (Martinez-Guzman et al, 2003). However, due to the fact that they are present in the virion (Overton *et al.*, 1992; Varnum *et al.*, 2004; Zhu *et al.*, 2005), they are released into the cytoplasm of host cells just after virus entry and play essential roles as innate host evasion proteins. Until recently, this conserved herpesviruses family of protein kinases did not have any assigned function. Further experiments, however, showed that the UL97 viral protein kinase was able to mimic cdc2 in infected cells by targeting the same phosphorylation site in eukaryotic elongation factor 1 delta (Kawaguchi *et al.*, 2003). In addition, ORF36 from KSHV was showed to be involved in the activation of c-jun N-terminal kinase (JNK) pathway (Hamza *et al.*, 2004). The ORF36 from MHV-68, a murine gamma-herpesvirus, was also found to phosphorylate histone H2AX during infection, suggesting that the virus actively initiates and benefits from the host DNA damage response (Tarakanova *et al.*, 2007b), a function that is only shared by BGLF4 and not by the other homologues. Recently, phosphorylation of H2AX has been shown to correlate with gamma-herpesviruses latency *in vivo* (Tarakanova *et al.*, 2010a).

More recently, however, ORF36 from the murine gamma-herpesvirus, MHV-68, has also been shown to suppress the host IFN mediated response by inhibiting the transcription factor IRF-3 (Hwang *et al.*, 2009). This function, although not requiring the conserved kinase domain, is shared by the other homologues. The ORF36 protein binds directly to IRF-3, in a region that is required for CBP binding to IRF-3. In the signaling pathway that leads to the activation of IFN-β, both CBP and Pol II are recruited to the promoter region, and when ORF36 is expressed, this recruitment, mediated by activated IRF-3, is impaired (Hwang *et al.*, 2009). The BGLF4 kinase was also shown to suppress the IRF-3 signaling pathway by inhibiting binding of IRF-3 to the IFN-β promoter (Wang *et al.*, 2009). In addition, studies by others (Jong *et al.*, 2010) have identified RNA helicase A (RHA) as an interacting partner of KSHV ORF36.

The principle focus of our work is on KSHV, which, as described above, has evolved many genes for the inhibition of type I IFN responses. Multiplicity of these genes reflects the importance of inhibiting IFN responses for virus survival. Specifically, we have screened the non-homologous genes for an inhibitory impact on the IFN response using reporter assays detecting activation of the critical transcription factors in particular conserved non-homologous herpesvirus genes, as they conservation suggests that their function must be important for virus survival and spreading. The ORF36 is indeed one such gene and, as already described, interacts directly with IRF-3 and inhibits IFN-β expression. When screened in ISRE and GAS reporter assays ORF36 inhibited both type I and type II IFN signaling cascades (Our unpublished results). The only other KSHV gene described so far to be interfering with the Jak-Stat signaling pathway is the IL-6 viral homologue, which play a role in the IL-6/STAT3 pathway. Our work raises the possibility that signaling through the type I and type II IFN receptors is inhibited by the ORF36 protein through a mechanism involving RHA and CBP. This is due to our observations that suggest that ORF36 does not impact directly on the STAT1 and STAT2 signaling transcription factors, but instead seems to be targeting a molecule downstream in the signaling cascade, perhaps one involved in the regulation/formation of the transcription complex at the promoter regions of both ISRE and GAS sequences, such as CBP or RHA.

We have also demonstrated that ORF36 of KSHV inhibited the expression of genes controlled through ISRE and GAS sequences in their promoter regions upon stimulation with IFN-α and IFN-γ, respectively. This inhibition was dependent on the kinase domain of ORF36, as its mutation reverted its inhibitory activity in both type I and type II IFN responses. As the STAT transcription factors are key regulators in this signaling pathway, we decided to investigate if the expression of ORF36 was interfering with the activation and subsequent nuclear translocation of STAT 1 and STAT2 after treatment of cells with IFN-α and IFN-γ. Both STATs were expressed at equal levels, and phosphorylated at specific residues in cells expressing ORF36 when compared to empty transfected cells after IFN treatment. However, the expression of the ORF36 protein did not alter the localization of the STATs proteins before or after treatment of the cells with type I and type II IFN. Thus both STAT1 and STAT2 similarly translocated to the nucleus upon IFN treatment in cells with and without expression of ORF36. These results suggest that the ORF36 protein may play a role in the nucleus, although this will have to be confirmed.

In conclusion, ORF36 is yet another multifunctional virus host evasion molecule which has impact at different stages of the virus replication cycle. Finally, a comprehensive understanding of herpesvirus mediated manipulation of interferon is far from complete, but will certainly provide a better understanding of the virus-host interactions, and a possible route to novel control strategies.

3. The cell cycle and DNA damage

3.1 Cell cycle progression

The eukaryotic cell cycle is operationally divided into four phases: G1, S, G2, and M. Quiescent cells, which are metabolically active but not dividing, are in the G0 phase, outside the cell cycle. The three DNA damage-induced cell cycle checkpoints, G1/S, intra-S, and G2/M, are critical points in the cell cycle that monitor the integrity of the genome, leading to repair or programmed cell death if DNA damage is detected. The DNA damage sensor molecules that activate the checkpoints and the signal transducer molecules, such as protein kinases and phosphatases, appear to be shared by the different checkpoints to varying degrees. The specificity of the checkpoint is due to the effector proteins, which inhibit phase transition (Sancar *et al.*, 2004).

The G1/S checkpoint prevents cells from entering the S phase in the presence of DNA damage by inhibiting the initiation of replication. In the case of double strand breaks, the kinase ATM initiates the checkpoint pathway by phosphorylation of Chk2, which, in turn, will phosphorylate Cdc25A, thereby causing its inactivation and consequent accumulation of the phosphorylated (inactive) form of Cdk2. If the DNA damage is caused by UV light, phosphorylation of Cdc25A is mediated by ATR-Chk1 proteins. In either case, this rapid response is followed by the p53-mediated maintenance of G1/S arrest. During this phase there is an ATM-mediated increase in the level of p53 due to an increase in protein stability, followed by posttranslational modifications, such as phosphorylation at amino acid residues 15 and 20, which regulate p53 functions. A key target for transcriptional activation of p53 is the cyclin-dependent kinase inhibitor, p21. The p53-dependent increase in p21 expression inhibits cyclin E and cyclin A-associated Cdk2 activities preventing G1-to-S phase progression (Lukas *et al.*, 2004; Sancar *et al.*, 2004).

The intra-S phase checkpoint is activated by damage encountered during the S phase or by unrepaired damage that escapes the G1/S checkpoint and leads to a block in replication. When double strand breaks are detected in S phase, the ATM-dependent pathway is activated leading to proteosome-mediated degradation of Cdc25A and consequently to the failure to maintain activation of cyclin-Cdk2 complexes and thus inhibition of DNA synthesis. A block of replication fork progression by intrinsic events or environmental insults, on the other hand, triggers an ATR-dependent pathway. In this latter case, members of the Rad family of checkpoint proteins function as DNA damage sensors and as scaffolds for the assembly of signaling complexes (Abraham, 2001).

The G2/M checkpoint prevents cells from undergoing mitosis in the presence of DNA damage, which could lead to the propagation of unrepaired DNA to the next generation. Double mutations of ATR and ATM completely eliminate G2 arrest following DNA damage, suggesting that both kinases are key regulators of this checkpoint. Thus, depending on the type of DNA damage, the ATM-Chk2 and/or ATR-Chk1 pathway is activated to arrest the cell cycle in G2 phase (Sancar *et al.*, 2004). Both pathways converge on the Cdc25C phosphatase. The Cdc2 catalityc subunit is inhibited by its phosphorylation at Thr14/Tyr15. Dephosphorylation of Cdc2 inhibitory sites by Cdc25C activates Cdc2-Cyclin B1 complex, allowing progression of cell cycle to mitosis. The activity of Cdc2 is also regulated by the availability of the cyclin B subunit. During S phase, cyclin B1 mRNA and protein begin to accumulate and their levels are maximal at G2/M. As cells pass through mitosis, cyclin B1 is ubiquitinated and degraded (Lou & Chen, 2005; Sancar *et al.*, 2004).

3.2 Herpesvirus modulation of the cell cycle

Replication of DNA viruses in host cells triggers a variety of cellular signaling cascades that regulate cell cycle, including the DNA damage response. It is generally accepted that viruses modulate the cell cycle to promote a transition through G1-S phase and achieve the cellular

environment for productive virus replication (Sato & Tsurumi, 2010). The herpesviruses genome, in contrast to other small DNA viruses, encodes a viral DNA polymerase and accessory factors, so it is not essential to promote entry into S phase of the cell cycle to exploit cellular genes involved in DNA replication. The interaction between herpesviruses and cell cycle regulatory mechanisms is more complex as some viral factors elicit cell cycle arrest while others promote cell cycle progression. Thus, it seems that herpesviruses induce cell cycle arrest, but they are able to block it in the cell cycle phase which most favors viral replication, perhaps to avoid competition with cellular DNA replication (Flemington, 2001).
Examples of cell cycle regulation by herpesviruses can be found in all three α-, β-, and γ-*herpesvirinae* subfamilies.
Herpes simplex virus type 1 (HSV-1) infection disrupts cell cycle progression in two different ways depending on the cell cycle phase. In quiescent cells, HSV-1 infection prevents G1 entry by inhibition of cyclin D/CDK4,6-specific and cyclin E/CDK2-specific phosphorylation of the retinoblastoma protein pRb. On the other hand, HSV-1 induces G1/S arrest in dividing cell cultures by inhibition of preexisting cyclin E/CDK2 and cyclin A/CDK2 activities (Ehmann *et al.*, 2000; Song *et al.*, 2000). The ability of HSV-1 to alter cellular environment in order to enhance viral replication has been related to the expression of immediate-early protein ICP0. Infection with a mutant virus in which ICP0 is the only IE protein expressed resulted in p53-independent cell cycle arrest in G1/S and G2/M phase. Although ICP27 also plays a key role in the activation of G1/S phase (Song *et al.*, 2001), infection with different mutant viruses demonstrated that the mitotic block requires ICP0 expression (Hobbs & DeLuca, 1999; Lomonte & Everett, 1999).
Similar to HSV-1, several studies demonstrated that HCMV infection leads to drastic and temporally coordinated alterations in the expression of host cell regulatory proteins, such as cyclins, resulting in cell cycle arrest at more than one phase (Bresnahan *et al.*, 1996; Dittmer & Mocarski, 1997; Jault *et al.*, 1995; Lu & Shenk, 1996). The cell cycle arrest was independent of the cell cycle phase (G0, G1, and S) at the moment of infection with HCMV (Salvant *et al.*, 1998). The immediate-early proteins IE1/IE2 and UL69 have been described as being able to block cell cycle in G1, suggesting that they may have a role in HCMV manipulation of cell cycle progression (Castillo *et al.*, 2005; Lu & Shenk, 1996; Wiebusch & Hagemeier, 1999). Infection with UV-irradiated HCMV virus resulted in G1 arrest when cells exit from G0, but it was unable to block the S phase entry in cycling cells, indicating that gene expression is required and excluding viral capsid proteins, such as UL69, function. Thus, it seems that under different conditions, these proteins may have a higher or lower impact on cell cycle regulation by HCMV (Wiebusch & Hagemeier, 1999).
The γ-herpesvirus EBV lytic program promotes its own specific cell cycle-associated activities involved in the progression from G1 to S phase, while at the same time inhibiting cellular DNA synthesis. Although the levels of p53 and CDK inhibitors remain unchanged throughout the lytic infection, there is an increase in the amounts of cyclin E/A and the hyperphosphorylated form of pRb. The resultant "quasi" S-phase cellular environment is essential for the transcription of viral immediate-early and early genes, probably due to the availability of transcription factors, such as E2F-1 and Sp1, which are expressed during S phase (Kudoh *et al.*, 2004; Kudoh *et al.*, 2003). The EBV gene which has a relevant role in cell cycle modulation is the immediate early transcription factor Zta, also known as ZEBRA or BZLF1. The Zta protein mediates the induction of three key cell cycle regulatory factors, p21, p27, and p53, resulting in G0/G1 cell cycle arrest in several epithelial cell lines (Cayrol &

Flemington, 1996). Interestingly, Zta mediates the induction of each one of these proteins, in part, through distinct pathways, a strategy which may have evolved to ensure that lytic replication occurs in a growth-arrested setting in different tissues in various states of differentiation (Rodriguez *et al.*, 1999). This emphasizes a fundamental aspect of pathogen-host evasion, the logical tailoring of the host evasion mechanism to the life style of the pathogen.

Recent studies with HHV-6A, one of the less studied β-herpesviruses, demonstrated that infection of T cells with HHV-6A results in cell cycle arrest at the G2/M phase. In this case, G2 arrest may serve to block the clonal expansion and proliferation of HHV-6A specific T cells to maintain immune suppression and evade the antiviral immune response (Li *et al.*, 2011). The mechanism that regulates the block in cell cycle progression by HHV-6A involves the inactivation of the cdc2-cyclin B1 complex and the increased expression of p21 protein in a p53-dependent manner. Manipulation of the cell cycle was also described for HHV-6B (Øster *et al.*, 2005) and HHV-6A infection in cord blood mononuclear cells (De Bolle *et al.*, 2004), but with different results, suggesting that the regulatory pathways and mechanisms induced by HHV-6 infection might be different according to the type of infected cells, once again correlating host evasion with host biology.

The regulation of cell cycle by herpesviruses is closely related to activation of the DNA damage response, including double strand break repair pathways. Viral infection confronts the host cell with large amounts of exogenous genetic material that might be recognized as abnormal and damaged DNA and so precipitates the premature apoptosis of the virus infected cells (Weitzman *et al.*, 2004). During replication, herpesvirus DNA is synthesized in a rolling-circle manner to produce head-to-tail concatemers that are subsequently cleaved into unit-length genomes. These too may be recognized as double strand breaks and trigger a DNA damage response (McVoy & Adler, 1994). Thus, in order to establish a productive infection, it is essential that viruses defend themselves from the host cell DNA damage response machinery. Paradoxically, recent reports indicate that such cellular responses may have a beneficial role in viral replication (Luo *et al.*, 2011).

Thus, during HSV-1 infection, RPA, RAD51, NBS1, and Ku86 components of the HR pathway are recruited to replication compartments, suggesting that homologous repair may play a role at the earliest stages of HSV-1 DNA replication. The phosphorylation of NBS1 and RPA indicates, in addition, that HSV-1 infection may activate components of the DNA damage response. Although siRNA-mediated "knock down" studies indicated that ATM is not absolutely required for HSV DNA replication and infectious virus production (Shirata *et al.*, 2005), another report has demonstrated that absence of specific DNA repair proteins, such as ATM or MRN complex, result in significant defects in viral replication, suggesting that a DNA damage response environment is beneficial for productive HSV-1 infection (Lilley *et al.*, 2005). Consistent with the HSV-1 infection studies, the mechanism of cell cycle arrest by ICP0 requires ATM and Chk2 proteins, and results from the activation of ATM-Chk2-Cdc25C DNA damage pathway (Li *et al.*, 2008).

The DNA damage response is also activated during HCMV replication, as indicated by the phosphorylation of ATM and H2AX and the downstream proteins Chk2 and p53. However, during HCMV infection, the localization of various checkpoint proteins, normally organized near the site of damage, is altered, inhibiting their normal function. Importantly, recent results indicate that the DNA damage response mediated by E2F1 transcription factor contributes to replication of HCMV (E *et al.*, 2011).

The EBV BGLF4 kinase may be relevant for EBV-induced DNA damage, as it induces H2AX phosphorylation. This function, conserved in the MHV-68 homolog (ORF36), is dependent of the kinase domain and is enhanced by ATM (Tarakanova *et al.*, 2007a). Recently, it has been demonstrated that ORF36 and H2AX have an important role in the establishment of MHV-68 latency, suggesting that γ-herpesviruses may exploit the components of DNA damage responses, not only during lytic replication, but also during latent infection *in vivo* (Tarakanova *et al.*, 2010b).

It is still not clear if virus-induced DNA damage involves the recognition of existing double strand breaks. Thus, it is possible that the trigger of herpesvirus-induced DNA damage response is not the recognition of viral DNA as double-strand breaks, or actual damage to DNA, but is the recruitment of DNA damage repair factors observed during viral infection.

Understanding the interaction between the DNA damage response machinery and virus infections will not only provide insights into viral pathology and persistence, but also new ideas for the development of antiviral and anti-tumour drugs. Moreover, knowledge of virus–host interactions can elucidate the mechanisms of key cellular control processes and help in identifying as yet unrecognized signaling pathways. Thus, the study of virus host evasion mechanisms can provide new tools to study recognition and repair of damaged DNA by cellular machinery.

3.3 The UL24 family: Multifunctional virus host evasion proteins

The UL24 gene is located in the unique long segment of HSV-1 genome, overlapping the thymidine kinase gene (McGeoch *et al.*, 1988). It is conserved not only in all three subfamilies of human herpesviruses, but also in other mammalian, avian, and reptilian herpesviruses, with exception of amphibians or fish, all of which have a distinct relationship to all subfamilies. Of the core herpesviruses genes, UL24 is the only one that remains unassigned to any functional category (Davison *et al.*, 2002); its universal presence in herpesviruses and lack of homology with cellular genes suggests that UL24 gene family has a relevant role in the viral life cycle and/or host evasion mechanisms. The UL24 homologues are generally expressed with late kinetics, although HSV-1 UL24 has a complex transcription pattern with leaky-late kinetics since its expression is not completely dependent on viral replication (Pearson & Coen, 2002). The HSV-2 UL24 and HCMV UL76 homologues, however, have unambiguously been identified as virion-associated proteins, and so they are found within the cell from the moment of infection (Hong-Yan *et al.*, 2001; Wang *et al.*, 2000). The alignment of the predicted amino acid sequences of UL24 homologues reveals five regions of strong sequence similarity (Jacobson *et al.*, 1989). Interestingly, a comparison of sequence profiles, enriched by predicted secondary structure, has identified UL24 as a novel PD-(D/E)XK endonuclease belonging to a large superfamily of restriction endonuclease-like fold proteins (Knizewski *et al.*, 2006). To date, however, no nuclease activity has been reported for UL24 or any of its homologues.

Deletion of the UL24 gene in HSV-1 resulted in a virus with significantly reduced plaque size and associated decreased viral yield, suggesting that the UL24 function, although not essential, is important for virus growth, at least in cell culture (Jacobson *et al.*, 1998; Jacobson *et al.*, 1989). Similar results were obtained for HSV-2 UL24 (Blakeney *et al.*, 2005), VZV ORF35 (Ito *et al.*, 2005), MHV-68 ORF20 (Nascimento & Parkhouse, 2007), and HCMV UL76 from AD169 strain (Yu *et al.*, 2003). Global functional analysis conducted using HCMV Towne complete genome, however, indicated that UL76 is an essential gene for viral replication (Dunn *et al.*, 2003). Virus strains with substitution mutations in the endonuclease motif of UL24 exhibited titers in the mouse eye model that were 10-fold lower than the wild-type virus and similar results were obtained in trigeminal ganglia. Furthermore, the percentage of virus reactivation was also significantly lower. These results are consistent with the endonuclease motif being important for the role of UL24 *in vivo* (Leiva-Torres et al., 2010). Further deletion studies revealed that absence of UL24 from HSV-1, HSV-2 and VZV leads to a syncytial plaque phenotype, similar to that observed for other HSV-1 viral proteins, suggesting that UL24, like UL20 and gK, may have a role in viral egress (Blakeney *et al.*, 2005; Ito *et al.*, 2005; Pearson & Coen, 2002), although the possible involvement of UL24 in assembly and egress of virus particles remains to be explored.

During viral infection, UL24 homologues are detected predominantly in the nucleus, and transiently localize in the nucleoli (Hong-Yan *et al.*, 2001; Nascimento & Parkhouse, 2007; Pearson & Coen, 2002; Wang *et al.*, 2000). Indeed, infection with HSV-1 results in dramatic alterations to nuclear structure and organization, including the morphology of nucleoli (Besse & Puvion-Dutilleul, 1996). Moreover, in cells infected with HSV-1, in contrast to the large, prominent spots observed within the nucleus of mock-infected cells, nucleolin had a diffuse distribution throughout the nucleus. Significantly, cells infected with two independent UL24-deficient viruses, UL24XB and UL24XG, retained the prominent punctate foci of nucleolin revealed by staining, although not absolutely identical to the distribution seen in uninfected cells.

Thus UL24 must contribute to the observed alteration of the nucleoli in HSV-1 infected cells (Lymberopoulos & Pearson, 2007), a conclusion reinforced by experiments demonstrating that expression of the N-terminal domain of UL24 alone is sufficient to induce the redistribution of nucleolin in the nucleus (Bertrand & Pearson, 2008). A similar impact of UL24 on nucleolar morphology was observed with B23, another abundant nucleolar protein, but not with fibrillarin, which also assumes a diffuse nuclear distribution as a consequence of HSV-1 infection, but in a UL24-independent manner (Callé *et al.*, 2008; Lymberopoulos *et al.*, 2011). Since UL24 is implicated in the redistribution of B23 and nucleolin, it is possible that it plays a role in nuclear egress through its effect on nucleoli, although how nucleolin affects HSV-1 nuclear egress is obscure. Finally, the fact that deletion of UL24 conserved homology domains, including the putative endonuclease motifs, resulted in loss of nucleolin and B23 dispersal activity, suggests that this function may be shared among all herpesviruses and must be relevant for the viral life cycle (Bertrand *et al.*, 2010; Bertrand & Pearson, 2008; Lymberopoulos *et al.*, 2011).

The first results that demonstrated UL24 involvement with cell cycle manipulation were obtained for ORF20 protein, the UL24 homologue from MHV-68 (Nascimento & Parkhouse, 2007). This virus is a particularly useful model for the study of herpesvirus *in vivo*. Similar to the human homologues, ORF20 is located in the nucleus and, when transiently expressed in human and murine cell lines, it induces cell cycle arrest at the G2/M phase, followed by apoptosis at later time points. During the G2 phase, the cyclin B/Cdc2 complex is inactive as the Cdc2 protein is in the phosphorylated form. Consistent with the observed G2 arrest, cells expressing MHV-68 ORF20 showed an increased phosphoryation of Cdc2 at the inhibitory site Tyr15 and a consequent inactivation of Cdc2-cyclin B complex was demonstrated (Nascimento & Parkhouse, 2007). As ORF20 belongs to UL24 gene family, the possibility that other homologues might have a role in cell cycle modulation was explored. In fact, the UL24 homologues from human herpesviruses representative of each subfamily

(HSV-1 UL24, HCMV UL76 and KSHV ORF20) also induced cell cycle arrest followed by apoptosis. Moreover, and as observed for MHV-68 ORF20, the UL24 homologues expression also resulted in Cdc2 phosphorylation at the Tyr-15 inactivation site and consequent inhibition of the mitotic cdc2-cyclin B complex (Nascimento *et al.*, 2009).

The precise mechanism of cell cycle arrest induced by UL24 homologues remains to be clarified. An interesting and possible explanation is the recent report that HCMV UL76 induces chromosomal aberrations and DNA damage (Siew *et al.*, 2009). Phosphorylation of ATM and γ-H2AX, accepted signals of DNA damage activation, were also observed for HSV-1 UL24 (our unpublished work), possibly revealing a conserved effect similar to the observed cell cycle arrest. It may be relevant that the number of cells with DNA damage breaks increased with increasing levels of the UL76 protein, a feature perhaps related to the putative endonuclease activity of the viral protein (Siew *et al.*, 2009).

Another example of this multi-functionality of virus host evasion proteins is the induction of the expression of interleukin-8 (IL-8) by the HCMV UL76 gene (our unpublished work). Thus the up-regulation of IL-8 observed in infections with HCMV (Murayama *et al.*, 1997), HSV-1 (Li *et al.*, 2006), KSHV (Lane *et al.*, 2002), and EBV (Klein *et al.*, 1996) is consistent with the properties of the conserved herpesvirus host evasion gene, UL24 gene family. The pro-inflammatory chemokine IL-8 is a member of the CXC chemokine family that binds with high affinity to two chemokine receptors, CXCR1 and CXCR2 (Zlotnik & Yoshie, 2000) and is predominantly chemotactic for neutrophils. Following infection, HCMV spreads via the bloodstream to various organs. During this phase, infectious HCMV is detected in all major leukocyte populations, with neutrophils being the most frequent reservoirs of viral DNA.

Although the virus may not replicate within them, neutrophils play an important role in the dissemination of HCMV throughout the body. Significantly, IL-8 expression is up-regulated in HCMV infected cells (Craigen *et al.*, 1997), and its secretion has direct consequences as it increases the production of infectious virus (Murayama *et al.*, 1994). Thus the stimulation of IL-8 expression appears to be a virus strategy evolved to enhance virus dissemination and survival, playing a key role in the pathogenesis of the infection. In summary, it is interesting that activation of DNA damage by UL76, a single viral gene, without cellular homology, yet conserved in all herpesviruses, has two very different activities, cell cycle manipulation and IL-8 induction, both very important for HCMV life cycle and host evasion. Whether these two activities are the consequence of two entirely different functional domains, or are in some way related, remains to be seen.

To further understand the role of UL24 on viral pathogenesis *in vivo,* we constructed two independent ORF20 deletion mutant MHV-68 viruses. Since MHV-68 infects both outbred and inbred mice, MHV-68 is a useful model to study the lytic and latent phase of herpesvirus infection and consequent pathogenesis *in vivo*. After intranasal inoculation of mice, MHV-68 replicates in lung epithelial cells. This lytic phase of infection is resolved within 10-12 days in mice infected with wild-type virus. In contrast, in mice infected with the two independent mutants for ORF20, the virus titers in the lungs were still elevated after ten days post-infection, whereas it was almost undetectable, at the same time point in the mice infected with wild-type MHV-68 and revertant viruses. However, fifteen days after infection, the lytic phase in mice infected with ORF20 deficient viruses was resolved and the virus established latency in the spleen. The fundamental cause of the extended viraemia in mice infected with ORF20-mutant viruses remains to be elucidated. After the initial lytic virus replication in the lungs, MHV-68 establishes latency in B lymphocytes in the spleen. In contrast to the extended acute phase of ORF20 mutant viruses, no major difference was found in the reactivation from latency of mutant virus compared to MHV-68 wild type infection (Nascimento *et al.*, 2011).

Other studies *in vivo,* using UL24 homologues from HSV-2 or VZV, also suggest a critical role for UL24 in viral pathogenesis. Intravaginal inoculation of BALB/c mice and Hartley guinea pigs with a UL24 deletion mutant of HSV-2 virus resulted in delayed disease kinetics and minimal disease progression, and the mutant virus was avirulent at higher doses compared to the parental virus (Blakeney *et al.*, 2005). Deletion mutant VZV virus infection of skin and T cells xenografts *in vivo* also indicated that ORF35 is a determinant of VZV virulence (Ito *et al.*, 2005). It would be important to analyze the ORF20 mutant MHV-68 pathogenesis in its natural host, the wood mice (members of the genus *Apodemus*) (Ehlers *et al.*, 2007), as a recent comparative analysis revealed that MHV-68 infection of BALB/c (*M. musculus*) and laboratory-bred wood mice are markedly different (Hughes *et al.*, 2010).

In conclusion, manipulation of the DNA damage response is a major target of herpesviruses, and one that in turn may determine a variety of significant outcomes to favor the virus, with cell cycle arrest and induction of IL-8 now identified.

4. Conclusion

Many virus genes that manipulate host defense mechanisms are recognized by their homology to cellular genes. Viruses, however, contain many genes without any homology or known function in the now vast sequences database. As all the structural proteins and most of the enzymes of herpesvirus are now known, it is likely that a considerable number of their non-assigned, non-homologous genes have evolved for host manipulation, thus offering opportunities for other novel strategies for control of virus infection, such as construction of a gene deletion, avirulent virus vaccines. Indeed, as we report here, the UL24 gene family, which is conserved in all herpesviruses, and has no cellular homologue, combines the dual function of inhibiting cell cycle progression and inducing IL-8 expression.

Significantly, both UL24 and the kinase ORF36 are genes conserved in α-, β- and γ-herpesviruses, and both share the function of activating the DNA damage pathway. At the same time, both UL24 and ORF36 impact on innate immunity, the first inducing expression of IL-8, and the second inhibiting IFN responses. Thus UL24, like many other virus host evasion genes, is multifunctional, impacting on two cellular activities, the cell cycle and IL-8 expression. Although at first site this particular combination of targets for one viral gene is not an obviously rational one, future studies may provide the logical mechanistic link for many more multifunctional virus host evasion genes.

In conclusion, non-homologous virus genes may be an Aladdin's cave of "ready-made tools" for the manipulation of cell biology and immune responses, and the multi-functionality of virus host evasion genes may provide important tools to unravel the complex interactions underlying the regulation of intracellular signaling.

5. Acknowledgment

The authors thank the FCT (SFRH/BD/8929/2002, SFRH/ BD/27677/2006, PTDC/SAU-MII/69290/2006, PTDC/SAU-MIC/110316/2009), for supporting their work.

6. References

Abate, D. A., Watanabe, S. & Mocarski, E. S. (2004). Major human cytomegalovirus structural protein pp65 (ppUL83) prevents interferon response factor 3 activation in the interferon response. *J Virol* 78, 10995-11006.

Abraham, R. T. (2001). Cell cycle checkpoint signaling through the ATM and ATR kinases. *Genes Dev* 15, 2177-2196.

Ahmad, H., Gubbels, R., Ehlers, E., Meyer, F., Waterbury, T., Lin, R. & Zhang, L. (2011). Kaposi sarcoma-associated herpesvirus degrades cellular Toll-interleukin-1 receptor domain-containing adaptor-inducing beta-interferon (TRIF). *J Biol Chem* 286, 7865-7872.

Ahn, J. H., Brignole, E. J., 3rd & Hayward, G. S. (1998). Disruption of PML subnuclear domains by the acidic IE1 protein of human cytomegalovirus is mediated through interaction with PML and may modulate a RING finger-dependent cryptic transactivator function of PML. *Mol Cell Biol* 18, 4899-4913.

Ahn, J. H. & Hayward, G. S. (1997). The major immediate-early proteins IE1 and IE2 of human cytomegalovirus colocalize with and disrupt PML-associated nuclear bodies at very early times in infected permissive cells. *J Virol* 71, 4599-4613.

Ankel, H., Westra, D. F., Welling-Wester, S. & Lebon, P. (1998). Induction of interferon-alpha by glycoprotein D of herpes simplex virus: a possible role of chemokine receptors. *Virology* 251, 317-326.

Arnheiter, H., Frese, M., Kambadur, R., Meier, E. & Haller, O. (1996). Mx transgenic mice--animal models of health. *Curr Top Microbiol Immunol* 206, 119-147.

Asai, R., Ohno, T., Kato, A. & Kawaguchi, Y. (2007). Identification of proteins directly phosphorylated by UL13 protein kinase from herpes simplex virus 1. *Microbes Infect* 9, 1434-1438.

Bach, E. A., Aguet, M. & Schreiber, R. D. (1997). The IFN gamma receptor: a paradigm for cytokine receptor signaling. *Annu Rev Immunol* 15, 563-591.

Barnes, B. J., Moore, P. A. & Pitha, P. M. (2001). Virus-specific activation of a novel interferon regulatory factor, IRF-5, results in the induction of distinct interferon alpha genes. *J Biol Chem* 276, 23382-23390.

Bertrand, L., Leiva-Torres, G. A., Hyjazie, H. & Pearson, A. (2010). Conserved residues in the UL24 protein of herpes simplex virus 1 are important for dispersal of the nucleolar protein nucleolin. *J Virol* 84, 109-118.

Bertrand, L. & Pearson, A. (2008). The conserved N-terminal domain of herpes simplex virus 1 UL24 protein is sufficient to induce the spatial redistribution of nucleolin. *J Gen Virol* 89, 1142-1151.

Besse, S. & Puvion-Dutilleul, F. (1996). Distribution of ribosomal genes in nucleoli of herpes simplex virus type 1 infected cells. *Eur J Cell Biol* 71, 33-44.

Bisson, S. A., Page, A. L. & Ganem, D. (2009). A Kaposi's sarcoma-associated herpesvirus protein that forms inhibitory complexes with type I interferon receptor subunits, Jak and STAT proteins, and blocks interferon-mediated signal transduction. *J Virol* 83, 5056-5066.

Blakeney, S., Kowalski, J., Tummolo, D., DeStefano, J., Cooper, D., Guo, M., Gangolli, S., Long, D., Zamb, T., Natuk, R. J. & Visalli, R. J. (2005). Herpes simplex virus type 2 UL24 gene is a virulence determinant in murine and guinea pig disease models. *J Virol* 79, 10498-10506.

Boehme, K. W., Singh, J., Perry, S. T. & Compton, T. (2004). Human cytomegalovirus elicits a coordinated cellular antiviral response via envelope glycoprotein B. *J Virol* 78, 1202-1211.

Bresnahan, W. A., Boldogh, I., Thompson, E. A. & Albrecht, T. (1996). Human cytomegalovirus inhibits cellular DNA synthesis and arrests productively infected cells in late G1. *Virology* 224, 150-160.

Burysek, L. & Pitha, P. M. (2001). Latently expressed human herpesvirus 8-encoded interferon regulatory factor 2 inhibits double-stranded RNA-activated protein kinase. *J Virol* 75, 2345-2352.

Burysek, L., Yeow, W. S., Lubyova, B., Kellum, M., Schafer, S. L., Huang, Y. Q. & Pitha, P. M. (1999). Functional analysis of human herpesvirus 8-encoded viral interferon regulatory factor 1 and its association with cellular interferon regulatory factors and p300. *J Virol* 73, 7334-7342.

Callé, A., Ugrinova, I., Epstein, A. L., Bouvet, P., Diaz, J. J. & Greco, A. (2008). Nucleolin is required for an efficient herpes simplex virus type 1 infection. *J Virol* 82, 4762-4773.

Cassady, K. A. (2005). Human cytomegalovirus TRS1 and IRS1 gene products block the double-stranded-RNA-activated host protein shutoff response induced by herpes simplex virus type 1 infection. *J Virol* 79, 8707-8715.

Cassady, K. A., Gross, M. & Roizman, B. (1998). The herpes simplex virus US11 protein effectively compensates for the gamma1(34.5) gene if present before activation of protein kinase R by precluding its phosphorylation and that of the alpha subunit of eukaryotic translation initiation factor 2. *J Virol* 72, 8620-8626.

Castillo, J. P., Frame, F. M., Rogoff, H. A., Pickering, M. T., Yurochko, A. D. & Kowalik, T. F. (2005). Human cytomegalovirus IE1-72 activates ataxia telangiectasia mutated kinase and a p53/p21-mediated growth arrest response. *J Virol* 79, 11467-11475.

Cayrol, C. & Flemington, E. K. (1996). The Epstein-Barr virus bZIP transcription factor Zta causes G0/G1 cell cycle arrest through induction of cyclin-dependent kinase inhibitors. *EMBO J* 15, 2748-2759.

Chee, A. V., Lopez, P., Pandolfi, P. P. & Roizman, B. (2003). Promyelocytic leukemia protein mediates interferon-based anti-herpes simplex virus 1 effects. *J Virol* 77, 7101-7105.

Chuluunbaatar, U., Roller, R., Feldman, M. E., Brown, S., Shokat, K. M. & Mohr, I. (2010). Constitutive mTORC1 activation by a herpesvirus Akt surrogate stimulates mRNA translation and viral replication. *Genes Dev* 24, 2627-2639.

Cloutier, N. & Flamand, L. (2010). Kaposi sarcoma-associated herpesvirus latency-associated nuclear antigen inhibits interferon (IFN) beta expression by competing with IFN regulatory factor-3 for binding to IFNB promoter. *J Biol Chem* 285, 7208-7221.

Colamonici, O. R., Domanski, P., Krolewski, J. J., Fu, X. Y., Reich, N. C., Pfeffer, L. M., Sweet, M. E. & Platanias, L. C. (1994). Interferon alpha (IFN alpha) signaling in cells expressing the variant form of the type I IFN receptor. *J Biol Chem* 269, 5660-5665.

Cooray, S., Bahar, M. W., Abrescia, N. G., McVey, C. E., Bartlett, N. W., Chen, R. A., Stuart, D. I., Grimes, J. M. & Smith, G. L. (2007). Functional and structural studies of the vaccinia virus virulence factor N1 reveal a Bcl-2-like anti-apoptotic protein. *J Gen Virol* 88, 1656-1666.

Craigen, J. L., Yong, K. L., Jordan, N. J., MacCormac, L. P., Westwick, J., Akbar, A. N. & Grundy, J. E. (1997). Human cytomegalovirus infection up-regulates interleukin-8 gene expression and stimulates neutrophil transendothelial migration. *Immunology* 92, 138-145.

Daikoku, T., Shibata, S., Goshima, F., Oshima, S., Tsurumi, T., Yamada, H., Yamashita, Y. & Nishiyama, Y. (1997). Purification and characterization of the protein kinase encoded by the UL13 gene of herpes simplex virus type 2. *Virology* 235, 82-93.

Darwich, L., Coma, G., Pena, R., Bellido, R., Blanco, E. J., Este, J. A., Borras, F. E., Clotet, B., Ruiz, L., Rosell, A., Andreo, F., Parkhouse, R. M. & Bofill, M. (2009). Secretion of interferon-gamma by human macrophages demonstrated at the single-cell level after costimulation with interleukin (IL)-12 plus IL-18. *Immunology* 126, 386-393.

Davison, A. J., Dargan, D. J. & Stow, N. D. (2002). Fundamental and accessory systems in herpesviruses. *Antiviral Res* 56, 1-11.

De Bolle, L., Hatse, S., Verbeken, E., De Clercq, E. & Naesens, L. (2004). Human herpesvirus 6 infection arrests cord blood mononuclear cells in G(2) phase of the cell cycle. *FEBS Lett* 560, 25-29.

Dittmer, D. & Mocarski, E. S. (1997). Human cytomegalovirus infection inhibits G1/S transition. *J Virol* 71, 1629-1634.

Dunn, W., Chou, C., Li, H., Hai, R., Patterson, D., Stolc, V., Zhu, H. & Liu, F. (2003). Functional profiling of a human cytomegalovirus genome. *Proc Natl Acad Sci U S A* 100, 14223-14228.

E, X., Pickering, M. T., Debatis, M., Castillo, J., Lagadinos, A., Wang, S., Lu, S. & Kowalik, T. F. (2011). An E2F1-mediated DNA damage response contributes to the replication of human cytomegalovirus. *PLoS Pathog* 7, e1001342.

Ehlers, B., Küchler, J., Yasmum, N., Dural, G., Voigt, S., Schmidt-Chanasit, J., Jäkel, T., Matuschka, F. R., Richter, D., Essbauer, S., Hughes, D. J., Summers, C., Bennett, M., Stewart, J. P. & Ulrich, R. G. (2007). Identification of novel rodent herpesviruses, including the first gammaherpesvirus of Mus musculus. *J Virol* 81, 8091-8100.

Ehmann, G. L., McLean, T. I. & Bachenheimer, S. L. (2000). Herpes simplex virus type 1 infection imposes a G(1)/S block in asynchronously growing cells and prevents G(1) entry in quiescent cells. *Virology* 267, 335-349.

Eidson, K. M., Hobbs, W. E., Manning, B. J., Carlson, P. & DeLuca, N. A. (2002). Expression of herpes simplex virus ICP0 inhibits the induction of interferon-stimulated genes by viral infection. *J Virol* 76, 2180-2191.

Flemington, E. K. (2001). Herpesvirus lytic replication and the cell cycle: arresting new developments. *J Virol* 75, 4475-4481.

Flint, S. J., Enquist, L.W., Racaniello, V.R. and Skalka, A.M. (2004). *Principles of Virology*.

Fuld, S., Cunningham, C., Klucher, K., Davison, A. J. & Blackbourn, D. J. (2006). Inhibition of interferon signaling by the Kaposi's sarcoma-associated herpesvirus full-length viral interferon regulatory factor 2 protein. *J Virol* 80, 3092-3097.

Garcia, M. A., Gil, J., Ventoso, I., Guerra, S., Domingo, E., Rivas, C. & Esteban, M. (2006). Impact of protein kinase PKR in cell biology: from antiviral to antiproliferative action. *Microbiol Mol Biol Rev* 70, 1032-1060.

Gershburg, E. & Pagano, J. S. (2008). Conserved herpesvirus protein kinases. *Biochim Biophys Acta* 1784, 203-212.

Hakki, M. & Geballe, A. P. (2005). Double-stranded RNA binding by human cytomegalovirus pTRS1. *J Virol* 79, 7311-7318.

Haller, O., Arnheiter, H., Gresser, I. & Lindenmann, J. (1981). Virus-specific interferon action. Protection of newborn Mx carriers against lethal infection with influenza virus. *J Exp Med* 154, 199-203.

Haller, O., Kochs, G. & Weber, F. (2007). Interferon, Mx, and viral countermeasures. *Cytokine Growth Factor Rev* 18, 425-433.

Hamza, M. S., Reyes, R. A., Izumiya, Y., Wisdom, R., Kung, H. J. & Luciw, P. A. (2004). ORF36 protein kinase of Kaposi's sarcoma herpesvirus activates the c-Jun N-terminal kinase signaling pathway. *J Biol Chem* 279, 38325-38330.

He, B., Gross, M. & Roizman, B. (1998). The gamma134.5 protein of herpes simplex virus 1 has the structural and functional attributes of a protein phosphatase 1 regulatory subunit and is present in a high molecular weight complex with the enzyme in infected cells. *J Biol Chem* 273, 20737-20743.

He, Z., He, Y. S., Kim, Y., Chu, L., Ohmstede, C., Biron, K. K. & Coen, D. M. (1997). The human cytomegalovirus UL97 protein is a protein kinase that autophosphorylates on serines and threonines. *J Virol* 71, 405-411.

Hefti, H. P., Frese, M., Landis, H., Di Paolo, C., Aguzzi, A., Haller, O. & Pavlovic, J. (1999). Human MxA protein protects mice lacking a functional alpha/beta interferon system against La crosse virus and other lethal viral infections. *J Virol* 73, 6984-6991.

Hiscott, J., Nguyen, T. L., Arguello, M., Nakhaei, P. & Paz, S. (2006). Manipulation of the nuclear factor-kappaB pathway and the innate immune response by viruses. *Oncogene* 25, 6844-6867.

Hobbs, W. E. & DeLuca, N. A. (1999). Perturbation of cell cycle progression and cellular gene expression as a function of herpes simplex virus ICP0. *J Virol* 73, 8245-8255.

Holzerlandt, R., Orengo, C., Kellam, P. & Albà, M. M. (2002). Identification of new herpesvirus gene homologs in the human genome. *Genome Res* 12, 1739-1748.

Honda, K., Takaoka, A. & Taniguchi, T. (2006). Type I interferon [corrected] gene induction by the interferon regulatory factor family of transcription factors. *Immunity* 25, 349-360.

Hong-Yan, Z., Murata, T., Goshima, F., Takakuwa, H., Koshizuka, T., Yamauchi, Y. & Nishiyama, Y. (2001). Identification and characterization of the UL24 gene product of herpes simplex virus type 2. *Virus Genes* 22, 321-327.

Hughes, D. J., Kipar, A., Sample, J. T. & Stewart, J. P. (2010). Pathogenesis of a model gammaherpesvirus in a natural host. *J Virol* 84, 3949-3961.

Huh, Y. H., Kim, Y. E., Kim, E. T., Park, J. J., Song, M. J., Zhu, H., Hayward, G. S. & Ahn, J. H. (2008). Binding STAT2 by the acidic domain of human cytomegalovirus IE1 promotes viral growth and is negatively regulated by SUMO. *J Virol* 82, 10444-10454.

Hwang, S., Kim, K. S., Flano, E., Wu, T. T., Tong, L. M., Park, A. N., Song, M. J., Sanchez, D. J., O'Connell, R. M., Cheng, G. & Sun, R. (2009). Conserved herpesviral kinase promotes viral persistence by inhibiting the IRF-3-mediated type I interferon response. *Cell Host Microbe* 5, 166-178.

Ito, H., Sommer, M. H., Zerboni, L., Baiker, A., Sato, B., Liang, R., Hay, J., Ruyechan, W. & Arvin, A. M. (2005). Role of the varicella-zoster virus gene product encoded by open reading frame 35 in viral replication in vitro and in differentiated human skin and T cells in vivo. *J Virol* 79, 4819-4827.

Izumiya, Y., Izumiya, C., Van Geelen, A., Wang, D. H., Lam, K. S., Luciw, P. A. & Kung, H. J. (2007). Kaposi's sarcoma-associated herpesvirus-encoded protein kinase and its interaction with K-bZIP. *J Virol* 81, 1072-1082.

Jacobson, J. G., Chen, S. H., Cook, W. J., Kramer, M. F. & Coen, D. M. (1998). Importance of the herpes simplex virus UL24 gene for productive ganglionic infection in mice. *Virology* 242, 161-169.

Jacobson, J. G., Martin, S. L. & Coen, D. M. (1989). A conserved open reading frame that overlaps the herpes simplex virus thymidine kinase gene is important for viral growth in cell culture. *J Virol* 63, 1839-1843.

James, S. H., Hartline, C. B., Harden, E. A., Driebe, E. M., Schupp, J. M., Engelthaler, D. M., Keim, P. S., Bowlin, T. L., Kern, E. R. & Prichard, M. N. (2011). Cyclopropavir Inhibits the Normal Function of the Human Cytomegalovirus UL97 Kinase. *Antimicrob Agents Chemother.*

Jault, F. M., Jault, J. M., Ruchti, F., Fortunato, E. A., Clark, C., Corbeil, J., Richman, D. D. & Spector, D. H. (1995). Cytomegalovirus infection induces high levels of cyclins, phosphorylated Rb, and p53, leading to cell cycle arrest. *J Virol* 69, 6697-6704.

Johnson, K. E. & Knipe, D. M. (2010). Herpes simplex virus-1 infection causes the secretion of a type I interferon-antagonizing protein and inhibits signaling at or before Jak-1 activation. *Virology* 396, 21-29.

Johnson, K. E., Song, B. & Knipe, D. M. (2008). Role for herpes simplex virus 1 ICP27 in the inhibition of type I interferon signaling. *Virology* 374, 487-494.

Jong, J. E., Park, J., Kim, S. & Seo, T. (2010). Kaposi's sarcoma-associated herpesvirus viral protein kinase interacts with RNA helicase a and regulates host gene expression. *J Microbiol* 48, 206-212.

Joo, C. H., Shin, Y. C., Gack, M., Wu, L., Levy, D. & Jung, J. U. (2007). Inhibition of interferon regulatory factor 7 (IRF7)-mediated interferon signal transduction by the Kaposi's sarcoma-associated herpesvirus viral IRF homolog vIRF3. *J Virol* 81, 8282-8292.

Kawaguchi, Y. & Kato, K. (2003). Protein kinases conserved in herpesviruses potentially share a function mimicking the cellular protein kinase cdc2. *Rev Med Virol* 13, 331-340.

Kawaguchi, Y., Kato, K., Tanaka, M., Kanamori, M., Nishiyama, Y. & Yamanashi, Y. (2003). Conserved protein kinases encoded by herpesviruses and cellular protein kinase cdc2 target the same phosphorylation site in eukaryotic elongation factor 1delta. *J Virol* 77, 2359-2368.

Klein, S. C., Kube, D., Abts, H., Diehl, V. & Tesch, H. (1996). Promotion of IL8, IL10, TNF alpha and TNF beta production by EBV infection. *Leuk Res* 20, 633-636.

Knizewski, L., Kinch, L., Grishin, N. V., Rychlewski, L. & Ginalski, K. (2006). Human herpesvirus 1 UL24 gene encodes a potential PD-(D/E)XK endonuclease. *J Virol* 80, 2575-2577.

Korioth, F., Maul, G. G., Plachter, B., Stamminger, T. & Frey, J. (1996). The nuclear domain 10 (ND10) is disrupted by the human cytomegalovirus gene product IE1. *Exp Cell Res* 229, 155-158.

Kudoh, A., Daikoku, T., Sugaya, Y., Isomura, H., Fujita, M., Kiyono, T., Nishiyama, Y. & Tsurumi, T. (2004). Inhibition of S-phase cyclin-dependent kinase activity blocks expression of Epstein-Barr virus immediate-early and early genes, preventing viral lytic replication. *J Virol* 78, 104-115.

Kudoh, A., Fujita, M., Kiyono, T., Kuzushima, K., Sugaya, Y., Izuta, S., Nishiyama, Y. & Tsurumi, T. (2003). Reactivation of lytic replication from B cells latently infected with Epstein-Barr virus occurs with high S-phase cyclin-dependent kinase activity while inhibiting cellular DNA replication. *J Virol* 77, 851-861.

Kwong, A. D. & Frenkel, N. (1989). The herpes simplex virus virion host shutoff function. *J Virol* 63, 4834-4839.

Lane, B. R., Liu, J., Bock, P. J., Schols, D., Coffey, M. J., Strieter, R. M., Polverini, P. J. & Markovitz, D. M. (2002). Interleukin-8 and growth-regulated oncogene alpha mediate angiogenesis in Kaposi's sarcoma. *J Virol* 76, 11570-11583.

Lefort, S., Soucy-Faulkner, A., Grandvaux, N. & Flamand, L. (2007). Binding of Kaposi's sarcoma-associated herpesvirus K-bZIP to interferon-responsive factor 3 elements modulates antiviral gene expression. *J Virol* 81, 10950-10960.

Leiva-Torres, G. A., Rochette, P. A. & Pearson, A. (2010). Differential importance of highly conserved residues in UL24 for herpes simplex virus 1 replication in vivo and reactivation. *J Gen Virol* 91, 1109-1116.

Li, H., Baskaran, R., Krisky, D. M., Bein, K., Grandi, P., Cohen, J. B. & Glorioso, J. C. (2008). Chk2 is required for HSV-1 ICP0-mediated G2/M arrest and enhancement of virus growth. *Virology* 375, 13-23.

Li, H., Zhang, J., Kumar, A., Zheng, M., Atherton, S. S. & Yu, F. S. (2006). Herpes simplex virus 1 infection induces the expression of proinflammatory cytokines, interferons and TLR7 in human corneal epithelial cells. *Immunology* 117, 167-176.

Li, L., Gu, B., Zhou, F., Chi, J., Wang, F., Peng, G., Xie, F., Qing, J., Feng, D., Lu, S. & Yao, K. (2011). Human herpesvirus 6 suppresses T cell proliferation through induction of cell cycle arrest in infected cells in the G2/M phase. *J Virol* 85, 6774-6783.

Lilley, C. E., Carson, C. T., Muotri, A. R., Gage, F. H. & Weitzman, M. D. (2005). DNA repair proteins affect the lifecycle of herpes simplex virus 1. *Proc Natl Acad Sci U S A* 102, 5844-5849.

Lin, R., Genin, P., Mamane, Y. & Hiscott, J. (2000). Selective DNA binding and association with the CREB binding protein coactivator contribute to differential activation of alpha/beta interferon genes by interferon regulatory factors 3 and 7. *Mol Cell Biol* 20, 6342-6353.

Lin, R., Genin, P., Mamane, Y., Sgarbanti, M., Battistini, A., Harrington, W. J., Jr., Barber, G. N. & Hiscott, J. (2001). HHV-8 encoded vIRF-1 represses the interferon antiviral response by blocking IRF-3 recruitment of the CBP/p300 coactivators. *Oncogene* 20, 800-811.

Littler, E., Stuart, A. D. & Chee, M. S. (1992). Human cytomegalovirus UL97 open reading frame encodes a protein that phosphorylates the antiviral nucleoside analogue ganciclovir. *Nature* 358, 160-162.

Lomonte, P. & Everett, R. D. (1999). Herpes simplex virus type 1 immediate-early protein Vmw110 inhibits progression of cells through mitosis and from G(1) into S phase of the cell cycle. *J Virol* 73, 9456-9467.

Lou, Z. & Chen, J. (2005). Mammalian DNA damage response pathway. *Adv Exp Med Biol* 570, 425-455.

Lu, M. & Shenk, T. (1996). Human cytomegalovirus infection inhibits cell cycle progression at multiple points, including the transition from G1 to S. *J Virol* 70, 8850-8857.

Lukas, J., Lukas, C. & Bartek, J. (2004). Mammalian cell cycle checkpoints: signalling pathways and their organization in space and time. *DNA Repair (Amst)* 3, 997-1007.

Luo, Y., Chen, A. Y. & Qiu, J. (2011). Bocavirus infection induces a DNA damage response that facilitates viral DNA replication and mediates cell death. *J Virol* 85, 133-145.

Lymberopoulos, M. H., Bourget, A., Abdeljelil, N. B. & Pearson, A. (2011). Involvement of the UL24 protein in herpes simplex virus 1-induced dispersal of B23 and in nuclear egress. *Virology* 412, 341-348.

Lymberopoulos, M. H. & Pearson, A. (2007). Involvement of UL24 in herpes-simplex-virus-1-induced dispersal of nucleolin. *Virology* 363, 397-409.

Marie, I., Durbin, J. E. & Levy, D. E. (1998). Differential viral induction of distinct interferon-alpha genes by positive feedback through interferon regulatory factor-7. *EMBO J* 17, 6660-6669.

Marschall, M., Marzi, A., aus dem Siepen, P., Jochmann, R., Kalmer, M., Auerochs, S., Lischka, P., Leis, M. & Stamminger, T. (2005). Cellular p32 recruits cytomegalovirus kinase pUL97 to redistribute the nuclear lamina. *J Biol Chem* 280, 33357-33367.

Matis, J. & Kudelova, M. (2001). Early shutoff of host protein synthesis in cells infected with herpes simplex viruses. *Acta Virol* 45, 269-277.

McGeoch, D. J., Dalrymple, M. A., Davison, A. J., Dolan, A., Frame, M. C., McNab, D., Perry, L. J., Scott, J. E. & Taylor, P. (1988). The complete DNA sequence of the long unique region in the genome of herpes simplex virus type 1. *J Gen Virol* 69 (Pt 7), 1531-1574.

McVoy, M. A. & Adler, S. P. (1994). Human cytomegalovirus DNA replicates after early circularization by concatemer formation, and inversion occurs within the concatemer. *J Virol* 68, 1040-1051.

Melroe, G. T., DeLuca, N. A. & Knipe, D. M. (2004). Herpes simplex virus 1 has multiple mechanisms for blocking virus-induced interferon production. *J Virol* 78, 8411-8420.

Michel, D. & Mertens, T. (2004). The UL97 protein kinase of human cytomegalovirus and homologues in other herpesviruses: impact on virus and host. *Biochim Biophys Acta* 1697, 169-180.

Mogensen, K. E., Lewerenz, M., Reboul, J., Lutfalla, G. & Uze, G. (1999). The type I interferon receptor: structure, function, and evolution of a family business. *J Interferon Cytokine Res* 19, 1069-1098.

Moore, P. S., Boshoff, C., Weiss, R. A. & Chang, Y. (1996). Molecular mimicry of human cytokine and cytokine response pathway genes by KSHV. *Science* 274, 1739-1744.

Mossman, K. L., Macgregor, P. F., Rozmus, J. J., Goryachev, A. B., Edwards, A. M. & Smiley, J. R. (2001). Herpes simplex virus triggers and then disarms a host antiviral response. *J Virol* 75, 750-758.

Murayama, T., Kuno, K., Jisaki, F., Obuchi, M., Sakamuro, D., Furukawa, T., Mukaida, N. & Matsushima, K. (1994). Enhancement human cytomegalovirus replication in a human lung fibroblast cell line by interleukin-8. *J Virol* 68, 7582-7585.

Murayama, T., Ohara, Y., Obuchi, M., Khabar, K. S., Higashi, H., Mukaida, N. & Matsushima, K. (1997). Human cytomegalovirus induces interleukin-8 production by a human monocytic cell line, THP-1, through acting concurrently on AP-1- and NF-kappaB-binding sites of the interleukin-8 gene. *J Virol* 71, 5692-5695.

Naranatt, P. P., Krishnan, H. H., Svojanovsky, S. R., Bloomer, C., Mathur, S. & Chandran, B. (2004). Host gene induction and transcriptional reprogramming in Kaposi's sarcoma-associated herpesvirus (KSHV/HHV-8)-infected endothelial, fibroblast, and B cells: insights into modulation events early during infection. *Cancer Res* 64, 72-84.

Nascimento, R., Costa, H., Dias, J. D. & Parkhouse, R. M. (2011). MHV-68 Open Reading Frame 20 is a nonessential gene delaying lung viral clearance. *Arch Virol* 156, 375-386.

Nascimento, R., Dias, J. D. & Parkhouse, R. M. (2009). The conserved UL24 family of human alpha, beta and gamma herpesviruses induces cell cycle arrest and inactivation of the cyclinB/cdc2 complex. *Arch Virol* 154, 1143-1149.

Nascimento, R. & Parkhouse, R. M. (2007). Murine gammaherpesvirus 68 ORF20 induces cell-cycle arrest in G2 by inhibiting the Cdc2-cyclin B complex. *J Gen Virol* 88, 1446-1453.

Novick, D., Cohen, B. & Rubinstein, M. (1994). The human interferon alpha/beta receptor: characterization and molecular cloning. *Cell* 77, 391-400.

Overton, H. A., McMillan, D. J., Klavinskis, L. S., Hope, L., Ritchie, A. J. & Wong-kai-in, P. (1992). Herpes simplex virus type 1 gene UL13 encodes a phosphoprotein that is a component of the virion. *Virology* 190, 184-192.

Paladino, P. & Mossman, K. L. (2009). Mechanisms employed by herpes simplex virus 1 to inhibit the interferon response. *J Interferon Cytokine Res* 29, 599-607.

Park, J., Lee, D., Seo, T., Chung, J. & Choe, J. (2000). Kaposi's sarcoma-associated herpesvirus (human herpesvirus-8) open reading frame 36 protein is a serine protein kinase. *J Gen Virol* 81, 1067-1071.

Paulus, C., Krauss, S. & Nevels, M. (2006). A human cytomegalovirus antagonist of type I IFN-dependent signal transducer and activator of transcription signaling. *Proc Natl Acad Sci U S A* 103, 3840-3845.

Pearson, A. & Coen, D. M. (2002). Identification, localization, and regulation of expression of the UL24 protein of herpes simplex virus type 1. *J Virol* 76, 10821-10828.

Preston, C. M., Harman, A. N. & Nicholl, M. J. (2001). Activation of interferon response factor-3 in human cells infected with herpes simplex virus type 1 or human cytomegalovirus. *J Virol* 75, 8909-8916.

Randall, R. E. & Goodbourn, S. (2008). Interferons and viruses: an interplay between induction, signalling, antiviral responses and virus countermeasures. *J Gen Virol* 89, 1-47.

Rodriguez, A., Armstrong, M., Dwyer, D. & Flemington, E. (1999). Genetic dissection of cell growth arrest functions mediated by the Epstein-Barr virus lytic gene product, Zta. *J Virol* 73, 9029-9038.

Salvant, B. S., Fortunato, E. A. & Spector, D. H. (1998). Cell cycle dysregulation by human cytomegalovirus: influence of the cell cycle phase at the time of infection and effects on cyclin transcription. *J Virol* 72, 3729-3741.

Sancar, A., Lindsey-Boltz, L. A., Unsal-Kaçmaz, K. & Linn, S. (2004). Molecular mechanisms of mammalian DNA repair and the DNA damage checkpoints. *Annu Rev Biochem* 73, 39-85.

Sanchez, R. & Mohr, I. (2007). Inhibition of cellular 2'-5' oligoadenylate synthetase by the herpes simplex virus type 1 Us11 protein. *J Virol* 81, 3455-3464.

Sato, Y. & Tsurumi, T. (2010). Noise cancellation: viral fine tuning of the cellular environment for its own genome replication. *PLoS Pathog* 6, e1001158.

Shirata, N., Kudoh, A., Daikoku, T., Tatsumi, Y., Fujita, M., Kiyono, T., Sugaya, Y., Isomura, H., Ishizaki, K. & Tsurumi, T. (2005). Activation of ataxia telangiectasia-mutated DNA damage checkpoint signal transduction elicited by herpes simplex virus infection. *J Biol Chem* 280, 30336-30341.

Shuai, K., Stark, G. R., Kerr, I. M. & Darnell, J. E., Jr. (1993). A single phosphotyrosine residue of Stat91 required for gene activation by interferon-gamma. *Science* 261, 1744-1746.

Siew, V. K., Duh, C. Y. & Wang, S. K. (2009). Human cytomegalovirus UL76 induces chromosome aberrations. *J Biomed Sci* 16, 107.

Silverman, R. H. (2007). Viral encounters with 2',5'-oligoadenylate synthetase and RNase L during the interferon antiviral response. *J Virol* 81, 12720-12729.

Song, B., Liu, J. J., Yeh, K. C. & Knipe, D. M. (2000). Herpes simplex virus infection blocks events in the G1 phase of the cell cycle. *Virology* 267, 326-334.

Song, B., Yeh, K. C., Liu, J. & Knipe, D. M. (2001). Herpes simplex virus gene products required for viral inhibition of expression of G1-phase functions. *Virology* 290, 320-328.

Stark, G. R., Kerr, I. M., Williams, B. R., Silverman, R. H. & Schreiber, R. D. (1998). How cells respond to interferons. *Annu Rev Biochem* 67, 227-264.

Sun, R., Lin, S. F., Gradoville, L., Yuan, Y., Zhu, F. & Miller, G. (1998). A viral gene that activates lytic cycle expression of Kaposi's sarcoma-associated herpesvirus. *Proc Natl Acad Sci U S A* 95, 10866-10871.

Takeuchi, O. & Akira, S. (2007). Recognition of viruses by innate immunity. *Immunol Rev* 220, 214-224.

Tan, J. C., Avdic, S., Cao, J. Z., Mocarski, E. S., White, K. L., Abendroth, A. & Slobedman, B. (2011). Inhibition of 2',5'-oligoadenylate synthetase expression and function by the human cytomegalovirus ORF94 gene product. *J Virol* 85, 5696-5700.

Tang, X., Gao, J. S., Guan, Y. J., McLane, K. E., Yuan, Z. L., Ramratnam, B. & Chin, Y. E. (2007). Acetylation-dependent signal transduction for type I interferon receptor. *Cell* 131, 93-105.

Tarakanova, V. L., Leung-Pineda, V., Hwang, S., Yang, C. W., Matatall, K., Basson, M., Sun, R., Piwnica-Worms, H., Sleckman, B. P. & Virgin, H. W. (2007a). Gamma-herpesvirus kinase actively initiates a DNA damage response by inducing phosphorylation of H2AX to foster viral replication. *Cell Host Microbe* 1, 275-286.

Tarakanova, V. L., Leung-Pineda, V., Hwang, S., Yang, C. W., Matatall, K., Basson, M., Sun, R., Piwnica-Worms, H., Sleckman, B. P. & Virgin, H. W. t. (2007b). Gamma-herpesvirus kinase actively initiates a DNA damage response by inducing phosphorylation of H2AX to foster viral replication. *Cell Host Microbe* 1, 275-286.

Tarakanova, V. L., Stanitsa, E., Leonardo, S. M., Bigley, T. M. & Gauld, S. B. (2010a). Conserved gammaherpesvirus kinase and histone variant H2AX facilitate gammaherpesvirus latency in vivo. *Virology* 405, 50-61.

Tarakanova, V. L., Stanitsa, E., Leonardo, S. M., Bigley, T. M. & Gauld, S. B. (2010b). Conserved gammaherpesvirus kinase and histone variant H2AX facilitate gammaherpesvirus latency in vivo. *Virology* 405, 50-61.

Taylor, R. T. & Bresnahan, W. A. (2005). Human cytomegalovirus immediate-early 2 gene expression blocks virus-induced beta interferon production. *J Virol* 79, 3873-3877.

Varnum, S. M., Streblow, D. N., Monroe, M. E., Smith, P., Auberry, K. J., Pasa-Tolic, L., Wang, D., Camp, D. G., 2nd, Rodland, K., Wiley, S., Britt, W., Shenk, T., Smith, R. D. & Nelson, J. A. (2004). Identification of proteins in human cytomegalovirus (HCMV) particles: the HCMV proteome. *J Virol* 78, 10960-10966.

Verpooten, D., Ma, Y., Hou, S., Yan, Z. & He, B. (2009). Control of TANK-binding kinase 1-mediated signaling by the gamma(1)34.5 protein of herpes simplex virus 1. *J Biol Chem* 284, 1097-1105.

Vider-Shalit, T., Fishbain, V., Raffaeli, S. & Louzoun, Y. (2007). Phase-dependent immune evasion of herpesviruses. *J Virol* 81, 9536-9545.

Wang, J. T., Doong, S. L., Teng, S. C., Lee, C. P., Tsai, C. H. & Chen, M. R. (2009). Epstein-Barr virus BGLF4 kinase suppresses the interferon regulatory factor 3 signaling pathway. *J Virol* 83, 1856-1869.

Wang, S. K., Duh, C. Y. & Chang, T. T. (2000). Cloning and identification of regulatory gene UL76 of human cytomegalovirus. *J Gen Virol* 81, 2407-2416.

Watanabe, N., Sakakibara, J., Hovanessian, A. G., Taniguchi, T. & Fujita, T. (1991). Activation of IFN-beta element by IRF-1 requires a posttranslational event in addition to IRF-1 synthesis. *Nucleic Acids Res* 19, 4421-4428.

Wathelet, M. G., Lin, C. H., Parekh, B. S., Ronco, L. V., Howley, P. M. & Maniatis, T. (1998). Virus infection induces the assembly of coordinately activated transcription factors on the IFN-beta enhancer in vivo. *Mol Cell* 1, 507-518.

Weitzman, M. D., Carson, C. T., Schwartz, R. A. & Lilley, C. E. (2004). Interactions of viruses with the cellular DNA repair machinery. *DNA Repair (Amst)* 3, 1165-1173.

Wiebusch, L. & Hagemeier, C. (1999). Human cytomegalovirus 86-kilodalton IE2 protein blocks cell cycle progression in G(1). *J Virol* 73, 9274-9283.

Wilkinson, G. W., Kelly, C., Sinclair, J. H. & Rickards, C. (1998). Disruption of PML-associated nuclear bodies mediated by the human cytomegalovirus major immediate early gene product. *J Gen Virol* 79 (Pt 5), 1233-1245.

Yu, D., Silva, M. C. & Shenk, T. (2003). Functional map of human cytomegalovirus AD169 defined by global mutational analysis. *Proc Natl Acad Sci U S A* 100, 12396-12401.

Yu, Y., Wang, S. E. & Hayward, G. S. (2005). The KSHV immediate-early transcription factor RTA encodes ubiquitin E3 ligase activity that targets IRF7 for proteosome-mediated degradation. *Immunity* 22, 59-70.

Zhu, F. X., Chong, J. M., Wu, L. & Yuan, Y. (2005). Virion proteins of Kaposi's sarcoma-associated herpesvirus. *J Virol* 79, 800-811.

Zhu, F. X., King, S. M., Smith, E. J., Levy, D. E. & Yuan, Y. (2002). A Kaposi's sarcoma-associated herpesviral protein inhibits virus-mediated induction of type I interferon by blocking IRF-7 phosphorylation and nuclear accumulation. *Proc Natl Acad Sci U S A* 99, 5573-5578.

Zhu, F. X. & Yuan, Y. (2003). The ORF45 protein of Kaposi's sarcoma-associated herpesvirus is associated with purified virions. *J Virol* 77, 4221-4230.

Zlotnik, A. & Yoshie, O. (2000). Chemokines: a new classification system and their role in immunity. *Immunity* 12, 121-127.

Øster, B., Bundgaard, B. & Höllsberg, P. (2005). Human herpesvirus 6B induces cell cycle arrest concomitant with p53 phosphorylation and accumulation in T cells. *J Virol* 79, 1961-1965.

2

Optimal Gene Expression for Efficient Replication of Herpes Simplex Virus Type 1 (HSV-1)

Jun Nakabayashi
University of Tokyo
Japan

1. Introduction

Herpesviridae is a large class of animal viruses. Herpes simplex virus type 1 (HSV-1) is a prototypic virus in this taxonomic group. HSV-1 belongs to the *Alphaherpesviridae* which are most frequently responsible for cold-sore lesions around the lips and mouth. HSV-1 is extensively studied not only as a causative agent of human disease but also as a general model system for the gene expression. In the lytic replication cycle of HSV-1, temporally ordered viral gene expression is typically observed, that is, immediate early, early and late gene (Boehmer & Lehman, 1997; Boehmer & Nimonkar, 2003) . This classification of viral gene is based on the expression timing from the start of the infection. The immediate early gene is expressed within 30 minutes from the infection. The expression of the immediate early gene is introduced by the cooperation between the host transcription factor and VP-16 which is packed in the tegmentum of HSV-1 particle. The protein complex, composed of the host transcription factor and VP-16, binds to the immediate early gene promoter and then activates the immediate early gene expression (Wysocka & Herr, 2003). Immediate early genes encode the transcription factors. Under the control of the immediate early gene products, other viral genes are expressed (Weir, 2001; Yamamoto et al., 2006). 2~3 hours after infection, the early gene is expressed, delayed from the immediate early gene and proceeding to the late gene. Finally, the late gene expression has started after 8 hours after infection. Both the early and the late gene expression are regulated by the immediate early gene products such as ICP4 (Kim et al., 2002). The difference of the expression timing between the early and late gene is caused by the structural difference of the early and the late gene promoter as shown in Fig.1.

In the early gene promoter, many binding sites to the immediate early gene products are tandemly repeated. On the other hand, the number of repeat binding sites in the late gene promoter is fewer than that in the early gene promoter. The binding affinity of the early gene promoter to the immediate early gene products is higher as compared with the late gene promoter. Therefore the expression of the early gene proceeds to that of the late gene. The mechanism regulating the temporally ordered viral gene expression of HSV-1 is clarified as mentioned above. But the function of this expression pattern is not clear yet. The functional meaning of the expression profile of the HSV-1 gene is theoretically studied (Nakabayashi & Sasaki, 2009). In this chapter, the function of the temporally ordered viral gene expression of HSV-1 is considered from the point of view of the efficiency of the replication of HSV-1. Further, evolution of the temporal expression profile of the viral gene is taken into consideration. From the genome structure of HSV-1, the evolutionary process of HSV-1 is estimated (Umene & Sakaoka, 1999). Here, the evolution of HSV-1 is evaluated by the efficiency of the replication but not the genome structure. The regulatory system for the efficient replication of virus is developed through the evolutionary process. The HSV-1 genotype whose gene expression is optimally regulated to maximize the virion production is selected through the evolutionary process. It is considered that not only viral replication, but many biological systems, are optimized through the evolutionary process. It is shown that the optimality principle is valid and feasible to understand the mechanism of the biological system (Khanin et al., 2004; Tyurin & Khanin, 2005, 2006). It is confirmed how viral gene expression is temporally regulated to maximize the virion production by using the evolutionary simulation. The obtained expression pattern obtained from the evolutionary simulation is compared with the observed expression profile of HSV-1 gene.

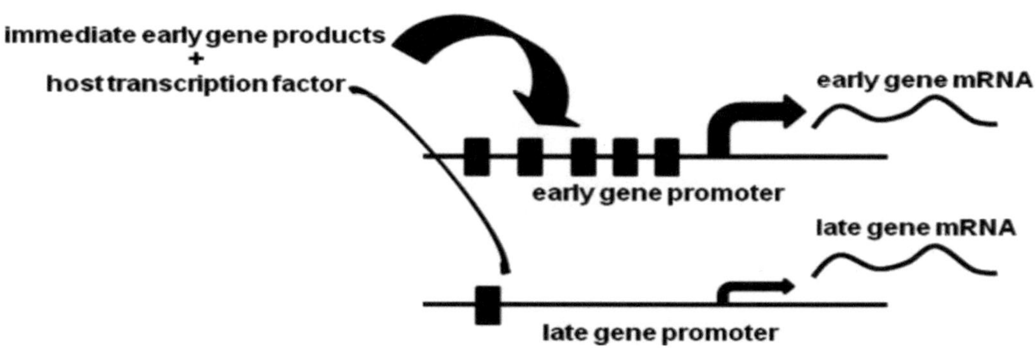

Fig. 1. The structural difference between the early and the late gene promoter. The expression timing of the early and late gene is determined by the structure of their promoters. In the early gene promoter, binding sites for the transcription factor are tandemly repeated. The number of binding sites in the late gene promoter is fewer than that in the early gene promoter.

2. Function of temporally ordered viral gene expression

The preceding expression of the early gene is necessary for the efficient replication of HSV-1. Though the classification of viral gene is based on the expression timing after infection, the protein function of viral gene is clearly distinguished between the early and the late gene (Nishiyama, 2004). Early genes encode the enzymes contributing to the DNA replication, while late genes encode the structural proteins of the HSV-1 particle (Cann, 2000). It is theoretically shown that the preceding DNA replication to the assembly of virion is appropriate for the efficient replication of HSV-1. The replication process is schematically shown in Fig. 2.

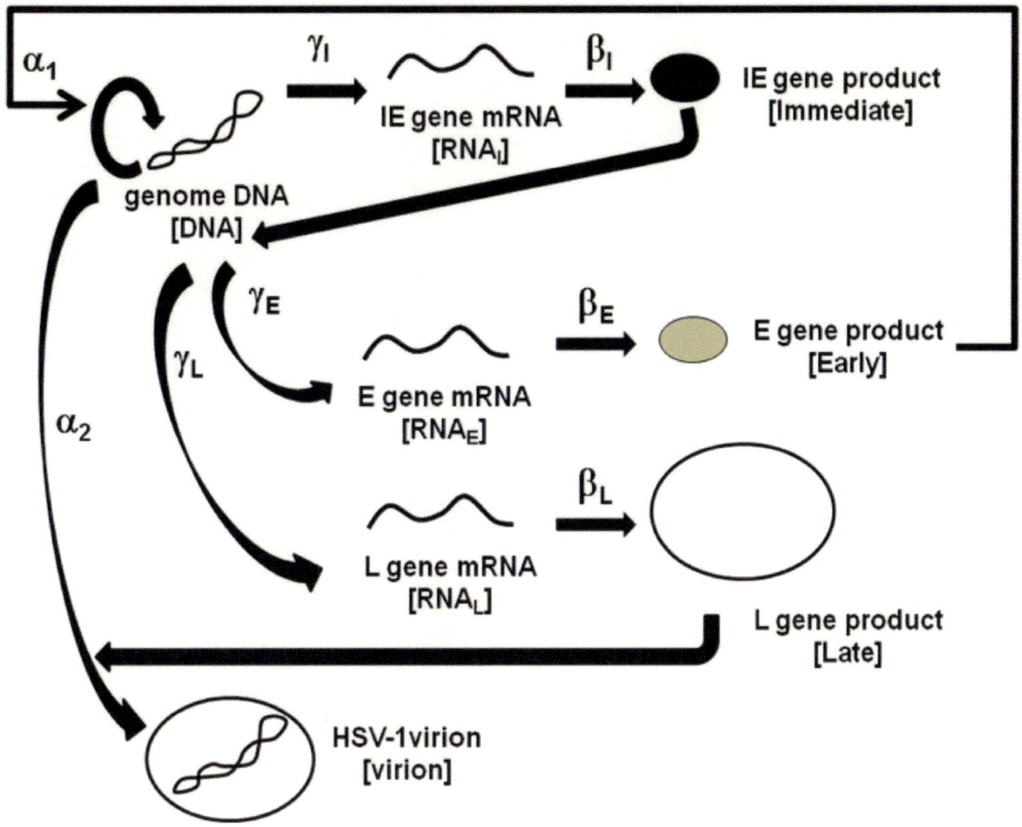

Fig. 2. The intracellular replication cycle of HSV-1. The replication of HSV-1 has started when the genome DNA of HSV-1 invades into the cell. First, the immediate early gene is expressed within 30 min. after infection. Under the control of the immediate early gene, both the early and the late gene are expressed. Early and late gene products contribute to the genome DNA replication and virion assembly, respectively. Finally, the complete virion is newly produced.

The replication process of HSV-1 is described as a chemical reaction equation as follows:

$$
\begin{aligned}
&[\mathrm{DNA}] \xrightarrow{\gamma_I} [\mathrm{DNA}] + [\mathrm{RNA_I}] \\
&[\mathrm{RNA_I}] \xrightarrow{\beta_I} [\mathrm{Immediate}] \\
&[\mathrm{RNA_I}] \xrightarrow{\delta_{RNA_I}} \mathrm{degradation} \\
&[\mathrm{Immediate}] \xrightarrow{\delta_I} \mathrm{degradation} \\
&[\mathrm{DNA}] + [\mathrm{Immediate}] \xrightarrow{\gamma_E} [\mathrm{DNA}] + [\mathrm{Immediate}] + [\mathrm{RNA_E}] \\
&[\mathrm{RNA_E}] \xrightarrow{\beta_E} [\mathrm{Early}] \\
&[\mathrm{RNA_E}] \xrightarrow{\delta_{RNA_E}} \mathrm{degradation} \\
&[\mathrm{Early}] \xrightarrow{\delta_E} \mathrm{degradation} \\
&[\mathrm{DNA}] + [\mathrm{Early}] \xrightarrow{a_1} 2[\mathrm{DNA}] + [\mathrm{Early}] \\
&[\mathrm{DNA}] + [\mathrm{Immediate}] \xrightarrow{\gamma_L} [\mathrm{DNA}] + [\mathrm{Immediate}] + [\mathrm{RNA_L}] \\
&[\mathrm{RNA_L}] \xrightarrow{\beta_L} [\mathrm{Late}] \\
&[\mathrm{RNA_L}] \xrightarrow{\delta_{RNA_L}} \mathrm{degradation} \\
&[\mathrm{Late}] \xrightarrow{\delta_L} \mathrm{degradation} \\
&[\mathrm{DNA}] + [\mathrm{Late}] \xrightarrow{a_2} [\mathrm{virion}] \\
&[\mathrm{virion}] \xrightarrow{\delta_v} \mathrm{degradation}
\end{aligned}
$$

The time change of each viral component is given according to law of mass action.

$$
\begin{aligned}
\frac{d[\mathrm{DNA}]}{dt} &= a_1[\mathrm{DNA}][\mathrm{Early}] - a_2[\mathrm{DNA}][\mathrm{Late}] - \delta_{DNA}[\mathrm{DNA}] \\
\frac{d[\mathrm{RNA_I}]}{dt} &= \gamma_I[\mathrm{DNA}] - \delta_{RNA_I}[\mathrm{RNA_I}] \\
\frac{d[\mathrm{Immediate}]}{dt} &= \beta_I[\mathrm{RNA_I}] - \delta_I[\mathrm{Immediate}] \\
\frac{d[\mathrm{RNA_E}]}{dt} &= \gamma_E[\mathrm{DNA}][\mathrm{Immediate}] - \delta_{RNA_E}[\mathrm{RNA_E}] \\
\frac{d[\mathrm{Early}]}{dt} &= \beta_E[\mathrm{RNA_E}] - \delta_E[\mathrm{Early}] \\
\frac{d[\mathrm{RNA_L}]}{dt} &= \gamma_L[\mathrm{DNA}][\mathrm{Immediate}] - \delta_{RNA_L}[\mathrm{RNA_L}] \\
\frac{d[\mathrm{Late}]}{dt} &= \beta_L[\mathrm{RNA_L}] - a_2[\mathrm{DNA}][\mathrm{Late}] - \delta_L[\mathrm{Late}] \\
\frac{d[\mathrm{virion}]}{dt} &= a_2[\mathrm{DNA}][\mathrm{Late}] - \delta_v[\mathrm{virion}]
\end{aligned} \tag{1}
$$

Notations used in the model (1) are summarized in Table1.

	Immediate Early	Early	Late
mRNA	[RNA_I]	[RNA_E]	[RNA_L]
Protein	[Immediate]	[Early]	[Late]
Transcription rate	γ_I	γ_E	γ_L
mRNA degradation rate	δ_{RNA_I}	δ_{RNA_E}	δ_{RNA_L}
Translation rate	β_I	β_E	β_L
Protein degradation rate	δ_I	δ_E	δ_L

Table 1. Notations used in the model (1).

The time course of HSV-1 replication is calculated from this mathematical model (1). The dependence of the intracellular dynamics of virion on the expression rates of the early and the late gene respectively designated by γ_E and γ_L is investigated. As a result, when the expression ratio γ_E/γ_L exceeds a certain threshold, HSV-1 virion is continuously reproduced. On the other hand, when the ratio γ_E/γ_L is smaller than a certain threshold level, HSV-1 replication is arrested. To understand this switching mechanism of the HSV-1 replication, model (1) is simplified for the theoretical analysis.
Model (1) is simplified under a certain constraints as follows:

$$\begin{aligned}
\frac{d[\text{DNA}]}{dt} &= a_1[\text{DNA}][\text{Early}] - a_2[\text{DNA}][\text{Late}] \\
\frac{d[\text{Immediate}]}{dt} &= \frac{\beta_I\gamma_I}{\delta_{RNA_I}}[\text{DNA}] \\
\frac{d[\text{Early}]}{dt} &= \frac{\beta_E\gamma_E}{\delta_{RNA_E}}[\text{DNA}][\text{Immediate}] \\
\frac{d[\text{Late}]}{dt} &= \frac{\beta_L\gamma_L}{\delta_{RNA_L}}[\text{DNA}][\text{Immediate}] - a_2[\text{DNA}][\text{Late}] \\
\frac{d[\text{virion}]}{dt} &= a_2[\text{DNA}][\text{Late}]
\end{aligned} \tag{2}$$

The diagram of the simplified model (2) is shown in Fig. 3.
Time dependent solutions of [DNA], [Early] and [Late] are obtained as a function of [Immediate] as follows:

$$\begin{aligned}
D &= D_0 + \frac{\xi_L}{a_2}[\text{Immediate}] - \frac{\xi_L}{2\xi_I}[\text{Immediate}]^2 + \frac{a_1\xi_E}{6{\xi_I}^2}[\text{Immediate}]^3 + \frac{\xi_I\xi_L}{{a_2}^2}\left(-1 + e^{-\frac{a_2}{\xi_I}[\text{Immediate}]}\right) \\
[\text{Early}] &= \frac{\xi_E}{2\xi_I}[\text{Immediate}]^2 \\
[\text{Late}] &= \frac{\xi_L}{\left({a_2}^2\xi_I\right)}\left(-1 + e^{-\frac{a_2}{\xi_I}[\text{Immediate}]}\right)
\end{aligned} \tag{3}$$

Here, $\xi_I = \frac{\gamma_I \beta_I}{\delta_{RNA_I}}, \xi_E = \frac{\gamma_E \beta_E}{\delta_{RNA_E}}, \xi_L = \frac{\gamma_L \beta_L}{\delta_{RNA_L}},$. D_0 is an initial condition for [DNA]. To investigate the trajectory of [DNA] as a function of [Immediate], the threshold for the continuous replication of HSV-1 without an arrest is analytically obtained as $\gamma_E/\gamma_L > \alpha_1/\alpha_2$ from the simplified model (2) and (3). Here α_1 and α_2 indicate the reaction rate constant of genome DNA replication and the virion assembly, respectively. Therefore $\gamma_E\alpha_1$ and $\gamma_L\alpha_2$ indicate the net genome DNA replication and virion assembly, respectively. This continuous replication of HSV-1 is caused by the effect of the positive feedback in the replication cycle. When the replication of genome DNA exceeds the virion assembly, the viral gene expression is further increased from the replicated viral DNA. Inversely, when the virion assembly exceeds the genome DNA replication, DNA of HSV-1 is consumed by the virion assembly. When all of the HSV-1 genome is consumed, HSV-1 replication is arrested because the template of the replication is absent. This result indicates that the temporally ordered viral gene expression, preceding expression of the early gene to the late gene, is necessary for the efficient replication of HSV-1 without an arrest.

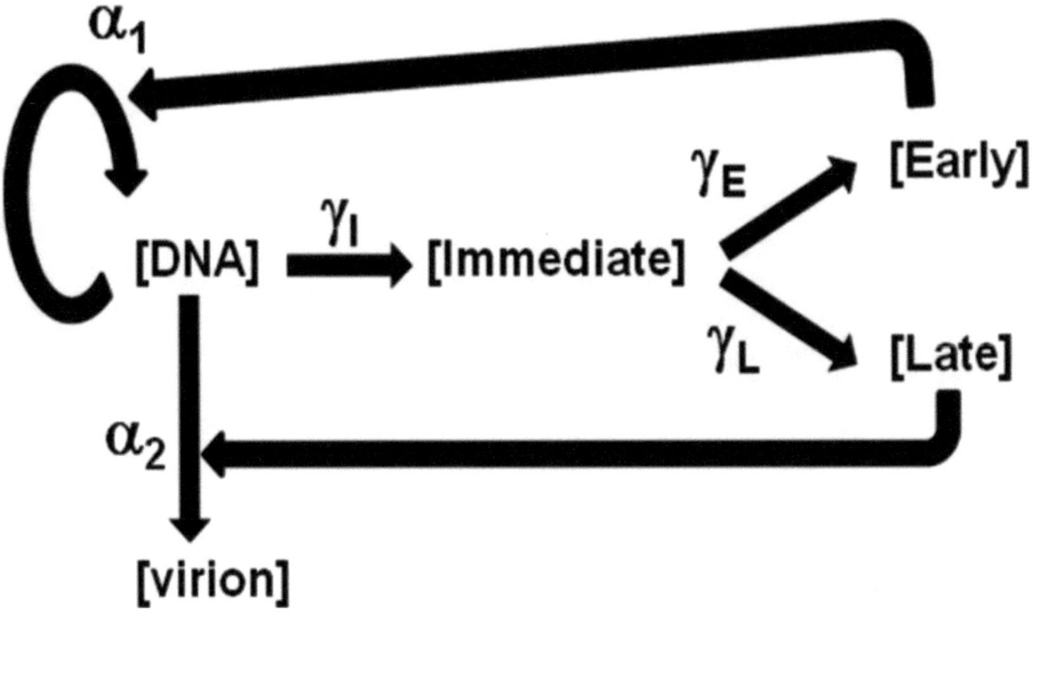

Fig. 3. The diagram of the simplified model (2).

3. Evolutionary process of HSV-1 gene expression

In this section, the evolution of the regulatory mechanism of HSV-1 gene expression is considered. The temporal profile of HSV-1 gene expression is determined by the structure of the promoter region on the HSV-1 genome. The structure of the HSV-1 promoter is changed by the mutation. For example, binding site is newly produced or lost by the point mutation in the promoter region. In the previous section, it is shown that the replication of HSV-1 is critically affected by the expression pattern of the viral gene. If the expression rate of the early gene is affected by the mutation in the promoter region of the early gene, replication dynamics of this mutant is changed as compared with that of the wild type. It is considered that the mutant with large expression rate of early gene becomes advantageous because of the continuous and efficient replication. It is considered that the frequency of the mutant with large expression rate of the early gene increases through the evolutionary process because of the improvement of the efficiency of the replication. It is hypothesized that the temporally ordered expression pattern of viral genes autonomously evolves through such an evolutionary process to maximize the efficiency of the replication of HSV-1. This hypothesis is confirmed by the evolutionary simulation.

3.1 Evolutionary simulation of the viral gene expression

Here, the procedure of the evolutionary simulation is briefly explained. Many genotypes of HSV-1 with various expression rates of the early and late genes are generated by drawing the random number. The production of virion of genotype j until a certain waiting time for the virion release designated by $v^{(j)}(\tau)$ is calculated according to the model (1). The frequency of each genotype is determined by the relative virion production designated by $\frac{v_j(\tau)}{\sum_{i=1}^{N} v_i(\tau)}$. This process means that the frequency of HSV-1 genotype with gene expression rate increasing the virion production increases its frequency. Mutation is reproduced by adding the random number to the expression rate $\gamma_E^{(j)}$ and $\gamma_L^{(j)}$. These processes are iterated over and over. After sufficient iterations, HSV-1 genotype with optimum gene expression rate maximizing the virion production is selected. The procedure of the evolutionary simulation is summarized in Fig. 4.

The initial condition of viral gene expression is set that the expression rate of the early gene is equal to that of the late gene. It is shown by the evolutionary simulation that HSV-1 genotype with large γ_E and small γ_L is selected through the evolutionary process. The frequency of HSV-1 genotype with large γ_E and small γ_L increases. The mean values of γ_E and γ_L increase and decrease, respectively. This result indicates that the temporally ordered gene expression of HSV-1 autonomously evolves to maximize the replication.

This result indicates that the preceding expression of the early gene to that of the late gene autonomously evolves from the initial condition when the expression rate of the early gene is equal to that of the late gene to maximize the efficiency of the virion production. If the new binding site to the transcription factor is newly created by the mutation in the early gene promoter, the mutant with large expression rate of the early gene becomes advantageous and increases its frequency. As a result, tandemly repeated binding sites observed in the early gene promoter are created. Inversely, a new binding site in the late gene prevents the efficient replication of HSV-1, because genome DNA of HSV-1 is consumed by the excessively expressed late gene product. HSV-1 replication stops because of the absence of the template of the replication. The binding site in the late gene cannot increase. The structural difference between the early gene promoter and the late gene promoter is reasonable from the view of the optimization of HSV-1 replication.

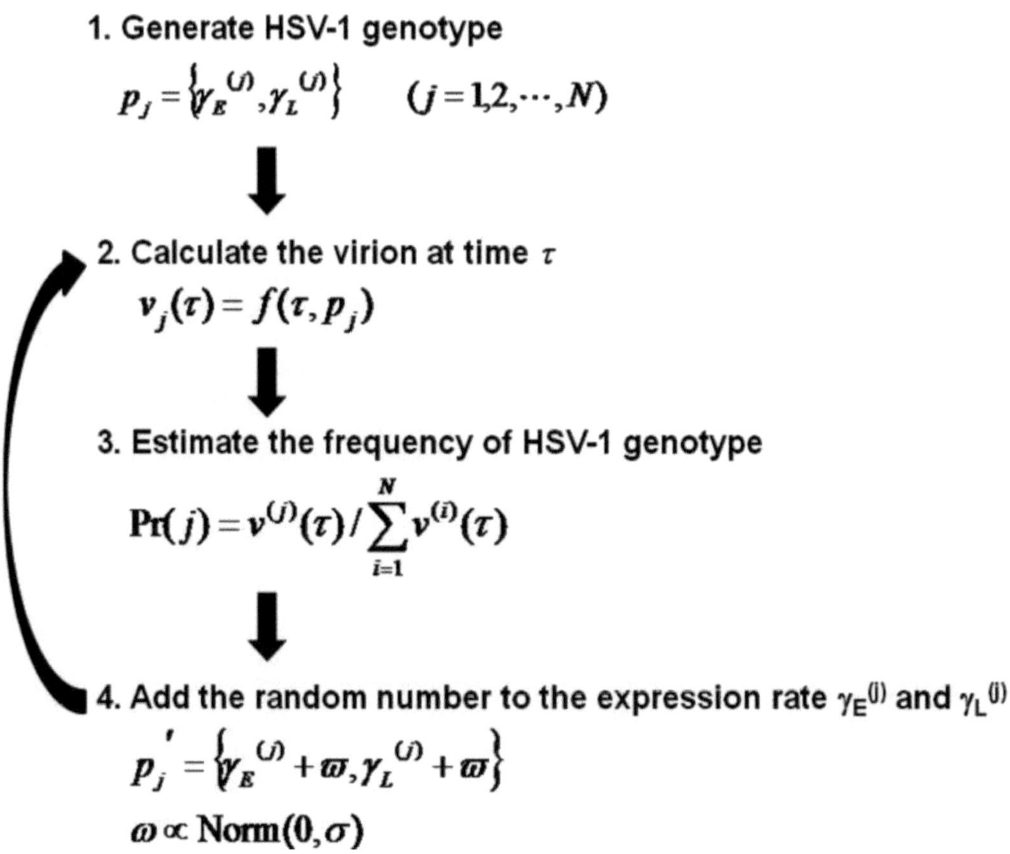

Fig. 4. The procedure of the evolutionary simulation.

But the genotype of HSV-1 with large γ_E and or small γ_L is not always advantageous. There is a condition for the evolution of the temporally ordered HSV-1 gene expression. It is also shown by the evolutionary simulation that the long waiting time for the virion release is necessary to evolve the preceding expression of the early gene to that of the late gene. Waiting time designated by τ is the period when HSV-1 replicates its copy in the infected cell until the newly produced virion is released from the infected cell. When waiting time for the virion release is small, HSV-1 genotype with small γ_E and large γ_L increases its frequency as shown in Fig. 6.

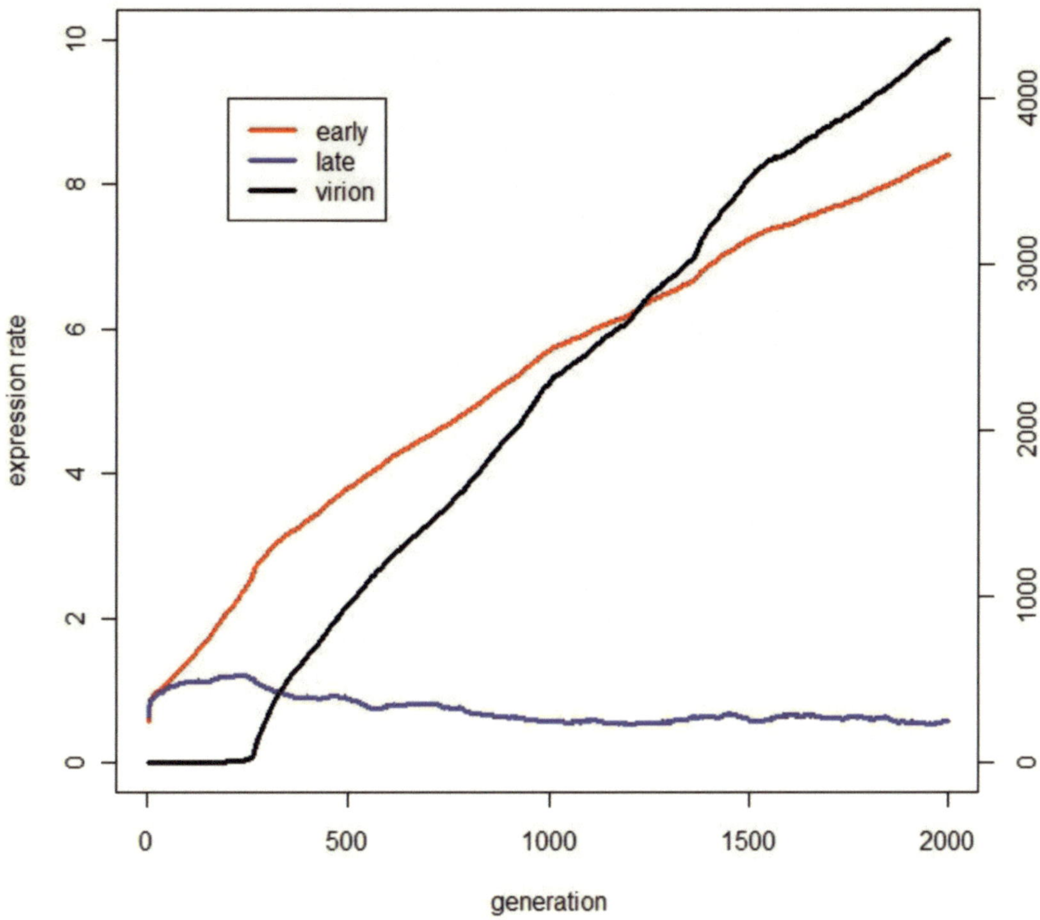

Fig. 5. A sample path of the evolutionary simulation. The mean expression rate of the early (red), late (blue) and mean value of virion (black) of 1000 HSV-1 genotypes are plotted. The initial expression rate of the early gene is equal to that of the late gene. The HSV-1 genotype with large γ_E increases its frequency as generation proceeds. The virion production rapidly increases when the expression ratio of the early gene to the late gene is larger than a certain threshold level.

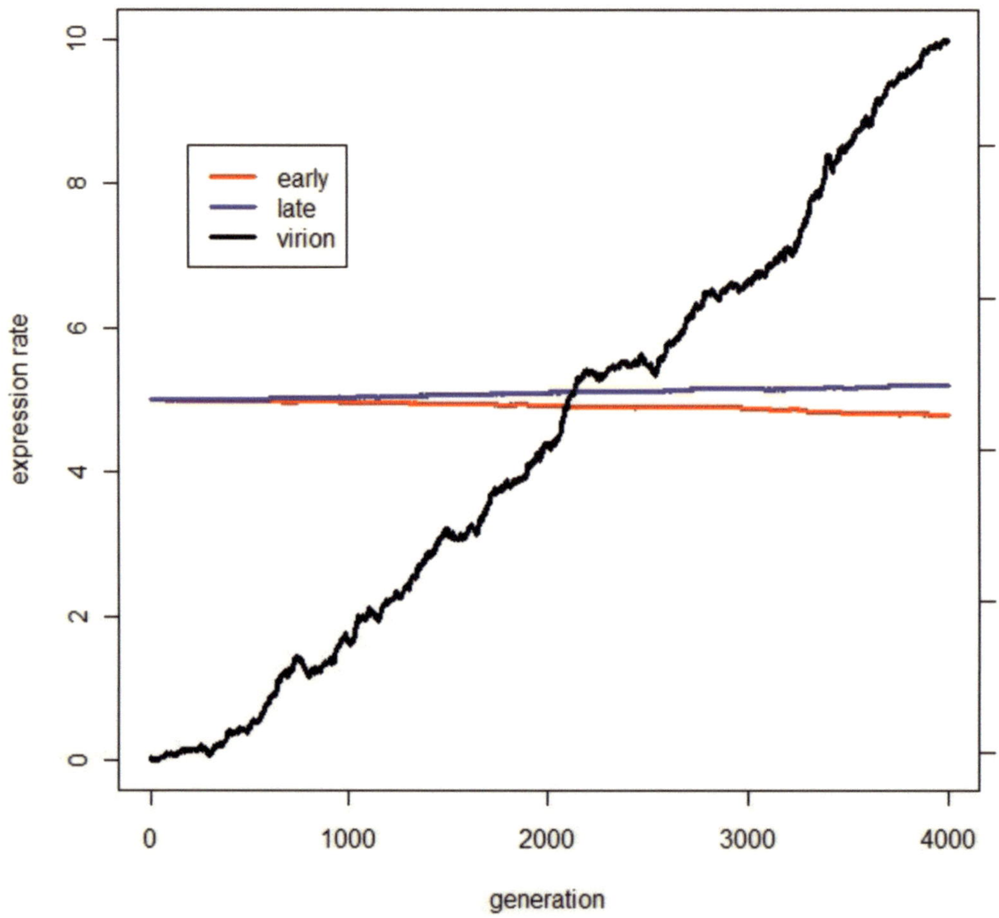

Fig. 6. A sample path of the evolutionary simulation with small waiting time τ. HSV-1 genotype with small γ_E (red) and large γ_L (blue) increases its frequency as generation proceeds. The virion production (black) slightly increases. Amount of virion remains at a small level as compared with the case when waiting time for the virion release is large.

The virion production of HSV-1 genotype with large γ_E and small γ_L is delayed in the initial phase of the replication as compared with HSV-1 genotype with small γ_E and large γ_L. As a result, when waiting time for the virion release from the infected cell is small, HSV-1 genotype with small γ_E and large γ_L becomes advantageous in spite of the fact that the replication of the HSV-1 genotype with small γ_E and large γ_L is arrested after sufficiently long time has passed after infection. Preceding expression of the early gene to that of the late gene cannot autonomously evolve. This result indicates that there is a trade-off between the initial speed and the final amount of virion production. When the expression of early gene becomes large, virion is continuously produced by the positive feedback in the replication cycle. But it takes much time to produce the virion. Inversely, when the late gene expression is large, virion is reproduced faster. But the replication cycle stops after sufficiently long time has passed because the positive feedback of the replication cannot function. To compare the virion production indicated by right-hand side axis in Fig. 5 and 6, the virion production remains small when τ is small. From the results of the evolutionary simulations, it is suggested that HSV-1 develops the efficient replication system with preceding expression of the early gene to that of the late gene under the condition that the waiting time for the virion release from the infected cell is large.

4. Conclusion

The function and the evolution of temporally ordered viral gene expression is investigated from the point of view of the efficiency of the replication. The preceding expression of the early gene to that of the late gene is advantageous for the continuous replication of HSV-1 without an arrest. Continuous replication of HSV-1 is caused by the effect of the positive feedback in the replication cycle. When the expression ratio γ_E/γ_L exceeds a certain threshold level, the positive feedback can function.

The expression timing of the viral genes is determined by the structure of their promoters. It is suggested by the evolutionary simulation that the tandemly repeated binding sites to the transcription factor in the early gene promoter autonomously evolves through the evolutionary process to maximize the virion production. As the promoter activity of the early gene increases, the efficiency of HSV-1 replication is improved. But large expression rate of the early gene is not always advantageous for the replication. The sufficiently long waiting time for the virion release is necessary to increase the frequency of HSV-1 genotype with large expression ratio of the early gene to the late gene. When waiting time for the virion release is small, the HSV-1 genotype with small γ_E and large γ_L that faster, but restrictedly, replicates its copy becomes advantageous. Preceding expression of the early gene to that of the late gene can evolve when the waiting time for the virion release is sufficiently long.

5. References

Boehmer, P. E.; & Lehman, I. R. (1997). Herpes simplex virus DNA replication. *Annual Review of Biochemistry* 66, pp347-384.

Boehmer, P. E.; & Nimonkar, A. V. (2003). Herpes virus replication. *IUBMB Life* 55 (1), pp13-22.

Cann, A. J. (2000). *DNA virus replication* Oxford University Press 0199637121 America

Khanin, M. A.; Lobanov, A. N. & Kaufman, H. (2004). Apoptosis: an optimization approach. *Computers in Biology and Medicine* 34(5), pp449-459.

Kim, D.B.; Zabierowski, S. & DeLuca, N. A. (2002). The initiator element in a herpes simplex virus type 1 late-gene promoter enhances activation by ICP4 resulting in abundant late-gene expression. *Journal of Virology* 76(4), pp1548-1558.

Nishiyama, Y. (2004). Herpes simplex virus gene products: the accessories reflect her lifestyle well. *Reviews in medical virology* 14(1), pp33-46.

Nakabayashi, J.; & Sasaki, A. (2009). The function of temporally ordered viral gene expression in the intracellular replication of herpes simplex virus type 1 (HSV-1). *Journal of Theoretical Biology* 261, pp156-164.

Pande, N. T.; Petroski, M. D. & Wagner, E. K. (1998). Functional modules important for activated expression of early genes of herpes simplex virus type 1 are clustered upstream of the TATA box. *Virology* 246, pp145-157.

Tyurin, K. V. & Khanin, M. A. (2005). Optimality principle and determination of kinetic constants for biochemical reactions. *Mathematical Medicine and Biology* 22(1), pp1-14.

Tyurin, K. V. & Khanin, M. A. (2006). Hemostasis as an optimal system. *Mathematical Bioscience* 204(2), pp167-184.

Umene, K. & Sakaoka, H. (1999). Evolution of herpes simplex virus type 1 under herpesviral evolutionary processes. *Archives of Virology* 144, pp637-656.

Weir, J. P. (2001). Regulation of herpes simplex virus gene expression. *Gene* 271(2), pp117-130.

Wysocka, J.; & Herr, W. (2003). The herpes simplex virus VP16-induced complex: the makings of a regulatory switch. *Trends in Biochemical Science* 28 (6), pp294-304.

Yamamoto, S.; Decker, L. A.; Kasai, K.; Chiocca, E. A.; & Saeki, Y. (2006). Imaging immediate-early and strict late promoter activity during oncolytic herpes simplex virus type 1 infection and replication in tumors. *Gene Therapy* 13(24), pp1731-1736.

3

Trojan Horses and Fake Immunity Idols: Molecular Mimicry of Host Immune Mediators by Human Cytomegalovirus

Juliet V. Spencer
University of San Francisco
United States of America

1. Introduction

Over the past 20 years, a fundamental shift has occurred in the study of virus-host relations. As scientists first began to identify and appreciate the clever tricks viral pathogens used to hide from the immune system, the terms **immune evasion** and **immune avoidance** became prevalent in the literature. More recently, we began to recognize and appreciate just how sophisticated and cunning some of these clever little tricks were, and the term **immune modulation** took center stage. This implies, correctly, that viruses are not just cowering in dark corners to avoid immune detection by the host, but rather that they are actively manipulating host conditions to create situations that favor virus persistence and make virus clearance difficult or even impossible.

1.1 Human cytomegalovirus and its bag of tricks

Once known as "salivary gland virus", HCMV was first isolated from the salivary glands and kidneys of a dying infant with greatly enlarged cells, or cytomegalic inclusion bodies, in affected tissues (Brennan, 2001). A member of the beta subgroup of the *Herpesviridae* family, HCMV is composed of a large double-stranded DNA genome surrounded by an icosahedral capsid. The linear genome of approximately 230 kb has terminal repeats flanking two unique segments, designated unique long (UL) and unique short (US), with open reading frames in each segment numbered sequentially. The nucleocapsid is covered by a protein layer termed the tegument, and the entire particle, approximately 200 nm in diameter, is enclosed by a membrane envelope featuring numerous glycoprotein spikes. HCMV infects multiple cell types, including epithelial cells, fibroblasts, monocytes, macrophages, and lymphocytes. The virus is transmitted between individuals via all body fluids (saliva, blood, breast milk, semen), as well as through bone marrow and solid organ transplants.

Infection with HCMV is often asymptomatic in the healthy host and a large percentage of the general population is seropositive (Staras et al., 2006). In contrast, serious disease frequently occurs in the immune suppressed. Diagnoses of life-threatening HCMV pneumonitis and retinitis are increasing among transplant recipients and persons living with AIDS (de la Hoz et al., 2002). Congenital HCMV infection is the leading viral cause of deafness and mental retardation in newborn infants (Damato and Winnen, 2002).

Like other herpesviruses, at some point following initial infection, HCMV establishes latent infection. Latency may be defined as the inability to detect infectious virus, despite the presence of viral DNA. All of the specific sites for HCMV latency are not well characterized, but myeloid progenitor cells in the bone marrow are believed to be the main reservoir of latent virus (Sinclair, 2008). Latent genomes have been detected in mononuclear cells in the peripheral blood, but not in neutrophils and other peripheral blood cells (Taylor-Wiedeman et al., 1993; Taylor-Wiedeman et al., 1991).

HCMV encodes over 180 genes, but only a subset of these is required for basic replication and generation of infectious progeny virions (Yu et al., 2003). The remaining viral genes have roles in mediating various aspects of the interaction between the virus and the host. Cellular processes that are affected by CMV gene products include the cell cycle, apoptosis, and immune recognition and response.

HCMV has developed numerous mechanisms for manipulating the host immune system (Scalzo et al., 2007). The virally encoded US2, US3, US6 and US11 gene products all interfere with antigen processing and presentation, resulting in reduced major histocompatibility complex (MHC) class I presentation (Ahn et al., 1996). This causes decreased recognition by cytotoxic T lymphocytes, which was recently found to enable superinfection by multiple virus strains in the same individual (Hansen et al., 2010). In addition, the UL18 gene product is a homolog of the MHC class I protein that is postulated to act as a decoy on the cell surface to assist in the evasion of natural killer cells (Beck and Barrell, 1988).

This chapter will focus on four HCMV genes: UL111A, UL144, UL146, and US28 (Figure 1). These genes encode a viral cytokine, cytokine receptor, chemokine, and chemokine receptor, respectively. Before expanding on each of these viral genes, an introduction to the human cytokine and chemokine system and its importance in immune responses is briefly discussed.

1.2 Cytokines, chemokines, and their receptors – Critical immune mediators

During World War II, the United States used the Navajo language to keep military communications from being intercepted by the enemy. Because the Navajo language had never been written down, it was virtually indecipherable without the help of a native speaker. The human immune system, on the other hand, relies on a system of secreted proteins to mediate the interactions required to coordinate and mount an effective immune response. Hundreds of different cytokines are constantly being secreted to regulate, stimulate, suppress, and control the many aspects of cell development, inflammation, and immunity.

Cytokines are produced by a wide variety of cell types , including monocytes, macrophages, lymphocytes, fibroblasts, mast cells, platelets, and the endothelial cells lining the walls of the blood vessels. Release of cytokines is an effective way to send information to multiple cells simultaneously, and only cells with the appropriate receptor can receive the signal, usually by binding to the cytokine at the plasma membrane and then transmitting the signal inside the cell via cellular pathways. Chemokines are a subtype of cytokine that function mainly as chemoattractants to induce migration of immune cells; in fact, the name is a contraction of the term "*chemo*tactic cyto*kine*". When released into the bloodstream, chemokines help to recruit monocytes, neutrophils, and other immune effector cells to sites of infection or damage. Chemokine receptors on target cells have seven transmembrane domains and belong to the G-protein coupled receptor superfamily.

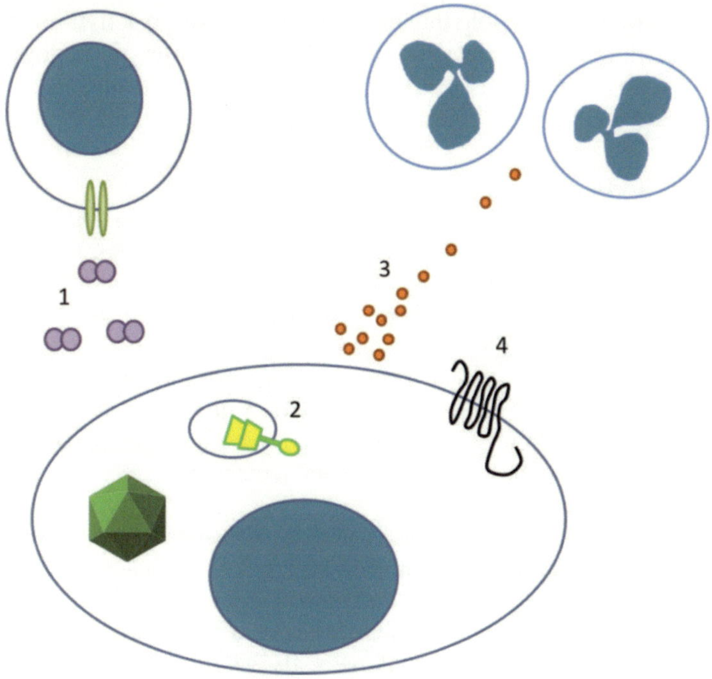

Fig. 1. An HCMV-infected cell displaying immunomodulatory viral proteins. 1) The UL111A gene product, cmvIL-10, is secreted from infected cells and binds to the cellular IL-10 receptor as a dimer. 2) The UL144 gene product is a TNF receptor homolog found primarily inside the cell. 3) The UL146 gene product, vCXC-1, is secreted and acts as an α-chemokine to attract neutrophils. 4) The US28 gene product is a seven-transmembrane chemokine receptor. A green icosahedron represents a virus nucleocapsid.

Despite its many complexities, the human cytokine system is not nearly as effective as the Navajo language was at confounding the enemy. Viruses like HCMV have not only broken the code, they produce their own cytokines, chemokines, and receptors during the course of infection to claim victory. Or, in viral terms, they render host immune responses ineffective and maintain persistent infection.

2. The UL111A gene product: CMV IL-10

Human cellular interleukin-10 (IL-10) is a pleiotropic cytokine that is important to the regulation of the immune response (Mosser and Zhang, 2008). Although stimulatory effects on the proliferation of B cells and mast cells have been reported, the primary function of IL-10 appears to be limiting the inflammatory response, in part by opposing interferon gamma (IFNγ) mediated effects. While IL-10 has effects on many cell types, monocytes in particular are a major target for IL-10 activity. IL-10 inhibits production of many cytokines by activated monocytes, including IL-1α, IL-1β, IL-6, TNFα, and even IL-10 itself (de Waal Malefyt et al., 1991a). Inhibition of IL-1 and TNFα are crucial to the anti-inflammatory effect, as these cytokines can have synergistic effects on other inflammatory pathways. Various cell surface molecules are also down-regulated by IL-10, including class II MHC and co-stimulatory molecules (de Waal Malefyt et al., 1991b), contributing to decreased T cell effector activity. A virally controlled IL-10 would enable the virus to direct immune activity to its advantage by inhibiting inflammation and evading T cell detection, thus providing a window of opportunity in which more virus could be produced and transmitted to other cells (Slobedman et al., 2009).

2.1 Gene structure and expression

The UL111 gene was originally designated as the coding region for ORF79, a 79 amino acid protein (Chee et al., 1990a). Another protein product from this region of the viral genome was later identified through searches for possible homologs to human IL-10 (Kotenko et al., 2000; Lockridge et al., 2000). Three exons separated by intervening sequences were identified and found to give rise to a 175 amino acid protein product with 27% identity to human IL-10 which has been designated cmvIL-10 (Figure 2). Interestingly, a homolog of IL-10 was identified in the genome of Epstein-Barr Virus a decade earlier, but the BCRF1 gene lacked introns and gave rise to a protein with 90% amino acid sequence identity to human IL-10 (Hsu et al., 1990). The human IL-10 gene, which is located on chromosome 1, is comprised of four introns and five exons.

The UL111A gene was found to be expressed with late kinetics in productively infected cells (Lockridge et al., 2000). The cmvIL-10 protein is secreted at sufficient levels to induce serum antibody responses in infected individuals (de Lemos Rieper et al., 2011). In addition to the full length cmvIL-10 protein, an alternative transcript is also produced from the UL111A gene, giving rise to a 139 amino acid protein (Jenkins et al., 2004). The smaller protein, designated LAcmvIL-10, results from read-through of the second intron and then premature termination. LAcmvIL-10 is co-linear with cmvIL-10 for the first 127 residues, then diverges in sequence at C-terminal domain (Figure 3). The name LAcmvIL-10 was based on the observation that this

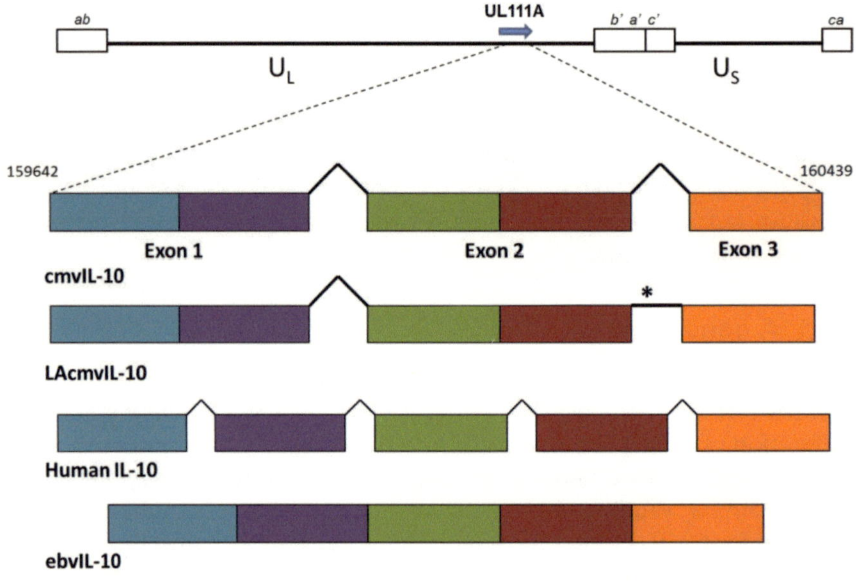

Fig. 2. Structure of the UL111A gene. The UL111A gene has two introns, but the organization is similar to the human IL-10 gene, which has four introns, and the ebvIL-10 gene, which has no introns. Also shown is the transcript for the LAcmvIL-10 gene, which reads through the second intron and encounters a stop codon, indicated by the asterisk (*).

shorter transcript was initially detected during latent infection of granulocyte-macrophage progenitors (and was therefore latency associated). However, it was subsequently found that LAcmvIL-10 is expressed during productive infection as well (Jenkins et al., 2008a). While the transcript encoding full length cmvIL-10 is expressed with late kinetics during infection, the transcript encoding LAcmvIL-10 is expressed with early kinetics during productive infection and continues to be expressed during latent infection.

2.2 Cell signaling

Despite having only 27% sequence identity to human IL-10, cmvIL-10 binds to the cellular IL-10 receptor and displays many of the immune suppressive functions of cellular IL-10 (Slobedman et al., 2009; Spencer et al., 2002). IL-10 effects are mediated via interaction with the cellular IL-10 receptor, a member of the interferon receptor superfamily, which consists of two subunits, a ligand binding subunit (IL-10R1) and a signaling subunit (IL-10R2), as shown in Figure 4. The IL-10/IL-10R interaction engages the Janus-family tyrosine kinases Jak1 and Tyk2, which are constitutively associated with IL-10R1 and IL-10R2, respectively. Ligand-induced oligomerization results in Jak1 activation leading to phosphorylation of the intercellular IL-10R1 chains. The transcription factor Stat (signal transducer and activator of transcription) is then recruited to the receptor complexes based on specific interaction of Stat SH2 domains with phosphotyrosine motifs in the receptor. Stats become phosphorylated, dissociate from receptor, form homo-or heterodimers, and translocate to the nucleus. IL-10 binding induces activation of Stat3, leading to suppression of IFNγ-inducible genes, such as those encoding class II MHC antigens (Donnelly et al., 1999; Mosser and Zhang, 2008).

CmvIL-10 engagement of the IL-10 receptors also leads to Stat3 activation (Spencer, 2007). Downstream immunomodulatory effects include inhibition of PBMC proliferation and inflammatory cytokine production, down-regulation of class I and class II MHC molecules, and impaired dendritic cell maturation (Chang et al., 2009; Chang et al., 2004; Raftery et al., 2001; Raftery et al., 2004; Spencer et al., 2002). Although Stat3 phosphorylation is mediated by Jak1, inhibition of cytokine synthesis also involves signaling through the phosphatidylinositol 3-kinase (PI3K) pathway (Spencer, 2007). Additional studies have shown that cmvIL-10 can inhibit NF-κB signaling in monocytes (Nachtwey and Spencer, 2008). Like human IL-10, the cmvIL-10 protein forms a dimer, and evidence suggests that cmvIL-10 can form heterodimers with human IL-10 that actually enhance Stat3 phosphorylation (Lin et al., 2008).

cmvIL-10

^{125}QCPLLGCGDKSVISRLSQEAERKSDNGTRKGLSELDTLFSRLEEYLHSRK

^{125}QCVSVSVAALSAQR

LA-cmvIL-10

Fig. 3. Amino acid sequence comparison of the C-terminal domain of full length cmvIL-10 and LAcmvIL-10. The proteins are identical from amino acids 1-127. Identical residues are shown in blue; residues that contact the cellular IL-10 receptor are shown in red.

LAcmvIL-10 retains some but not all of the immune suppressive properties of full length cmvIL-10 (Jenkins et al., 2008b; Spencer et al., 2008). LAcmvIL-10 can trigger down-regulation of class II MHC from the surface of monocytes and granulocyte-macrophage progenitor cells; however, this effect does not involve Stat3 phosphorylation and is independent of the IL-10 receptor. In addition, LAcmvIL-10 failed to inhibit maturation of dendritic cells and had no impact on the expression of co-stimulatory molecules (Jenkins et al., 2008b).

2.3 Role in infection

The UL111A gene is not required for virus replication *in vitro,* which supports the notion that cmvIL-10 and LAcmvIL-10 probably function in modifying host immune responses *in vivo* (Avdic et al., 2011). Studies with a UL111A deletion mutant virus have shown up-regulation of cytokines involved in dendritic cell formation and a higher proportion of myeloid dendritic cells compared to wild type virus. The results suggest that the UL111A gene products actively limit the ability of the host to respond to infection and clear virus, which is consistent with the observations of other groups that IL-10 is a key determinant of virus persistence (Brooks et al., 2008; Brooks et al., 2006). Vaccination studies of rhesus macaques also support the notion that the IL-10 pathway plays an important role in virus clearance (Barry, 2011). The Rhesus CMV genome also encodes an IL-10 homolog, designated RhcmvIL-10 (Lockridge et al., 2000). Uninfected rhesus macaques were immunized with a strategy designed to prevent engagement of the cellular IL-10 receptor by RhcmvIL-10 (Barry, 2011). Upon challenge with RhCMV, vaccinated animals had significantly fewer infected cells and infiltrate at the inoculation site, as well as reduced levels of virus in saliva and urine compared to control animals. Therapeutic strategies that neutralize cmvIL-10 activity hold great potential for enhancing the control or elimination of this persistent pathogen.

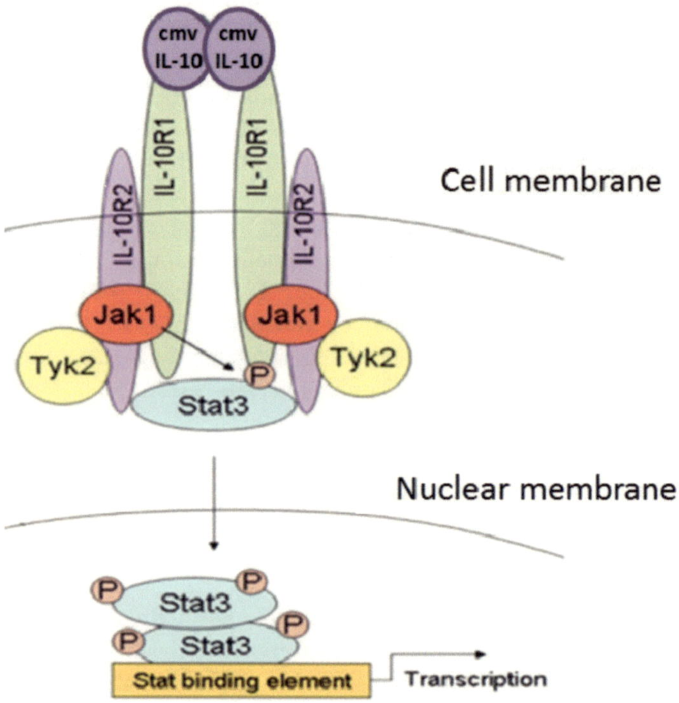

Fig. 4. Depiction of cmvIL-10 signaling through the cellular IL-10 receptor. The viral cytokine binds as a dimer, pulling together receptor chains to create a functional tetrameric receptor complex. The receptor associated kinase JAK1 phosphorylates Stat3, which then dimerizes and translocates to the nucleus to stimulate gene transcription.

2.4 Role in latent infection

Expression of the UL111A gene plays a role in maintaining a reservoir of virus by protecting latently infected cells from $CD4^+$ T cell recognition (Cheung et al., 2009). A UL111A deletion mutant virus was able to establish latent infection in myeloid progenitor cells and also reactivate from latency just as effectively as wild type virus. However, cells infected with the deletion mutant expressed higher levels of class II MHC on the cell surface. This effect was confirmed to be due to the lack of viral IL-10, since the addition of recombinant IL-10 (both full length cmvIL-10 and LAcmvIL-10) resulted in lower levels of class II MHC expression that was comparable to that of cells infected with wild type virus. Reduced class II expression correlated with diminished CD4 T cell responses, as measured by proliferation and interferon-γ production by purified allogeneic CD4 T cells co-cultured with the infected cells. CD4+T cells cultured with cells infected with the UL111A deletion virus exhibited significantly higher levels of proliferation and cytokine production, suggesting that UL111A gene products limit recognition of HCMV-infected cells by CD4+ T cells, thereby enhancing the pool of latently infected cells.

2.5 Role in cancer

The possible relationship between HCMV and cancer has been investigated for some time. The development of more sensitive detection methods has recently shown a very strong link between HCMV infection and glioblastoma and prostate cancer (Cobbs et al., 2002; Cobbs et al., 2007; Mitchell et al., 2008; Samanta et al., 2003). While HCMV is not generally regarded as an oncogenic virus, the term oncomodulation has been proposed to describe the increased malignancy associated with HCMV-infected tumor cells (Michaelis et al., 2009). The possible molecular mechanisms for oncomodulation include altered cell cycle regulation by immediate early proteins IE1 and IE2 (Sanchez and Spector, 2008), which promote entry into S phase, as well as the activity of the UL97 protein, which phosphorylates and inactivates tumor suppressor Rb (Hume et al., 2008). In addition, the UL36, UL37, and UL38 gene products all interfere with caspase function and convey resistance to apoptosis (McCormick, 2008; Skaletskaya et al., 2001). HCMV-infected neuroblastoma cells have been observed to down-regulate adhesion molecules and exhibit increased motility (Blaheta et al., 2004). In infected prostate cancer and glioma cells, HCMV infection resulted in increased migration and invasion that was dependent on phosphorylation of focal adhesion kinase (FAK) (Blaheta et al., 2006; Cobbs et al., 2007). Most recently, evidence points to a role of cmvIL-10 in promoting cancer progression.

HCMV has been shown to infect both glioma cancer stem cells (gCSCs) and macrophage/migroglial populations present in malignant gliomas (Dziurzynski et al., 2011). Production of cmvIL-10 by the gCSCs may convert peripheral blood monocytes into an immune suppressive, tumor-promoting cell type. The cmvIL-10 present in gCSC conditioned medium was shown to trigger activation of Stat3 and production of immune suppressive cytokines (Dziurzynski et al., 2011). At this point, the tumor promoting role of cmvIL-10 is largely associated with activation of Stat3. The Stat3 pathway is known to be active in a number of cell types in the tumor microenvironment and contributes to general immune suppression hindering anti-tumor responses (Kortylewski et al., 2005). In a murine model of glioma, Stat3 has been demonstrated to promote an influx of macrophages, which correlated negatively with survival (Kong et al., 2010). In addition, Stat3 activation is associated with poor prognosis in ovarian cancer and considered a key factor in metastasis formation and chemo-resistance (Zhang et al., 2010). This is one of the most exciting new areas of research involving cmvIL-10, and additional studies are currently underway to define the role of cmvIL-10 in potentiating tumor progression.

3. The UL144 gene product: TNF receptor homolog

Tumor necrosis factor (TNF) is an inflammatory cytokine that exists in both a membrane-bound and soluble form (Caminero et al., 2011). The biological effects of this cytokine are mediated through interactions with two receptors, TNF receptor 1 (TNFR1) and TNF receptor 2 (TNFR2). TNFR1 is expressed in a wide variety of cell types whereas TNFR2 is expressed only in cells of the immune system. Ligand-binding induces receptor trimerization and conformational changes that lead to dissociation of the inhibitory protein suppressor of death domain (SODD) followed by association of TRADD, or TNFR associated death domain protein (Wajant et al., 2003). Following TRADD binding, there are several possible outcomes, including activation of the NF-κB pathway, activation of the MAPK pathway, or induction of apoptosis. Both HSV-1 and HCMV target the TNF pathway (Figure 5); HSV-1 through glycoprotein D (Montgomery et al., 1996) and a TNFR homolog, HVEM (herpesvirus entry mediator) and HCMV through the UL144 gene product, also a TNFR homolog (Benedict et al., 1999; Cheung et al., 2005).

3.1 Gene structure and expression

The UL144 gene is one contiguous open reading frame located in the ULb' region of the HCMV genome (Figure 6). This region contains 19 ORFs first identified in the Toledo strain that are found in other clinical isolates yet deleted from laboratory strains (Cha et al., 1996). The UL144 gene product was identified through database searches and has regions of homology with the TNF receptor superfamily, especially the herpesvirus entry mediator, HVEM (Benedict et al., 1999), although the UL144 protein does not facilitate entry by HSV-1. UL144 is expressed early in HCMV infection with protein detected four hours post-infection (Benedict et al., 1999). Transcription from the UL144 gene is complex, with at least four differentially regulated transcripts expressed (He et al., 2011). One of these transcripts encompasses UL142 through UL145, and all transcripts contain both UL144 and UL145. Recent evidence also suggests that the UL144 gene is expressed by specific viral strains during experimental models of latency (Poole, 2011).

3.2 Cell signaling

The UL144 gene gives rise to a 176 amino acid protein with a transmembrane domain and short cytoplasmic tail. Despite the presence of an N-terminal signal sequence and multiple N-linked glycosylation sites in the ectodomain, the protein appears to be retained in an intracellular compartment (Benedict et al., 1999). Retention is mediated by tyrosine based sorting motif at the C-terminus of the protein (aa 173-176, YRTL), as demonstrated by a Y173A mutant expressed in 293T cells that displayed significantly higher levels of cell surface protein. The protein also contains two cysteine rich domains (CRDs) which are characteristic of TNFR family members, although many family members have as many as four CRDs. The CRD-2 region of the UL144 protein also shares significant homology with the ligand binding domain of another TNFR family member, TRAIL-R2. Although no TNF family ligands have been found to bind to the UL144 receptor, a member of the immunoglobulin superfamily known as BLTA, for B and T lymphocyte attenuator, was identified as a ligand for UL144 (Cheung et al., 2005). Presumably the UL144 protein would have to present on the cell surface in order to mediate this signaling. Despite its apparent intracellular localization, the UL144 protein must be exposed at some point during the infection since antibodies to this protein can be detected in HIV and HCMV co-infected individuals (Benedict et al., 1999).

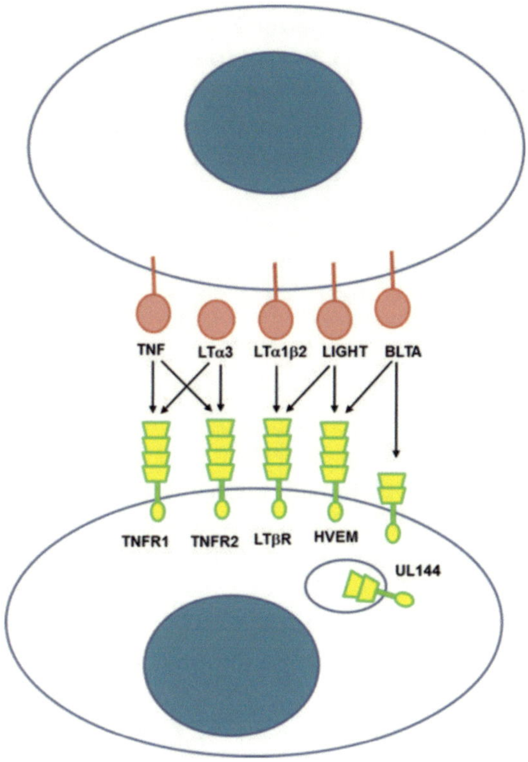

Fig. 5. TNF receptor superfamily members and their ligands. HVEM is the herpesvirus entry mediator of HSV-1. The UL144 gene product of HCMV is predominantly found inside the cell, but could interact with BLTA if present on the cell surface. Yellow trapezoids represent the CRD (cysteine rich domains) conserved throughout the TNFR superfamily.

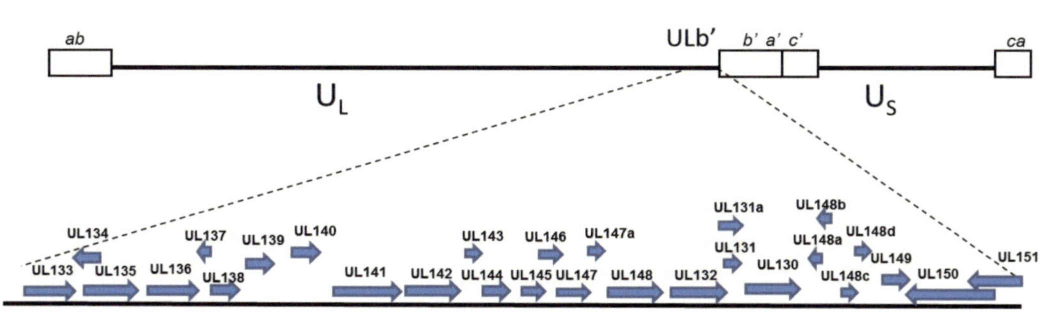

Fig. 6. Organization of the ULb' region of the HCMV Toledo strain genome.

3.3 Role in infection

In addition to the inhibitory effects on T-cell activation through engagement of BLTA (Cheung et al., 2005), UL144 also serves as an immune modulator during infection by triggering production of CCL22/MDC (or macrophage-derived chemokine) (Poole et al., 2008; Poole et al., 2006). CCL22 was detected in the supernatants from cells infected with a Toledo strain virus, but not in supernatants from cells infected with AD169, which lacks the ULb′ region. This effect was found to be mediated by NF-κB and is dependent on TRAF (TNFR associated factor). Induction of CCL22, which attracts Th2 and regulatory T cells expressing the CCR4 receptor (Yoshie et al., 2001), may aid in thwarting host immune responses by antagonizing the more effective TH1 antiviral response. The LMP1 protein of EBV also induces CCL2 expression (Nakayama et al., 2004), suggesting yet another common mechanism for manipulation of host responses among herpesviruses.

3.4 Polymorphisms as a measure of virulence

There have been conflicting reports regarding the correlation between UL144 genotype and clinical outcome. Genes in the ULb′ region, and the UL144 gene in particular, show a high level of variability among clinical strains. Three main genotypes have been described based on the extracellular region of the UL144 protein: type A, type B, and type C (Arav-Boger et al., 2006; Lurain et al., 1999). While some groups found that polymorphisms in the UL144 gene were not predictive of clinical outcome (Bale et al., 2001; Heo et al., 2008), others have found that types A and C do correlate with higher viral load and clinical sequelae (Arav-Boger et al., 2006; Waters et al., 2010). Differences in outcome may be attributable to sample size and population. Additionally, to date studies have been conducted only on congenitally infected infants, and so it is not clear how UL144 strain polymorphisms correlate with disease in other patient populations, such as transplant recipients or persons with HIV/AIDS.

4. The UL146 gene product: α-chemokine vCXC-1

Chemokines are a family of small soluble proteins that are secreted by immune cells in response to infection (Salazar-Mather and Hokeness, 2006). Members of the chemokine family fall mainly into one of two categories: α-chemokines or β-chemokines. The β-chemokines induce migration of monocytes, natural killer cells, and dendritic cells; they have two adjacent cysteines near the amino terminus of the protein and are also known as CC chemokines. In contrast, α-chemokines induce chemotaxis of neutrophils; they have the two cysteines separated by one amino acid and are known as CXC chemokines. CXC chemokines also generally have an ELR motif (glutamic acid - leucine - arginine) before the first cysteine. Interleukin-8 was the first CXC chemokine discovered, although its systemic designation is CXCL8. It is produced mainly by monocytes and lymphocytes, and it functions to induce neutrophil chemotaxis and degranulation through the chemokine receptors CXCR1 and CXCR2. Chemokines are important for controlling virus infection because they direct immune cells to sites of infection. However, for viruses that infect immune cells, chemokines may provide a vehicle for attracting host cells, or for directing infected cells to distribute virus to other parts of the body (Lusso, 2000; Murphy, 2001).

4.1 Gene structure, expression, and signaling

The UL146 gene, which is also located in the ULb′ region of the HCMV genome (Figure 6), encodes a functional α-chemokine (Penfold et al., 1999). The UL146 gene is expressed with late kinetics during infection and gives rise to a 117 amino acid protein. The protein contains an N-terminal signal sequence as well as the ELRCXC motif found in IL-8 that is known to be important for neutrophil binding and activation (Clark-Lewis et al., 1991). The UL146 gene product, which is also known as vCXC-1, was found to induce calcium flux and migration of neutrophils (Penfold et al., 1999). Since neutrophils express both CXCR1 and CXCR2, cells expressing each receptor separately were employed to dissect which receptor was mediating the effects of vCXC-1. While the initial studies identified CXCR2 as the primary receptor (Penfold et al., 1999), subsequent studies have found that vCXC-1 also binds to and effectively signals through the CXCR1 receptor (Luttichau, 2010). Although the adjacent gene, UL147, has a CXC motif, it lacks the ELR sequence and has not been shown to elicit signaling through human chemokine receptors (Penfold et al., 1999).

4.2 Role in infection

The UL146 gene product has been shown to encode a potent α-chemokine that induces neutrophil migration, calcium mobilization, and degranulation (Luttichau, 2010; Penfold et al., 1999). While it has been suggested that UL146 may function to recruit neutrophils to sites of infection to provide a vehicle for virus dissemination to distant sites in the body (Figure 7), this has yet to be examined in the context of virus infection *in vivo*, mainly because the species specificity of HCMV remains a barrier to its use with animal models. As discussed earlier, there is one model system that is particularly well-suited for investigating CMV-host interactions; the natural infection of Rhesus macaques (*Macaca mulatta*) by RhCMV (Powers and Fruh, 2008).

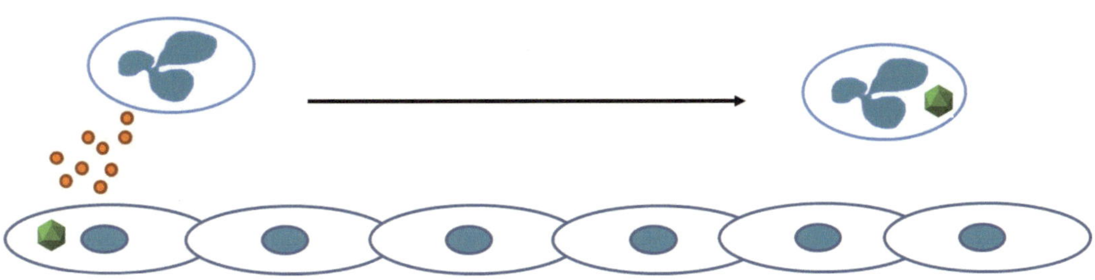

Fig. 7. Possible role for vCXC-1 in virus dissemination. Virus infected cells attract neutrophils via secretion of vCXC-1. Neutrophils could either become infected or phagocytose infected cells, then travel through the bloodstream, transporting virus to distant sites in the body.

The human and rhesus macaque genomes share about 95% sequence similarity. The complete genome of RhCMV strain 68.1 was sequenced in 2003, revealing 230 potential open reading frames, of which 138 were homologous to known HCMV proteins (Hansen et al., 2003). A more pathogenic isolate, RhCMV strain 180.92, was subsequently sequenced, revealing 10 additional open reading frames (Rivailler et al., 2006). A consensus map of both strains reveals that they each contain open reading frame designated Rh157.4, which was identified as having some homology to HCMV UL146 (Oxford et al., 2008). Most recently, RhCMV strains isolated from naturally infected macaques have recently been found to contain an additional genome segment not found in laboratory strains (Oxford et al., 2008). This segment, located between the Rh157.4 gene and the Rh161 gene, contains three open reading frames encoding proteins that exhibit 21-44% amino acid sequence identity with human IL-8 and/or HCMV UL146. Each of these three genes contains the ELRCXC motif (or a closely related sequence). Interestingly, these new genes (designated Rh161a, b, and c) also have homology to Rh161, which itself has low-level homology with human IL-8, suggesting that a gene duplication event may have occurred. Including RhUL146 and RhUL147 (rh158), this makes a total of 6 genes with homology to α-chemokines encoded by RhCMV. It is unclear why the virus would require six α-chemokine genes; however, such gene duplication events have been reported, notably in the case of the RhCMV US28 locus, where only one of the five genes was found to encode a functional receptor (Penfold et al., 2003). Additional studies are ongoing to determine which of these RhCMV genes encode functional chemokines and to discern their role in virus infection *in vivo*.

4.3 Polymorphisms as a measure of virulence

Like the UL144 gene, divergence of the UL146 has been noted in a large number of clinical strains (Aguayo et al., 2010; Arav-Boger et al., 2008; Bradley et al., 2008; He et al., 2006; Heo et al., 2008). In two of these studies, no connection between UL146 polymorphisms and clinical disease was noted (He et al., 2006; Heo et al., 2008). Arav-Boger et al developed an artificial neural network system to analyze variability of four different CMV genes (US28, UL144, UL146, and UL147) from congenitally infected infants in the Unites States and Italy (Arav-Boger et al., 2008). The results showed that UL144 and UL146 predicted the outcome of CMV disease in more than 80% of cases, when used separately, and specific nucleotide positions played a key role in these analyses. Despite the high degree of sequence variation noted for UL146, chemokine functionality is generally retained (Prichard et al., 2001).

5. The US28 gene product: Chemokine receptor

Chemokine receptors belong to the GPCR superfamily, one of the largest families of cell surface receptors. Receptors of this type relay signals from the cell surface to intracellular effectors and are found in all eukaryotic cells, from yeast to man. The human genome encodes over a thousand GPCRs, including receptors in the visual, olfactory, and gustatory (taste) systems, as well as many neurotransmitter, hormone, and chemokine receptors (Pierce et al., 2002). Members of this superfamily interact with heterotrimeric intracellular G proteins comprising α, β, and γ-subunits. In the inactive state, the Gα subunit binds to GDP (Gether, 2000). However, upon ligand binding, a conformational change occurs that promotes association of the intracellular domain of the receptor with a G-protein and catalyzes the exchange of GTP for bound GDP in the Gα subunit. Following receptor activation, the GTP-Gα subunit dissociates from both the receptor and the βγ subunits, which bind to each other very tightly. Each subunit can then interact with and activate specific downstream cellular effectors, depending on the nature of the receptor-ligand interaction. Intrinsic GTPase activity in the Gα subunit converts it to the inactive GDP-bound form, and re-association of the heterotrimeric complex terminates the signal and restores the receptor to its resting state. In addition to ligand dependent signaling, some GPCR, including HCMV US28, have been shown to signal in a ligand-independent, constitutive manner (Casarosa et al., 2001; Vischer et al., 2006a; Waldhoer et al., 2002).

5.1 Gene structure and expression

Of the four genes described here, only US28 was identified in the initial sequencing of the genome of HCMV strain AD169 (Chee et al., 1990a). Found within the unique short region of the HCMV genome, US28 is one of four genes with homology to the cellular G-protein coupled receptor (GPCR) superfamily (Chee et al., 1990b). Of the four HCMV GPCR (UL33, UL78, US27, and US28), only US28 has been shown to be a bona fide chemokine receptor. US28 has been extensively studied and is the subject of numerous reviews (Beisser et al., 2008; Vischer andLeurs and Smit, 2006a; Vischer et al., 2006b; Vomaske et al., 2009); only a brief overview of the current literature on US28 is provided here.

Expression of US28 transcripts occurs throughout the infection cycle, at immediate early, early, and late time points (Bodaghi et al., 1998; Zipeto et al., 1999), as well as during latency in THP-1 monocytes (Beisser et al., 2001). Although no homologs of this receptor exist in the genomes of rodent CMVs, five tandem homologs of US28 have been identified in the genome of Rhesus CMV (Penfold et al., 2003).

Because US27 and US28 are directly adjacent to one another in the HCMV genome and share 31% sequence identity, there has been some speculation that the two are a result of a gene duplication event. There is evidence for expression of both proteins in infected cells (Fraile-Ramos et al., 2001; Fraile-Ramos et al., 2002), suggesting that each receptor may have evolved (or is evolving) a distinct role in viral pathogenesis. US28 is expressed throughout the lytic and latent infection cycle, while US27 is expressed late in lytic infection only (Beisser et al., 2001; Welch et al., 1991), indicating that the two genes are independently regulated.

5.2 Cell signaling

US28 has been shown to bind to several human chemokines, including CX3CL/fractalkine, CCL5/RANTES, CCL3/MIP-1α, CCL2/MCP-1, and CCL7/MCP-3 (Beisser et al., 2002; Gao and Murphy, 1994; Neote et al., 1993). In addition, US28 is promiscuous in G protein coupling and has been shown to signal through $G\alpha_q$, $G\alpha_{i/o}$, $G\alpha_{12}$, and $G\alpha_{16}$ (Billstrom et al., 1998; Casarosa et al., 2001; Melnychuk et al., 2004). Chemokine binding to US28 induces a wide range of intracellular responses, including calcium mobilization, MAP kinase activation, cell migration, and activation of transcription factors such as NFAT, CREB, and NF-κB (Billstrom et al., 1998; Casarosa et al., 2001; Gao and Murphy, 1994; Streblow et al., 2003; Vieira et al., 1998). NF-κB activation has been shown to stimulate IL-6 production followed by a cascade including Stat3 phosphorylation and VEGF production (Figure 7) (Slinger et al., 2010).

Ligand-independent signaling has been found to include constitutive phospholipase C activation and inositol phosphate (IP_3) production (Casarosa et al., 2001; Minisini et al., 2003). US28 can also promote cell-cell fusion (Pleskoff et al., 1998) and was found to serve as a co-factor for entry of HIV into $CD4^+$ cells (Pleskoff et al., 1997).

For some types of GPCR, most notably the γ-aminobutyric acid (GABA) receptor, dimerization has been documented to be critical for effector activation and signaling (Kaupmann et al., 1998; Kuner et al., 1999; White et al., 1998). Chemokine receptors have also been shown to form functional dimers and oligomers that affect different aspects of receptor physiology, such as ligand affinity and signal transduction (Kramp et al., 2011; Mellado et al., 2001). Recent evidence suggests that US28 forms multimers with other GPCR (Tschische et al., 2011). UL33 and UL78 were both able to block US28-mediated activation of the transcription factor NF-κB, although constitutive signaling via the Gαq/phospholipase C pathway by US28 was not affected by receptor heteromerization (Tschische et al., 2011).

5.3 Role in infection

Despite the extensive in vitro characterization of US28, discerning a role for this protein in vivo during infection has been difficult since rodent CMVs do not encode a US28 homolog. However, murine CMV does encode homologs of two other HCMV GPCR, UL33 and UL78 (M33 and M78, respectively), suggesting that perhaps these genes were hijacked from an ancient host by an ancestral virus. Recent studies have shown that MCMV mutants lacking M33 exhibit a replication defect resulting in a significant reduction in virus replication in the salivary gland, as well as reduced reactivation from tissue explants (Farrell et al., 2011). Interestingly, HCMV US28 was found to complement the M33 mutant virus and restore both salivary gland replication and explant reactivation. These findings support the widely held view that the US28 receptor aids in virus dissemination by enabling infected cells to respond to chemokines and transport virus to distant sites in the body.

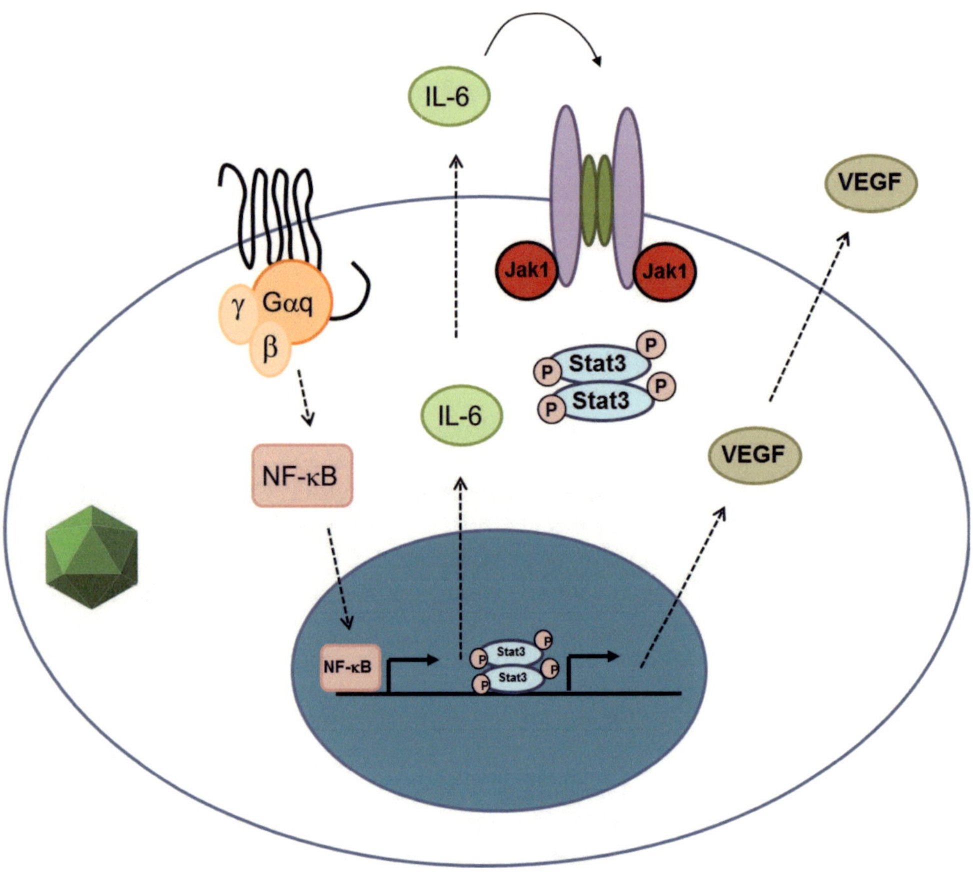

Fig. 8. US28 activates NF-kB inducing IL-6 expression. IL-6 can bind to its receptor in either an autocrine manner, as shown above, or act on nearby cells in a paracrine manner, to stimulate Stat3 and induce VEGF.

5.4 Role in atherosclerosis and cancer

The formation of atherosclerotic plaques resembles a chronic inflammatory response characterized by infiltration of monocytes, macrophages, and T lymphocytes recruited to the site via the secretion of chemokines from the vascular endothelium (Gautier et al., 2009; Zernecke and Weber, 2010). Both molecular and epidemiological data strongly links HCMV infection to atherosclerosis (Cheng et al., 2009; Epstein et al., 2009; Froberg et al., 2001; Gredmark-Russ et al., 2009; Hendrix et al., 1990; Hosenpud, 1999; Mattila et al., 1998; Straat et al., 2009; Streblow et al., 2008; Streblow et al., 2001a; Yi et al., 2008). Significant evidence now supports the notion that US28 may exacerbate atherosclerotic plaque formation by enhancing smooth muscle cell migration, and this subject has been reviewed elsewhere (Melnychuk et al., 2004; Streblow et al., 2001b; Streblow et al., 2007; Streblow et al., 1999; Streblow et al., 2003; Vischer andLeurs and Smit, 2006a).

In addition to a potential role in cardiovascular disease, HCMV infection has also been implicated in several types of cancer (see section 2.5). In particular, US28-expressing cells have been shown to promote tumorigenesis when injected into mice (Maussang et al., 2006). Activation of NF-κB by US28 contributed to increased expression of cyclooxygenase-2 (COX-2), an inflammatory mediator that plays a central role in several types of cancer (Maussang et al., 2009). Activation of Stat3 via the same pathway also has implications for cancer development, as previously discussed. Therapeutics blocking US28 activity may have utility for a number of diseases.

6. Conclusion

HCMV is endemic in the human population and may be associated with various human diseases. Most of the time, however, the virus peacefully co-exists with its human host. This interaction is governed by viral gene products that take an active role in establishing latency and modifying host immune responses in favor of virus persistence. Like the mythical Trojan horse that enabled the Greeks to conquer Troy, HCMV encodes many genes that seem innocuous, yet may have the power to decisively determine the outcome of virus infection.

7. References

Aguayo, F., Murayama, T., and Eizuru, Y. (2010). UL146 variability among clinical isolates of human cytomegalovirus from Japan. *Biol Res* 43(4), 475-80.

Ahn, K., Angulo, A., Ghazal, P., Peterson, P. A., Yang, Y., and Fruh, K. (1996). Human cytomegalovirus inhibits antigen presentation by a sequential multistep process. *Proc Natl Acad Sci U S A* 93(20), 10990-5.

Arav-Boger, R., Battaglia, C. A., Lazzarotto, T., Gabrielli, L., Zong, J. C., Hayward, G. S., Diener-West, M., and Landini, M. P. (2006). Cytomegalovirus (CMV)-encoded UL144 (truncated tumor necrosis factor receptor) and outcome of congenital CMV infection. *J Infect Dis* 194(4), 464-73.

Arav-Boger, R., Boger, Y. S., Foster, C. B., and Boger, Z. (2008). The use of artificial neural networks in prediction of congenital CMV outcome from sequence data. *Bioinform Biol Insights* 2, 281-9.

Avdic, S., Cao, J. Z., Cheung, A. K., Abendroth, A., and Slobedman, B. (2011). Viral Interleukin-10 Expressed by Human Cytomegalovirus during the Latent Phase of

Infection Modulates Latently Infected Myeloid Cell Differentiation. *J Virol* 85(14), 7465-71.

Bale, J. F., Jr., Petheram, S. J., Robertson, M., Murph, J. R., and Demmler, G. (2001). Human cytomegalovirus a sequence and UL144 variability in strains from infected children. *J Med Virol* 65(1), 90-6.

Barry, P. A., M. Eberhardt, and M. Walter (2011). Targeting the IL-10 Signaling Pathway as a Vaccine Strategy for HCMV. *In* "13th International CMV/Betaherpesvirus Workshop", Nuremburg, Germany.

Beck, S., and Barrell, B. G. (1988). Human cytomegalovirus encodes a glycoprotein homologous to MHC class-I antigens. *Nature* 331(6153), 269-72.

Beisser, P. S., Goh, C. S., Cohen, F. E., and Michelson, S. (2002). Viral chemokine receptors and chemokines in human cytomegalovirus trafficking and interaction with the immune system. CMV chemokine receptors. *Curr Top Microbiol Immunol* 269, 203-34.

Beisser, P. S., Laurent, L., Virelizier, J. L., and Michelson, S. (2001). Human cytomegalovirus chemokine receptor gene US28 is transcribed in latently infected THP-1 monocytes. *J Virol* 75(13), 5949-57.

Beisser, P. S., Lavreysen, H., Bruggeman, C. A., and Vink, C. (2008). Chemokines and chemokine receptors encoded by cytomegaloviruses. *Curr Top Microbiol Immunol* 325, 221-42.

Benedict, C. A., Butrovich, K. D., Lurain, N. S., Corbeil, J., Rooney, I., Schneider, P., Tschopp, J., and Ware, C. F. (1999). Cutting edge: a novel viral TNF receptor superfamily member in virulent strains of human cytomegalovirus. *J Immunol* 162(12), 6967-70.

Billstrom, M. A., Johnson, G. L., Avdi, N. J., and Worthen, G. S. (1998). Intracellular signaling by the chemokine receptor US28 during human cytomegalovirus infection. *J Virol* 72(7), 5535-44.

Blaheta, R. A., Weich, E., Marian, D., Bereiter-Hahn, J., Jones, J., Jonas, D., Michaelis, M., Doerr, H. W., and Cinatl, J., Jr. (2006). Human cytomegalovirus infection alters PC3 prostate carcinoma cell adhesion to endothelial cells and extracellular matrix. *Neoplasia* 8(10), 807-16.

Bodaghi, B., Jones, T. R., Zipeto, D., Vita, C., Sun, L., Laurent, L., Arenzana-Seisdedos, F., Virelizier, J. L., and Michelson, S. (1998). Chemokine sequestration by viral chemoreceptors as a novel viral escape strategy: withdrawal of chemokines from the environment of cytomegalovirus-infected cells. *J Exp Med* 188(5), 855-66.

Bradley, A. J., Kovacs, I. J., Gatherer, D., Dargan, D. J., Alkharsah, K. R., Chan, P. K., Carman, W. F., Dedicoat, M., Emery, V. C., Geddes, C. C., Gerna, G., Ben-Ismaeil, B., Kaye, S., McGregor, A., Moss, P. A., Pusztai, R., Rawlinson, W. D., Scott, G. M., Wilkinson, G. W., Schulz, T. F., and Davison, A. J. (2008). Genotypic analysis of two hypervariable human cytomegalovirus genes. *J Med Virol* 80(9), 1615-23.

Brennan, D. C. (2001). Cytomegalovirus in renal transplantation. *J Am Soc Nephrol* 12(4), 848-55.

Brooks, D. G., Lee, A. M., Elsaesser, H., McGavern, D. B., and Oldstone, M. B. (2008). IL-10 blockade facilitates DNA vaccine-induced T cell responses and enhances clearance of persistent virus infection. *J Exp Med* 205(3), 533-41.

Brooks, D. G., Trifilo, M. J., Edelmann, K. H., Teyton, L., McGavern, D. B., and Oldstone, M. B. (2006). Interleukin-10 determines viral clearance or persistence in vivo. *Nat Med* 12(11), 1301-9.

Caminero, A., Comabella, M., and Montalban, X. (2011). Tumor necrosis factor alpha (TNF-alpha), anti-TNF-alpha and demyelination revisited: an ongoing story. *J Neuroimmunol* 234(1-2), 1-6.

Casarosa, P., Bakker, R. A., Verzijl, D., Navis, M., Timmerman, H., Leurs, R., and Smit, M. J. (2001). Constitutive signaling of the human cytomegalovirus-encoded chemokine receptor US28. *J Biol Chem* 276(2), 1133-7.

Cha, T. A., Tom, E., Kemble, G. W., Duke, G. M., Mocarski, E. S., and Spaete, R. R. (1996). Human cytomegalovirus clinical isolates carry at least 19 genes not found in laboratory strains. *J Virol* 70(1), 78-83.

Chang, W. L., Barry, P. A., Szubin, R., Wang, D., and Baumgarth, N. (2009). Human cytomegalovirus suppresses type I interferon secretion by plasmacytoid dendritic cells through its interleukin 10 homolog. *Virology* 390(2), 330-7.

Chang, W. L., Baumgarth, N., Yu, D., and Barry, P. A. (2004). Human cytomegalovirus-encoded interleukin-10 homolog inhibits maturation of dendritic cells and alters their functionality. *J Virol* 78(16), 8720-31.

Chee, M. S., Bankier, A. T., Beck, S., Bohni, R., Brown, C. M., Cerny, R., Horsnell, T., Hutchison, C. A., 3rd, Kouzarides, T., Martignetti, J. A., and et al. (1990a). Analysis of the protein-coding content of the sequence of human cytomegalovirus strain AD169. *Curr Top Microbiol Immunol* 154, 125-69.

Chee, M. S., Satchwell, S. C., Preddie, E., Weston, K. M., and Barrell, B. G. (1990b). Human cytomegalovirus encodes three G protein-coupled receptor homologues. *Nature* 344(6268), 774-7.

Cheng, J., Ke, Q., Jin, Z., Wang, H., Kocher, O., Morgan, J. P., Zhang, J., and Crumpacker, C. S. (2009). Cytomegalovirus infection causes an increase of arterial blood pressure. *PLoS Pathog* 5(5), e1000427.

Cheung, A. K., Gottlieb, D. J., Plachter, B., Pepperl-Klindworth, S., Avdic, S., Cunningham, A. L., Abendroth, A., and Slobedman, B. (2009). The role of the human cytomegalovirus UL111A gene in down-regulating CD4+ T-cell recognition of latently infected cells: implications for virus elimination during latency. *Blood* 114(19), 4128-37.

Cheung, T. C., Humphreys, I. R., Potter, K. G., Norris, P. S., Shumway, H. M., Tran, B. R., Patterson, G., Jean-Jacques, R., Yoon, M., Spear, P. G., Murphy, K. M., Lurain, N. S., Benedict, C. A., and Ware, C. F. (2005). Evolutionarily divergent herpesviruses modulate T cell activation by targeting the herpesvirus entry mediator cosignaling pathway. *Proc Natl Acad Sci U S A* 102(37), 13218-23.

Clark-Lewis, I., Schumacher, C., Baggiolini, M., and Moser, B. (1991). Structure-activity relationships of interleukin-8 determined using chemically synthesized analogs. Critical role of NH2-terminal residues and evidence for uncoupling of neutrophil chemotaxis, exocytosis, and receptor binding activities. *J Biol Chem* 266(34), 23128-34.

Cobbs, C. S., Harkins, L., Samanta, M., Gillespie, G. Y., Bharara, S., King, P. H., Nabors, L. B., Cobbs, C. G., and Britt, W. J. (2002). Human cytomegalovirus infection and expression in human malignant glioma. *Cancer Res* 62(12), 3347-50.

Cobbs, C. S., Soroceanu, L., Denham, S., Zhang, W., Britt, W. J., Pieper, R., and Kraus, M. H. (2007). Human cytomegalovirus induces cellular tyrosine kinase signaling and promotes glioma cell invasiveness. *J Neurooncol* 85(3), 271-80.

Damato, E. G., and Winnen, C. W. (2002). Cytomegalovirus infection: perinatal implications. *J Obstet Gynecol Neonatal Nurs* 31(1), 86-92.

de la Hoz, R. E., Stephens, G., and Sherlock, C. (2002). Diagnosis and treatment approaches of CMV infections in adult patients. *J Clin Virol* 25 Suppl 2, S1-12.

de Lemos Rieper, C., Galle, P., Pedersen, B. K., and Hansen, M. B. (2011). Characterization of specific antibodies against cytomegalovirus (CMV)-encoded interleukin 10 produced by 28 % of CMV-seropositive blood donors. *J Gen Virol* 92(Pt 7), 1508-18.

de Waal Malefyt, R., Abrams, J., Bennett, B., Figdor, C. G., and de Vries, J. E. (1991a). Interleukin 10(IL-10) inhibits cytokine synthesis by human monocytes: an autoregulatory role of IL-10 produced by monocytes. *J Exp Med* 174(5), 1209-20.

de Waal Malefyt, R., Haanen, J., Spits, H., Roncarolo, M. G., te Velde, A., Figdor, C., Johnson, K., Kastelein, R., Yssel, H., and de Vries, J. E. (1991b). Interleukin 10 (IL-10) and viral IL-10 strongly reduce antigen-specific human T cell proliferation by diminishing the antigen-presenting capacity of monocytes via downregulation of class II major histocompatibility complex expression. *J Exp Med* 174(4), 915-24.

Donnelly, R. P., Dickensheets, H., and Finbloom, D. S. (1999). The interleukin-10 signal transduction pathway and regulation of gene expression in mononuclear phagocytes. *J Interferon Cytokine Res* 19(6), 563-73.

Dziurzynski, K., Wei, J., Qiao, W., Hatiboglu, M. A., Kong, L. Y., Wu, A., Wang, Y., Cahill, D., Levine, N. B., Prabhu, S., Rao, G., Sawaya, R., and Heimberger, A. B. (2011). Glioma-associated cytomegalovirus mediates subversion of the monocyte lineage to a tumor propagating phenotype. *Clin Cancer Res.*

Epstein, S. E., Zhu, J., Najafi, A. H., and Burnett, M. S. (2009). Insights into the role of infection in atherogenesis and in plaque rupture. *Circulation* 119(24), 3133-41.

Farrell, H. E., Abraham, A. M., Cardin, R. D., Sparre-Ulrich, A. H., Rosenkilde, M. M., Spiess, K., Jensen, T. H., Kledal, T. N., and Davis-Poynter, N. (2011). Partial functional complementation between human and mouse cytomegalovirus chemokine receptor homologues. *J Virol* 85(12), 6091-5.

Fraile-Ramos, A., Kledal, T. N., Pelchen-Matthews, A., Bowers, K., Schwartz, T. W., and Marsh, M. (2001). The human cytomegalovirus US28 protein is located in endocytic vesicles and undergoes constitutive endocytosis and recycling. *Mol Biol Cell* 12(6), 1737-49.

Fraile-Ramos, A., Pelchen-Matthews, A., Kledal, T. N., Browne, H., Schwartz, T. W., and Marsh, M. (2002). Localization of HCMV UL33 and US27 in endocytic compartments and viral membranes. *Traffic* 3(3), 218-32.

Froberg, M. K., Adams, A., Seacotte, N., Parker-Thornburg, J., and Kolattukudy, P. (2001). Cytomegalovirus infection accelerates inflammation in vascular tissue overexpressing monocyte chemoattractant protein-1. *Circ Res* 89(12), 1224-30.

Gao, J. L., and Murphy, P. M. (1994). Human cytomegalovirus open reading frame US28 encodes a functional beta chemokine receptor. *J Biol Chem* 269(46), 28539-42.

Gautier, E. L., Jakubzick, C., and Randolph, G. J. (2009). Regulation of the migration and survival of monocyte subsets by chemokine receptors and its relevance to atherosclerosis. *Arterioscler Thromb Vasc Biol* 29(10), 1412-8.

Gether, U. (2000). Uncovering molecular mechanisms involved in activation of G protein-coupled receptors. *Endocr Rev* 21(1), 90-113.

Gredmark-Russ, S., Dzabic, M., Rahbar, A., Wanhainen, A., Bjorck, M., Larsson, E., Michel, J. B., and Soderberg-Naucler, C. (2009). Active cytomegalovirus infection in aortic smooth muscle cells from patients with abdominal aortic aneurysm. *J Mol Med* 87(4), 347-56.

Hansen, S. G., Powers, C. J., Richards, R., Ventura, A. B., Ford, J. C., Siess, D., Axthelm, M. K., Nelson, J. A., Jarvis, M. A., Picker, L. J., and Fruh, K. (2010). Evasion of CD8+ T cells is critical for superinfection by cytomegalovirus. *Science* 328(5974), 102-6.

Hansen, S. G., Strelow, L. I., Franchi, D. C., Anders, D. G., and Wong, S. W. (2003). Complete sequence and genomic analysis of rhesus cytomegalovirus. *J Virol* 77(12), 6620-36.

He, R., Ma, Y., Qi, Y., Wang, N., Li, M., Ji, Y., Sun, Z., Jiang, S., and Ruan, Q. (2011). Characterization of the Transcripts of Human Cytomegalovirus UL144. *Virol J* 8(1), 299.

He, R., Ruan, Q., Qi, Y., Ma, Y. P., Huang, Y. J., Sun, Z. R., and Ji, Y. H. (2006). Sequence variability of human cytomegalovirus UL146 and UL147 genes in low-passage clinical isolates. *Intervirology* 49(4), 215-23.

Hendrix, M. G., Salimans, M. M., van Boven, C. P., and Bruggeman, C. A. (1990). High prevalence of latently present cytomegalovirus in arterial walls of patients suffering from grade III atherosclerosis. *Am J Pathol* 136(1), 23-8.

Heo, J., Petheram, S., Demmler, G., Murph, J. R., Adler, S. P., Bale, J., and Sparer, T. E. (2008). Polymorphisms within human cytomegalovirus chemokine (UL146/UL147) and cytokine receptor genes (UL144) are not predictive of sequelae in congenitally infected children. *Virology* 378(1), 86-96.

Hosenpud, J. D. (1999). Coronary artery disease after heart transplantation and its relation to cytomegalovirus. *Am Heart J* 138(5 Pt 2), S469-72.

Hsu, D. H., de Waal Malefyt, R., Fiorentino, D. F., Dang, M. N., Vieira, P., de Vries, J., Spits, H., Mosmann, T. R., and Moore, K. W. (1990). Expression of interleukin-10 activity by Epstein-Barr virus protein BCRF1. *Science* 250(4982), 830-2.

Hume, A. J., Finkel, J. S., Kamil, J. P., Coen, D. M., Culbertson, M. R., and Kalejta, R. F. (2008). Phosphorylation of retinoblastoma protein by viral protein with cyclin-dependent kinase function. *Science* 320(5877), 797-9.

Jenkins, C., Abendroth, A., and Slobedman, B. (2004). A Novel Viral Transcript with Homology to Human Interleukin-10 Is Expressed during Latent Human Cytomegalovirus Infection. *J Virol* 78(3), 1440-7.

Jenkins, C., Garcia, W., Abendroth, A., and Slobedman, B. (2008a). Expression of a human cytomegalovirus latency-associated homolog of interleukin-10 during the productive phase of infection. *Virology* 370(2), 285-94.

Jenkins, C., Garcia, W., Godwin, M. J., Spencer, J. V., Stern, J. L., Abendroth, A., and Slobedman, B. (2008b). Immunomodulatory properties of a viral homolog of human interleukin-10 expressed by human cytomegalovirus during the latent phase of infection. *J Virol* 82(7), 3736-50.

Kaupmann, K., Malitschek, B., Schuler, V., Heid, J., Froestl, W., Beck, P., Mosbacher, J., Bischoff, S., Kulik, A., Shigemoto, R., Karschin, A., and Bettler, B. (1998). GABA(B)-receptor subtypes assemble into functional heteromeric complexes. *Nature* 396(6712), 683-7.

Kong, L. Y., Wu, A. S., Doucette, T., Wei, J., Priebe, W., Fuller, G. N., Qiao, W., Sawaya, R., Rao, G., and Heimberger, A. B. (2010). Intratumoral mediated immunosuppression is prognostic in genetically engineered murine models of glioma and correlates to immunotherapeutic responses. *Clin Cancer Res* 16(23), 5722-33.

Kortylewski, M., Kujawski, M., Wang, T., Wei, S., Zhang, S., Pilon-Thomas, S., Niu, G., Kay, H., Mule, J., Kerr, W. G., Jove, R., Pardoll, D., and Yu, H. (2005). Inhibiting Stat3 signaling in the hematopoietic system elicits multicomponent antitumor immunity. *Nat Med* 11(12), 1314-21.

Kotenko, S. V., Saccani, S., Izotova, L. S., Mirochnitchenko, O. V., and Pestka, S. (2000). Human cytomegalovirus harbors its own unique IL-10 homolog (cmvIL-10). *Proc Natl Acad Sci U S A* 97(4), 1695-700.

Kramp, B. K., Sarabi, A., Koenen, R. R., and Weber, C. (2011). Heterophilic chemokine receptor interactions in chemokine signaling and biology. *Exp Cell Res* 317(5), 655-63.

Kuner, R., Kohr, G., Grunewald, S., Eisenhardt, G., Bach, A., and Kornau, H. C. (1999). Role of heteromer formation in GABAB receptor function. *Science* 283(5398), 74-7.

Lin, Y. L., Chang, P. C., Wang, Y., and Li, M. (2008). Identification of novel viral interleukin-10 isoforms of human cytomegalovirus AD169. *Virus Res* 131(2), 213-23.

Lockridge, K. M., Zhou, S. S., Kravitz, R. H., Johnson, J. L., Sawai, E. T., Blewett, E. L., and Barry, P. A. (2000). Primate cytomegaloviruses encode and express an IL-10-like protein. *Virology* 268(2), 272-80.

Lurain, N. S., Kapell, K. S., Huang, D. D., Short, J. A., Paintsil, J., Winkfield, E., Benedict, C. A., Ware, C. F., and Bremer, J. W. (1999). Human cytomegalovirus UL144 open reading frame: sequence hypervariability in low-passage clinical isolates. *J Virol* 73(12), 10040-50.

Lusso, P. (2000). Chemokines and viruses: the dearest enemies. *Virology* 273(2), 228-40.

Luttichau, H. R. (2010). The cytomegalovirus UL146 gene product vCXCL1 targets both CXCR1 and CXCR2 as an agonist. *J Biol Chem* 285(12), 9137-46.

Mattila, K. J., Valtonen, V. V., Nieminen, M. S., and Asikainen, S. (1998). Role of infection as a risk factor for atherosclerosis, myocardial infarction, and stroke. *Clin Infect Dis* 26(3), 719-34.

Maussang, D., Langemeijer, E., Fitzsimons, C. P., Stigter-van Walsum, M., Dijkman, R., Borg, M. K., Slinger, E., Schreiber, A., Michel, D., Tensen, C. P., van Dongen, G. A., Leurs, R., and Smit, M. J. (2009). The human cytomegalovirus-encoded chemokine receptor US28 promotes angiogenesis and tumor formation via cyclooxygenase-2. *Cancer Res* 69(7), 2861-9.

Maussang, D., Verzijl, D., van Walsum, M., Leurs, R., Holl, J., Pleskoff, O., Michel, D., van Dongen, G. A., and Smit, M. J. (2006). Human cytomegalovirus-encoded chemokine receptor US28 promotes tumorigenesis. *Proc Natl Acad Sci U S A* 103(35), 13068-73.

McCormick, A. L. (2008). Control of apoptosis by human cytomegalovirus. *Curr Top Microbiol Immunol* 325, 281-95.

Mellado, M., Rodriguez-Frade, J. M., Vila-Coro, A. J., Fernandez, S., Martin de Ana, A., Jones, D. R., Toran, J. L., and Martinez, A. C. (2001). Chemokine receptor homo- or heterodimerization activates distinct signaling pathways. *Embo J* 20(10), 2497-507.

Melnychuk, R. M., Streblow, D. N., Smith, P. P., Hirsch, A. J., Pancheva, D., and Nelson, J. A. (2004). Human cytomegalovirus-encoded G protein-coupled receptor US28 mediates smooth muscle cell migration through Galpha12. *J Virol* 78(15), 8382-91.

Michaelis, M., Doerr, H. W., and Cinatl, J. (2009). The story of human cytomegalovirus and cancer: increasing evidence and open questions. *Neoplasia* 11(1), 1-9.

Minisini, R., Tulone, C., Luske, A., Michel, D., Mertens, T., Gierschik, P., and Moepps, B. (2003). Constitutive inositol phosphate formation in cytomegalovirus-infected human fibroblasts is due to expression of the chemokine receptor homologue pUS28. *J Virol* 77(8), 4489-501.

Mitchell, D. A., Xie, W., Schmittling, R., Learn, C., Friedman, A., McLendon, R. E., and Sampson, J. H. (2008). Sensitive detection of human cytomegalovirus in tumors and peripheral blood of patients diagnosed with glioblastoma. *Neuro Oncol* 10(1), 10-8.

Montgomery, R. I., Warner, M. S., Lum, B. J., and Spear, P. G. (1996). Herpes simplex virus-1 entry into cells mediated by a novel member of the TNF/NGF receptor family. *Cell* 87(3), 427-36.

Mosser, D. M., and Zhang, X. (2008). Interleukin-10: new perspectives on an old cytokine. *Immunol Rev* 226, 205-18.

Murphy, P. M. (2001). Viral exploitation and subversion of the immune system through chemokine mimicry. *Nat Immunol* 2(2), 116-22.

Nachtwey, J., and Spencer, J. V. (2008). HCMV IL-10 suppresses cytokine expression in monocytes through inhibition of nuclear factor-kappaB. *Viral Immunol* 21(4), 477-82.

Nakayama, T., Hieshima, K., Nagakubo, D., Sato, E., Nakayama, M., Kawa, K., and Yoshie, O. (2004). Selective induction of Th2-attracting chemokines CCL17 and CCL22 in human B cells by latent membrane protein 1 of Epstein-Barr virus. *J Virol* 78(4), 1665-74.

Neote, K., DiGregorio, D., Mak, J. Y., Horuk, R., and Schall, T. J. (1993). Molecular cloning, functional expression, and signaling characteristics of a C-C chemokine receptor. *Cell* 72(3), 415-25.

Oxford, K. L., Eberhardt, M. K., Yang, K. W., Strelow, L., Kelly, S., Zhou, S. S., and Barry, P. A. (2008). Protein coding content of the UL)b' region of wild-type rhesus cytomegalovirus. *Virology* 373(1), 181-8.

Penfold, M. E., Dairaghi, D. J., Duke, G. M., Saederup, N., Mocarski, E. S., Kemble, G. W., and Schall, T. J. (1999). Cytomegalovirus encodes a potent alpha chemokine. *Proc Natl Acad Sci U S A* 96(17), 9839-44.

Penfold, M. E., Schmidt, T. L., Dairaghi, D. J., Barry, P. A., and Schall, T. J. (2003). Characterization of the rhesus cytomegalovirus US28 locus. *J Virol* 77(19), 10404-13.

Pierce, K. L., Premont, R. T., and Lefkowitz, R. J. (2002). Seven-transmembrane receptors. *Nat Rev Mol Cell Biol* 3(9), 639-50.

Pleskoff, O., Treboute, C., and Alizon, M. (1998). The cytomegalovirus-encoded chemokine receptor US28 can enhance cell-cell fusion mediated by different viral proteins. *J Virol* 72(8), 6389-97.

Pleskoff, O., Treboute, C., Brelot, A., Heveker, N., Seman, M., and Alizon, M. (1997). Identification of a chemokine receptor encoded by human cytomegalovirus as a cofactor for HIV-1 entry. *Science* 276(5320), 1874-8.

Poole, E., Atkins, E., Nakayama, T., Yoshie, O., Groves, I., Alcami, A., and Sinclair, J. (2008). NF-kappaB-mediated activation of the chemokine CCL22 by the product of the human cytomegalovirus gene UL144 escapes regulation by viral IE86. *J Virol* 82(9), 4250-6.

Poole, E., K. Raven, M. Reeves, J. Sinclair (2011). UL144 is expressed during latency but in a strain specific manner. *In* "13th International CMV/Betaherpesvirus Workshop", Nuremberg, Germany.

Poole, E., King, C. A., Sinclair, J. H., and Alcami, A. (2006). The UL144 gene product of human cytomegalovirus activates NFkappaB via a TRAF6-dependent mechanism. *Embo J* 25(18), 4390-9.

Powers, C., and Fruh, K. (2008). Rhesus CMV: an emerging animal model for human CMV. *Med Microbiol Immunol* 197(2), 109-15.

Prichard, M. N., Penfold, M. E., Duke, G. M., Spaete, R. R., and Kemble, G. W. (2001). A review of genetic differences between limited and extensively passaged human cytomegalovirus strains. *Rev Med Virol* 11(3), 191-200.

Raftery, M. J., Schwab, M., Eibert, S. M., Samstag, Y., Walczak, H., and Schonrich, G. (2001). Targeting the function of mature dendritic cells by human cytomegalovirus: a multilayered viral defense strategy. *Immunity* 15(6), 997-1009.

Raftery, M. J., Wieland, D., Gronewald, S., Kraus, A. A., Giese, T., and Schonrich, G. (2004). Shaping phenotype, function, and survival of dendritic cells by cytomegalovirus-encoded IL-10. *J Immunol* 173(5), 3383-91.

Rivailler, P., Kaur, A., Johnson, R. P., and Wang, F. (2006). Genomic sequence of rhesus cytomegalovirus 180.92: insights into the coding potential of rhesus cytomegalovirus. *J Virol* 80(8), 4179-82.

Salazar-Mather, T. P., and Hokeness, K. L. (2006). Cytokine and chemokine networks: pathways to antiviral defense. *Curr Top Microbiol Immunol* 303, 29-46.

Samanta, M., Harkins, L., Klemm, K., Britt, W. J., and Cobbs, C. S. (2003). High prevalence of human cytomegalovirus in prostatic intraepithelial neoplasia and prostatic carcinoma. *J Urol* 170(3), 998-1002.

Sanchez, V., and Spector, D. H. (2008). Subversion of cell cycle regulatory pathways. *Curr Top Microbiol Immunol* 325, 243-62.

Scalzo, A. A., Corbett, A. J., Rawlinson, W. D., Scott, G. M., and Degli-Esposti, M. A. (2007). The interplay between host and viral factors in shaping the outcome of cytomegalovirus infection. *Immunol Cell Biol* 85(1), 46-54.

Sinclair, J. (2008). Human cytomegalovirus: Latency and reactivation in the myeloid lineage. *J Clin Virol* 41(3), 180-5.

Skaletskaya, A., Bartle, L. M., Chittenden, T., McCormick, A. L., Mocarski, E. S., and Goldmacher, V. S. (2001). A cytomegalovirus-encoded inhibitor of apoptosis that suppresses caspase-8 activation. *Proc Natl Acad Sci U S A* 98(14), 7829-34.

Slinger, E., Maussang, D., Schreiber, A., Siderius, M., Rahbar, A., Fraile-Ramos, A., Lira, S. A., Soderberg-Naucler, C., and Smit, M. J. (2010). HCMV-encoded chemokine receptor US28 mediates proliferative signaling through the IL-6-STAT3 axis. *Sci Signal* 3(133), ra58.

Slobedman, B., Barry, P. A., Spencer, J. V., Avdic, S., and Abendroth, A. (2009). Virus-encoded homologs of cellular interleukin-10 and their control of host immune function. *J Virol* 83(19), 9618-29.

Spencer, J. V. (2007). The cytomegalovirus homolog of interleukin-10 requires phosphatidylinositol 3-kinase activity for inhibition of cytokine synthesis in monocytes. *J Virol* 81(4), 2083-6.

Spencer, J. V., Cadaoas, J., Castillo, P. R., Saini, V., and Slobedman, B. (2008). Stimulation of B lymphocytes by cmvIL-10 but not LAcmvIL-10. *Virology* 374(1), 164-9.

Spencer, J. V., Lockridge, K. M., Barry, P. A., Lin, G., Tsang, M., Penfold, M. E., and Schall, T. J. (2002). Potent immunosuppressive activities of cytomegalovirus-encoded interleukin-10. *J Virol* 76(3), 1285-92.

Staras, S. A., Dollard, S. C., Radford, K. W., Flanders, W. D., Pass, R. F., and Cannon, M. J. (2006). Seroprevalence of cytomegalovirus infection in the United States, 1988-1994. *Clin Infect Dis* 43(9), 1143-51.

Straat, K., de Klark, R., Gredmark-Russ, S., Eriksson, P., and Soderberg-Naucler, C. (2009). Infection with human cytomegalovirus alters the MMP-9/TIMP-1 balance in human macrophages. *J Virol* 83(2), 830-5.

Streblow, D. N., Dumortier, J., Moses, A. V., Orloff, S. L., and Nelson, J. A. (2008). Mechanisms of cytomegalovirus-accelerated vascular disease: induction of paracrine factors that promote angiogenesis and wound healing. *Curr Top Microbiol Immunol* 325, 397-415.

Streblow, D. N., Orloff, S. L., and Nelson, J. A. (2001a). Do pathogens accelerate atherosclerosis? *J Nutr* 131(10), 2798S-2804S.

Streblow, D. N., Orloff, S. L., and Nelson, J. A. (2001b). The HCMV chemokine receptor US28 is a potential target in vascular disease. *Curr Drug Targets Infect Disord* 1(2), 151-8.

Streblow, D. N., Orloff, S. L., and Nelson, J. A. (2007). Acceleration of allograft failure by cytomegalovirus. *Curr Opin Immunol* 19(5), 577-82.

Streblow, D. N., Soderberg-Naucler, C., Vieira, J., Smith, P., Wakabayashi, E., Ruchti, F., Mattison, K., Altschuler, Y., and Nelson, J. A. (1999). The human cytomegalovirus chemokine receptor US28 mediates vascular smooth muscle cell migration. *Cell* 99(5), 511-20.

Streblow, D. N., Vomaske, J., Smith, P., Melnychuk, R., Hall, L., Pancheva, D., Smit, M., Casarosa, P., Schlaepfer, D. D., and Nelson, J. A. (2003). Human cytomegalovirus chemokine receptor US28-induced smooth muscle cell migration is mediated by focal adhesion kinase and Src. *J Biol Chem* 278(50), 50456-65.

Taylor-Wiedeman, J., Hayhurst, G. P., Sissons, J. G., and Sinclair, J. H. (1993). Polymorphonuclear cells are not sites of persistence of human cytomegalovirus in healthy individuals. *J Gen Virol* 74 (Pt 2), 265-8.

Taylor-Wiedeman, J., Sissons, J. G., Borysiewicz, L. K., and Sinclair, J. H. (1991). Monocytes are a major site of persistence of human cytomegalovirus in peripheral blood mononuclear cells. *J Gen Virol* 72 (Pt 9), 2059-64.

Tschische, P., Tadagaki, K., Kamal, M., Jockers, R., and Waldhoer, M. (2011). Heteromerization of human cytomegalovirus encoded chemokine receptors. *Biochem Pharmacol*.

Vieira, J., Schall, T. J., Corey, L., and Geballe, A. P. (1998). Functional analysis of the human cytomegalovirus US28 gene by insertion mutagenesis with the green fluorescent protein gene. *J Virol* 72(10), 8158-65.

Vischer, H. F., Leurs, R., and Smit, M. J. (2006a). HCMV-encoded G-protein-coupled receptors as constitutively active modulators of cellular signaling networks. *Trends Pharmacol Sci* 27(1), 56-63.

Vischer, H. F., Vink, C., and Smit, M. J. (2006b). A viral conspiracy: hijacking the chemokine system through virally encoded pirated chemokine receptors. *Curr Top Microbiol Immunol* 303, 121-54.

Vomaske, J., Nelson, J. A., and Streblow, D. N. (2009). Human Cytomegalovirus US28: a functionally selective chemokine binding receptor. *Infect Disord Drug Targets* 9(5), 548-56.

Wajant, H., Pfizenmaier, K., and Scheurich, P. (2003). Tumor necrosis factor signaling. *Cell Death Differ* 10(1), 45-65.

Waldhoer, M., Kledal, T. N., Farrell, H., and Schwartz, T. W. (2002). Murine cytomegalovirus (CMV) M33 and human CMV US28 receptors exhibit similar constitutive signaling activities. *J Virol* 76(16), 8161-8.

Waters, A., Hassan, J., De Gascun, C., Kissoon, G., Knowles, S., Molloy, E., Connell, J., and Hall, W. W. (2010). Human cytomegalovirus UL144 is associated with viremia and infant development sequelae in congenital infection. *J Clin Microbiol* 48(11), 3956-62.

Welch, A. R., McGregor, L. M., and Gibson, W. (1991). Cytomegalovirus homologs of cellular G protein-coupled receptor genes are transcribed. *J Virol* 65(7), 3915-8.

White, J. H., Wise, A., Main, M. J., Green, A., Fraser, N. J., Disney, G. H., Barnes, A. A., Emson, P., Foord, S. M., and Marshall, F. H. (1998). Heterodimerization is required for the formation of a functional GABA(B) receptor. *Nature* 396(6712), 679-82.

Yi, L., Wang, D. X., and Feng, Z. J. (2008). Detection of human cytomegalovirus in atherosclerotic carotid arteries in humans. *J Formos Med Assoc* 107(10), 774-81.

Yoshie, O., Imai, T., and Nomiyama, H. (2001). Chemokines in immunity. *Adv Immunol* 78, 57-110.

Yu, D., Silva, M. C., and Shenk, T. (2003). Functional map of human cytomegalovirus AD169 defined by global mutational analysis. *Proc Natl Acad Sci U S A* 100(21), 12396-401.

Zernecke, A., and Weber, C. (2010). Chemokines in the vascular inflammatory response of atherosclerosis. *Cardiovasc Res.*

Zhang, X., Liu, P., Zhang, B., Wang, A., and Yang, M. (2010). Role of STAT3 decoy oligodeoxynucleotides on cell invasion and chemosensitivity in human epithelial ovarian cancer cells. *Cancer Genet Cytogenet* 197(1), 46-53.

Zipeto, D., Bodaghi, B., Laurent, L., Virelizier, J. L., and Michelson, S. (1999). Kinetics of transcription of human cytomegalovirus chemokine receptor US28 in different cell types. *J Gen Virol* 80 (Pt 3), 543-7.

4

Contributions of the EBNA1 Protein of Epstein-Barr Virus Toward B-Cell Immortalization and Lymphomagenesis

Amber T. Washington and Ashok Aiyar
LSU Health Sciences Center, New Orleans
United States of America

1. Introduction

Epstein-Barr Virus (EBV) is a human herpesvirus, infecting 95% of humans, that is causally associated with the benign B-cell proliferative disorder, infectious mononucleosis. EBV has also been etiologically associated with several cancers, such as Burkitt's lymphoma, AIDS-related immunoblastic lymphomas, post-transplant lymphomas, nasopharyngeal carcinoma, and gastric carcinoma. Very few viral genes are expressed in these malignancies and infectious virus is rarely released, defining a state of infection termed latency. Many EBV-associated malignancies respond poorly to treatment with large variability in success rates dependent on disease stage, viral gene expression patterns, and concurrent immunosuppressive therapy. Developing broadly effective strategies to suppress cell proliferation induced by EBV requires careful consideration of viral factors common to many malignancy types. One interesting viral therapeutic target is the viral protein Epstein-Barr nuclear antigen 1 (EBNA1), which is expressed in all EBV-associated malignancies and has been extensively characterized. Upon association with a region on EBV's genome, termed *oriP*, EBNA1 facilitates the licensed replication and mitotic segregation of EBV genomes in proliferating tumor cells. EBNA1 bound to *oriP* also activates transcription from two major EBV promoters. Finally, EBNA1 is known to suppress apoptosis of EBV-positive tumor cells. In this review, we have described the molecular mechanisms by which EBNA1's functions are operant.

2. Malignancies associated with Epstein-Barr virus (EBV)

EBV is a double-stranded lymphotropic gammaherpesvirus with a 172-kb linear DNA genome that is widely distributed in the human population (Kieff and Rickinson 2007; Rickinson and Kieff 2007). EBV was discovered through its association with B-cell lymphomas in children and young adults in sub-Saharan Africa. These tumors, now termed Burkitt's lymphoma, were recognized by Denis Burkitt, a British surgeon, as occurring at an unusually high rate in regions of Africa where malaria was endemic. Postulating that an infectious agent was the cause, Burkitt provided tumor biopsies to Anthony Epstein and Yvonne Barr, who screened them for the presence of viral-like particles using electron microscopy (Epstein, Achong et al. 1964). EBV subsequently became the first virus to be isolated from human cancer (Henle, Henle et al. 1968). Soon after this discovery, epidemiological studies revealed that a primary acute infection with EBV was causally associated with the development of infectious mononucleosis in adolescence and adulthood (Niederman, McCollum et al. 1968). Similar studies revealed a causal association between EBV and Burkitt's lymphoma (de-The, Geser et al. 1978). Molecular studies conducted since 1975 have revealed EBV genomes and expressed genes to be present in several other malignancies.

EBV is currently associated with Hodgkin's lymphoma, non-Hodgkin's lymphoma, AIDS-related immunoblastic lymphomas, primary effusion lymphomas, post-transplant lymphomas, CNS lymphomas, gastric carcinoma, and nasopharyngeal carcinoma (Crawford, Thomas et al. 1980; Purtilo and Klein 1981; Ernberg and Altiok 1989; Glaser, Lin et al. 1997; Dockrell, Strickler et al. 1998; Taylor, Marcus et al. 2005; Navarro and Kaplan 2006). Indeed, together with Kaposi's sarcoma, lymphomas caused by EBV were the first malignancies identified as AIDS-defining clinical conditions (1987). In Figure 1, we have depicted a brief overview of the EBV life-cycle. During primary infection, EBV is transmitted by saliva to oral epithelial cells in which it replicates lytically (Kieff and Rickinson 2007; Rickinson and Kieff 2007). Released virus infects circulating B-lymphocytes using the B-cell surface proteins MHC class II and complement receptor 2 (CR2/CD21) as viral receptors (Fingeroth, Weis et al. 1984; Li, Spriggs et al. 1997). A small subset of viral genes, including EBNA1, are expressed in these infected B-cells that concurrently home to the closest lymphoid tissue, such as the Waldeyer's tonsillar ring, where they proliferate (Laichalk, Hochberg et al. 2002). These latently infected B-cells proliferate rapidly, a process driven by the expression of viral proteins that are described in the next section.

It is pertinent to note that these infected B-cells are latently infected; while they express viral genes that drive cell proliferation, they do not express the large number of viral genes required for production of infectious virus. Cytokines released by rapidly proliferating infected B-cells promote a strong primary CTL response that suppresses their proliferation (Rickinson, Lee et al. 1996; Steven, Leese et al. 1996). Infected B-cells that are not deleted by the CTL response exist in peripheral circulation as quiescent memory B-cells in which EBNA1 is typically the only viral protein expressed (Babcock, Decker et al. 1999). With a very low frequency, EBV's lytic replication is activated in these latently infected cells, releasing virus that is ultimately transmitted through oral mucosa (Laichalk, Hochberg et al. 2002). If EBV-positive memory B-cells transit to a regional lymph node or back to the tonsils, they can return to a highly proliferative state (*ibid*). When this occurs, a strong secondary CTL response limits their proliferation.

Under immunosuppressive conditions, such as a prior malarial infection, HIV-disease, or post-transplantation immunosuppressive therapy, an impaired CTL response permits the unimpeded proliferation of EBV-infected cells (Rickinson, Lee et al. 1996; Kieff and Rickinson 2007). Mutations in cellular genes caused by errors in DNA replication initially result in oligoclonal proliferative disorders, such as post-transplant lymphoproliferative disease; the progressive acquisition of additional mutations ultimately results in clonal malignancies, such as Burkitt's lymphoma (Hammerschmidt 2011; Vereide and Sugden 2011)

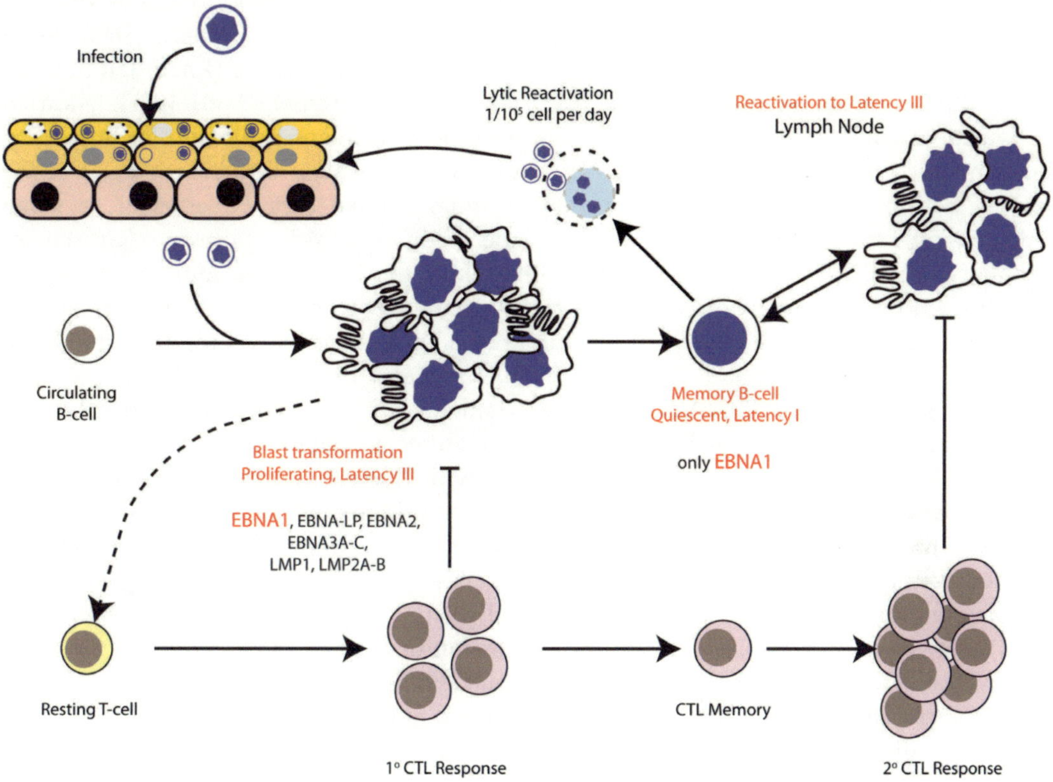

After lytic replication in epithelial cells, the virus is transmitted to circulating B-cells that undergo blast transformation in the nearest lymphoid tissue. A subset of viral genes, including EBNA1, is expressed in these proliferating blasts. A primary CTL response limits blast proliferation, and the surviving cells reside as quiescent, memory B-cells in the peripheral circulation. EBNA1 is the only viral protein expressed in EBV-positive memory B-cells. Additional details are in the text.

Fig. 1. Schematic overview of the EBV life-cycle.

2.1 EBV genes necessary for B-cell immortalization and patterns of viral gene expression

The capacity of EBV to drive unfettered B-cell proliferation is recapitulated during infections of naive B-cells in cell culture. EBV efficiently immortalizes naive B-cells to yield cell-lines termed lymphoblastoid cell-lines (LCLs) (Sugden and Mark 1977). Genetic studies have been used to identify the viral proteins required to immortalize naive B-cells in cell culture. Although the EBV genome encodes for approximately 90 proteins, only eight of these proteins are expressed when EBV infects naive B-cells (Mark and Sugden 1982). Of these, only six are required for naive B-cells' immortalization (Kieff and Rickinson 2007). Five of these genes are nuclear proteins, collectively referred to as the Epstein-Barr nuclear antigens (EBNAs). The five proteins are expressed from the same EBNA1-responsive viral promoter (Woisetschlaeger, Strominger et al. 1989). The sixth protein is membrane-associated, and termed latent membrane protein 1 (LMP1) that is also expressed from an EBNA1-responsive promoter (Abbot, Rowe et al. 1990).

The EBV proteins expressed during immortalization have numerous functions that are described briefly here. LMP1 is a homolog of the B-cell membrane protein CD40. While CD40 requires a ligand to be activated, LMP1 is constitutively active (Kaye, Izumi et al. 1993; Zimber-Strobl, Kempkes et al. 1996; Gires, Zimber-Strobl et al. 1997). Akin to activated CD40, it activates NFκB, AP-1, and JNK pathways, and their cellular targets, to sustain B-cell proliferation (Laherty, Hu et al. 1992; Mosialos, Birkenbach et al. 1995; Kieser, Kaiser et al. 1999). The five EBNA proteins have distinct, as well as some overlapping, functions. EBNA2 subverts the cellular Notch pathway (Grossman, Johannsen et al. 1994; Henkel, Ling et al. 1994). Like the intracellular domain of Notch, Notch-IC, EBNA2 associates with the transcription repressor human suppressor of hairless (hSH) converting it into an activator. This complex activates transcription from the same two viral promoters activated by EBNA1, and the cellular Enhancer of Split complex genes. While EBNA-LP greatly augments the efficiency with which EBV immortalizes naive B-cells, it is not required for immortalization (Hammerschmidt and Sugden 1989). In either event, it acts in concert with EBNA2 at specific viral promoters (Harada and Kieff 1997; Ling, Peng et al. 2005; Peng, Moses et al. 2005). EBNA3A and EBNA3C are similar in sequence and have some overlapping functions. They can both act to modulate the activation of hSH-responsive genes by EBNA2 by interacting with hSH (Robertson, Lin et al. 1996; Zhao, Marshall et al. 1996; Dalbies-Tran, Stigger-Rosser et al. 2001). However, only EBNA3C alters the expression of the metastatic suppressor Nm23-H1 (Murakami, Kaul et al. 2009). Finally, recent evidence indicates that EBNA3A and EBNA3C can individually, and cooperatively, down-modulate the expression of the pro-apoptotic cellular protein Bim (Paschos, Smith et al. 2009).

Latency Type	Active Promoter(s)	Genes Expressed	Condition(s)
0	Qp	EBNA1 (upon cell division)	Memory B-cells
I	Qp	EBNA1, EBERs, BARTs	Burkitt's lymphoma
II	Qp, LMP1p, LMP2p	EBNA1, LMP1, LMP2A, LMP2B, EBERs, BARTs	nasopharyngeal carcinoma, T-cell lymphoma
III	Wp, Cp, LMP1p, LMP2p	EBNA1, EBNA2, EBNA3A, EBNA3B, EBNA3C, EBNA-LP, LMP1, LMP2A, LMP2B, EBERs, BARTs	PTL, AIDS-related immunoblastic lymphoma, CNS lymphoma

Subsets of viral genes are expressed in cells infected latently with EBV. Different viral promoters are used to express EBNA1 in Type III and Type 0/I/II latency. The EBERs and BARTs are expressed from their own promoters that are not listed above.

Table 1. EBV gene expression programs in latency.

In addition to the five EBNA proteins and LMP1, there are three other EBV proteins expressed during latent infection. These proteins are EBNA3B, LMP2A and LMP2B (Kieff and Rickinson 2007; Rickinson and Kieff 2007). Two non-coding RNAs, termed EBER1 and EBER2, as well as a variable number of viral microRNAs, are also expressed during latency (*ibid*). The six proteins required for immortalization (EBNA1, EBNA2, EBNA3A, EBNA3C, EBNA-LP, LMP1) are expressed in four distinct programs termed Latency types 0, I, II, and III (*ibid*). These programs, indicated in Table I, are associated with specific cellular phenotypes. All six proteins are expressed in type III latency, which is a gene expression pattern observed in lymphoblastoid cell lines immortalized by EBV. Type III latency is also observed in post-transplant lymphomas and AIDS-related immunoblastic lymphomas. A more restricted pattern of gene expression is observed during the other latency types. Only EBNA1 is expressed in most Burkitt's lymphoma cells, which is a pattern termed type I latency. Latency type 0 is observed in infected memory B-cells where only EBNA1 expression is detected, and that too only when cells divide. No other viral proteins are expressed during latency type 0. Finally, latency type II is observed in rare T-cell lymphomas and EBV-associated carcinomas. In this pattern, the expression of EBNA1, LMP1, LMP2A, and LMP2B is detected.

The differential expression of the EBNA proteins in these latency types results from the use of two different promoters for the expression of EBNA1. During latency type III, the chromatin conformation and epigenetic markup of the viral genome favors the activation of the viral BamHI-C promoter (BamHI-Cp) by EBNA1 and EBNA2 (Day, Chau et al. 2007; Tempera, Klichinsky et al. 2011). All the six EBNA proteins are expressed from spliced transcripts that originate at BamHI-Cp. During latency type I, an alternative conformation and markup represses BamHI-Cp (*ibid*). When this occurs, the viral BamHI-Q promoter (BamHI-Qp) is activated; splicing of BamHI-Qp transcripts permits the expression of EBNA1 but not the other EBNAs (*ibid*). Irrespective of the promoter used, EBNA1 is the only viral protein expressed in all four latency types, rendering it an excellent target for therapies directed against EBV-infected cells.

3. EBNA1, its domains, and their functions

A schematic representation of EBNA1 is shown in Figure 2. EBNA1 from the prototypic B95-8 strain of EBV is 641 amino-acids (a.a.) long, and can be divided into several functional domains. EBNA1 associates with several cognate binding sites on the EBV genome through its DNA binding and dimerization domain (DBD), which lies from a.a. 451-641 (Ambinder, Shah et al. 1990; Ambinder, Mullen et al. 1991). The capacity of this domain, when expressed by itself, to bind EBNA1 binding sites was first demonstrated by the studies of Ambinder and Hayward (Ambinder, Shah et al. 1990) . While sufficient to bind EBNA1 binding sites, DBD alone does not support the replication & mitotic segregation of EBV genomes, nor can it activate EBNA1-responsive EBV promoters (Kirchmaier and Sugden 1997; Aiyar and Sugden 1998; Sears, Ujihara et al. 2004) . Indeed, when co-expressed with wild-type EBNA1, DBD functions as a dominant-negative by displacing EBNA1 from its binding sites (Kirchmaier and Sugden 1997).

The DBD is also the only domain of EBNA1 whose structure has been determined (Bochkarev, Barwell et al. 1995); it has a beta-barrel core region that is used for dimerization, flanked by a long alpha-helix that extends into the major groove of the binding site (Bochkarev, Barwell et al. 1996). Surprisingly, this structure is remarkably close to the structure of the DNA binding domain of the E2 protein (E2DBD) from bovine papilomavirus (BPV) (Hegde, Grossman et al. 1992), despite a lack of sequence conservation. In this context, it should be noted that BPV, a small DNA virus, is very distantly related to EBV, and the related structure of DBD and E2DBD is proposed to result from convergent evolution (Grossman and Laimins 1996). The modular nature of the DBD is reflected by several observations. Sugden and co-workers demonstrated that the DBD could be substituted by DNA-binding domain from the yeast GAL4 protein (Mackey, Middleton et al. 1995; Mackey and Sugden 1997). The chimeric protein displayed several biochemical properties of EBNA1 when bound to GAL4 binding sites. In a similar observation, we have shown that a chimeric protein in which a.a. 1-450 of EBNA1 was fused to E2DBD activated transcription from a cluster of E2 binding sites in a manner similar to WT EBNA1 (Aras, Singh et al. 2009). We have also demonstrated that a chimeric protein in which a strong heterologous acidic activation domain was fused to DBD activated transcription with the characteristics of the heterologous activation domain (*ibid*).

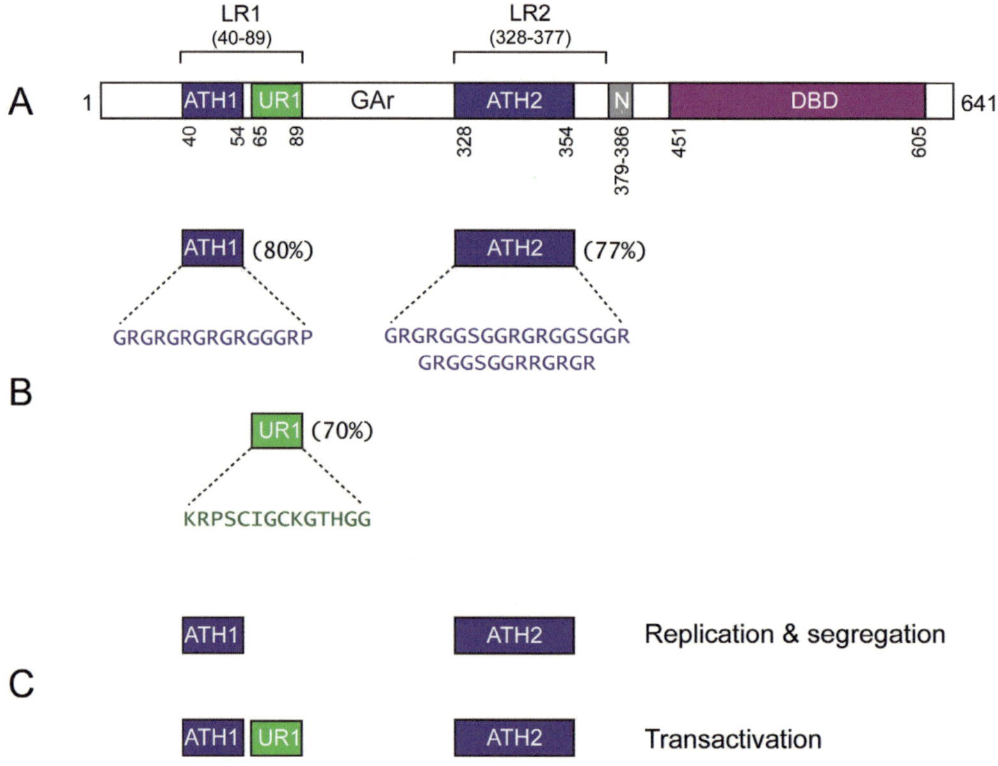

(A) EBNA1 is 641 a.a. in length. ATH1 and ATH2 are two AT-hooks, and UR1 is a domain necessary for transactivation. The GAr is a repeat of glycine and alanine, which can vary in length between EBV isolates. The DBD is used to bind defined sites on EBV's genome. N represents EBNA1's NLS. (B) ATH1 and ATH2 are highly conserved, 80% and 77% respectively, in EBNA1 orthologs from other EBV-like gammaherpesviruses. These regions have a repeated sequence of glycine and arginine. A portion of UR1 is also highly conserved in EBNA1 orthologs. UR1 contains a conserved cys-x-x-cys motif. (C) In addition to DBD, genome replication and segregation requires ATH1 and ATH2. For transactivation, EBNA1 needs both AT-hooks and UR1.

Fig. 2. Schematic diagram of EBNA1 and its domains.

EBNA1 contains at least one nuclear localization sequence (NLS) between a.a. 379-386. When fused to a cytoplasmic protein, the NLS is sufficient to render it nuclear (Ambinder, Mullen et al. 1991). Consistent with its function, the NLS interacts with the nuclear transporters karyopherin alpha1 and alpha2 (Fischer, Kremmer et al. 1997; Kim, Maher et al. 1997). However, an EBNA1 NLS mutant that is substantially reduced in its association with the karyopherins remains nuclear and is functional (Kim, Maher et al. 1997). Therefore, it is likely that EBNA1 has additional NLS signals that are currently unknown.

While B95-8 EBNA1 is 641 a.a. long, EBNA1 proteins from other EBV strains and isolates vary in size. This difference in size arises from differences in the length of a central glycine-alanine repeat region (GAr) (Falk, Gratama et al. 1995). Reductions in the length of the GAr to just 15 a.a. have no effect on the efficiency of B-cell immortalization by EBV (Lee, Diamond et al. 1999), EBNA1's capacity to activate transcription (Aiyar and Sugden 1998), or its ability to support replication and mitotic segregation of EBV genomes (Yates, Warren et al. 1985). It is now appreciated that the GAr reduces the efficiency with which EBNA1 epitopes are presented on the surface of EBV-infected cells. This reduction in efficiency is either a consequence of the GAr affecting processing by the proteosome (Levitskaya, Sharipo et al. 1997), or by reducing the efficiency with which EBNA1 is translated (Yin, Manoury et al. 2003; Apcher, Komarova et al. 2009; Apcher, Daskalogianni et al. 2010). Peculiarly, while cell-culture studies indicate that long GAr sequences substantially reduce proteosome processing and EBNA1 translation, the presence of a long GAr reduces the recognition of EBV-infected cells by EBNA1-specific CTLs by 50% or less (Lee, Brooks et al. 2004). Therefore, the conservation of long GArs in various EBV isolates may reflect other GAr functions, in addition to reduced epitope presentation, that are not recapitulated in cell culture.

The GAr is flanked by positively charged domains. These domains were originally termed linking regions 1 and 2 (LR1/LR2) (Figure 2) because they had the capacity to link DNAs bound by EBNA1 into large multimeric complexes (Mackey, Middleton et al. 1995; Mackey and Sugden 1997; Mackey and Sugden 1999) . Linking is dependent on the capacity of LR1 and LR2 to directly bind nucleic acids. LR1 and LR2 contain within them repeats of glycine and arginine (GR repeats) that can associate specifically with AT-rich DNA and G-quadruplex RNA (Sears, Ujihara et al. 2004; Norseen, Thomae et al. 2008) . These nucleic acid binding properties are observed for cellular AT-hook proteins that also contain GR repeats (Huth, Bewley et al. 1997; Reeves 2001; Norseen, Thomae et al. 2008). For this reason, the GR repeats of EBNA1 are referred to as AT-hook 1 and 2 (ATH1, ATH2) in this review. Deletion of ATH1 or ATH2 reduces the capacity of EBNA1 to transactivate EBV promoters and to support genome replication/segregation (Sears, Ujihara et al. 2004; Singh, Aras et al. 2009). Deletion of both ATH1 and ATH2 eliminates both functions (Sears, Kolman et al. 2003). A chimeric protein in which ATH1 and ATH2 are replaced by the cellular AT-hook protein HMGA1 supports transactivation and genome replication/segregation when bound to EBNA1 binding sites (Hung, Kang et al. 2001; Sears, Kolman et al. 2003). In contrast, a chimeric protein in which EBNA1's AT-hooks were replaced by a non-sequence specific cellular DNA binding protein, HMG1, does not support either function (Sears, Kolman et al. 2003). Therefore, an association between EBNA1's AT-hooks and specific nucleic acids, such as AT-rich DNA or G-quadruplex RNA, is necessary for EBNA1's functions.

While initially considered to be a single positively-charged domain, it is now appreciated that LR1 contains two distinct domains: 1) ATH1; and 2) A short unique region (UR1) that lies between ATH1 and GAr (Figure 2) (Kennedy and Sugden 2003; Singh, Aras et al. 2009). Deletion mutagenesis has revealed that UR1 is essential for EBNA1 to transactivate, but is not required for EBNA1 to support genome replication/segregation (Kennedy and Sugden 2003). Recent studies have revealed that UR1 contains a short sequence with a cys-x-x-cys motif that is conserved in the EBNA1 orthologs from other EBV-like primate gammaherpesviruses (Aras, Singh et al. 2009). Mutation of the conserved cysteines is sufficient to abrogate EBNA1's capacity to activate transcription, emphasizing the importance of the conserved cys-x-x-cys motif (*ibid*).

EBNA1's ability to transactivate EBV promoters and to support EBV genome replication/segregation is dependent upon its association with two clusters of cognate binding sites on the EBV genome (Figure 3). The organization of these two clusters is critical to EBNA1's EBV-specific functions and therefore is detailed below.

4. *OriP*, the family of repeats (FR), and the dyad symmetry element (DS)

Adams observed that akin to eukaryotic chromosomes, EBV genomes are replicated once per cell-cycle during latency, by a process termed licensed DNA replication (Lindner and Sugden 2007). This pattern of genome replication in which genomes are precisely duplicated during S phase had not been observed previously for other DNA viruses such as polyomaviruses, papilomaviruses, and alphaherpesviruses. EBV's unique mode of replication, coupled with an efficient segregation mechanism, permits viral genomes to be distributed equally to daughter cells when latently infected cells proliferate (Figure 4) (Sears, Kolman et al. 2003; Sears, Ujihara et al. 2004; Nanbo, Sugden et al. 2007; Norseen, Thomae et al. 2008). To identify EBV sequences necessary for licensed replication and mitotic segregation, Yates and Sugden screened for EBV fragments that conferred these properties to small plasmids introduced into EBV-positive cells (Yates, Warren et al. 1984). Their screen identified a fragment with 24 similar sequences arranged in two clusters. This fragment was termed *oriP* and is depicted in Figure 3. Upon determining *oriP* to be sufficient for the licensed replication and mitotic segregation of plasmids in EBV-positive cells, these investigators identified EBNA1 as the sole EBV protein necessary for licensed replication and mitotic segregation of *oriP*-plasmids (Yates, Warren et al. 1985). Later, it was determined that EBNA1 bound each of the repeated sequences within *oriP* as a dimer (Rawlins, Milman et al. 1985; Ambinder, Shah et al. 1990; Ambinder, Mullen et al. 1991). The repeats in *oriP* are arranged in two clusters (Figure 3): 1) A cluster with 20 EBNA1-binding sites, termed the Family of Repeats (FR); and 2) A cluster with four EBNA1-binding sites arranged as a dyad (DS) (Lupton and Levine 1985; Reisman, Yates et al. 1985).

Deletion and complementation experiments revealed that EBNA1 bound to FR and DS has distinct functions. Plasmids containing only DS undergo DNA replication in cells expressing EBNA1, but are mitotically unstable and lost within 1-2 cell-cycles. Plasmids containing FR alone are distributed as EBNA1-expressing cells divide, but do not replicate, and therefore ultimately diluted out of a proliferating culture (Yates, Camiolo et al. 2000). These studies indicate that DS functions primarily as a licensed replication origin, and FR functions as an element similar to a chromosomal centromere in that it permits newly-replicated *oriP*-plasmids to be mitotically stable and segregated (Wysokenski and Yates 1989; Aiyar, Tyree et al. 1998). The studies of Calos and co-workers reiterate these functional assignations (Krysan, Haase et al. 1989; Krysan and Calos 1993). Similar to DS-only plasmids, plasmids containing putative chromosomal replication origins undergo licensed replication but are mitotically unstable and lost within 1-2 cell cycles. Introducing FR into these plasmids permitted them to undergo licensed replication and become mitotically stable in EBNA1-expressing cells (*ibid*).

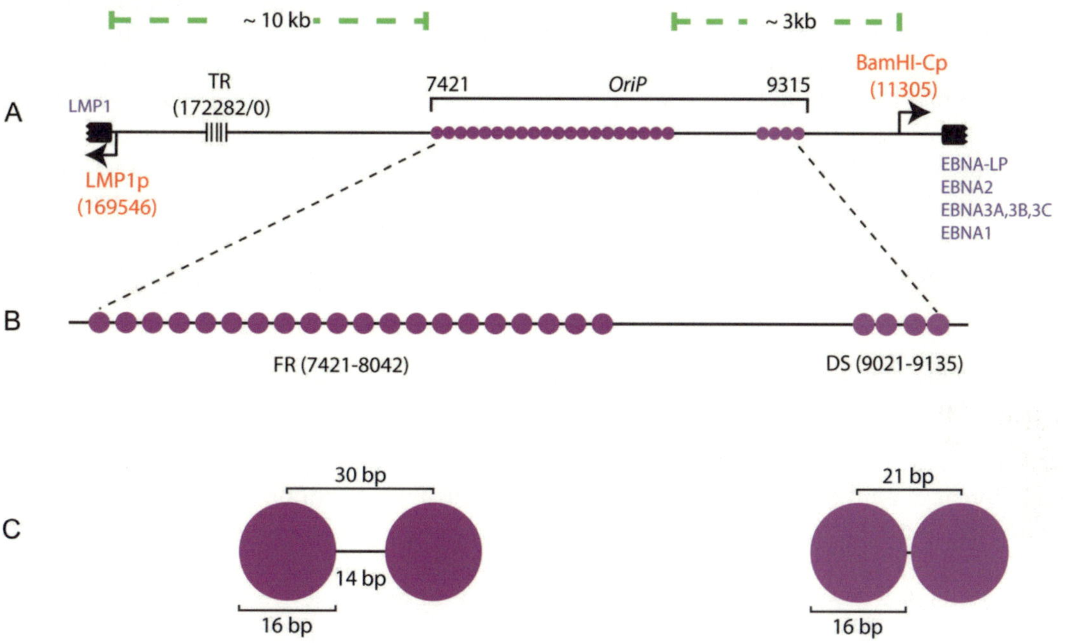

(A) *OriP* contains two clusters of EBNA1 binding sites, represented by the purple and pink filled circles. *OriP* is approximately 3 kb removed from the BamHI-C promoter, which is used to transcribe all the EBNA proteins, and 10 kb removed from the LMP1 promoter that is used to transcribe LMP1. (B) An expanded view of the two clusters of EBNA1 binding sites with *oriP*. The family of repeats (FR) contains 20 high-affinity binding sites, and is approximately 1 kb removed from the dyad symmetry element (DS) that contains four low-affinity binding sites. (C) Each EBNA1 binding site is 16 bp is length, and represented by a purple or pink filled circle. The distance between adjacent binding sites in FR is 14 bp, and therefore EBNA1 dimers bound to adjacent sites are on the same phase of the DNA double helix. The four sites in DS are configured as two pairs of two sites. The EBNA1 binding sites within each pair are 5 bp apart, and this distance is essential for DS to function as a replication origin.

Fig. 3. Schematic representation of *OriP*, and the two EBV promoters transactivated by EBNA1 bound to *OriP*.

Although FR contains 20 EBNA1-binding sites, numerous studies by others and us have revealed that it must contain a minimum of 7 EBNA1-binding sites to provide mitotic stability in EBNA1-expressing cells. These studies also revealed that plasmids with a modified FR, which only contained 10 EBNA1-binding sites, were more stable than plasmids containing a wild-type FR (Wysokenski and Yates 1989; Hebner, Lasanen et al. 2003). This is because EBNA1 dimers bound to 20 contiguous EBNA1-binding sites in FR impede, but do not completely abrogate, the migration of replication forks through FR (Aiyar, Aras et al. 2009). 10 contiguous EBNA1-binding sites are not an effective replication fork-block; therefore, replication initiating from DS is completed efficiently (*ibid*). Because EBV isolates contain a minimum of 20 EBNA1-binding sites, it is likely that the capacity of 20 or more contiguous binding sites to limit genome replication is of importance to EBV.

The four EBNA1-binding sites in DS are of lower affinity than the binding sites in FR (Ambinder, Shah et al. 1990). The four sites are arranged in two pairs in which the distance between the centers of the two sites in each pair is 21 base-pairs (bp) (Figure 3). Either pair is sufficient for DS to function as an origin, but alterations of the spacing between them blocks origin function (Harrison, Fisenne et al. 1994; Bashaw and Yates 2001). When EBNA1 binds the sites in DS, it induces a large symmetrical bend in the DNA and forms a structure necessary for the cellular licensed DNA replication machinery to function at DS (Bashaw and Yates 2001). There is an additional sequence juxtaposed 3' to DS, termed Rep*, which can associate with EBNA1 (Kirchmaier and Sugden 1998). The non-canonical EBNA1 binding sites in Rep* are also 21 bp apart, and multiple copies of Rep* can substitute for DS for the licensed replication of *oriP*-plasmids (Wang, Lindner et al. 2006).

5. Contributions of EBNA1 to the licensed replication and segregation of oriP-plasmids

Although it bends DS, DBD alone is not sufficient to support replication from DS (Kirchmaier and Sugden 1998). The latter requires contributions from other EBNA1 domains, particularly ATH1 and ATH2. Investigations into the mechanism by which DS functions as a cell-cycle controlled licensed replication origin have revealed it is similar to the mechanism that restricts chromosomal replication origins to "fire" only once per cell-cycle (Lindner and Sugden 2007). During licensed replication of chromosomal DNA, the cellular origin recognition complex (ORC) marks replication origins throughout the cell-cycle. Late in mitosis or early in G1, the cellular minichromosome maintenance complex (MCM) associates with ORC. Phosphorylation events at the G1/S boundary convert the MCM complex into an active helicase that opens the replication origin and permits DNA polymerase α/primase to be recruited to the origin. MCM functions as the leading strand helicase and can reassociate with ORC only at the end of mitosis. The inability for MCM to be re-used during S phase prevents any single origin from being used more than once in a single cell-cycle. Studies by the groups of Dutta, Lieberman, Schepers, and Yates have provided insights into the mechanism which DS functions as an origin through (Chaudhuri, Xu et al. 2001; Dhar, Yoshida et al. 2001; Schepers, Ritzi et al. 2001; Ritzi, Tillack et al. 2003; Zhou, Chau et al. 2005; Norseen, Thomae et al. 2008). It is now clear that EBNA1 recruits ORC to DS, with the subsequent cell-cycle dependent recruitment of MCM, thus ensuring that *oriP* is subject to the same cell-cycle controlled replication as cellular chromosomes. Studies from several groups, including ours, indicated that EBNA1's AT-hooks were essential to recruit ORC to DS (Sears, Ujihara et al. 2004; Norseen, Thomae et al. 2008). This conclusion has been reiterated by our observations that chimeric proteins in which ATH1 and ATH2 were substituted by cellular AT-hook proteins support licensed replication from DS (Sears, Kolman et al. 2003; Kelly, Singh et al. 2011). Lieberman and co-workers have demonstrated that EBNA1 uses its AT-hooks to recruit the ORC complex to DS via a G-quadruplex RNA intermediate, underscoring a critical role for these domains in *oriP*-replication (Norseen, Thomae et al. 2008).

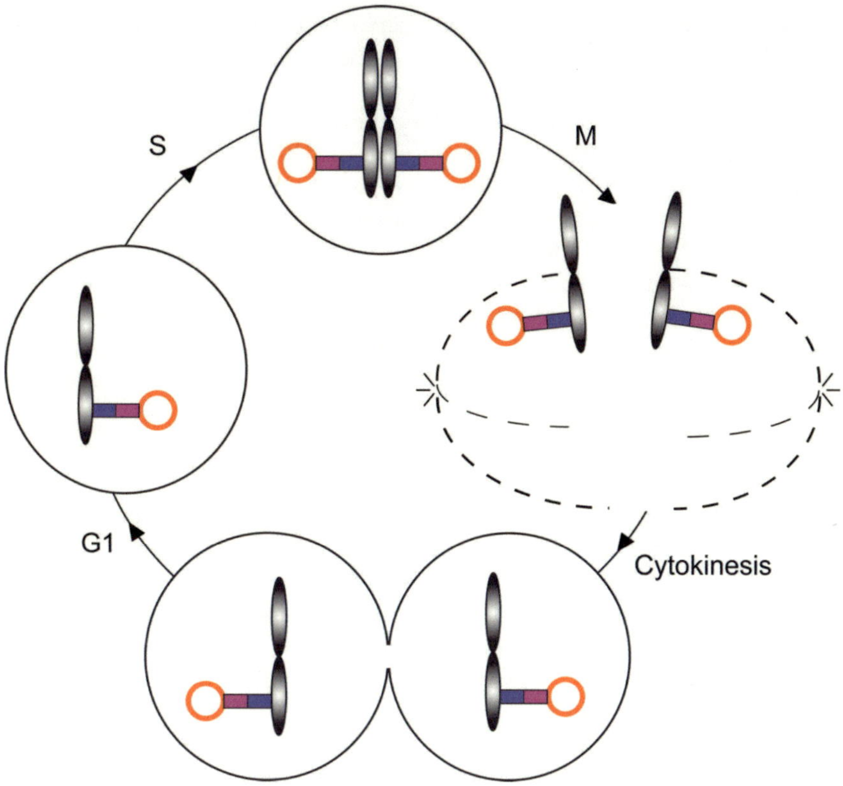

EBV genomes, represented by an orange circle, are tethered by EBNA1 to cellular chromosomes. The AT-hooks of EBNA1 are shown in blue, and the DBD in purple. EBNA1 recruits ORC/MCM to permit duplication of EBV genomes in S-phase. Replicated genomes are tethered to sister chromatids by EBNA1 and piggy-back on the mitotic spindle to partition into daughter cells.

Fig. 4. Model for piggy-back partitioning of EBV genomes.

ATH1 and ATH2 are also essential for the mitotic stability and partitioning of newly-replicated *oriP*-plasmids (Sears, Kolman et al. 2003; Sears, Ujihara et al. 2004). The studies of Miller and co-workers were the first to indicate that EBNA1 associates with mitotic chromosomes in a punctate manner (Grogan, Summers et al. 1983). This observation, which has been recapitulated by others and us, is used as the basis of the piggy-back partitioning model depicted in Figure 4 (Sears, Kolman et al. 2003; Sears, Ujihara et al. 2004; Nanbo, Sugden et al. 2007). In this model, *oriP*-plasmids are proposed to be tethered to cellular chromosomes throughout the cell-cycle. Tethered plasmids are duplicated during chromosomal replication, and distributed to sister chromatids after replication. Plasmids then piggy-back on chromatids being partitioned by the mitotic apparatus. The association of EBNA1 with chromosomes is central to this model. Two alternative mechanisms have been proposed for this association. In the first, it was observed using a yeast two-hybrid screen that the ATH2 domain of EBNA1 associates with the cellular nucleolar protein EBP2/p40 (Shire, Ceccarelli et al. 1999). Expression of human EBP2 in budding yeast permitted EBNA1 to partition FR-containing plasmids in yeast, suggesting a role for EBP2 in partitioning of *oriP*-plasmids in human cells (Kapoor, Shire et al. 2001). The second model relies on the nucleic acid binding properties of ATH1 and ATH2. EBNA1 mutants in which either ATH1 or ATH2 is deleted retain the capacity to bind mitotic chromosomes and support the segregation of *oriP*-plasmids (Sears, Ujihara et al. 2004). Further, both ATH1 and ATH2 can be substituted by cellular AT-hook proteins, and the resulting chimeras associate with mitotic chromosomes and support segregation of *oriP*-plasmids (Hung, Kang et al. 2001; Sears, Kolman et al. 2003; Kelly, Singh et al. 2011). Because both ATH1 and ATH2 function equivalently to support *oriP*-plasmid segregation, but only ATH2 associates with EBP2/p40, it is likely that EBP2 does not mediate the partitioning of *oriP*-plasmids or EBV genomes. This interpretation is supported strongly by recent observations examining the segregation of *oriP*-plasmids in live cells. Derivatives of EBNA1 lacking ATH2 were found to segregate *oriP*-plasmids in a mechanism that could not be distinguished from the function of wild-type EBNA1 (Nanbo, Sugden et al. 2007). It remains to be determined whether an association with AT-rich DNA or G-quadruplex RNA underlies EBNA1's binding of cellular chromosomes.

5.1 Transcription activation by EBNA1

Shortly after identification of *oriP*, it was recognized that FR functioned as an enhancer when placed 5' to a promoter-luciferase reporter in cells that expressed EBNA1, but not control cells (Reisman and Sugden 1986). Transactivation by FR-bound EBNA1 is not restricted to specific promoters from EBV, but has also been observed for multiple heterologous promoters when they are juxtaposed to FR (*ibid*). In the context of the EBV genome and promoter-reporter constructs, EBNA1 bound to FR transactivates EBV's BamHI-C promoter (BamHI-Cp) that is approximately 3 kb distal to FR, and the LMP1 promoter (LMP1p), which is more than 10 kb removed from FR (Figure 3) (Gahn and Sugden 1995; Puglielli, Woisetschlaeger et al. 1996). All the proteins necessary for EBV to immortalize naive B-cells are expressed from these two promoters, and therefore EBNA1's capacity to transactivate is essential for B-cell immortalization (Altmann, Pich et al. 2006).

The failure to find cellular co-activators that bound EBNA1 led to the proposal that EBNA1's capacity to "transactivate" reflected its capacity to retain FR-containing plasmids or the EBV genome, in the nuclei of proliferating cells. In this model, retention of FR-containing plasmids in nuclei provides additional transcription templates and therefore increased reporter activity. The plasmid retention model was tested by querying whether EBNA1 could transactivate a chromosomally integrated FR-dependent reporter (Kennedy and Sugden 2003; Sears, Kolman et al. 2003). The outcome from these studies indicated that EBNA1 transactivated the integrated reporter (*ibid*). Further, EBNA1 mutants that are replication/segregation competent, but transactivation defective, do not transactivate the integrated reporter or episomal reporters (*ibid*). While it is now accepted that EBNA1 is a genuine transactivator, the precise mechanism of transactivation remains to be clearly defined. Nevertheless, recent studies identifying domains of EBNA1 necessary for transactivation, and the regulation of transactivation, have provided glimpses into this mechanism. These studies, detailed below, support a structural role for EBNA1 in the activation of transcription, similar to the formation of enhanceosomes by the cellular AT-hook protein, HMGA1.

In addition to DBD, two other EBNA1 domains are necessary to activate FR-dependent transcription: 1) The AT-hooks (ATH1/ATH2); and 2) UR1. Deletion of either ATH1 or ATH2 reduces transactivation by about 50% (Aras, Singh et al. 2009; Singh, Aras et al. 2009); deletion of both ATH1 and ATH2 reduced transactivation to 5% of wild-type EBNA1 (*ibid*).

Similarly, deletion of UR1 reduced transactivation to 5% of WT EBNA1 (Kennedy and Sugden 2003; Aras, Singh et al. 2009; Singh, Aras et al. 2009). These studies also indicate that UR1 and the AT-hooks are individually insufficient to activate transcription; deletion of either domain eliminates the capacity of the remaining domain to promote transactivation (Singh, Aras et al. 2009). Studies using chimeric proteins indicate the nucleic-acid binding properties of ATH1/ATH2 are critical for EBNA1 to transactivate. The chimeric protein HMGA1-UR1-DBD, in which ATH1/ATH2 are replaced by the cellular AT-hook protein, HMGA1, can transactivate when bound to FR (Altmann, Pich et al. 2006).

The UR1-deleted EBNA1 mutant was used to establish definitively that EBNA1's capacity to transactivate was necessary for EBV to immortalize naive B-cells. A recombinant EBV in which WT EBNA1 was replaced by this protein established latent infection in transformed B-cell lymphomas, but failed to immortalize naive B-cells (Altmann, Pich et al. 2006). Consistent with immortalization requiring both AT-hooks and UR1, a recombinant EBV in which WT EBNA1 was replaced by HMGA1-UR1-DBD was competent to immortalize naive B-cells (*ibid*).

5.2 AT-hooks and transactivation

Cellular AT-hook proteins function as architectural proteins in transactivation. This structural function was first revealed for the cellular AT-hook protein, HMGA1, at the ®-interferon enhancer by the studies of Thanos and Maniatis (Kim and Maniatis 1997; Yie, Liang et al. 1997; Yie, Merika et al. 1999). The β-interferon enhancer contains sites bound by the transactivators ATF2, NFκB, and IRF1, and contains four short AT-rich sites bound by HMGA1, previously referred to as HMG-I(Y) (Kim and Maniatis 1997; Yie, Merika et al. 1999). A basal level of transcription was observed during *in vitro* transcription reactions in which ATF2, NFκB, and IRF1 were provided individually, or as a combination of all three. Similarly, addition of HMGA1 alone also resulted in basal transcription. However, a dramatic increase in transcription was observed when all four factors were provided at the same time. DNA phasing experiments were used to establish a structural role for HMGA1 in transactivation. A six bp deletion that changed the phasing between two HMGA1-binding sites by a half-turn of DNA double helix decreased transactivation by 50%. In contrast, a 10 bp deletion, which restored the original DNA phasing, also restored transactivation (*ibid*). On this basis, it was proposed that structural changes imposed in the enhancer by HMGA1-induced DNA bending, and HMGA1 self-association, formed a transactivation complex termed an "enhanceosome" (Maniatis, Falvo et al. 1998). Other proteins that bind the β-interferon enhancer, namely ATF2, IRF1, and NFκB, recruited transcription co-activators only in the context of this enhanceosome (Merika, Williams et al. 1998). The role of HMGA1 at the β-interferon enhanceosome has been recapitulated at other promoters, such as the early promoter of human papilomavirus type 18 (Bouallaga, Massicard et al. 2000; Bouallaga, Teissier et al. 2003). Six bp deletions or insertions between HMGA1 binding sites at this promoter reduce transcription by about 50%. In contrast, no change in transcription is observed consequent to 10 bp deletions or insertions (Bouallaga, Massicard et al. 2000). At this enhanceosome as well, HMGA1 is necessary to recruit transcription co-activators (Bouallaga, Teissier et al. 2003).

The unusual property of phasing dependent transactivation that was previously observed only for HMGA1 has been observed for EBNA1 (Hebner, Lasanen et al. 2003). The center-to-center distance between adjacent EBNA1-binding sites in FR is 30 bp, or three turns of the

DNA double-helix (Figure 3). Reduction of this distance to 24 bp alters transactivation by 50% without affecting EBNA1's capacity to bind adjacent sites (*ibid*). EBNA1's phasing-dependent transactivation provided the first indication that it functions as an architectural transactivator. Studies with inhibitors indicate the AT-rich DNA binding property of ATH1/ATH2 to be critical for EBNA1 to transactivate. The peptidomimetic netropsin, which displaces AT-hook proteins from AT-rich DNA (Wartell, Larson et al. 1974; Freyer, Buscaglia et al. 2007), also reduces the capacity of EBNA1 to transactivate at BamHI-Cp (Sears, Ujihara et al. 2004). Deletion of ATH1 reduces transactivation to 50% of WT EBNA1, and the reduction is reversed when ATH1 is substituted by AT-hooks from HMGA1 (Singh, Aras et al. 2009). While it is apparent that EBNA1's AT-hooks are necessary for transactivation, how they function bears clarification. AT-hook proteins typically bind AT-rich sequences that are close to the transcription start-site. Although AT-rich sequences are found juxtaposed to BamHI-Cp, and increase BamHI-Cp activity in reporter assays (Walls and Perricaudet 1991), it is yet to be determined if this increase is EBNA1-dependent and if EBNA1 associates with these sequences.

5.3 The role of UR1 in transactivation

Because the UR1-deleted EBNA1 mutant is transactivation defective, efforts have focused on cellular transcription co-activators that associate with UR1. However, several yeast two-hybrid screens (Fischer, Kremmer et al. 1997; Kim, Maher et al. 1997; Aiyar, Tyree et al. 1998), and proteomic analyses, have failed to identify co-activators that bind EBNA1. It has been reported recently that the chromatin remodeling protein Brd4 interacts with EBNA1 in yeast (Lin, Wang et al. 2008). While both over-expression and depletion of Brd4 reduced EBNA1's capacity to transactivate (*ibid*), these conditions also cause a striking reduction in cell viability (Schweiger, Ottinger et al. 2007). Therefore, it is currently not possible to assign a role for Brd4 in EBNA1's capacity to transactivate.

K	R	P	S	C	I	G	C	K	G	T	EBV (B95-8)
K	R	R	S	C	V	G	C	K	G	G	YP_067973
K	R	R	S	C	I	G	C	R	G	G	BAB03281
K	R	R	S	C	V	G	C	K	G	G	AAA66373
K	R	S	T	C	I	G	C	K	A	T	NP_001087694
K	R	S	T	C	I	G	C	R	A	V	CAM46996
K	R	S	T	C	I	G	C	K	A	L	XP_001641357
K	K	A	S	C	I	G	C	K	S	L	XP_002008314
R	R	N	C	C	I	G	C	R	T	V	P28340

UR1 is highly conserved in the EBNA1 orthologs from other gammaherpesviruses, whose Genbank accession numbers are in blue. The conserved domain closely matches one-half a zinc finger from the DNA polymerase δ active subunit from many eukaryotic species, whose accession numbers are shown in orange

Fig. 5. The UR1 domain of EBNA1.

During our studies to identify co-activators that associated with UR1, we observed that a sub-sequence within UR1 was highly conserved in the UR1 domains of EBNA1 orthologs from other EBV-like gammaherpesviruses (Aras, Singh et al. 2009). The conserved sequence, KRPSCIGCK, also resembles one-half of a C4 zinc-finger present in the catalytic subunit of DNA polymerase δ from multiple eukaryotes (Figure 5). In zinc fingers, the group 12 metal zinc is coordinated between two cys-x-x-cys containing sequences of a protein, bringing these two segments together. Because EBNA1 and its orthologs do not contain another pair of cysteines in a cys-x-x-cys configuration, it is unlikely that zinc is coordinated by a single molecule of EBNA1. Sometimes, zinc coordination between dicysteine motifs in two separate proteins is used to mediate an association between the two proteins. This is exemplified by the interaction between the C-terminal cytoplasmic tail of CD4 or CD8α with the Lck kinase (Huse, Eck et al. 1998; Lin, Rodriguez et al. 1998; Kim, Sun et al. 2003). Therefore, we postulated, and experimentally confirmed, that: 1) UR1 bound zinc; and 2) Zinc coordination resulted in UR1 self-association (Aras, Singh et al. 2009). The role of the cys-x-x-cys motif within UR1 for both properties was confirmed by replacing both cysteines with serines. This mutant UR1 did not bind zinc or self-associate (*ibid*).

Zinc is essential for EBNA1 to transactivate. Chelation of zinc using the cell-permeable zinc chelator **N,N,N',N'-tetrakis(2-pyridylmethyl)ethylenediamine** (TPEN) severely reduced EBNA1's capacity to transactivate without affecting levels of EBNA1 or cell viability (*ibid*). The specific effect of TPEN on EBNA1-dependent transactivation was confirmed by determining it had no effect on transcription from EBNA1-independent promoters, on the function of zinc-independent transactivators. Consistent with the chelation studies, an EBNA1 mutant in which both UR1 cysteines were altered to serine transactivates as poorly as UR1-deleted EBNA1 (*ibid*). Biochemical studies indicate that zinc is coordinated intermolecularly between adjacent EBNA1 dimers bound to adjacent sites in FR, rather than intramolecularly within an EBNA1 dimer bound to a single site in FR (*ibid*). Intermolecular coordination results in a large structured array of EBNA1 at FR that is essential for EBNA1 to transactivate cooperatively. Confirming this conclusion, the EBNA1 mutant in which UR1 cysteines were changed to serines does not transactivate cooperatively. On this basis, it is proposed that a zinc-coordinated array of EBNA1 at FR creates a structured complex within which EBNA1's AT-hooks can form an enhanceosome at promoter proximal sequences (Aras, Singh et al. 2009; Singh, Aras et al. 2009). The model mechanistically explains the co-dependent roles of UR1 and the AT-hooks in transactivation. In the absence of UR1, EBNA1's AT-hooks cannot form a structured complex at promoter proximal AT-rich sequences. In the absence of the AT-hooks, EBNA1 bound to FR lacks the domains necessary to bind such sequences. This model also explains why alteration of phasing between adjacent EBNA1-binding sites in FR affects transactivation. Adjacent EBNA1 dimers bound to sites that lie on opposite sides of DNA will coordinate zinc with different kinetics than dimers bound to adjacent sites on the same side of DNA. This in turn will alter the structure necessary for effective enhanceosome formation, as observed previously for the function of HMGA1 in enhanceosomes (Kim and Maniatis 1997; Bouallaga, Massicard et al. 2000).

5.4 Regulation of transactivation by phosphorylation

EBNA1 contains multiple serine and threonine residues in sequence contexts that resemble recognition sites for protein kinases including cAMP-dependent protein kinase, protein kinase C, glycogen synthase kinase, and mitogen activated protein kinase (PKA)

(Duellman, Thompson et al. 2009). Indeed, a sequence recognized by PKA, KRxS, is conserved in UR1 (Figure 5), and the conserved serine is phosphorylated *in vivo* (*ibid*). Because this sequence is juxtaposed to the critical cys-x-x-cys motif within UR1, we created three mutants of EBNA1 in which this serine was altered to alanine, aspartic acid, or threonine (Singh, Aras et al. 2009). These substitutions were chosen because alanine resembles an unphosphorylated serine, aspartic acid resembles a phosphorylated serine, and threonine restores a PKA recognition site. All three substitutions did not affect the half-life of EBNA1, its nuclear localization, or the efficiency of transactivation (*ibid*). Therefore, although this site is phosphorylated *in vivo*, phosphorylation does not affect any property or function of EBNA1. Subsequent to our analysis, Duellman and Burgess created a mutant derivative of EBNA1 in which all 10 serines known to be phosphorylated were simultaneously substituted by alanine (Duellman, Thompson et al. 2009). This mutant EBNA1 displayed no defects in half-life, expression level, or nuclear localization. There were minor reductions in the efficiency of replication/segregation of *oriP*-plasmids and transactivation (*ibid*). Therefore, it appears unlikely that phosphorylation is a major mechanism that regulates the activities of EBNA1. This conclusion was also drawn from studies in which activators and inhibitors of various kinases were observed to not affect EBNA1's capacity to transactivate.

5.5 Transactivation is sensitive to oxidative stress and regulated by cellular redox effectors

Many viral and mammalian transactivators, including AP-1, NFκB, the Tat protein of human immunodeficiency virus (HIV), and the E2 protein of papillomavirus, are regulated by redox (Hutchison, Matic et al. 1991; Xanthoudakis and Curran 1992; Xanthoudakis, Miao et al. 1992; Huang and Adamson 1993; Mitomo, Nakayama et al. 1994; Xanthoudakis and Curran 1996; Jayaraman, Murthy et al. 1997; Okamoto, Tanaka et al. 1999; Kalantari, Narayan et al. 2008; Wan, Ottinger et al. 2008; Washington, Singh et al. 2010). These proteins contain one or several cysteine residues susceptible to oxidation, whose redox status regulates the capacity to transactivate, due to the effect of oxidative stress on protein structure. Upon exposure to superoxide and hydroxyl radicals, the thiol groups of cysteine can either be oxidized to form a disulfide bond, or progressively oxidized to form sulfenic acid, sulfinic acid, and finally sulfonic acid via the Fenton reaction (Held, Sylvester et al. 1996). Proteins containing zinc fingers essential for their function are especially sensitive to oxidative stress because the thiol group, but not oxidized thiol adducts, can coordinate zinc (Kiley and Storz 2004). In light of EBNA1's UR1 domain containing two conserved cysteines that are critical for transactivation, we tested whether transactivation was susceptible to oxidative stress or alterations in environmental oxygen tension (Aras, Singh et al. 2009; Washington, Singh et al. 2010). Exposure of EBNA1-expressing cells to low levels of agents that generate intracellular hydroxyl and superoxide radicals, such as menadione and paraquat, dramatically reduced transactivation without substantially affecting cell survival or proliferation. In contrast, lowering the oxygen tension by placing EBNA1 expressing cells in hypoxic conditions extended the half-life of transactivation (*ibid*). The latter result suggests that although EBNA1 is very stable, the critical cysteines within UR1 are subject to intracellular oxidative stress, reducing EBNA1's capacity to transactivate over time. Hypoxic conditions reduce the generation of intracellular oxidative radicals, and therefore prolong the activity of EBNA1 as a transactivator (*ibid*).

Cellular and viral transactivators with redox-sensitive cysteines are often regulated by cellular redox effectors such as thioredoxin, thioredoxin reductase and the bifunctional enzyme AP-endonuclease 1 (APE1) (Hutchison, Matic et al. 1991; Xanthoudakis and Curran 1992; Xanthoudakis, Miao et al. 1992; Huang and Adamson 1993; Mitomo, Nakayama et al. 1994; Xanthoudakis and Curran 1996; Jayaraman, Murthy et al. 1997; Okamoto, Tanaka et al. 1999; Kalantari, Narayan et al. 2008; Wan, Ottinger et al. 2008; Washington, Singh et al. 2010). Thioredoxin and thioredoxin reductase can reduce disulfide bridges that result from cysteine oxidation, and therefore function similarly to small molecules such as b-mercaptoethanol (b-ME) and dithiothreitol (DTT) (Lothrop, Ruggles et al. 2009). APE1 is a bifunctional enzyme with two activities: 1) It is an AP-endonuclease that participates in DNA damage repair (Bhakat, Mantha et al. 2009); and 2) It can reduce the oxidized cysteine adduct sulfenic acid back to a thiol (*ibid*). Therefore, oxidized cysteine adducts reduced by APE1 are not acted on by b-ME and DTT.

We determined that treating cells with b-ME or DTT did not alter EBNA1's ability to transactivate, or ameliorate the effect of oxidative stress on transactivation (Washington, Singh et al. 2010). Therefore, it is unlikely that oxidative stress reduces EBNA1's ability to transactivate by creating intra- or intermolecular disulfide bridges. Consistent with this, over-expression of thioredoxin or thioredoxin reductase also did not increase transactivation, or rescue transactivation from intracellular oxidative stress generated by menadione or paraquat exposure (*ibid*). In striking contrast, over-expression of APE1 increases EBNA1's ability to transactivate, and curtails the effect of oxidative stress on EBNA1's function as a transactivator (Aras, Singh et al. 2009; Washington, Singh et al. 2010). It is relevant to note that cysteine residues regulated by APE1 are often adjacent to arginine or lysine residues, as observed for the cysteines in UR1 (Figure 5).

6. Functions of EBNA1 in EBV-positive lymphomas

Two patterns of gene expression predominate in EBV-positive lymphomas: 1) The type III latency pattern of gene expression; and 2) The type I latency pattern of gene expression, in which EBNA1 is the only viral protein expressed. In type III lymphomas, EBNA1 drives the expression of other EBV genes necessary for cell proliferation and facilitates virus genome replication/segregation into daughter cells. It is not clear what functions are provided by EBNA1 in type I lymphomas. It is possible that EBNA1 itself provides functions necessary for cell survival and proliferation. One function indicated by the studies of Kennedy and Sugden is that EBNA1 can inhibit or reduce p53-dependent apoptosis (Kennedy, Komano et al. 2003). In addition, it is possible that by facilitating genome replication/segregation, EBNA1 permits the expression of EBV microRNAs in type I lymphoma cells (Cai, Schafer et al. 2006; Choy, Siu et al. 2008; Pratt, Kuzembayeva et al. 2009). Finally, as described in the next section, several studies indicate that EBNA1 can transactivate some cellular genes, and it is possible that one or a combination of these genes is necessary for lymphoma survival/proliferation (Wood, O'Neil et al. 2007; Baumforth, Birgersdotter et al. 2008; Flavell, Baumforth et al. 2008; O'Neil, Owen et al. 2008; Gruhne, Sompallae et al. 2009).

In either event, it is of interest that introduction of a dominant-negative derivative of EBNA1 into EBV-positive Burkitt's lymphoma cells severely decreases their rate of proliferation, and dramatically increases their apoptosis, reiterating the utility of devising therapies against EBNA1 (Kennedy, Komano et al. 2003; Nasimuzzaman, Kuroda et al. 2005).

6.1 Modulation of cellular gene expression by EBNA1

Recent studies show that EBNA1 alters the transcriptional pattern of several cellular genes (Dawson, Rickinson et al. 1990; Falk, Gratama et al. 1995; Wood, O'Neil et al. 2007; Baumforth, Birgersdotter et al. 2008; Flavell, Baumforth et al. 2008; O'Neil, Owen et al. 2008). These include increasing the expression of STAT1 and AP-1 family transcription factors c-Jun and ATF2. EBNA1 has been demonstrated to bind the promoters of the latter two genes in carcinoma cells (Wood, O'Neil et al. 2007; O'Neil, Owen et al. 2008). If these genes are also activated in the context of an EBV infection, they may contribute to the proliferation of cells transformed by EBV and the immortalization of naive B-cells by EBV. One pro-oncogenic function of EBNA1 is predicted by the recent observation that EBNA1 induces the expression of *NOX2*, resulting in the generation of reactive oxygen species (ROS) that cause genome instability (Gruhne, Sompallae et al. 2009). The cellular enzyme complex, nicotinamide adenine dinucleotide phosphate (NADPH) oxidase, produces ROS by transferring electrons from cytosolic NADPH to O_2 (Geiszt and Leto 2004). *NOX2* is the β-subunit of flavocytochrome b_{558}, which forms the catalytic core of NADPH oxidase (D'Autreaux and Toledano 2007). While all the components of NADPH oxidase are expressed in B-cells, *NOX2* is expressed at very low levels (Suzuki and Ono 1999). Therefore, by inducing *NOX2* expression, EBNA1 causes a significant increase in ROS production, which in turn causes pro-oncogenic DNA damage (Gruhne, Sompallae et al. 2009; Gruhne, Sompallae et al. 2009).

Several sequences bound by EBNA1's DBD have been identified in the human genome (Canaan, Haviv et al. 2009; Dresang, Vereide et al. 2009; Lu, Wikramasinghe et al. 2010), permitting the creation of a position-weighted matrix that has been used to predict additional binding sites (Dresang, Vereide et al. 2009). The relevance of EBNA1 binding to these sites is yet to be established because it does not transactivate any genes within 10 kb of the sites bound with highest affinity (*ibid*). Curiously, there are no sequences predicted to be recognized by EBNA1's DBD within the promoter/enhancer regions of genes that are transactivated by EBNA1, suggesting that EBNA1 may associate with these promoters without using its DBD. It is possible that EBNA1 associates with the promoters for these genes through its AT-hooks, similar to the association of HMGA1 with AT-rich sequences at several promoters (Skalnik and Neufeld 1992; Siddiqa, Sims-Mourtada et al. 2001; Martinez Hoyos, Fedele et al. 2004; Tesfaye, Di Cello et al. 2007; Henriksen, Stabell et al. 2010). In this context, it may be of relevance that HMGA1 binds to the *NOX2* promoter (Skalnik and Neufeld 1992).

7. Conclusions

In this review, we have focused on the biological functions and biochemical properties of the EBNA1 protein of EBV. Genetic studies have indicated that EBNA1 is essential for EBV to immortalize naive B-cells, and EBNA1 is the only EBV protein that is expressed in all cells infected latently by EBV, including lymphomas. EBNA1 provides two major functions necessary for EBV to immortalize naive B-cells: 1) It permits replication/segregation of virus genomes; and 2) It activates transcription from two critical viral promoters. Current therapies against EBV have severe side-effects, and recurrent tumors are often resistant to therapy (O'Reilly, Connors et al. 1997; Khanna, Moss et al. 1999; Gottschalk, Rooney et al. 2005; Heslop 2005; Mounier, Spina et al. 2006; Mounier, Spina et al. 2007; Spina, Simonelli et al. 2007). It is therefore desirable to develop new therapies that are specific to EBV-positive cells, and are highly effective at disrupting their proliferation and survival. Its unique expression pattern and critical functions render EBNA1 an excellent target for the development of such therapies.

Molecular and biochemical analyses have provided insights into the mechanisms by which EBNA1 functions to support replication/segregation and transactivate viral promoters. For both replication and transactivation, EBNA1 needs to bind the *oriP* region of EBV's genome. Therefore, small molecules that interfere with the capacity of DBD to bind its cognate binding sites are predicted to block EBNA1's functions, and indeed, several candidate inhibitors have already been identified (Li, Thompson et al. 2010). EBNA1 needs its AT-hook domains for replication, segregation and transactivation, and therefore these domains are good targets for therapies against EBV-positive lymphomas. Laemmli and co-workers have designed peptidomimetics that interfere with the function of specific AT-hook proteins in Drosophila, with three desirable properties: 1) high specificity; 2) low toxicity; and 3) oral delivery (Janssen, Cuvier et al. 2000; Janssen, Durussel et al. 2000; Blattes, Monod et al. 2006). They also provide a framework for the development of small molecules that disrupt the functions of EBNA1's AT-hooks.

8. Acknowledgements

This work was supported in part by NIH awards CA112564 and AI055172. AW was supported by NIH award CA150442.

9. References

Abbot, S. D., M. Rowe, et al. (1990). "Epstein-Barr virus nuclear antigen 2 induces expression of the virus-encoded latent membrane protein." *J Virol* 64(5): 2126-34.

Aiyar, A., S. Aras, et al. (2009). "Epstein-Barr Nuclear Antigen 1 modulates replication of oriP-plasmids by impeding replication and transcription fork migration through the family of repeats." *Virol J* 6: 29.

Aiyar, A. and B. Sugden (1998). "Fusions between Epstein-Barr viral nuclear antigen-1 of Epstein-Barr virus and the large T-antigen of simian virus 40 replicate their cognate origins." *J Biol Chem* 273(49): 33073-81.

Aiyar, A., C. Tyree, et al. (1998). "The plasmid replicon of EBV consists of multiple cis-acting elements that facilitate DNA synthesis by the cell and a viral maintenance element." *EMBO J* 17(21): 6394-403.

Altmann, M., D. Pich, et al. (2006). "Transcriptional activation by EBV nuclear antigen 1 is essential for the expression of EBV's transforming genes." *Proc Natl Acad Sci U S A* 103(38): 14188-93.

Ambinder, R. F., M. A. Mullen, et al. (1991). "Functional domains of Epstein-Barr virus nuclear antigen EBNA-1." *J Virol* 65(3): 1466-78.

Ambinder, R. F., W. A. Shah, et al. (1990). "Definition of the sequence requirements for binding of the EBNA-1 protein to its palindromic target sites in Epstein-Barr virus DNA." *J Virol* 64(5): 2369-79.

Apcher, S., C. Daskalogianni, et al. (2010). "Epstein Barr virus-encoded EBNA1 interference with MHC class I antigen presentation reveals a close correlation between mRNA translation initiation and antigen presentation." *PLoS Pathog* 6(10): e1001151.

Apcher, S., A. Komarova, et al. (2009). "mRNA translation regulation by the Gly-Ala repeat of Epstein-Barr virus nuclear antigen 1." *J Virol* 83(3): 1289-98.

Aras, S., G. Singh, et al. (2009). "Zinc coordination is required for and regulates transcription activation by Epstein-Barr nuclear antigen 1." *PLoS Pathogens*.

Babcock, G. J., L. L. Decker, et al. (1999). "Epstein-barr virus-infected resting memory B cells, not proliferating lymphoblasts, accumulate in the peripheral blood of immunosuppressed patients." *J Exp Med* 190(4): 567-76.

Bashaw, J. M. and J. L. Yates (2001). "Replication from oriP of Epstein-Barr virus requires exact spacing of two bound dimers of EBNA1 which bend DNA." *J Virol* 75(22): 10603-11.

Baumforth, K. R., A. Birgersdotter, et al. (2008). "Expression of the Epstein-Barr virus-encoded Epstein-Barr virus nuclear antigen 1 in Hodgkin's lymphoma cells mediates Up-regulation of CCL20 and the migration of regulatory T cells." *Am J Pathol* 173(1): 195-204.

Bhakat, K. K., A. K. Mantha, et al. (2009). "Transcriptional regulatory functions of mammalian AP-endonuclease (APE1/Ref-1), an essential multifunctional protein." *Antioxid Redox Signal* 11(3): 621-38.

Blattes, R., C. Monod, et al. (2006). "Displacement of D1, HP1 and topoisomerase II from satellite heterochromatin by a specific polyamide." *EMBO J* 25(11): 2397-408.

Bochkarev, A., J. A. Barwell, et al. (1996). "Crystal structure of the DNA-binding domain of the Epstein-Barr virus origin-binding protein, EBNA1, bound to DNA." *Cell* 84(5): 791-800.

Bochkarev, A., J. A. Barwell, et al. (1995). "Crystal structure of the DNA-binding domain of the Epstein-Barr virus origin-binding protein EBNA 1." *Cell* 83(1): 39-46.

Bouallaga, I., S. Massicard, et al. (2000). "An enhanceosome containing the Jun B/Fra-2 heterodimer and the HMG-I(Y) architectural protein controls HPV 18 transcription." *EMBO Rep* 1(5): 422-7.

Bouallaga, I., S. Teissier, et al. (2003). "HMG-I(Y) and the CBP/p300 coactivator are essential for human papillomavirus type 18 enhanceosome transcriptional activity." *Mol Cell Biol* 23(7): 2329-40.

Cai, X., A. Schafer, et al. (2006). "Epstein-Barr virus microRNAs are evolutionarily conserved and differentially expressed." *PLoS Pathog* 2(3): e23.

Canaan, A., I. Haviv, et al. (2009). "EBNA1 regulates cellular gene expression by binding cellular promoters." *Proc Natl Acad Sci U S A* 106(52): 22421-6.

Centers for Disease Control (1987). "Revision of the CDC surveillance case definition for acquired immunodeficiency syndrome. Council of State and Territorial Epidemiologists; AIDS Program, Center for Infectious Diseases." *MMWR Morb Mortal Wkly Rep* 36 Suppl 1: 1S-15S.

Chaudhuri, B., H. Xu, et al. (2001). "Human DNA replication initiation factors, ORC and MCM, associate with oriP of Epstein-Barr virus." *Proc Natl Acad Sci U S A* 98(18): 10085-9.

Choy, E. Y., K. L. Siu, et al. (2008). "An Epstein-Barr virus-encoded microRNA targets PUMA to promote host cell survival." *J Exp Med* 205(11): 2551-60.

Crawford, D. H., J. A. Thomas, et al. (1980). "Epstein Barr virus nuclear antigen positive lymphoma after cyclosporin A treatment in patient with renal allograft." *Lancet* 1(8182): 1355-6.

D'Autreaux, B. and M. B. Toledano (2007). "ROS as signalling molecules: mechanisms that generate specificity in ROS homeostasis." *Nat Rev Mol Cell Biol* 8(10): 813-24.

Dalbies-Tran, R., E. Stigger-Rosser, et al. (2001). "Amino acids of Epstein-Barr virus nuclear antigen 3A essential for repression of Jkappa-mediated transcription and their evolutionary conservation." *J Virol* 75(1): 90-9.

Dawson, C. W., A. B. Rickinson, et al. (1990). "Epstein-Barr virus latent membrane protein inhibits human epithelial cell differentiation." *Nature* 344(6268): 777-80.

Day, L., C. M. Chau, et al. (2007). "Chromatin profiling of Epstein-Barr virus latency control region." *J Virol* 81(12): 6389-401.

de-The, G., A. Geser, et al. (1978). "Epidemiological evidence for causal relationship between Epstein-Barr virus and Burkitt's lymphoma from Ugandan prospective study." *Nature* 274(5673): 756-61.

Dhar, S. K., K. Yoshida, et al. (2001). "Replication from oriP of Epstein-Barr virus requires human ORC and is inhibited by geminin." *Cell* 106(3): 287-96.

Dockrell, D. H., J. G. Strickler, et al. (1998). "Epstein-Barr virus-induced T cell lymphoma in solid organ transplant recipients." *Clin Infect Dis* 26(1): 180-2.

Dresang, L. R., D. T. Vereide, et al. (2009). "Identifying sites bound by Epstein-Barr virus nuclear antigen 1 (EBNA1) in the human genome: defining a position-weighted matrix to predict sites bound by EBNA1 in viral genomes." *J Virol* 83(7): 2930-40.

Duellman, S. J., K. L. Thompson, et al. (2009). "Phosphorylation sites of Epstein-Barr virus EBNA1 regulate its function." *J Gen Virol* 90(Pt 9): 2251-9.

Epstein, M. A., B. G. Achong, et al. (1964). "Virus Particles in Cultured Lymphoblasts from Burkitt's Lymphoma." *Lancet* 1(7335): 702-3.

Ernberg, I. and E. Altiok (1989). "The role of Epstein-Barr virus in lymphomas of HIV-carriers." *APMIS Suppl* 8: 58-61.

Falk, K., J. W. Gratama, et al. (1995). "The role of repetitive DNA sequences in the size variation of Epstein-Barr virus (EBV) nuclear antigens, and the identification of different EBV isolates using RFLP and PCR analysis." *J Gen Virol* 76 (Pt 4): 779-90.

Fingeroth, J. D., J. J. Weis, et al. (1984). "Epstein-Barr virus receptor of human B lymphocytes is the C3d receptor CR2." *Proc Natl Acad Sci U S A* 81(14): 4510-4.

Fischer, N., E. Kremmer, et al. (1997). "Epstein-Barr virus nuclear antigen 1 forms a complex with the nuclear transporter karyopherin alpha2." *J Biol Chem* 272(7): 3999-4005.

Flavell, J. R., K. R. Baumforth, et al. (2008). "Down-regulation of the TGF-beta target gene, PTPRK, by the Epstein-Barr virus encoded EBNA1 contributes to the growth and survival of Hodgkin lymphoma cells." *Blood* 111(1): 292-301.

Freyer, M. W., R. Buscaglia, et al. (2007). "Binding of netropsin to several DNA constructs: evidence for at least two different 1:1 complexes formed from an -AATT-containing ds-DNA construct and a single minor groove binding ligand." *Biophys Chem* 126(1-3): 186-96.

Gahn, T. A. and B. Sugden (1995). "An EBNA-1-dependent enhancer acts from a distance of 10 kilobase pairs to increase expression of the Epstein-Barr virus LMP gene." *J Virol* 69(4): 2633-6.

Geiszt, M. and T. L. Leto (2004). "The Nox family of NAD(P)H oxidases: host defense and beyond." *J Biol Chem* 279(50): 51715-8.

Gires, O., U. Zimber-Strobl, et al. (1997). "Latent membrane protein 1 of Epstein-Barr virus mimics a constitutively active receptor molecule." *EMBO J* 16(20): 6131-40.

Glaser, S. L., R. J. Lin, et al. (1997). "Epstein-Barr virus-associated Hodgkin's disease: epidemiologic characteristics in international data." *Int J Cancer* 70(4): 375-82.

Gottschalk, S., C. M. Rooney, et al. (2005). "Post-transplant lymphoproliferative disorders." *Annu Rev Med* 56: 29-44.

Grogan, E. A., W. P. Summers, et al. (1983). "Two Epstein-Barr viral nuclear neoantigens distinguished by gene transfer, serology, and chromosome binding." *Proc Natl Acad Sci U S A* 80(24): 7650-3.

Grossman, S. R., E. Johannsen, et al. (1994). "The Epstein-Barr virus nuclear antigen 2 transactivator is directed to response elements by the J kappa recombination signal binding protein." *Proc Natl Acad Sci U S A* 91(16): 7568-72.

Grossman, S. R. and L. A. Laimins (1996). "EBNA1 and E2: a new paradigm for origin-binding proteins?" *Trends Microbiol* 4(3): 87-9.

Gruhne, B., R. Sompallae, et al. (2009). "The Epstein-Barr virus nuclear antigen-1 promotes genomic instability via induction of reactive oxygen species." *Proc Natl Acad Sci U S A* 106(7): 2313-8.

Gruhne, B., R. Sompallae, et al. (2009). "Three Epstein-Barr virus latency proteins independently promote genomic instability by inducing DNA damage, inhibiting DNA repair and inactivating cell cycle checkpoints." *Oncogene* 28(45): 3997-4008.

Hammerschmidt, W. (2011). "What keeps the power on in lymphomas?" *Blood* 117(6): 1777-8.

Hammerschmidt, W. and B. Sugden (1989). "Genetic analysis of immortalizing functions of Epstein-Barr virus in human B lymphocytes." *Nature* 340(6232): 393-7.

Harada, S. and E. Kieff (1997). "Epstein-Barr virus nuclear protein LP stimulates EBNA-2 acidic domain-mediated transcriptional activation." *J Virol* 71(9): 6611-8.

Harrison, S., K. Fisenne, et al. (1994). "Sequence requirements of the Epstein-Barr virus latent origin of DNA replication." *J Virol* 68(3): 1913-25.

Hebner, C., J. Lasanen, et al. (2003). "The spacing between adjacent binding sites in the family of repeats affects the functions of Epstein-Barr nuclear antigen 1 in transcription activation and stable plasmid maintenance." *Virology* 311(2): 263-74.

Hegde, R. S., S. R. Grossman, et al. (1992). "Crystal structure at 1.7 A of the bovine papillomavirus-1 E2 DNA-binding domain bound to its DNA target." *Nature* 359(6395): 505-12.

Held, K. D., F. C. Sylvester, et al. (1996). "Role of Fenton chemistry in thiol-induced toxicity and apoptosis." *Radiat Res* 145(5): 542-53.

Henkel, T., P. D. Ling, et al. (1994). "Mediation of Epstein-Barr virus EBNA2 transactivation by recombination signal-binding protein J kappa." *Science* 265(5168): 92-5.

Henle, G., W. Henle, et al. (1968). "Relation of Burkitt's tumor-associated herpes-ytpe virus to infectious mononucleosis." *Proc Natl Acad Sci U S A* 59(1): 94-101.

Henriksen, J., M. Stabell, et al. (2010). "Identification of target genes for wild type and truncated HMGA2 in mesenchymal stem-like cells." *BMC Cancer* 10(1): 329.

Heslop, H. E. (2005). "Biology and treatment of Epstein-Barr virus-associated non-Hodgkin lymphomas." *Hematology Am Soc Hematol Educ Program*: 260-6.

Huang, R. P. and E. D. Adamson (1993). "Characterization of the DNA-binding properties of the early growth response-1 (Egr-1) transcription factor: evidence for modulation by a redox mechanism." *DNA Cell Biol* 12(3): 265-73.

Hung, S. C., M. S. Kang, et al. (2001). "Maintenance of Epstein-Barr virus (EBV) oriP-based episomes requires EBV-encoded nuclear antigen-1 chromosome-binding domains, which can be replaced by high-mobility group-I or histone H1." *Proc Natl Acad Sci U S A* 98(4): 1865-70.

Huse, M., M. J. Eck, et al. (1998). "A Zn2+ ion links the cytoplasmic tail of CD4 and the N-terminal region of Lck." *J Biol Chem* 273(30): 18729-33.

Hutchison, K. A., G. Matic, et al. (1991). "Redox manipulation of DNA binding activity and BuGR epitope reactivity of the glucocorticoid receptor." *J Biol Chem* 266(16): 10505-9.

Huth, J. R., C. A. Bewley, et al. (1997). "The solution structure of an HMG-I(Y)-DNA complex defines a new architectural minor groove binding motif." *Nat Struct Biol* 4(8): 657-65.

Janssen, S., O. Cuvier, et al. (2000). "Specific gain- and loss-of-function phenotypes induced by satellite-specific DNA-binding drugs fed to Drosophila melanogaster." *Mol Cell* 6(5): 1013-24.

Janssen, S., T. Durussel, et al. (2000). "Chromatin opening of DNA satellites by targeted sequence-specific drugs." *Mol Cell* 6(5): 999-1011.

Jayaraman, L., K. G. Murthy, et al. (1997). "Identification of redox/repair protein Ref-1 as a potent activator of p53." *Genes Dev* 11(5): 558-70.

Kalantari, P., V. Narayan, et al. (2008). "Thioredoxin reductase-1 negatively regulates HIV-1 transactivating protein Tat-dependent transcription in human macrophages." *J Biol Chem* 283(48): 33183-90.

Kapoor, P., K. Shire, et al. (2001). "Reconstitution of Epstein-Barr virus-based plasmid partitioning in budding yeast." *EMBO J* 20(1-2): 222-30.

Kaye, K. M., K. M. Izumi, et al. (1993). "Epstein-Barr virus latent membrane protein 1 is essential for B-lymphocyte growth transformation." *Proc Natl Acad Sci U S A* 90(19): 9150-4.

Kelly, B. L., G. Singh, et al. (2011). "Molecular and cellular characterization of an AT-hook protein from Leishmania." *PLoS One* 6(6): e21412.

Kennedy, G., J. Komano, et al. (2003). "Epstein-Barr virus provides a survival factor to Burkitt's lymphomas." *Proc Natl Acad Sci U S A* 100(24): 14269-74.

Kennedy, G. and B. Sugden (2003). "EBNA-1, a bifunctional transcriptional activator." *Mol Cell Biol* 23(19): 6901-8.

Khanna, R., D. J. Moss, et al. (1999). "Vaccine strategies against Epstein-Barr virus-associated diseases: lessons from studies on cytotoxic T-cell-mediated immune regulation." *Immunol Rev* 170: 49-64.

Kieff, E. D. and A. B. Rickinson (2007). Epstein-Barr Virus and Its Replication. *Fields Virology*. D. M. Knipe and P. M. Howley. 2: 2603-2653.

Kieser, A., C. Kaiser, et al. (1999). "LMP1 signal transduction differs substantially from TNF receptor 1 signaling in the molecular functions of TRADD and TRAF2." *EMBO J* 18(9): 2511-21.

Kiley, P. J. and G. Storz (2004). "Exploiting thiol modifications." *PLoS Biol* 2(11): e400.

Kim, A. L., M. Maher, et al. (1997). "An imperfect correlation between DNA replication activity of Epstein-Barr virus nuclear antigen 1 (EBNA1) and binding to the nuclear import receptor, Rch1/importin alpha." *Virology* 239(2): 340-51.

Kim, P. W., Z. Y. Sun, et al. (2003). "A zinc clasp structure tethers Lck to T cell coreceptors CD4 and CD8." *Science* 301(5640): 1725-8.

Kim, T. K. and T. Maniatis (1997). "The mechanism of transcriptional synergy of an in vitro assembled interferon-beta enhanceosome." *Mol Cell* 1(1): 119-29.

Kirchmaier, A. L. and B. Sugden (1997). "Dominant-negative inhibitors of EBNA-1 of Epstein-Barr virus." *J Virol* 71(3): 1766-75.

Kirchmaier, A. L. and B. Sugden (1998). "Rep*: a viral element that can partially replace the origin of plasmid DNA synthesis of Epstein-Barr virus." *J Virol* 72(6): 4657-66.

Krysan, P. J. and M. P. Calos (1993). "Epstein-Barr virus-based vectors that replicate in rodent cells." *Gene* 136(1-2): 137-43.

Krysan, P. J., S. B. Haase, et al. (1989). "Isolation of human sequences that replicate autonomously in human cells." *Mol Cell Biol* 9(3): 1026-33.

Laherty, C. D., H. M. Hu, et al. (1992). "The Epstein-Barr virus LMP1 gene product induces A20 zinc finger protein expression by activating nuclear factor kappa B." *J Biol Chem* 267(34): 24157-60.

Laichalk, L. L., D. Hochberg, et al. (2002). "The dispersal of mucosal memory B cells: evidence from persistent EBV infection." *Immunity* 16(5): 745-54.

Lee, M. A., M. E. Diamond, et al. (1999). "Genetic evidence that EBNA-1 is needed for efficient, stable latent infection by Epstein-Barr virus." *J Virol* 73(4): 2974-82.

Lee, S. P., J. M. Brooks, et al. (2004). "CD8 T cell recognition of endogenously expressed epstein-barr virus nuclear antigen 1." *J Exp Med* 199(10): 1409-20.

Levitskaya, J., A. Sharipo, et al. (1997). "Inhibition of ubiquitin/proteasome-dependent protein degradation by the Gly-Ala repeat domain of the Epstein-Barr virus nuclear antigen 1." *Proc Natl Acad Sci U S A* 94(23): 12616-21.

Li, N., S. Thompson, et al. (2010). "Discovery of selective inhibitors against EBNA1 via high throughput in silico virtual screening." *PLoS One* 5(4): e10126.

Li, Q., M. K. Spriggs, et al. (1997). "Epstein-Barr virus uses HLA class II as a cofactor for infection of B lymphocytes." *J Virol* 71(6): 4657-62.

Lin, A., S. Wang, et al. (2008). "The EBNA1 protein of Epstein-Barr virus functionally interacts with Brd4." *J Virol* 82(24): 12009-19.

Lin, R. S., C. Rodriguez, et al. (1998). "Zinc is essential for binding of p56(lck) to CD4 and CD8alpha." *J Biol Chem* 273(49): 32878-82.

Lindner, S. E. and B. Sugden (2007). "The plasmid replicon of Epstein-Barr virus: mechanistic insights into efficient, licensed, extrachromosomal replication in human cells." *Plasmid* 58(1): 1-12.

Ling, P. D., R. S. Peng, et al. (2005). "Mediation of Epstein-Barr virus EBNA-LP transcriptional coactivation by Sp100." *EMBO J* 24(20): 3565-75.

Lothrop, A. P., E. L. Ruggles, et al. (2009). "No selenium required: reactions catalyzed by mammalian thioredoxin reductase that are independent of a selenocysteine residue." *Biochemistry* 48(26): 6213-23.

Lu, F., P. Wikramasinghe, et al. (2010). "Genome-wide analysis of host-chromosome binding sites for Epstein-Barr Virus Nuclear Antigen 1 (EBNA1)." *Virol J* 7: 262.

Lupton, S. and A. J. Levine (1985). "Mapping genetic elements of Epstein-Barr virus that facilitate extrachromosomal persistence of Epstein-Barr virus-derived plasmids in human cells." *Mol Cell Biol* 5(10): 2533-42.

Mackey, D., T. Middleton, et al. (1995). "Multiple regions within EBNA1 can link DNAs." *J Virol* 69(10): 6199-208.

Mackey, D. and B. Sugden (1997). "Studies on the mechanism of DNA linking by Epstein-Barr virus nuclear antigen 1." *J Biol Chem* 272(47): 29873-9.

Mackey, D. and B. Sugden (1999). "The linking regions of EBNA1 are essential for its support of replication and transcription." *Mol Cell Biol* 19(5): 3349-59.

Maniatis, T., J. V. Falvo, et al. (1998). "Structure and function of the interferon-beta enhanceosome." *Cold Spring Harb Symp Quant Biol* 63: 609-20.

Mark, W. and B. Sugden (1982). "Transformation of lymphocytes by Epstein-Barr virus requires only one-fourth of the viral genome." *Virology* 122(2): 431-43.

Martinez Hoyos, J., M. Fedele, et al. (2004). "Identification of the genes up- and down-regulated by the high mobility group A1 (HMGA1) proteins: tissue specificity of the HMGA1-dependent gene regulation." *Cancer Res* 64(16): 5728-35.

Merika, M., A. J. Williams, et al. (1998). "Recruitment of CBP/p300 by the IFN beta enhanceosome is required for synergistic activation of transcription." *Mol Cell* 1(2): 277-87.

Mitomo, K., K. Nakayama, et al. (1994). "Two different cellular redox systems regulate the DNA-binding activity of the p50 subunit of NF-kappa B in vitro." *Gene* 145(2): 197-203.

Mosialos, G., M. Birkenbach, et al. (1995). "The Epstein-Barr virus transforming protein LMP1 engages signaling proteins for the tumor necrosis factor receptor family." *Cell* 80(3): 389-99.

Mounier, N., M. Spina, et al. (2006). "AIDS-related non-Hodgkin lymphoma: final analysis of 485 patients treated with risk-adapted intensive chemotherapy." *Blood* 107(10): 3832-40.

Mounier, N., M. Spina, et al. (2007). "Modern management of non-Hodgkin lymphoma in HIV-infected patients." *Br J Haematol* 136(5): 685-98.

Murakami, M., R. Kaul, et al. (2009). "Nucleoside diphosphate kinase/Nm23 and Epstein-Barr virus." *Mol Cell Biochem*.

Nanbo, A., A. Sugden, et al. (2007). "The coupling of synthesis and partitioning of EBV's plasmid replicon is revealed in live cells." *EMBO J* 26(19): 4252-62.

Nasimuzzaman, M., M. Kuroda, et al. (2005). "Eradication of Epstein-Barr virus episome and associated inhibition of infected tumor cell growth by adenovirus vector-mediated transduction of dominant-negative EBNA1." *Mol Ther* 11(4): 578-90.

Navarro, W. H. and L. D. Kaplan (2006). "AIDS-related lymphoproliferative disease." *Blood* 107(1): 13-20.

Niederman, J. C., R. W. McCollum, et al. (1968). "Infectious mononucleosis. Clinical manifestations in relation to EB virus antibodies." *JAMA* 203(3): 205-9.

Norseen, J., A. Thomae, et al. (2008). "RNA-dependent recruitment of the origin recognition complex." *EMBO J* 27(22): 3024-35.

O'Neil, J. D., T. J. Owen, et al. (2008). "Epstein-Barr virus-encoded EBNA1 modulates the AP-1 transcription factor pathway in nasopharyngeal carcinoma cells and enhances angiogenesis in vitro." *J Gen Virol* 89(Pt 11): 2833-42.

O'Reilly, S. E., J. M. Connors, et al. (1997). "Malignant lymphomas in the elderly." *Clin Geriatr Med* 13(2): 251-63.

Okamoto, K., H. Tanaka, et al. (1999). "Redox-dependent regulation of nuclear import of the glucocorticoid receptor." *J Biol Chem* 274(15): 10363-71.

Paschos, K., P. Smith, et al. (2009). "Epstein-barr virus latency in B cells leads to epigenetic repression and CpG methylation of the tumour suppressor gene Bim." *PLoS Pathog* 5(6): e1000492.

Peng, R., S. C. Moses, et al. (2005). "The Epstein-Barr virus EBNA-LP protein preferentially coactivates EBNA2-mediated stimulation of latent membrane proteins expressed from the viral divergent promoter." *J Virol* 79(7): 4492-505.

Pratt, Z. L., M. Kuzembayeva, et al. (2009). "The microRNAs of Epstein-Barr Virus are expressed at dramatically differing levels among cell lines." *Virology* 386(2): 387-97.

Puglielli, M. T., M. Woisetschlaeger, et al. (1996). "oriP is essential for EBNA gene promoter activity in Epstein-Barr virus-immortalized lymphoblastoid cell lines." *J Virol* 70(9): 5758-68.

Purtilo, D. T. and G. Klein (1981). "Introduction to Epstein-Barr virus and lymphoproliferative diseases in immunodeficient individuals." *Cancer Res* 41(11 Pt 1): 4209.

Rawlins, D. R., G. Milman, et al. (1985). "Sequence-specific DNA binding of the Epstein-Barr virus nuclear antigen (EBNA-1) to clustered sites in the plasmid maintenance region." *Cell* 42(3): 859-68.

Reeves, R. (2001). "Molecular biology of HMGA proteins: hubs of nuclear function." *Gene* 277(1-2): 63-81.

Reisman, D. and B. Sugden (1986). "trans activation of an Epstein-Barr viral transcriptional enhancer by the Epstein-Barr viral nuclear antigen 1." *Mol Cell Biol* 6(11): 3838-46.

Reisman, D., J. Yates, et al. (1985). "A putative origin of replication of plasmids derived from Epstein-Barr virus is composed of two cis-acting components." *Mol Cell Biol* 5(8): 1822-32.

Rickinson, A. B. and E. Kieff (2007). Epstein-Barr Virus. *Fields Virology*. D. M. Knipe and P. M. Howley. 2: 2656-2700.

Rickinson, A. B., S. P. Lee, et al. (1996). "Cytotoxic T lymphocyte responses to Epstein-Barr virus." *Curr Opin Immunol* 8(4): 492-7.

Ritzi, M., K. Tillack, et al. (2003). "Complex protein-DNA dynamics at the latent origin of DNA replication of Epstein-Barr virus." *J Cell Sci* 116(Pt 19): 3971-84.

Robertson, E. S., J. Lin, et al. (1996). "The amino-terminal domains of Epstein-Barr virus nuclear proteins 3A, 3B, and 3C interact with RBPJ(kappa)." *J Virol* 70(5): 3068-74.

Schepers, A., M. Ritzi, et al. (2001). "Human origin recognition complex binds to the region of the latent origin of DNA replication of Epstein-Barr virus." *EMBO J* 20(16): 4588-602.

Schweiger, M. R., M. Ottinger, et al. (2007). "Brd4-independent transcriptional repression function of the papillomavirus e2 proteins." *J Virol* 81(18): 9612-22.

Sears, J., J. Kolman, et al. (2003). "Metaphase chromosome tethering is necessary for the DNA synthesis and maintenance of oriP plasmids but is insufficient for transcription activation by Epstein-Barr nuclear antigen 1." *J Virol* 77(21): 11767-80.

Sears, J., M. Ujihara, et al. (2004). "The amino terminus of Epstein-Barr Virus (EBV) nuclear antigen 1 contains AT hooks that facilitate the replication and partitioning of latent EBV genomes by tethering them to cellular chromosomes." *J Virol* 78(21): 11487-505.

Shire, K., D. F. Ceccarelli, et al. (1999). "EBP2, a human protein that interacts with sequences of the Epstein-Barr virus nuclear antigen 1 important for plasmid maintenance." *J Virol* 73(4): 2587-95.

Siddiqa, A., J. C. Sims-Mourtada, et al. (2001). "Regulation of CD40 and CD40 ligand by the AT-hook transcription factor AKNA." *Nature* 410(6826): 383-7.

Singh, G., S. Aras, et al. (2009). "Optimal transactivation by Epstein-Barr nuclear antigen 1 requires the UR1 and ATH1 domains." *J Virol* 83(9): 4227-35.

Skalnik, D. G. and E. J. Neufeld (1992). "Sequence-specific binding of HMG-I(Y) to the proximal promoter of the gp91-phox gene." *Biochem Biophys Res Commun* 187(2): 563-9.

Spina, M., C. Simonelli, et al. (2007). "Phase II trial of CHOP plus rituximab in patients with HIV-associated non-Hodgkin's lymphoma." *J Clin Oncol* 25(6): e7.

Steven, N. M., A. M. Leese, et al. (1996). "Epitope focusing in the primary cytotoxic T cell response to Epstein-Barr virus and its relationship to T cell memory." *J Exp Med* 184(5): 1801-13.

Sugden, B. and W. Mark (1977). "Clonal transformation of adult human leukocytes by Epstein-Barr virus." *J Virol* 23(3): 503-8.

Suzuki, Y. and Y. Ono (1999). "Involvement of reactive oxygen species produced via NADPH oxidase in tyrosine phosphorylation in human B- and T-lineage lymphoid cells." *Biochem Biophys Res Commun* 255(2): 262-7.

Taylor, A. L., R. Marcus, et al. (2005). "Post-transplant lymphoproliferative disorders (PTLD) after solid organ transplantation." *Crit Rev Oncol Hematol* 56(1): 155-67.

Tempera, I., M. Klichinsky, et al. (2011). "EBV Latency Types Adopt Alternative Chromatin Conformations." *PLoS Pathog* 7(7): e1002180.

Tesfaye, A., F. Di Cello, et al. (2007). "The high-mobility group A1 gene up-regulates cyclooxygenase 2 expression in uterine tumorigenesis." *Cancer Res* 67(9): 3998-4004.

Vereide, D. T. and B. Sugden (2011). "Lymphomas differ in their dependence on Epstein-Barr virus." *Blood* 117(6): 1977-85.

Walls, D. and M. Perricaudet (1991). "Novel downstream elements upregulate transcription initiated from an Epstein-Barr virus latent promoter." *EMBO J* 10(1): 143-51.

Wan, L., E. Ottinger, et al. (2008). "Inactivation of the SMN complex by oxidative stress." *Mol Cell* 31(2): 244-54.

Wang, J., S. E. Lindner, et al. (2006). "Essential elements of a licensed, mammalian plasmid origin of DNA synthesis." *Mol Cell Biol* 26(3): 1124-34.

Wartell, R. M., J. E. Larson, et al. (1974). "Netropsin. A specific probe for A-T regions of duplex deoxyribonucleic acid." *J Biol Chem* 249(21): 6719-31.

Washington, A. T., G. Singh, et al. (2010). "Diametrically opposed effects of hypoxia and oxidative stress on two viral transactivators." *Virol J* 7: 93.

Woisetschlaeger, M., J. L. Strominger, et al. (1989). "Mutually exclusive use of viral promoters in Epstein-Barr virus latently infected lymphocytes." *Proc Natl Acad Sci U S A* 86(17): 6498-502.

Wood, V. H., J. D. O'Neil, et al. (2007). "Epstein-Barr virus-encoded EBNA1 regulates cellular gene transcription and modulates the STAT1 and TGFbeta signaling pathways." *Oncogene* 26(28): 4135-47.

Wysokenski, D. A. and J. L. Yates (1989). "Multiple EBNA1-binding sites are required to form an EBNA1-dependent enhancer and to activate a minimal replicative origin within oriP of Epstein-Barr virus." *J Virol* 63(6): 2657-66.

Xanthoudakis, S. and T. Curran (1992). "Identification and characterization of Ref-1, a nuclear protein that facilitates AP-1 DNA-binding activity." *EMBO J* 11(2): 653-65.

Xanthoudakis, S. and T. Curran (1996). "Redox regulation of AP-1: a link between transcription factor signaling and DNA repair." *Adv Exp Med Biol* 387: 69-75.

Xanthoudakis, S., G. Miao, et al. (1992). "Redox activation of Fos-Jun DNA binding activity is mediated by a DNA repair enzyme." *EMBO J* 11(9): 3323-35.

Yates, J., N. Warren, et al. (1984). "A cis-acting element from the Epstein-Barr viral genome that permits stable replication of recombinant plasmids in latently infected cells." *Proc Natl Acad Sci U S A* 81(12): 3806-10.

Yates, J. L., S. M. Camiolo, et al. (2000). "The minimal replicator of Epstein-Barr virus oriP." *J Virol* 74(10): 4512-22.

Yates, J. L., N. Warren, et al. (1985). "Stable replication of plasmids derived from Epstein-Barr virus in various mammalian cells." *Nature* 313(6005): 812-5.

Yie, J., S. Liang, et al. (1997). "Intra- and intermolecular cooperative binding of high-mobility-group protein I(Y) to the beta-interferon promoter." *Mol Cell Biol* 17(7): 3649-62.

Yie, J., M. Merika, et al. (1999). "The role of HMG I(Y) in the assembly and function of the IFN-beta enhanceosome." *EMBO J* 18(11): 3074-89.

Yin, Y., B. Manoury, et al. (2003). "Self-inhibition of synthesis and antigen presentation by Epstein-Barr virus-encoded EBNA1." *Science* 301(5638): 1371-4.

Zhao, B., D. R. Marshall, et al. (1996). "A conserved domain of the Epstein-Barr virus nuclear antigens 3A and 3C binds to a discrete domain of Jkappa." *J Virol* 70(7): 4228-36.

Zhou, J., C. M. Chau, et al. (2005). "Cell cycle regulation of chromatin at an origin of DNA replication." *EMBO J* 24(7): 1406-17.

Zimber-Strobl, U., B. Kempkes, et al. (1996). "Epstein-Barr virus latent membrane protein (LMP1) is not sufficient to maintain proliferation of B cells but both it and activated CD40 can prolong their survival." *EMBO J* 15(24): 7070-8.

5

Kaposi's Sarcoma-Associated Virus Governs Gene Expression Profiles Toward B Cell Transformation

Keiji Ueda[1], Emi Ito[2], Masato Karayama[3], Eriko Ohsaki[1], Kazushi Nakano[1] and Shinya Watanabe[2]
[1]*Division of Virology, Department of Microbiology and Immunology Osaka University Graduate School of Medicine*
[2]*Department of Clinical Genomics, Translational Research Center Fukushima Medical University*
[3]*Department of Infectious Diseases, Hamamatsu University School of Medicine Japan*

1. Introduction

Kaposi's sarcoma-associated herpesvirus (KSHV), also called human herpesvirus-8 (HHV-8) was found in patients' specimens as a causative agent of Kaposi's sarcoma by representational difference analysis (RDA) (Chang et al., 1994). Initially identified fragments by RDA were KS330Bam and KS631Bam, which showed a sequence similarity to a portion of the open reading frame (ORF) 26 open reading frame encoding the capsid protein VP23 of herpesvirus saimiri (HVS) and the amino acid sequence encoded by the corresponding BDLF1 ORF of Epstein-Barr virus (EBV), and to the tegment protein, ORF75 and also the tegment protein of EBV, BNRF1 (p140), respectively. The following full sequence analysis revealed that KSHV was belonging to the γ-herpesvirus subfamily, the genus rhadinovirus rather than lymphocryptic virus and could be a new oncogenic DNA virus (Moore et al., 1996; Russo et al., 1996).

KSHV is supposed to infect various kinds of tissue *in vitro* at least by using integrin αVβ3 as a receptor (Garrigues et al., 2008) and establishes latency in B cells (Chen and Lagunoff, 2005). KSHV has been reported to infect a primary endothelial cell and can transform it into a spindle cell which is a characteristic feature of the oncogenic activity of KSHV in endothelial cells (Lagunoff et al., 2002) However, it has not been revealed effective *in vitro* infection to primary peripheral blood mononuclear cells (PBMC), which of course include B cell, as EBV can form lymphoblastoid cell lines (LCL). Extensive studies so far have revealed that KSHV should be an etiologic agent for Kaposi's sarcoma (KS), multicentric Castleman's disease (MCD), and primary effusion lymphoma (PEL) (Hengge et al., 2002a; Hengge et al., 2002b).

It is quite a big question how oncogenic viruses are involved in their related cancers. Especially limited host ranges of viruses only infecting with humans make this question more unanswerable. One approach to get a hint about this question and solve it is to see gene expression profiles of viruses-associated tumors. Recently, we analyzed three types of typical lymphocyte-originated tumor cell lines-primary effusion lymphoma (PEL) cell lines,

T cell leukemia cell lines (TCL), Burkitt lymphoma (BL) cell lines-and two sets of PBMCs-in order to know how PEL was generated by searching characteristic gene expression profiles. Our approach, however, might be just to show typical gene expression profiles after establishment of PEL cell lines and it may be very difficult to account for viral pathogenesis only by gene expression profiles. Needless to say, we need an experimental model to observe the whole process from virus infection to cancer formation. In this chapter, we discuss about how KSHV is involved in PEL formation and what to do next to solve questions about viral oncogenesis.

2. Characteristic features of KSHV

KSHV is a γ-herpesvirus mentioned above and the genome is double stranded linearized DNA about 170kb long including GC-rich repetitious repeat called terminal sequences (TR), the unit of which is 801bp and repeated 30~50 times at the end of the genome though the sequence and the repeated unit might be different among clones. The unique region of the genome is about 140kb long and encodes more than 80 genes, most of which are lytic genes (Russo et al., 1996). The linearized genome is circularized at the TR after entry into cells and usually stealthies as an episome not going to full lytic replication.

2.1 KSHV life cycles

Like the other herpesviruses, KSHV has two typical life cycles called lytic infection (or reactivation from latency) and latent infection. Lytic infection/reactivation is a virus producing cycle and probably all viral genes are expressed from immediate early (IE), early (E) and late (L) genes in a cascade-like fashion. A key factor for lytic replication is Reactivation Transcription Activator (RTA) (Chen et al., 2001; Lukac et al., 1998; Sun et al., 1998). RTA is a very strong transactivator and trans-activates the other viral E genes such as *K-bZIP* (*K8*), *orf57*, *pan* including *kaposin* (*k12*), a latent gene, not only through specific binding sequences but also through an indirect mechanism (Sakakibara et al., 2001). When L genes are successfully expressed, it leads to explosive daughter virus production, which is a final end of the viral life cycle to disseminate viral infection and survive as its virus itself in nature.

On the other hand, latent infection is a viral stealthing state. The viral genome replicates according to the host cell cycle and is partitioned into divided cells at least in KSHV infected PEL cell lines (Ballestas, Chatis, and Kaye, 1999). The viral copy number per cell appears to be maintained at the same (Ueda et al., 2006). In this state, expressing viral genes are extremely limited to a few genes such latency-associated nuclear antigen (*lana*), viral cyclin (*v-cyc*), viral flip (*v-flip*), kaposin (*k12*) and viral interferon regulatory factor 3 (*v-irf-3*) (Paulose-Murphy et al., 2001). The former three genes are actually in one unit of gene (Fig. 1). *lana* and *v-cyc-v-flip* expression is regulated by alternative splicing. *v-cyc-v-flip* is in one transcript and v-FLIP is translated through internal ribosome entry site (IRES). Although *k12* is an independent gene, these four genes are present in one region and actively expressed. It remains to be solved how latent genes are regulated, since neighbor genes just upstream or downstream are tightly inactivated in a high density of genes in the genome. Epigenetic marking might be important to establish this state but it is unclear how such an effect itself is controlled (Toth et al., 2010). As for a virus, latency is a kind of poised state waiting for lytic replication, because it could be unfavorable for the virus to disseminate and expand its generation.

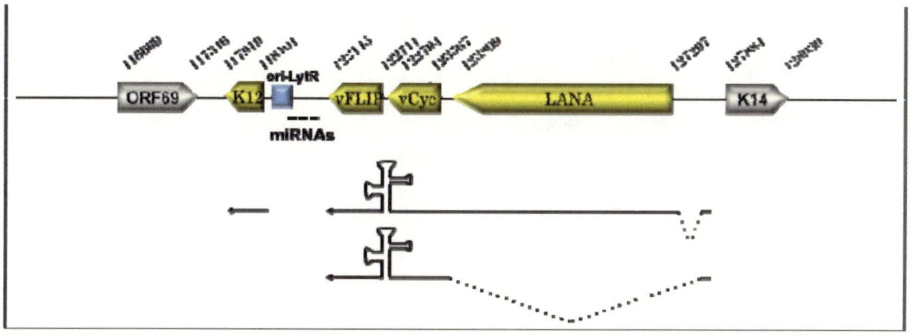

Fig. 1. The active gene locus around *lana*.

The viral latency might be the places for KSHV-associated malignancies mentioned below, since such malignancies usually show viral latent infection. And therefore, it seems to be quite important to understand what the viral latency is and it will give us hints to investigate functions of the viral latent genes products. Nevertheless, if the viral latenct genes products work for cellular immortalization and/or transformation, there may be more patients in KSHV infected people suffering from KSHV-associated malignancies. Thus, it should be kept in our mind to take this idea into consideration when thinking how KSHV is involved in cancer formation.

2.2 Latency-associated nuclear antigen (LANA)

LANA is one of the most actively produced viral factors and controls the viral latency. Though LANA seems to be a multifunctional protein, important functions of LANA in the latency are to support the viral genome replication, to partition the replicated viral genome and to maintain the same genome copy number per cell, and to regulate the viral genes expression (Han et al., 2010).

LANA has two binding sites called LANA binding sequences (LBS) in TR and replication origin of the KSHV genome in latency (ori-P) consists of the LBS and the following 32bp GC-rich segment (32GC) (Garber, Hu, and Renne, 2002; Garber et al., 2001). One of two LBS is required for the viral replication at least but it is not enough, i.e., 32GC is also required (Hu and Renne, 2005). Though it remains to be solved how the viral ori-P is determined among repeated TR sequences and how 32GC is functioning, LANA has been reported to interact with components of cellular replication machinery; origin recognition complex 1 to 6 (ORC1~ORC6) (Verma et al., 2006). Probably LANA binds with LBS and recruits ORCs on the ori-P to start replication. It is, however, very questionable whether LANA binds all ORCs at the same time. LANA also interacts with a histone acetyltransferase binding to ORC1 (HBO1) and epigenetic control around ori-P is may be more important (Stedman et al., 2004).

LANA is supposed to interact with a chromosome component, since the viral genomes are found in the vicinity of chromosomes and actually reported to bind with a histone such as H2B, and with Bub1, CENP-F and so on (Barbera et al., 2006; Xiao et al., 2010). Such interaction might account for the viral genome partition and maintenance, though the detail is unclear.

LANA regulates the viral genes expression and maybe cellular gene expression by interacting with components involved in heterochromatin formation such as heterochromatin protein 1 (HP1) and histone methyl transferase, suv39H1. LANA binds with LBS and recruits such

factors on the viral genome, which forms heterochromatin-like environment of the genome and as a whole inactive gene expression (Sakakibara et al., 2004).
Viral genes expressed in the latency might have oncogenic activities because KSHV-associated malignancies are usually in latency setting. Multifunctional LANA interacts with many cellular factors other than those mentioned above. Several mechanisms are thought how LANA works in the viral oncogenesis. LANA interacts with suppressive oncogenes such as p53 (Friborg et al., 1999) as the other oncogenic DNA viral genes products. We have confirmed that LANA interacts with p53 to degradade (Suzuki et al., 2010) but not pRb (our personal observation). It was also reported that LANA interacted with glycogen synthase kinase 3β (GSK3β) and blocked β-catenin degradation pathway that was promoted β-catenin phosphorylation by GSK3β (Liu et al., 2007). On the other hand, stably LANA expressing cells are, however, very difficult to establish, which means that LANA expression might give disadvantage for cell growth rather than cell growth promotion (our personal observation).

2.3 Viral cyclin (v-CYC)

KSHV encodes a cyclin D homologue termed v-cyclin, which is translated from alternatively spliced mRNA covering the *lana-v-cyc-v-flip* region (Li et al., 1997) (Fig. 1). v-CYC interacts with cyclin dependent kinase 6 (CDK6) and promotes G1-S progression (Godden-Kent et al., 1997; Swanton et al., 1997). The Cyclin D-CDK6 complex is to function to exit from G0 to G1 phase (Laman et al., 2001) and the v-cyc/CDK6 complex is resistant to inhibition by CDK inhibitors by p16, p21 and p27 (Jarviluoma et al., 2004). Thus, its real function has not been elucidated and it was reported that ectopic or overexpression of c-CYC evokes rather cell/DNA damage (Koopal et al., 2007).

2.4 Viral FLICE inhibitory protein (v-FLIP)

KSHV encoded *v-flip*, a homologue of cellular flip (*c-flip*) is expressed as co-transcript with *v-cyc* and translated via internal ribosome entry site (IRES). v-FLIP activates NF-kB to maintain PEL cell tumor phenotype (Guasparri, Keller, and Cesarman, 2004). Inhibition of NF-kB activity and knocking down v-FLIP lead to KSHV infected PEL cell death (Keller, Schattner, and Cesarman, 2000). NF-kB activity is also required for maintenance of KSHV latency (Ye et al., 2008) and v-FLIP, thus, may sustain the viral latency in B cells to stand by for oncogenic transformation and maintain the transformed phenotype (de Oliveira, Ballon, and Cesarman, 2010). Oncogenic activity of v-FLIP was also reported and in transgenic mice models, v-FLIP expression induces B cell transdifferentiation and tumorigenesis (Ballon et al., 2011). Furthermore, v-FLIP represses cell death with autophagy by interacting Atg3 (Lee et al., 2009).

2.5 Kaposin (K12)

Kaposin is a uniquely transcribed at the edge of the active transcription region of the KSHV genome (Li et al., 2002). There are three frames around this region and probably a major gene is so-called *kaposin B* whose C-terminal region is corresponding to K12 ORF. Open reading frame (ORF) of KAPOSIN B contains reiterated proline-rich, 23-amino acid direct repeats, since this region includes one of two ori-Lyt sequences (lytic replication origin) (Sadler et al., 1999). KAPOSIN B activates p38 mediated mitogen-activated protein kinase [MAPK]-associated protein kinase 2 (MK2) make AU-rich 3′ UTR containing mRNA stabilize (McCormick and Ganem, 2005). Activation of p38, on the other hand, was reported to induce lytic cycle of the virus (Yoo et al., 2010). Thus, although there is a conflict in KAPOSIN B function in the KSHV latency, a lot of transcripts including T0.7 polyA (-) RNA and k12 mRNA are generated in this region.

2.6 KSHV microRNAs

Importantly, the region between ori-LytR and v-flip ORF is the region for the KSHV microRNA cluster and supplies with 17 mature microRNAs that do something in the viral latency (Boss, Plaisance, and Renne, 2009). As the cellular genomes produce various kinds of microRNA, especially DNA viruses also do (Cullen, 2009). Among them, some of them are targeting cellular genes; miR-K12-11 to BACH1, miR-K12-6-3p to THBS1, miR-K12-4-5p to Rbl2 (Lu et al., 2010), miR-K12-6 and miR-K12-11 to MAF (Hansen et al., 2010) and miR-K9 to *rta* to tune lytic reactivation finely (Lin et al., 2011), though their accurate transcription units or mechanisms have not been cleared. From now on, micro deletion mutant viruses in which each microRNA is precisely deleted will be required to understand their real sufficiency and necessity for their function, because gross deletion might have an effect on gene expression program around it.

2.7 v-IRF3 (K10.5)

KSHV encodes four genes with homology to human interferon regulatory factors (IRFs) called vIRF-1, -2, -3, -4 whose genes are clustered totally different region far from a *lana* including locus. And interestingly, one of them, vIRF-3 is expressed in the KSHV latency (Fig. 2). vIRF-3 was reported to be required for the survival of KSHV infected PELs (Wies et al., 2008), suggesting that it is a growth promoting factor by disabling type I and II interferon responses (Schmidt, Wies, and Neipel, 2011) , PML-mediated transcriptional repression of suvivin (Marcos-Villar et al., 2009), and inhibiting p53 function (Rivas et al., 2001) as well.

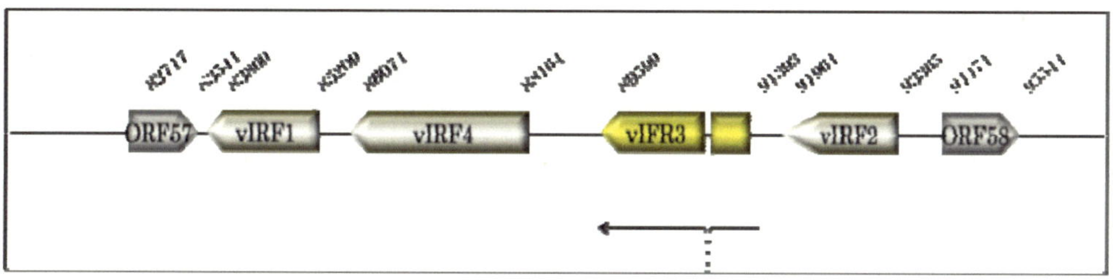

Fig. 2. vIRF region of the KSHV genome

2.8 Lytic viral genes and oncognesis

As mentioned, viral latency genes seems to have pivotal roles for the viral oncogenesis partly because the KSHV related malignancies usually happen in cells with the viral latency. Such genes products, however, do not have immortalizing and/or transforming activity either *in vitro* or *in vivo* except *v-flip* (Ballon et al., 2011). Putative KSHV oncogenes are rather encoded in lytic viral genes. KSHV *k1* and *v-gpcr* (*orf72*) showed real oncogenic activities (Mutlu et al., 2007). Thus, lytic genes should not be forgot and rather KSHV oncogenic activities should be considered on the pathway of reactivation from latency.

3. KSHV-associated malignancies

Since KHSV was found, extensive studies were performed to prove the involvement of KSHV in many cancers. Related diseases, however, are confined to a few cancers or cancer-like diseases; KS, MCD, and PEL. The other diseases such as multiple myeloma, sarcoidosis and primary pulmonary hypertension could not be KSHV-associated diseases. The former three diseases are certainly related to KSHV, though not hundred percent. Here, we would like to discuss about two B lymphocyte-originated tumors associated with KSHV infection.

3.1 Multicentric castleman's diesease (MCD)

MCD is a disease in which KSHV is involved. But KSHV is not necessarily associated in MCD and KSHV associated MCD is usually seen in AIDS setting (Dupin et al., 1999). KSHV-associated MCD is not associated with Epstein-Barr virus (EBV) (Oksenhendler et al., 1996). In contrast, PEL is usually coinfected with KSHV and EBV in vivo (Ansari et al., 1996). MCD is a B cell lymphoma morphologically resembling plasmablasts without undergoing a germinal center reaction (Parravicini et al., 2000). It is unclear how this disease is established but a KSHV viral load is a decisive factor for exacerbation of MCD (Grandadam et al., 1997) and thus KSHV should have a role in MCD pathogenesis.
High level interleukin 6 (IL-6) is a well-known fact in MCD and should do something in MCD pathogenesis (Oksenhendler et al., 1996). B cell markers, CD20 and the memory B cell marker CD27 are usually expressed, but B cell activation markers such as CD23, CD38 and CD30 are not. KSHV gene expression profiles are different from those in KS and PEL. It was reported that viral lytic genes; v-IRF-1 and v-IL-6 and ORF59 (a polymerase processivity factor, PF8) as well as a latent gene; LANA were expressed, suggesting that not a few cells in MCD are in the lytic phase.

3.2 Primary effusion lymphoma (PEL)

PEL is a rare B-cell originated lymphoma, most of which are infected with KSHV and usually emerges in patients suffering from acquired immunodeficiency syndrome (Carbone and Gloghini, 2008) by human immunodeficiency virus-1 (HIV-1) infection. PEL, used to be called body cavity-based lymphoma (BCBL), has been differentiated from the other lymphomas based on a *sine qua non* etiologic agent, KSHV. This rare lymphoma does not form a solid mass and is spreading along the serous membrane as PEL initially rises in one serous cavity such as a pleural cavity and a peritoneal cavity.
Cytologically, it is supposed that the tumor cells are derived from postgerminal center B cells and show a large cell immunobalstic plasmacytoid lymphoma and anaplastic large cell lymphoma and display a non-B, non-T phenotype (Brimo et al., 2007).
70 percent of PEL cases were co-infected with Epstein-Barr virus (EBV) in vivo (Ascoli et al., 1998). However, tightness with KSHV/HHV-8 infection suggests that KSHV/HHV-8 should have an important role for PEL pathogenesis with no doubt, taking into consideration that PEL frequently loses EBV but not KSHV after in vitro establishment of PEL cell lines.
Analyses on gene expression profiles of this rare tumor would give us a lot of information on how PEL was formed (Naranatt et al., 2004; Uetz et al., 2006) and we also analyzed three types of typical lymphocyte-originated tumor cell lines-primary effusion lymphoma (PEL) cell lines, T cell leukemia cell lines (TCL), Burkitt lymphoma (BL) cell lines and two sets of normal peripheral blood mononuclear cells (PBMCs)-in order to know how PEL was generated by searching characteristic gene expression profiles (Ueda et al., 2010). As a

result, these cell lines showed respective typical gene expression profiles and classified into clear four groups, PEL, TCL, BL and normal PBMCs. Two B lymphocyte-originated tumor cell lines, PEL and BL cell lines, clearly exhibited distinct gene expression profiles, respectively, which could be consistent with the fact that each was originated from different B-cell stages. KSHV seemed to govern the gene expression profile of the co-infected cell line, even though PEL is often co-infected with EBV in vivo and there was only one line that was co-infected with both KSHV and EBV. This suggests that existence of KSHV promotes PEL formation but not BL. Gene expression profiles of PEL were also distinct from those of KS, suggesting that cell environment affects a gene expression pattern. These data suggested not only that established typical tumor cell lines showed a distinct gene expression profile but also that this profile may be governed by a certain virus.

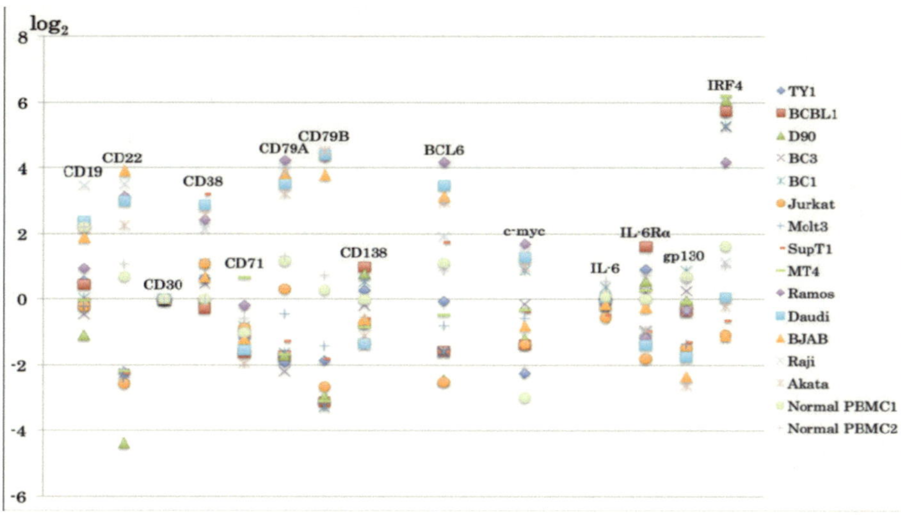

Fig. 3. Typical genes expression levels in PEL, BL and TCL

About sixty genes were prominently expressed in PEL cell lines, including Angiopoietin 1 (Ang-1, NM001146)), methyl CpG binding protein 1 (MBD1, NM015845), interleukin 2 receptor β (IL2Rβ, NM000878) and so on, compared with the other cell lines. The Ang-1 receptor, TIE-2 was not increased in PEL cell line, meaning that an autocrine loop could be unlikely but Ang-1 expression might take an effect in the AIDS environment. CD79A, B and BCL6 were remarkably reduced in PEL cell lines as reported (Du et al., 2002). CD138 (syndecan), CD22 and interferon regulatory factor 4 (IRF4) were relatively higher and CD38 and CD71 were lower in PEL cell lines and might reflect the difference between *in vitro* and *in vivo* (Fig. 3). c-myc was certainly higher in BL as BCL6, and IL-6 expression level was not so different but IL-6 receptor genes seemed to be more expressed in PEL and therefore, sensitivity to IL-6 could be higher in PEL.

4. Conclusion

It is very difficult to talking about viral oncogenesis, since we do not have a useful system for observation of the virus infection to pathogenesis, especially for high host-specific viruses. And our DNA array data suggest just that tumor cells show typical gene expression profiles after establishment of PEL cell lines at an RNA level and it is may be very difficult to account for viral pathogenesis only by gene expression profiles. Furthermore, lytic gene expression should be taken into consideration to understand how PEL is formed and thus, it would be meaningful to find what kinds of gene were typically induced in lytic induction and for much better understanding, convenient viral infection to oncogenesis models in which we can observe continuously.

5. Acknowledgement

We thank all Lab members to prepare this manuscript. We here apologize that we just list a very limited reference and could not take many references to show the facts obtained by researchers due to a limited space.

6. References

Ansari, M. Q., Dawson, D. B., Nador, R., Rutherford, C., Schneider, N. R., Latimer, M. J., Picker, L., Knowles, D. M., and McKenna, R. W. (1996). Primary body cavity-based AIDS-related lymphomas. *Am J Clin Pathol* 105(2), 221-9.

Ascoli, V., Mastroianni, C. M., Galati, V., Sirianni, M. C., Fruscalzo, A., Pistilli, A., and Lo Coco, F. (1998). Primary effusion lymphoma containing human herpesvirus 8 DNA in two AIDS patients with Kaposi's sarcoma. *Haematologica* 83(1), 8-12.

Ballestas, M. E., Chatis, P. A., and Kaye, K. M. (1999). Efficient persistence of extrachromosomal KSHV DNA mediated by latency-associated nuclear antigen. *Science* 284(5414), 641-4.

Ballon, G., Chen, K., Perez, R., Tam, W., and Cesarman, E. (2011). Kaposi sarcoma herpesvirus (KSHV) vFLIP oncoprotein induces B cell transdifferentiation and tumorigenesis in mice. *J Clin Invest* 121(3), 1141-53.

Barbera, A. J., Chodaparambil, J. V., Kelley-Clarke, B., Joukov, V., Walter, J. C., Luger, K., and Kaye, K. M. (2006). The nucleosomal surface as a docking station for Kaposi's sarcoma herpesvirus LANA. *Science* 311(5762), 856-61.

Boss, I. W., Plaisance, K. B., and Renne, R. (2009). Role of virus-encoded microRNAs in herpesvirus biology. *Trends Microbiol* 17(12), 544-53.

Brimo, F., Michel, R. P., Khetani, K., and Auger, M. (2007). Primary effusion lymphoma: a series of 4 cases and review of the literature with emphasis on cytomorphologic and immunocytochemical differential diagnosis. *Cancer* 111(4), 224-33.

Carbone, A., and Gloghini, A. (2008). KSHV/HHV8-associated lymphomas. *Br J Haematol* 140(1), 13-24.

Chang, Y., Cesarman, E., Pessin, M. S., Lee, F., Culpepper, J., Knowles, D. M., and Moore, P. S. (1994). Identification of herpesvirus-like DNA sequences in AIDS-associated Kaposi's sarcoma. *Science* 266(5192), 1865-9.

Chen, J., Ueda, K., Sakakibara, S., Okuno, T., Parravicini, C., Corbellino, M., and Yamanishi, K. (2001). Activation of latent Kaposi's sarcoma-associated herpesvirus by demethylation of the promoter of the lytic transactivator. *Proc Natl Acad Sci U S A* 98(7), 4119-24.

Chen, L., and Lagunoff, M. (2005). Establishment and maintenance of Kaposi's sarcoma-associated herpesvirus latency in B cells. *J Virol* 79(22), 14383-91.

Cullen, B. R. (2009). Viral and cellular messenger RNA targets of viral microRNAs. *Nature* 457(7228), 421-5.

de Oliveira, D. E., Ballon, G., and Cesarman, E. (2010). NF-kappaB signaling modulation by EBV and KSHV. *Trends Microbiol* 18(6), 248-57.

Du, M. Q., Diss, T. C., Liu, H., Ye, H., Hamoudi, R. A., Cabecadas, J., Dong, H. Y., Harris, N. L., Chan, J. K., Rees, J. W., Dogan, A., and Isaacson, P. G. (2002). KSHV- and EBV-associated germinotropic lymphoproliferative disorder. *Blood* 100(9), 3415-8.

Friborg, J., Jr., Kong, W., Hottiger, M. O., and Nabel, G. J. (1999). p53 inhibition by the LANA protein of KSHV protects against cell death. *Nature* 402(6764), 889-94.

Garber, A. C., Hu, J., and Renne, R. (2002). Latency-associated nuclear antigen (LANA) cooperatively binds to two sites within the terminal repeat, and both sites contribute to the ability of LANA to suppress transcription and to facilitate DNA replication. *J Biol Chem* 277(30), 27401-11.

Garrigues, H. J., Rubinchikova, Y. E., Dipersio, C. M., and Rose, T. M. (2008). Integrin alphaVbeta3 Binds to the RGD motif of glycoprotein B of Kaposi's sarcoma-associated herpesvirus and functions as an RGD-dependent entry receptor. *J Virol* 82(3), 1570-80.

Godden-Kent, D., Talbot, S. J., Boshoff, C., Chang, Y., Moore, P., Weiss, R. A., and Mittnacht, S. (1997). The cyclin encoded by Kaposi's sarcoma-associated herpesvirus stimulates cdk6 to phosphorylate the retinoblastoma protein and histone H1. *J Virol* 71(6), 4193-8.

Grandadam, M., Dupin, N., Calvez, V., Gorin, I., Blum, L., Kernbaum, S., Sicard, D., Buisson, Y., Agut, H., Escande, J. P., and Huraux, J. M. (1997). Exacerbations of clinical symptoms in human immunodeficiency virus type 1-infected patients with multicentric Castleman's disease are associated with a high increase in Kaposi's sarcoma herpesvirus DNA load in peripheral blood mononuclear cells. *J Infect Dis* 175(5), 1198-201.

Guasparri, I., Keller, S. A., and Cesarman, E. (2004). KSHV vFLIP is essential for the survival of infected lymphoma cells. *J Exp Med* 199(7), 993-1003.

Han, S. J., Hu, J., Pierce, B., Weng, Z., and Renne, R. (2010). Mutational analysis of the latency-associated nuclear antigen DNA-binding domain of Kaposi's sarcoma-associated herpesvirus reveals structural conservation among gammaherpesvirus origin-binding proteins. *J Gen Virol* 91(Pt 9), 2203-15.

Hansen, A., Henderson, S., Lagos, D., Nikitenko, L., Coulter, E., Roberts, S., Gratrix, F., Plaisance, K., Renne, R., Bower, M., Kellam, P., and Boshoff, C. (2010). KSHV-encoded miRNAs target MAF to induce endothelial cell reprogramming. *Genes Dev* 24(2), 195-205.

Hengge, U. R., Ruzicka, T., Tyring, S. K., Stuschke, M., Roggendorf, M., Schwartz, R. A., and Seeber, S. (2002a). Update on Kaposi's sarcoma and other HHV8 associated diseases. Part 1: epidemiology, environmental predispositions, clinical manifestations, and therapy. *Lancet Infect Dis* 2(5), 281-92.

Hengge, U. R., Ruzicka, T., Tyring, S. K., Stuschke, M., Roggendorf, M., Schwartz, R. A., and Seeber, S. (2002b). Update on Kaposi's sarcoma and other HHV8 associated diseases. Part 2: pathogenesis, Castleman's disease, and pleural effusion lymphoma. *Lancet Infect Dis* 2(6), 344-52.

Hu, J., and Renne, R. (2005). Characterization of the minimal replicator of Kaposi's sarcoma-associated herpesvirus latent origin. *J Virol* 79(4), 2637-42.

Jarviluoma, A., Koopal, S., Rasanen, S., Makela, T. P., and Ojala, P. M. (2004). KSHV viral cyclin binds to p27KIP1 in primary effusion lymphomas. *Blood* 104(10), 3349-54.

Keller, S. A., Schattner, E. J., and Cesarman, E. (2000). Inhibition of NF-kappaB induces apoptosis of KSHV-infected primary effusion lymphoma cells. *Blood* 96(7), 2537-42.

Klein, U., Gloghini, A., Gaidano, G., Chadburn, A., Cesarman, E., Dalla-Favera, R., and Carbone, A. (2003). Gene expression profile analysis of AIDS-related primary effusion lymphoma (PEL) suggests a plasmablastic derivation and identifies PEL-specific transcripts. *Blood* 101(10), 4115-21.

Koopal, S., Furuhjelm, J. H., Jarviluoma, A., Jaamaa, S., Pyakurel, P., Pussinen, C., Wirzenius, M., Biberfeld, P., Alitalo, K., Laiho, M., and Ojala, P. M. (2007). Viral oncogene-induced DNA damage response is activated in Kaposi sarcoma tumorigenesis. *PLoS Pathog* 3(9), 1348-60.

Lagunoff, M., Bechtel, J., Venetsanakos, E., Roy, A. M., Abbey, N., Herndier, B., McMahon, M., and Ganem, D. (2002). De novo infection and serial transmission of Kaposi's sarcoma-associated herpesvirus in cultured endothelial cells. *J Virol* 76(5), 2440-8.

Laman, H., Coverley, D., Krude, T., Laskey, R., and Jones, N. (2001). Viral cyclin-cyclin-dependent kinase 6 complexes initiate nuclear DNA replication. *Mol Cell Biol* 21(2), 624-35.

Lee, J. S., Li, Q., Lee, J. Y., Lee, S. H., Jeong, J. H., Lee, H. R., Chang, H., Zhou, F. C., Gao, S. J., Liang, C., and Jung, J. U. (2009). FLIP-mediated autophagy regulation in cell death control. *Nat Cell Biol* 11(11), 1355-62.

Li, H., Komatsu, T., Dezube, B. J., and Kaye, K. M. (2002). The Kaposi's sarcoma-associated herpesvirus K12 transcript from a primary effusion lymphoma contains complex repeat elements, is spliced, and initiates from a novel promoter. *J Virol* 76(23), 11880-8.

Li, M., Lee, H., Yoon, D. W., Albrecht, J. C., Fleckenstein, B., Neipel, F., and Jung, J. U. (1997). Kaposi's sarcoma-associated herpesvirus encodes a functional cyclin. *J Virol* 71(3), 1984-91.

Lin, X., Liang, D., He, Z., Deng, Q., Robertson, E. S., and Lan, K. (2011). miR-K12-7-5p encoded by Kaposi's sarcoma-associated herpesvirus stabilizes the latent state by targeting viral ORF50/RTA. *PLoS One* 6(1), e16224.

Liu, J., Martin, H., Shamay, M., Woodard, C., Tang, Q. Q., and Hayward, S. D. (2007). Kaposi's sarcoma-associated herpesvirus LANA protein downregulates nuclear glycogen synthase kinase 3 activity and consequently blocks differentiation. *J Virol* 81(9), 4722-31.

Lu, F., Stedman, W., Yousef, M., Renne, R., and Lieberman, P. M. (2010). Epigenetic regulation of Kaposi's sarcoma-associated herpesvirus latency by virus-encoded microRNAs that target Rta and the cellular Rbl2-DNMT pathway. *J Virol* 84(6), 2697-706.

Lukac, D. M., Renne, R., Kirshner, J. R., and Ganem, D. (1998). Reactivation of Kaposi's sarcoma-associated herpesvirus infection from latency by expression of the ORF 50 transactivator, a homolog of the EBV R protein. *Virology* 252(2), 304-12.

Mann, D. J., Child, E. S., Swanton, C., Laman, H., and Jones, N. (1999). Modulation of p27(Kip1) levels by the cyclin encoded by Kaposi's sarcoma-associated herpesvirus. *Embo J* 18(3), 654-63.

Marcos-Villar, L., Lopitz-Otsoa, F., Gallego, P., Munoz-Fontela, C., Gonzalez-Santamaria, J., Campagna, M., Shou-Jiang, G., Rodriguez, M. S., and Rivas, C. (2009). Kaposi's sarcoma-associated herpesvirus protein LANA2 disrupts PML oncogenic domains and inhibits PML-mediated transcriptional repression of the survivin gene. *J Virol* 83(17), 8849-58.

McCormick, C., and Ganem, D. (2005). The kaposin B protein of KSHV activates the p38/MK2 pathway and stabilizes cytokine mRNAs. *Science* 307(5710), 739-41.

Moore, P. S., Gao, S. J., Dominguez, G., Cesarman, E., Lungu, O., Knowles, D. M., Garber, R., Pellett, P. E., McGeoch, D. J., and Chang, Y. (1996). Primary characterization of a herpesvirus agent associated with Kaposi's sarcomae. *J Virol* 70(1), 549-58.

Mutlu, A. D., Cavallin, L. E., Vincent, L., Chiozzini, C., Eroles, P., Duran, E. M., Asgari, Z., Hooper, A. T., La Perle, K. M., Hilsher, C., Gao, S. J., Dittmer, D. P., Rafii, S., and Mesri, E. A. (2007). In vivo-restricted and reversible malignancy induced by human herpesvirus-8 KSHV: a cell and animal model of virally induced Kaposi's sarcoma. *Cancer Cell* 11(3), 245-58.

Naranatt, P. P., Krishnan, H. H., Svojanovsky, S. R., Bloomer, C., Mathur, S., and Chandran, B. (2004). Host gene induction and transcriptional reprogramming in Kaposi's sarcoma-associated herpesvirus (KSHV/HHV-8)-infected endothelial, fibroblast, and B cells: insights into modulation events early during infection. *Cancer Res* 64(1), 72-84.

Oksenhendler, E., Duarte, M., Soulier, J., Cacoub, P., Welker, Y., Cadranel, J., Cazals-Hatem, D., Autran, B., Clauvel, J. P., and Raphael, M. (1996). Multicentric Castleman's disease in HIV infection: a clinical and pathological study of 20 patients. *AIDS* 10(1), 61-7.

Parravicini, C., Chandran, B., Corbellino, M., Berti, E., Paulli, M., Moore, P. S., and Chang, Y. (2000). Differential viral protein expression in Kaposi's sarcoma-associated herpesvirus-infected diseases: Kaposi's sarcoma, primary effusion lymphoma, and multicentric Castleman's disease. *Am J Pathol* 156(3), 743-9.

Paulose-Murphy, M., Ha, N. K., Xiang, C., Chen, Y., Gillim, L., Yarchoan, R., Meltzer, P., Bittner, M., Trent, J., and Zeichner, S. (2001). Transcription program of human herpesvirus 8 (kaposi's sarcoma-associated herpesvirus). *J Virol* 75(10), 4843-53.

Rivas, C., Thlick, A. E., Parravicini, C., Moore, P. S., and Chang, Y. (2001). Kaposi's sarcoma-associated herpesvirus LANA2 is a B-cell-specific latent viral protein that inhibits p53. *J Virol* 75(1), 429-38.

Russo, J. J., Bohenzky, R. A., Chien, M. C., Chen, J., Yan, M., Maddalena, D., Parry, J. P., Peruzzi, D., Edelman, I. S., Chang, Y., and Moore, P. S. (1996). Nucleotide sequence of the Kaposi sarcoma-associated herpesvirus (HHV8). *Proc Natl Acad Sci U S A* 93(25), 14862-7.

Sadler, R., Wu, L., Forghani, B., Renne, R., Zhong, W., Herndier, B., and Ganem, D. (1999). A complex translational program generates multiple novel proteins from the latently expressed kaposin (K12) locus of Kaposi's sarcoma-associated herpesvirus. *J Virol* 73(7), 5722-30.

Sakakibara, S., Ueda, K., Chen, J., Okuno, T., and Yamanishi, K. (2001). Octamer-binding sequence is a key element for the autoregulation of Kaposi's sarcoma-associated herpesvirus ORF50/Lyta gene expression. *J Virol* 75(15), 6894-900.

Sakakibara, S., Ueda, K., Nishimura, K., Do, E., Ohsaki, E., Okuno, T., and Yamanishi, K. (2004). Accumulation of heterochromatin components on the terminal repeat sequence of Kaposi's sarcoma-associated herpesvirus mediated by the latency-associated nuclear antigen. *J Virol* 78(14), 7299-310.

Schmidt, K., Wies, E., and Neipel, F. (2011). Kaposi's Sarcoma-Associated Herpesvirus Viral Interferon Regulatory Factor 3 Inhibits IFN{gamma} and MHC II Expression. *J Virol.*

Stedman, W., Deng, Z., Lu, F., and Lieberman, P. M. (2004). ORC, MCM, and histone hyperacetylation at the Kaposi's sarcoma-associated herpesvirus latent replication origin. *J Virol* 78(22), 12566-75.

Sun, R., Lin, S. F., Gradoville, L., Yuan, Y., Zhu, F., and Miller, G. (1998). A viral gene that activates lytic cycle expression of Kaposi's sarcoma-associated herpesvirus. *Proc Natl Acad Sci U S A* 95(18), 10866-71.

Suzuki, T., Isobe, T., Kitagawa, M., and Ueda, K. (2010). Kaposi's sarcoma-associated herpesvirus-encoded LANA positively affects on ubiquitylation of p53. *Biochem Biophys Res Commun* 403(2), 194-7.

Swanton, C., Mann, D. J., Fleckenstein, B., Neipel, F., Peters, G., and Jones, N. (1997). Herpes viral cyclin/Cdk6 complexes evade inhibition by CDK inhibitor proteins. *Nature* 390(6656), 184-7.

Toth, Z., Maglinte, D. T., Lee, S. H., Lee, H. R., Wong, L. Y., Brulois, K. F., Lee, S., Buckley, J. D., Laird, P. W., Marquez, V. E., and Jung, J. U. (2010). Epigenetic analysis of KSHV latent and lytic genomes. *PLoS Pathog* 6(7), e1001013.

Ueda, K., Ito, E., Karayama, M., Ohsaki, E., Nakano, K., and Watanabe, S. (2010). KSHV-infected PEL cell lines exhibit a distinct gene expression profile. *Biochem Biophys Res Commun* 394(3), 482-7.

Ueda, K., Sakakibara, S., Ohsaki, E., and Yada, K. (2006). Lack of a mechanism for faithful partition and maintenance of the KSHV genome. *Virus Res* 122(1-2), 85-94.

Uetz, P., Dong, Y. A., Zeretzke, C., Atzler, C., Baiker, A., Berger, B., Rajagopala, S. V., Roupelieva, M., Rose, D., Fossum, E., and Haas, J. (2006). Herpesviral protein networks and their interaction with the human proteome. *Science* 311(5758), 239-42.

Verma, S. C., Choudhuri, T., Kaul, R., and Robertson, E. S. (2006). Latency-associated nuclear antigen (LANA) of Kaposi's sarcoma-associated herpesvirus interacts with origin recognition complexes at the LANA binding sequence within the terminal repeats. *J Virol* 80(5), 2243-56.

Wies, E., Mori, Y., Hahn, A., Kremmer, E., Sturzl, M., Fleckenstein, B., and Neipel, F. (2008). The viral interferon-regulatory factor-3 is required for the survival of KSHV-infected primary effusion lymphoma cells. *Blood* 111(1), 320-7.

Xiao, B., Verma, S. C., Cai, Q., Kaul, R., Lu, J., Saha, A., and Robertson, E. S. (2010). Bub1 and CENP-F can contribute to Kaposi's sarcoma-associated herpesvirus genome persistence by targeting LANA to kinetochores. *J Virol* 84(19), 9718-32.

Ye, F. C., Zhou, F. C., Xie, J. P., Kang, T., Greene, W., Kuhne, K., Lei, X. F., Li, Q. H., and Gao, S. J. (2008). Kaposi's sarcoma-associated herpesvirus latent gene vFLIP inhibits viral lytic replication through NF-kappaB-mediated suppression of the AP-1 pathway: a novel mechanism of virus control of latency. *J Virol* 82(9), 4235-49.

Yoo, J., Kang, J., Lee, H. N., Aguilar, B., Kafka, D., Lee, S., Choi, I., Lee, J., Ramu, S., Haas, J., Koh, C. J., and Hong, Y. K. (2010). Kaposin-B enhances the PROX1 mRNA stability during lymphatic reprogramming of vascular endothelial cells by Kaposi's sarcoma herpes virus. *PLoS Pathog* 6(8).

Part 2

Infection in Humans

6

Human Herpesviruses in Hematologic Diseases

Márta Csire[1] and Gábor Mikala[2]
[1]*Division of Virology, National Center for Epidemiology, Budapest,*
[2]*Department of Hematology and Stem Cell Transplantation,*
Szt. István and Szt. László Hospital of Budapest,
Hungary

1. Introduction

The members of the *Herpesvirales* containing more than 130 different herpesviruses have already been isolated from all animal species representing the higher steps of evolution. According to our knowledge, eight herpesviruses are classified as human herpesviruses: Herpes simplex virus 1 (Human herpesvirus 1, HHV-1), Herpes simplex virus 2 (Human herpesvirus 2, HHV-2), Varicella-zoster virus (Human herpesvirus 3, HHV-3), Epstein-Barr virus (Human herpesvirus 4, HHV-4), Cytomegalovirus (Human herpesvirus 5, HHV-5), Human herpesvirus 6 (HHV-6A and HHV-6B), Human herpesvirus 7 (HHV-7), and Human herpesvirus 8 (HHV-8 or Kaposi's sarcoma associated herpesvirus, KSHV).

It is a characteritic of herpesviral infections that after the frequently fulminant initial infection, they persist in the neurons or the B- and T-cells of the body throughout life. Sometimes they reactivate. With respect to lymphotropic human herpesviruses, HHV-4 and HHV-8 reproduce mainly in the B-cells, while HHV-5, HHV-6 and HHV-7 reproduce in T-cells. HHV-4 causes most of the infectious mononucleosis cases and can immortalize B-lymphocytes. HHV-5 can also cause infectious mononucleosis. A significant part of primary infections occurs in an asymptomatic way. Immunsuppression makes virus reproduction easier.

A wide range of diseases may appear in an immunodeficient state. HHV-6 was first described in 1986 and was isolated from patients suffering from lymphoproliferative disease. It infects CD4+ T-lymphocytes and it reproduces in them. Two variants of it, HHV-6A and HHV-6B, are known. Variant B is the pathogen of exanthema subitum (roseola infantum) and it can also cause latent infection with fever, diarrhoea, neural symptoms, and hepatitis. After transplantation, HHV-6 can reactivate and it is able to replicate in liver-cells. HHV-6 can activate the replication of HHV-4; it reduces or increases the replication of HIV, and accelerates the expression of antigens coded by HPV. HHV-7 was isolated from CD4+ cells in 1990 and was purified from a healthy patient. It is the pathogen of pityriasis rosea, but it can also cause exanthema subitum. Additionally, it can create latent infection in T-lymphocytes and productive infection in salivary gland epithelial cells. During pregnancy, viremia is more frequent and may adopt urogenital, perigenital and congenital transmission.

HHV-7 may play a role in cases of immunodeficient patients; in the case of immunosuppression HHV-6 and HHV-7 play the role of cofactor in states accompanied by pneumonia. HHV-8 is the latest identified human tumorvirus; since its discovery in 1994 it has been in the limelight of research. It plays a critical role in the AIDS-associated body cavity B-cell lymphoma (BCBL). The new virus was named Kaposi's sarcoma associated herpesvirus (KSHV). Four clinical forms of Kaposi's sarcoma are known: 1. classical type (described by Kaposi), 2. epidemic-African type, 3. iatrogen, and 4. AIDS associated type. It is possible that KSHV plays a direct or indirect stimulating role: in BCBL in elderly patients or ones suffering from AIDS, and in Castleman disease.

Viral infections are important causes of morbidity and mortality for patients with haematological diseases and haematological malignancies. However, the true incidence and consequences of human herpesviral infections for these patients who undergo conventional nontransplantant therapy are poorly defined. The difference in incidence and outcome of viral infections among patient groups is wide, but dependent upon the infections among the intensity and duration of T-cell-mediated immune suppression. Infections are caused mainly by cytomegalovirus (CMV), herpes simplex virus (HSV), varicella-zoster virus (VZV) and less Epstein-Barr virus (EBV), human herpesvirus 6, 7, 8 (HHV-6, HHV-7, HHV-8).

Fortunately, a growing number of antiviral medications and vaccines are allowing for more effective prophylaxis against these pathogens.

Modern virology diagnostics use multiple methods for detecting viral infections. These include viral isolation in culture, cytologic staining, detection of viral antigens, nucleic acids, and viral antibodies.

Science has been examining the role of herpesviruses in haematologic malignant cases and in plasma-cell dyscrasias for decades now. Plasma-cell diseases (monoclonal gammopathies) are multiple myeloma (MM), Waldenstörm macroglobulinaemia (WM), and monoclonal gammopathy with unknown significance (MGUS). A potential role of HHV-8 has emerged in the pathogenesis of these diseases.

The increase in the number of histiocytes is characteristic of eosinophil granuloma (Langerhans cell histiocytosis, LCH). The causal role of lymphotropic herpesviruses has also been suggested in the pathogenesis of LCH. The rate of HHV-8 reactivation in patients suffering from monoclonal gammopathies significantly exceeds that of those suffering from Non-Hodgkins lymphoma. HHV-8 reactivation may refer to immunological lesion in patients suffering from monoclonal gammopathies. During its pathogenesis, HHV-8 might play a role in the formation of pathographies. HHV-4 is proportionately present in haematological pathographies. The data also indicate that in addition to HHV-8, the transient reactivation of HHV-4 might also play a role in the pathogenesis of monoclonal gammopathies.

2. Epidemiology, diagnosis and prevention of human herpesviruses infections in hematologic diseases

2.1 Human herpesvirus 1 (HHV-1) and human herpesvirus 2 (HHV-2) [Herpes simplex virus 1 (HSV-1) and herpes simplex virus 2 (HSV-2)]

Herpes simplex viruses were the first of the human herpesviruses to be discovered and are among the most intensively investigated of all viruses. Herpes simplex virus (HSV) was first isolated by Lowenstein (Lowenstein, 1919). The ability of HSV to establish a life-long latent infection in its human host is one of the most intellectually challenging aspects of HSV biology.

Herpes simplex virus (HSV) belongs to the *Simplexvirus* genus of the *Alphaherpesvirinae* subfamily of the *Herpesviridae* family. It has two serotypes, HSV-1 and HSV-2. It was classified into two serologically distinct types by Schneweiss (Schneweiss, 1962). HSV-1 and HSV-2 are phylogenetically ancient viruses that have evolved together with their human host (Davison, 2002). In humans, latent virus is reactivated after local stimuli such as injury to tissues innervated by neurons harboring latent virus, or by systemic stimuli (e.g., physical or emotional stress, hyperthermia, exposure to UV light, menstruation, or hormonal imbalance), which may reactivate virus simultaneously in neurons of diverse ganglia (e.g., trigeminal and sacral).

Transmission of HSV depends on intimate, personal contact between a susceptible individual (namely, one who is seronegative) and someone excreting HSV. Thus, virus must come in contact with mucosal surfaces or abraded skin for infection to be initiated. Following oropharyngeal infection, usually caused by HSV-1, the trigeminal ganglion becomes colonized and harbors latent virus. Acquisition of HSV-2 infection is usually the consequence of transmission by genital contact. The epidemiology and clinical characteristics of primary infection are distinctly different from those associated with recurrent infection. HSV-1 causes acute gingivostomatitis, recurrent herpes labialis (cold sores), keratoconjunctivitis, blepharitis, iridocyclitis, encephalitis, tracheobroncitis, pneumonia, esophagitis, pharingitis, disseminalt infections, mucocutaneus lesions, herpetic whitlow, herpes gladiatorum, genital disease, neonatal infectio, and meningitis. HSV-2 causes genital disease, anal and perianal infection, proctitis, neonatal herpes, meningitis, mucocutaneus lesions, herpetic whitlow, oral disease, keratoconjunctivitis, esophagitis, pharingitis, and encephalitis.

A reappearance of HSV, known as recurrent infection, results in a limited number of vesicular lesions as occurs with HSV labialis or recurrent HSV genitalis. Reinfection with a different strain of HSV occurs, but it is uncommon in the normal host. Herpes simplex virus disease ranges from the usual case of mild illness, nondiscernible in most individuals, to sporadic, severe, and life-threatening disease in a few infants, children, and adults. Although HSV-1 and HSV-2 are usually transmitted via different routes and involve different areas of the body, much overlap is seen between the epidemiology and clinical manifestations of these two viruses. Historically, primary HSV-1 infections usually occurred in the young child, less than 5 years of age, and were most often asymptomatic. When the oropharynx is involved, the mouth and lips are the most common sites of HSV-1 infections, causing gingivostomatitis; however, any organ can become infected with this virus. Primary infection in young adults has been associated with only pharyngitis and a mononucleosis-like syndrome (McMillan et al., 1993). Genital herpes can be caused by either HSV-1 or 2. As infections with HSV-2 are usually acquired through sexual contact, antibodies to this virus are rarely found before ages of onset of sexual activity. Recurrent HSV-2 infection, as with HSV-1, can be either symptomatic or asymptomatic.

HSV-1 accounts for the majority of nongenital HSV-induced infections in humans, with 45% to 98% of the world population and 40% to 63% of the people in the United States reported HSV-1 seropositive (Ribes et al., 2001). Worldwide HSV-1 prevalence varies with age, race, geographic location, and socioeconomic status; a higher rate of seropositivity has been reported for less industrialized countries (Fatahzadeh & Schwartz, 2007; Chayavichitsilp et al., 2009). By the age of sixty, 60% to 85% of adults in the United States demonstrate HSV-1 seroconversion. Incidence is not seasonal. Over the past thirty years, HSV-2 seroprevalence

has increased dramatically, with 20% to 25% of US adults tested positive for HSV-2 antibodies by the age of forty (Fleming et al., 1997).
Risk factors for HSV-2 infection include older age, female gender, black race, poor socioeconomic status, low level of education, prior sexually transmitted disease, early age at first intercourse, and a higher number of lifetime sexual partners (Corey & Handsfield, 2000). Prepubertal detection of HSV-2 antibodies is rare. Prevalence of HSV2 seropositivity is strongly correlated with sexual maturity and promiscuity. Prevalence of HSV-2 antibodies is reported to be higher in women (Hettmann et al., 2008).
Patients compromised by immunosuppressive therapy, underlying disease, or malnutrition are at increased risk of severe HSV infections. Renal, hepatic, bone marrow, and cardiac recipients are all at a particular risk of increased severity of transplant HSV infection.

2.1.1 Epidemiology

HSV-1 and HSV-2 commonly cause mucocutaneus lesions in patients with haematological malignancies, but HSV-1 is more frequent (Gnann, 2003). Up to 80% of adult patients with leukemia are HSV seropositive. The rate of HSV reactivation among HSV seropositive allo-Stem Cell Transplant recipients was reported to be approximately 80%, with the majority of these infections occurring during the first four weeks after transplant. They are also common, ranging from 15% among CLL (chronic lymphocytic leukemia) patients treated with fludarabine to 90% of patients with acute leukemia (Sandherr et al., 2006; Anaisse et al., 1998). Most individuals undergoing conventional chemotherapy are at low risk of HSV reactivation; however, those receiving T-cell depleting agents (e.g. fludarabine, alemtuzumab) or proteasome inhibitors are at high risk of reactivation of both HSV-1 and HSV-2 (Sandherr et al., 2006).
The greatest risk of reactivation is seen in individuals with CD4 T-cell counts <50 cells/mm^3, and other contribuiting risk factors are corticosteroid use, prolonged neutropenia, renal insufficiency, and age above 65 years.

2.1.2 Clinical manifestations

HSV reactivation in leukemic patients is usually associated with localizated mucocutaneous disease in the orofacial region (85-90%), and less frequently in the genital area (10-15%). The diagnosis of oropharyngeal HSV disease clinically can be difficult when severe mucositis is present. Mucositis and mucocutaneous ulcerations are common following high doses of chemotherapy, and occur at the same time as oral disease. Another frequent manifestation of HSV reactivations is esophageal disease. HSV esophagitis was found in about 10% of patients in studies of patients with leukaemia and other neoplastic disorders who had gastrointestinal symptoms. Uncommon HSV disease manifestations are pneumonia (2-3%), hepatitis, meningitis, and encephalitis (Kaufman et al., 1997; Angarone, 2011).
Recurrent HSV infection is a major cause of morbidity and occasional mortality in the immunosuppressed patient who experiences frequent, persistent and severe recurrences of HSV-1 and HSV-2 infection.

2.1.3 Monitoring and laboratory diagnosis of HSV infections

An important characteristic of modern diagnostic virology is the use of multiple methods for detecting viral infections. These include viral isolation in culture, cytologic staining for viral infection with the Tzanck smear (Tzanck & Aron-Brunietiere, 1949), detection of viral antigens, nucleic acids, and viral antibodies, which are all used to diagnose current viral infection. Light microscopy is used to detect the effect of viral infection in tissue and to define the role of viral infection in producing disease. Clinicians may wish to utilize laboratory tests to establish definitive diagnosis when clinical presentation of HSV infections is atipical. Virus isolation remains the definitive diagnostic method; however, polymerase chain reaction (PCR) detection of viral DNA is gaining increased acceptance even for routine skin infections. If skin lesions are present, skin vesicles should be scraped and transferred in appropriate virus transport media to a diagnostic virology laboratory. Virus may be isolated from various samples including skin lesions, cerebrospinal fluid (CSF), ocular fluid, swabs from mucocutaneous lesions, blood, stool, urine, throat, nasopharynx, conjunctivae and cornea. The experience with PCR indicates that it is an especially useful tool for diagnosis of HSV encephalitis in cerebrospinal fluid (CSF).

The Tzanck smear is a rapid and reasonably priced diagnostic test that can confirm the presence of HSV infection. Although the test can confirm the presence of HSV or VZV, it cannot differentiate between the two herpes simplex serotypes and, therefore, cannot diagnose HSV-1 or HSV-2 infection definitively. The Tzanck smear has decreased in popularity as a diagnostic alternative to the direct fluorescent antibody assay (DFA) technique. In addition, DFA may be employed to serotype the HSV infection. Because DFA testing is rapid, inexpensive, and virally selective, it is often used to substantiate clinical suspicion and determine serotype. The biopsied cells are observed microscopically to detect degenerative cytopathologic changes commonly associated with the infection. The degenerative changes present in cells infected with HSV-1 and HSV-2 also are observed in cells infected with VZV. Thus, the specificity of the technique is low, and it cannot be used to serotype the infection.

As HSV PCR becomes more readily available and less expensive, it has the potential to become the most widely used means of detecting HSV for all types of infection because it is rapid, highly reliable, and valid. Serologic assay is employed to detect the presence of HSV antibodies when other techniques are impractical or ineffective. Such assay takes longer to complete than other techniques and should be considered primarily for diagnosing recurrent infections, in the presence of healing lesions and the absence of active lesions, or when partners of a person who has clinical herpes are at risk. Sera are collected at two sepatate times. Acute serum is obtained within three to four days after the onset of initial symptoms, and convalescent serum is gathered several weeks after the symptoms have abted. To confirm a diagnosis of primary HSV infection, the acute sample should be devoid of HSV-positive antibodies due to the delayed humoral response, and the convalescent sample should demonstrate the presence of both immunoglobulin G and M antibodies to HSV proteins. If any quantities of antibodies are observed in the acute sample, primary infection is ruled out and the diagnosis is recurrent herpes infection. Measurement of antiviral antibodies was one of the first methods used for the specific diagnosis of viral infections and it remains an important tool in the diagnostic virology laboratory.

The role of serology can be for the diagnosis of acute or current infection or for the determination of immune status to specific viruses. Serologic diagnosis of HSV infection is clinically valuable in the counseling of patients. Therapeutic decisions do not depend on the results of serologic studies. Immunoglobulin M (IgM) and IgG humoral responses have been well characterized. Antibodies [as detected by immunofluorescence assay (IFA), Enzyme immunoassay (EIA), enzyme-linked immunosorbent assays (ELISA)] are specific for HSV.

Serological tests are used for identification of seropositive patients before chemotherapy or hematopoietic stem cell transplantation (HSCT), but are not helpful in confirming the diagnosis of HSV reactivation. Routine surveillance for HSV reactivation could be done by culture or PCR, single (sPCR), nested PCR (n-PCR) and real-time or quantitative PCR (RT-PCR or Q-PCR). PCR for HSV DNA in CFS is indicated in the diagnosis of HSV meningitis and encephalitis.

2.1.4 Prevention of HSV diseases

Vaccination remains the ideal method for prevention of viral infection; however, prevention of HSV infections introduces unique problems because of recurrences in the presence of humoral immunity. Nevertheless, protection from life-threatening infection can be achieved in animal models with avirulent, inactivated, or subunit glycoprotein vaccines, each of which has unique differences. Future study of the immune response induced by natural HSV infections in both adults and neonates is needed to provide insight into the requirements for vaccination against acute disease and recurrences. Attempts to produce an effective vaccine against HSV have been largely unsuccessful. Perhaps a most effective vaccine will be needed to stimulate most, if not all, key parameters of innate and adaptive immunity, both systematic and mucosal (Jones & Cunningham, 2004; Stanberry, 2004).

HSV seronegative patients should attempt to prevent exposure to HSV. Early studies of intravenosus acyclovir in hematopetic stem cell transplantation recipients clearly documented its clinical efficacy: 0% to 2.5% of patients treated with acyclovir versus 50% to 70% of those treated with placebo developed HSV lesions (Lundgren et al., 1985; Angarone & Ison, 2008).

HSV seropositive patients: Based on the data, most cancer centers routinely use antiviral prophylaxis against HSV reactivation for leukemia patients' chemotherapy, especially those at high risk of ractivation such as those treated with purine analogs or alemtuzumab (Styczynski et al., 2009). Antiviral agents are routinely used as prophylaxis against HSV reactivation, using either i.v. acyclovir, oral acyclovir or valacyclovir, until three–five weeks after chemotherapy has been stopped (Angarone, 2011).

2.1.5 Therapy of HSV diseases

Advances in the treatment of HSV infections have led the way in the development of antiviral therapeutics. In the 1970s, vidarabine (adenine arabinoside) became the first licensed antiviral therapeutic for the treatment for herpes simplex encephalitis and neonatal HSV infections. Quickly, however, vidarabine was replaced by acyclovir in the the treatment of all HSV infections. Today acyclovir, valacyclovir, penciclovir, famciclovir, ganciclovir, valganciclovir, cidofovir and foscarnet are the most useful and widely used therapeutics for the treatment of HSV-1 and HSV-2 infections (Knipe & Howley, 2007; Gilbert et al., 2010; Jancel & Penzak, 2009; Angarone, 2011).

2.2 Human herpesvirus 3 (HHV-3) [Varicella-zoster virus (VZV)]

Varicella-zoster virus (VZV) is a human alphaherpesvirus, which belongs to the *Varicellovirus* genus of the *Alphaherpesvirinae* subfamily of the *Herpesviridae* family. It causes varicella, commonly called chickenpox, during primary infection. Varicella, which is characterized by fever and a generalized, pruritic vesicular rash, is most prevalent in childhood. Varicella is highly contagious, producing annual epidemics among susceptible individuals during winter and spring in temperate climates. Among the alphaherpesviruses, VZV is unique in its tropism for T lymphocytes, which allows dissemination of the virus to skin. VZV also infects and establishes latency in cells of the dorsal root ganglia. Its reactivation from latency produces herpes zoster, commonly referred to as shingles, an illness observed most often in older adults and immunocompromised patients of any age. The vesicular rash of herpes zoster is largely confined to regions of the skin served by a single sensory dermatome. Unlike varicella, herpes zoster infections are associated with acute pain that can be severe and prolonged. Pain that persists after the onset of herpes zoster for more than 30 days is called postherpetic neuralgia (PHN).

Varicella and herpes zoster were described in very early medical literature. Once thought to be the same disorder, Heberden distinguished smallpox and varicella as two diseases in 1867. In 1892, Bokay suggested an infectious etiology for varicella and herpes zoster and postulated that they were related (von Bokay, 1909), an idea supported by the demonstration that varicella occurs in children following inoculation with vesicular fluid from herpes zoster lesions and that virions from varicella and herpes zoster vesicle fluids are identical in appearance by electron microscopy (Almeida, 1962). The isolation of VZV in tissue culture was reported by Weller in 1953 (Weller, 1953). Primary VZV infection is presumed to be initiated by inhalation of respiratory droplets or by contact with infectious vesicular fluid from an infected individual. The potential for aerosol transmission is suggested by epidemiologic reports, and VZV DNA is detected in air samples from rooms occupied by patients with varicella or disseminated herpes zoster (Sawyer, 1994).

Varicella-zoster virus latency is established during primary infection. VZV persists in sensory nerve ganglia. VZV can access neural tissues, either hematogenously or by centripetal neural transport from mucocutaneous lesions.

Varicella-zoster virus reactivation, although possibly asymptomatic at times, typically presents as herpes zoster, a vesicular rash that is usually confined to the dermatomal distribution of a single sensory nerve. Because herpes zoster is caused by the reactivation of latent virus, susceptibility requires previous primary VZV infection. Given the high incidence of varicella, most adults are at risk of VZV reactivation. Herpes zoster is rare in childhood, but varicella during the first year of life, or VZV infection acquired by intrauterine transmission, are associated with an increased risk.

The attack rate for previously uninfected household or day care center contacts exposed to varicella is about 90%. Varicella pneumonia in healthy adults presents with fever, cough, tachypnea, and dyspnea and may be associated with cyanosis, pleuritic chest pain, or hemoptysis. Varicella pneumonia is often transient, resolving completely within 24 to 72 hours, but interstitial pneumonitis with severe hypoxemia progresses rapidly to cause respiratory failure in severe cases.

Varicella hepatitis can occur subclinically, although it may be associated with severe vomiting. Aspirin is contraindicated in children with varicella because it predisposes to liver damage (Reye's syndrome). Patients with encephalitis typically have a sudden onset of seizures and altered sensorium, whereas those with cerebellar disease show a gradual progression of irritability, nystagmus, and gait and speech disturbances. Some patients have fever, headache, and meningismus, only without any altered consciousness or seizures. Acute thrombocytopenia causes petechiae and purpuric skin lesions, hemorrhage into the varicella vesicles, epistaxis, hematuria, and gastrointestinal bleeding. Hemorrhagic complications are usually transient. Purpura fulminans, caused by arterial thrombosis and hemorrhagic gangrene, is a rare but life-threatening complication. Postinfectious thrombocytopenia occurs from 1 to 2 weeks or longer after varicella. Varicella nephritis causes hematuria, proteinuria, diffuse oedema, and decreased renal function, with or without hypertension. A few cases of nephrotic syndrome and hemolytic-uremic syndrome have been reported in children with varicella. Varicella arthritis is rare; it resolves spontaneously, with no residual joint disease. Other unusual complications of varicella include myocarditis, pericarditis, pancreatitis, and orchitis. Varicella vesicles are common on eyelids and conjunctivae, but eye disease is unusual.

Reactivation of VZV in the trigeminal ganglion can produce ophthalmic disease, including conjunctivitis, dendritic keratitis, anterior uveitis, iridocyclitis with secondary glaucoma, and panophthalmitis. Loss of vision associated with herpes zoster is predominantly caused by retrobulbar neuritis and optic atrophy.

2.2.1 Epidemiology

The high incidence of herpes zoster in elderly and immunocompromised patients suggests that waning host immune responses to the virus have a significant impact on whether reactivation occurs and whether it will lead to symptomatic disease. Herpes zoster in young children after intrauterine or early postnatal varicella and the short interval between primary and recurrent VZV infections in children with HIV infection probably reflect their development of suboptimal cell-mediated immunity. Diminished in vitro T-cell proliferation to VZV antigens in elderly patients and in patients receiving immunosuppressive therapy correlates with higher susceptibility to herpes zoster.

The incidence of VZV infection ranges from 2% among patients with chronic myelogenous leukemia (CML) receiving imatinib mesylate, to 10-15% in patients with chronic lymphocytic leukemia (CLL) receiving flurdarabine or alemtuzumab, to 25% of patients with Hodgkin lymphoma, myeloma treated with bortezomib or autologous stem cell transplant recipients, and to 45-60% among allogenic stem cell transplant recipients (Locksley et al., 1985; Anaisse et al., 1998; Sandherr et al., 2006; Wade, 2006). Infection risk is the greatest within the first twelve months following treatment or transplant. The majority of VZV infections in adult patients with a hematological malignancy are reactivation infections and 80% with localized disease (Locksley et al., 1985). After exposure to an individual with VZV infection (varicella or herpes zoster) seronegative leukemia patients and HSCT recipients are at risk of developing varicella, wich can be very severe. After HSCT, the risk of varicella is the highest in the first 24 months, or beyond this time if undergoing immunsuppressive therapy and having chronic graft-versus-host-disease (GVHD). Other risk factors include the pretransplantant diagnosis of leukemia and other lymphoproliferative disorders.

2.2.2 Clinical manifestations

Varicella manifests as a generalized, pruritic, vesicular rash. In leukemic patients and in those following HSCT, there is a risk of progressive severe varicella characterized by continuous eruptions of lesions, high fever, visceral dissemination, encephalitis, hepatitis, pneumonia, nausea, vomiting and diarrhea. Hemorrhagic varicella may sometimes occur.

In herpes zoster, grouped painful vesicular lesions appear in the distribution of one to three dermatomes in the immuncompetent patients. In leukemia patients and HSCT recipients, varicella zoster may disseminate to several more dermatomes or throughout the whole body, with the risk of visceral involvement, which may prove fatal. This visceral dissemination may sometimes occur without skin vesicles, which makes diagnosis difficult.

2.2.3 Laboratory diagnosis

Laboratory diagnosis is not necessary for the clinical management of most VZV infections in the immunocompetent host, but rapid diagnostic techniques are useful to guide decisions about antiviral treatment, especially for high-risk patients.

The differentiation of the VZV infections from HSV and bullous dermatitis is an important indication for virological diagnosis. VZV infections of pregnant women and of newborn infants, atypical infections of immunodeficient patients, and suspected VZV infections of the central nervous system must be confirmed by laboratory diagnosis.

VZV can be isolated in tissue culture, but it is not as easy as for HSV. Tzanck smear cannot differentiate between HSV and VZV. Nucleic acids are readily detected by PCR and detection of VZV antigens by immunohistochemical assays of cells from cutaneous lesions allows rapid diagnosis. The most sensitive methods are the fluorescent-antibody membrane antigen assay (FAMA) (Gershon et al., 1999). Latex agglutination methods provide a useful, sensitive alternative to FAMA (Steinberg & Gershon, 1991).

Assays for VZV IgG antibodies are most useful for determining the immune status of individuals whose clinical history of varicella is unknown or equivocal. The enzyme-linked immunosorbent assay (ELISA) and the immunfluorescence technique are especially suited for the detection of VZV specific immunglobulin of classes IgG, IgM and IgA. Detection of IgM and high titered IgA anti-VZV antibodies usually indicates a reactivated VZV infection regardless of whether lesions are visible or not (Gross et al., 2003).

PCR techniques (sPCR, n-PCR, RT- PCR or Q-PCR) for VZV DNA are considered the best diagnostic tools because they are very specific and sensitive and can detect viral DNA in vesicle samples, crusts, and throat swabs from patients with varicella or herpes zoster. PCR can be used for tissue specimens as well. VZV encephalitis following HSCT is diagnosed by PCR of cerebrospinal fluid. PCR of blood samples (serum, plasma) can document VZV DNA viremia in an HSCT recipient with herpes zoster, and quantitative monitoring (RT-PCR or Q-PCR) of circulating VZV DNA may be useful for the diagnosis and for assessing the response to treatment of visceral VZV infection without skin manifestation. PCR can also distinguish vaccine strain from wild-type VZV in clinical specimens (Kalpoe et al., 2006).

2.2.4 Prevention

The live attenuated Oka varicella vaccine is the first human herpesvirus vaccine licensed for clinical use in several countries. Its development and initial clinical evaluation were first reported by Takahashi in 1974 (Takahashi et al., 1974). The vaccine virus derived from a clinical isolate of VZV, the Oka strain; was isolated from a healthy Japanese child with varicella and atteunated by serial passage in cell culture; initially propagated in guinea pig embryo fibroblasts, and then in WI38 human cells. Clinical studies in Japan demonstrated the safety, immunogenicity, and clinical efficacy of Oka vaccine, which protected susceptibile immuncompetent and immuncompromissed children against varicella, even when administered shortly after exposure. Oka vaccine also boosted VZV specific cell-mediated immunity in immunocompetent and immunocompromised adults. Varicella vaccine (Varivax; Merck) was licensed by the US Food and Drug Administration (FDA) in 1995. Zoster vaccine (Zostavax; Merck) was licenced by the FDA in 2005. Recent development of genetic analysis of VZV Oka strains isolated from vaccine-associated rashes and cases of herpes zoster may help identify specific single nucleotid polymorphisms (SNPs) that differentiate Oka vaccine from wild-type strains of VZV, and which contribute to attenuation of the vaccine and the pathogenicity of wild type VZV (Oxman, 2010).

Oka vaccine is the most attenuated of all currently licensed live, attenuated virus vaccines, and it has been safely administered to VZV-susceptible children and VZV-seropositive children and adults, including susceptible children with human immunodeficiency virus 1 infection and leukemia. Oka vaccine strain of VZV is fully susceptible to acyclovir, famciclovir, and valacyclovir; thus, effective antiviral therapy is available if complications involving vaccine virus replication occur.

Inactivated zoster vaccines for administration to immuncompromised patients are potentially beneficial. Heat-inactivated VZV vaccine has been safely administrated to autologous bone marrow transplant recipients, in whom it accelerated recovery of VZV-cell mediated immunity and reduced the occurence of herpes zoster (Hata et al., 2002). Encouraged by these results, several groups are exploring the development of inactivated VZV vaccines, with and without adjuvants, to permit immunization of profundly immunsuppressed patients.

2.2.4.1 Passive antibody prophylaxis

Varicella zoster immune globulin (VZIG) and the related product are made from high-titer immune human serum. VZV antibody prophylaxis is recommended for passive immunization of individuals at high risk of serious varicella who were recently exposed to people with acute varicella or herpes zoster.

2.2.4.2 VZV seronegative patients

Fortunately, VZV can be prevented by minimizing exposure, passive immunization, and antiviral prophilaxis. VZV seronegative family members and contacts of HSCT candidates should be vaccinated against VZV no later than four weeks before conditioning begins. Contact with patients after vaccination must be avoided, especially if post-vaccination eczema occurs. In VZV seronegative patients, who have been in contact with varicella or herpes zoster and hence potentially contagious, airborne precautions should be instituted seven days after the first contact and continued until 21 days after the last exposure or 28 days post-exposure if the patient received passive immunization against VZV (VZIG-varicella-zoster immune globulin or ZIG-zoster immune globulin). Prior to the start of chemotherapy, VZV serologies should be evaluated and, if negative, exposure should be minimized. The role of direct prophylaxis and duration of that has yet to be tested in clinical trials (Wade, 2006; Styczynski et al., 2009).

2.2.4.3 VZV seropositive patients

Most HSCT recipients are VZV seropositive, following varicella in their childhood or following immunization with varicella vaccine, and are at risk of virus reactivation. There have been several retrospective studies of the use of acyclovir prophylaxis to prevent VZV reactivation in HSCT recipients. Arguments for the use of passive immunisation for VZV-seropositive leukemia and HSCT recipients include the theoretical potential for supplementing immunity against VZV. The arguments against include scarity of VZIG and ZIG, their cost, the low incidence of reinfection, lack of proven efficiency in VZV-seropositive recipients, and the possible adverse effect and discomfort associated with passive immunization (Weinstock et al., 2004).

2.2.5 Therapy

Treatment of VZV disease should include the early institution of antiviral therapy (valacyclovir, acyclovir or famciclovir). Acyclovir therapy diminishes the clinical severity of varicella in immunocompromised children by ensuring that cell-associated viremia is terminated efficiently despite the impaired host response. Early antiviral therapy prevents progressive varicella and visceral dissemination. Acyclovir and valacyclovir are highly effective. Yet, despite its efficiency in preventing disease, antiviral prophylaxis is not routinely recommended by many of the clinical care guidelines (Sandherr et al, 2006).
In addition to preventing life-threatening dissemination, early acyclovir therapy minimizes cutaneous disease, which may reduce the risk of secondary bacterial infections. Immunocompromised patients who have pneumonia, hepatitis, thrombocytopenia, or encephalitis require immediate treatment with intravenous acyclovir. Oral acyclovir can be used to diminish varicella symptoms in healthy children, adolescents, and adults when administered within 24 hours after the appearance of the initial cutaneous lesions. Adults with varicella pneumonia, including pregnant women, require immediate treatment with intravenous acyclovir. Acyclovir is effective for the treatment of recurrent VZV infection in healthy and immunocompromised patients. Among healthy individuals, the period of continued new lesions in the involved dermatome was shortened, as was the time to complete healing.
Acyclovir treatment is especially important in patients who are immunocompromised because of their risk of disseminated disease, and it is important in healthy adults with ophthalmic zoster because of their risk of developing acute uveitis and chronic keratitis. Acute neuropathic pain is reduced by early treatment with acyclovir, valacyclovir, or famciclovir, but effects on rates of subsequent PHN are less obvious. Acyclovir is given intravenously to immunocompromised patients who are at high risk of disseminated disease. Daily acyclovir (or suitable alternative) appears to be effective at preventing herpes zoster virus in patients with myeloma who are receiving bortezomib, with or without corticosteroids (Vickrey et al., 2009). Acyclovir prophylaxis effectively prevented VZV disease after allogenic transplantation. This regimen is highly effective, safe, inexpensive, and does not appear to interfere with VZV specific immune reconstruction (Boeckh et al., 2006). At present, acyclovir prophylaxis is not a universal practice in all transplant centers, because the prompt initiation of acyclovir for the treatment of recurrent VZV infections is effective (Weinstock et al., 2004) and long-term use can be associated with emergence of drug-resistant VZV mutants.

2.3 Human herpesvirus 4 (HHV-4) [Epstein-Barr virus (EBV)]

The discovery of Epstein-Barr virus (EBV) by Epstein, Achong, and Barr, reported in 1964 (Epstein et al., 1964), was stimulated by Denis Burkitt's recognition of novel African childhood lymphoma and his postulation that an infectious agent was involved in the tumor etiology. Human herpesvirus 4 (HHV-4 or EBV) was classified as belonging to the *Lymphocryptovirus* genus within the subfamily *Gammaherpesvirinae* of the *Herpesviridae* family. With respect to biology, it causes two types of infection: primary infection, mainly in children and adolescents, and reactivation of latent infection. The syndrome caused by primary infection includes infectious mononucleosis, chronic active EBV infection and X-linked lymphoproliferative syndrome. Most EBV reactivations are subclinical and require no therapies; however, it may be manifest as encephalitis, myelitis, pneumonia, and hepatitis. HHV-4 associated tumors (reactivation syndromes) include lymphoproliferative disease (LPD), Burkitt's lymphoma, non-Hodgkin's lymphoma, nasopharyngeal carcinoma, natural killer (NK)-cell leukemia, Hodgkin's disease, hemophagocytic lymphohistiocytosis, and angioblastic T-cell lymphoma (Ambinder, 2007; Delecluse et al., 2007).

2.3.1 Epidemiology

EBV infection occurs in more than 90% of the normal population, and immuncompromised patients are predominantly at risk of disease due to EBV reactivation. The incidence of PTLD (post-transplant lymphoprolifertaive disease) varies with the organ transplanted, and ranges from 1% for renal to 14% small bowel transplant recipients.

2.3.2 Clinical manifestations

A significant number (at least 25%) of serologically confirmed primary infections in adolescence or early adult life are manifested as infectious mononucleosis, as they are a small number of infections in childhood. Symptoms can range from mild transient fever to several weeks of pharyngitis, lymphodenopathy, and general malaise. The period of acute disease correlates much more closely with that of CD8 T lymphocytosis than with high virus shedding and, indeed, treating patients using infectious mononucleosis with oral acyclovir to block virus shedding brings little if any clinical benefit.

The main manifestation of EBV infection after allogenic HSCT is the development of post-transplant lymphoprolifertaive disease (PTLD) in the presence of reactivated infection, which has a very poor prognosis. The clinical manifestation of EBV-associated PLTD may include fever, lymphadenopathy, tonsillitis, hepatosplenomegaly, and symptoms and signs from other affected organs. Although the incidence is low (0.5-2.0 %), it may rise as high as 20% in the presence of three or more risk factors. The morbidity risk is highest during the six months post HSCT (Islam et al., 2010). Risk factors for developing EBV related PLTD are: *ex vivo* T-cell depletion, treatment with antithymocyte globulin for preventing or treating GVHD, anti-CD3 antibodies for GVHD therapy, and unrelated or HLA-mismatched transplant.

2.3.3 Laboratory diagnosis

Viral detection and *in situ* hybridization techniques fall into the former category whereas immunohistochemistry is useful for distinguishing latent from replicative infection and for identifying the prevailing from of EBV latency. Fluorecence *in situ* hybridisation (FISH) is the method of choice for visualisation of viral nucleotide sequences in the infected cells, interphase nuclei or on chromosomes (Wilson & May 2001). Using PCR with this sensitivity can be used to quantitate absolute numbers of infected cells in a given population. Virus can be isolated on cell line.

The serologic profile, therefore, can be a useful marker of past infection. Because patients who are B-cell deficient do not naturally acquire EBV, we have no direct information from clinical observation about the biological importance of the antibody response. Antibodies to VCA, EA, and the EBNAs target intracellular antigen complexes and, therefore, seem unlikely to play any major effector role in controlling virally infected cells *in vivo*.

EBV reactivation prospective monitoring of EBV viraemia by Q-PCR is recommended after high risk allo HSCT. Screening for EBV DNA should start at the day of HSCT, and last for three months with frequency of at least once a week in high-risk cases.

Diagnosis of LPD or PTLD must be based on symptoms and/or signs consistent with lympoproloferative processdeveloping after HSCT, together with detection of EBV by an appropriate method applied to specimen from the involved tissue. EBV detection in a biopsy specimen requires detection of viral antigen or *in situ* hibridization for the EBER (Epstein-Barr-encoded RNA).

2.3.4 Prevention

The sheer range of EBV-associated diseases emphasizes the importance of developing either prophylactic vaccines to reduce disease burden or therapeutic strategies that specifically target virus-positive lesions. A number of approaches are currently being pursued. The first clinical testing of a gp350-expressing recombinant viral vaccine, based on the Chinese Tien Tan strain of vaccinia virus, was carried out on small groups of EBV-seronegative and EBV-seropositive children (Gu et al., 1995). Phase I and II trials of a gp350 subunit vaccine in young adults have induced a neutralizing antibody response; this did not prevent primary infection within the vaccinated group, but it did significantly reduce the incidence of infectious mononucleosis symptoms compared with the placebo controls.

2.3.4.1 EBV seronegative patients

Seronegative individuals should undertake behaviour that minimizes the likelihood of EBV exposure. If a patient is found seronegative, the risk of PTLD is higher. Also, HSCT donors should be tested before transplantation for EBV serology. When there is choice, the selection of a seronegative donor might be beneficial as EBV might be transmitted with the graft. Prevention of PTLD has focused on EBV DNA monitoring and use of the donor-derived cytotoxic T-cells.

2.3.4.2 EBV seropositive patients

Reactivation of EBV is common after allo-HSCT, but rarely causes significant problems through direct viral end-organ disease. The important complication of EBV replication is PTLD. Poor or negative data are available regarding EBV prophylaxis. Ganciclovir can reduce EBV replication, but neither ganciclovir and foscarnet nor cidofovir therapy and prophylaxis have any impact on the development of PTLD.

2.3.5 Therapy

Anti-CD20 antibodies (rituximab), reduction of immunsuppression or adoptive immunotherapy are recommended as a first-line therapy for PTLD. Four to eight doses of rituximab are needed to obtain clincal improvement and reduce the EBV DNA load. Chemotherapy is a second-line option.

2.4 Human herpesvirus 5 (HHV-5) [Cytomegalovirus (CMV)]

Human herpesvirus 5 (HHV-5 or CMV) was classified as belonging to the *Cytomegalovirus* genus within the subfamily *Betaherpesvirinae* of the *Herpesviridae* family. The virus usually infects the population in early childhood, and later, at the time of sexual activity. The primary infection of immuncompetent patients is generally symptomless, or causes self-limiting diseases, such as certain cases of infectious mononucleosis. The primary CMV infections of seronegative pregnant women's transplacental transmission during pregnancy leading to fetal damage may cause severe congenital damage in the neonates, including deafness and mental retardation. Reactivation or primary CMV infection in immunocompromised patients can give rise to a wide range of complications in many organs of the host. Ho provides a comprehensive summary of work leading to the recognition of CMV as a separate medically important herpesvirus subfamily (Ho, 1991).

By the early 1950s, cytomegalic inclusion disease was diagnosed based on the presence of inclusion-bearing cells in urine, and viral etiology was predicted based on the detection of approximately 100 nm viruslike particles with low-resolution electron microscopy (EM). The unrelenting efforts of Margaret Smith, which led to isolation of this virus from urine of congenitally damaged newborns, followed her earlier success isolating the related mouse salivary gland virus (now called murine CMV) commonly used a viral strain that bears her name (Knipe & Howley, 2007). As with all herpesviruses, CMV latency is likely to be maintained in everyone who experiences primary infection. The propensity of virus to reactivate following immunosuppression or immunodeficiency is an important factor leading to CMV-associated diseases. CMV also remains medically prominent as an opportunistic infection in the immunocompromised host and this drives initiatives for therapeutic intervention.

CMV reactivation remains a significant cause of morbidity and mortality due to the extended period of immunodeficiency after allogenis HSTC. The CMV status of the recipients before HSCT has strong influence on HSCT outcome (Zhou et al., 2009).

2.4.1 Epidemiology

CMV has a worldwide distribution and infects up to 50-85% of the population in industrialized countries. CMV is predictably transmitted in settings where susceptible persons have contact with body fluids from persons excreting virus. Transmission appears to require direct contact with infectious material; spread by the airborne route or through aerosols does not occur. Following initial acquisition of CMV, infectious virus is present in urine, saliva, tears, semen, and cervical secretions for months to years. Two types of exposures have consistently been linked with horizontal transmission of CMV: sexual activity and contact with young children. Vertical transmission from mother to fetus or newborn not only occurs but is common and plays an important role in maintaining infection in the population. In this context, CMV is spread by three routes: transplacental, intrapartum, and via human milk.

Immuncompromised hosts are at elevated risk of serious CMV disease following primary infection, reinfection, or reactivation of latent virus (Sandherr et al., 2006). CMV is a leading infectious cause of morbidity and mortality in patients after HSCT and solid organ transplantation, and is an emerging problem in adults with leukaemia. CMV infection occurs in 60-70% of allogenic HSCT recipients when patient or donor are CMV seropositive, and is documented in about 50-60% of CMV seropositive autograph recipients. Other predisposing factors include the occurrence of acute GVHD, HLA-mismatched transplant, and a positive CMV serology of the graft donor in seronegative patients (Ng et al. 2005). The majority of CMV infections occur during the first three to four months after transplant largely controlled by preventive strategies using antiviral drugs; CMV infection remains a significant problem in this setting because of breakthrough disease in high risk patients, late onset disease, and indirect effects that adversely affect outcome.

2.4.2 Clinical manifestations

CMV infection is manifested clinically in the normal host. The illness is similar to mononucleosis that occurs with EBV infection. Estimates indicate that CMV is responsible for 20% to 50% of heterophile-negative mononucleosis and that it accounts for approximately 8% of all cases of mononucleosis. It is characterized by fever for more than 10 days, malaise, myalgias, headache, and fatigue. Splenomegaly, hepatomegaly, adenopathy, and rash are present in some patients. Compared to EBV-induced mononucleosis, pharyngitis, adenopathy, and splenomegaly are noted less commonly with CMV.

CMV disease manifestation includes pneumonia, enteritis, encephalitis, retinitis, hepatitis, cholangitis, cystitis, nephritis, sinusitis, and marrow suppression. CMV pneumonia was also increased among patients with lymphoma and acute leukemia. CMV-attributable mortality for these patients ranged from 30% to 60%.

Primary CMV infection is when CMV is detected in a previously CMV seronegative patient. Recurrent CMV infection is when CMV is detected in a CMV seropositive patient. At symptomatic CMV infection, patients develop symptoms (fever with or without bone marrow suppression) and carry detectable CMV virions, antigens or nucleic acid, but with no sign of CMV endorgan disease. CMV disease is when CMV can be detected by test with appropriate sensitivity and specificity in an organ, in a biopsy, or in samples from other invasive procedures, bronco-alveolar lavage (BAL), cerebrospinal fluid (CSF) together with symptoms and/or sings from the affected organ. For CMV retinitis, typical findings by ophtalmologic examination are sufficient.

2.4.3 Laboratory diagnosis

Several techniques exist allowing rapid diagnosis of CMV with high sensitivity. Serologic tests for antibody to CMV are useful for determining whether a patient had CMV infection in the past, a determination of great clinical importance for organ and blood donors, and in the pretransplant evaluation of prospective transplant recipients. The avidity of IgG antibody increases with time after initial infection and demonstration of low CMV-IgG avidity can improve the accuracy of identification of recent primary infection. Antibody tests are not useful in the diagnosis of CMV disease in the immunocompromised host. Serology determination of either IgG or IgM has no place in the diagnosis of CMV infection or disease but is useful to determine the risk of subsequent CMV infection. The most commonly used tests for diagnosis of CMV infection are the detection of antigen (pp65 antigenaemia assay), DNA, or mRNA. Use of a quantitative assay (Q-PCR) gives additional information valuable for patient management. CMV gastrointestinal disease is the combination of clinical symptoms, findings of macroscopic mucosal lesions on endoscopy, and demonstration of CMV by culture, histopathologic testing, immunohistochemistry or *in situ* hybridization in a biopsy specimen. PCR on biopsy material is insufficient for the diagnosis of CMV gastrointestinal disease.

2.4.4 Prevention

The different preventive strategies for CMV disease include the use of antiviral agents, such as chemoprophylaxis, pre-emptive therapy or treatment of symptomatic CMV infection. The currently available aniviral agents for prevention of CMV infection and disease are ganciclovir, valganciclovir, foscarnet and cidofovir (Ljungman et al.,2008).

CMV seronegative patients have low risk of contracting CMV infection. To reduce the risk of CMV transmission, blood product from CMV seronegative donors or leukocyte-depleted blood product should be used. CMV seronegative patients with CMV seronegative stem-cell donors have a lower risk of post transplant complications both from CMV and from the effect of CMV associated immunsuppression with its concomitant increased risk of bacterial and fungal infections.

Hyperimmune globulin preparations with high levels of antibody to CMV (CMVIG) have been evaluated for prevention of CMV disease in organ transplant recipients, premature newborns at risk for postnatal infection and pregnant women. Although attempts to develop a vaccine for prevention of maternal and congenital CMV have been pursued for more than 25 years, no vaccine is currently licensed or near licensure. Improved understanding of the role of specific viral proteins in eliciting protective immune responses and recent recognition of the potential benefit to society and cost-effectiveness of CMV vaccines, however, are stimulating development of new vaccines. Investigational vaccines using different formats have been evaluated in clinical trials; these include attenuated live virus, a recombinant protein in a fowl pox vector, a DNA vaccine, and a recombinant protein given with a new adjuvant (Sung & Schleiss, 2010).

2.4.4.1 CMV seropositive patients

The use of preemptive monitoring for CMV reactivation in patients receiving alemtuzumab for at least two months following the receipt of chemotherapy is recommended. Once CMV reactivation is recognized, either oral valganciclovir or intravenous ganciclovir may be used.

2.4.5 Therapy

The four antiviral agents (Ganciclovir, Valganiclovir, Foscarnet, and Cidofovir) are currently approved for treatment of CMV disease (Fellay et al. 2005; Knipe & Howley, 2007). Antiviral agents are commonly used in transplant medicine to prevent CMV disease, either as a daily prophylactic regimen or in a preemptive approach in which laboratory surveillance for CMV in blood is used to identify patients for antiviral therapy (Reusser 2002).

2.5 Human herpesvirus 6 (HHV-6)

Human herpesvirus 6 (HHV-6) belongs to the *Roseolovirus* genus of the *Betaherpesvirinae* subfamily of the *Herpesviridae* family. HHV-6 was first isolated in 1986 from B-lymphocytes of patients infected with HIV, HTLV, and lymphoproliferative disorders (Salahuddin et al., 1986). Because of tropism to B lymphocytes, the virus was first named human B-lymphotropic virus, but was later found mainly to infect and replicate in lymphocytes of the T-cell lineage. HHV-6 isolates are classified into two closely related groups, variants A (HHV-6A) and B (HHV-6B). HHV-6B is the major causative agent of exanthem subitum (roseola infantum), which is characterized by high fever, diarrhoea, and a mild skin rash along the trunk, neck, and face (Yamanishi et al., 1988). HHV-6A has been associated with several adult diseases, including cofactor in AIDS progression, and various neurological disorders including encephalitis, ataxia, seizure, liver disfunction, and chronic fatigue syndrome; however, the causal link between human diseases and virus infection remains to be fully elucidated (De Bolle et al., 2005; Ablashi et al, 2010).

Following primary infection, the genome of herpesviruses establishes latency as a nuclear circular episome. The *in vivo* and *in vitro* integration of HHV-6A and HHV-6B into the telomers of human chromosomaes during latency was demonstrated by Arbuckle et al. (Arbuckle et al., 2010; Arbuckle & Medveczky 2011). The integrate HHV-6 genome was also found to be vertically transmitted from parent to child in the germ-line. Characterisation of the integration sites in tumor samples and long-term follow up studies may elucidate the relationship between integration and leukemogenesis (Minarovits et al., 2007)

2.5.1 Epidemiology

Seroprevalence of HHV-6 decreases at five months of age, as maternal antibody wanes. Beginning at about 6 months, seroprevalence increases rapidly, with almost all children becoming positive by 2 years of age. Internationally, HHV-6 seroprevalence is high in almost all areas, but ranges from approximately 39% to nearly 100% among some ethnically diverse adult populations.

HHV-6 genomes and antigens are detectable in lymph nodes of patients with sinus histiocytosis with massive lymphadenopathy tubular epithelial cells, endothelial cells and histiocytes in kidney salivary glands and central nervous system tissues, where viral gene products have been localized to neurons and oligodendrocytes (Levine et al., 1992; Kurata et al., 1990). HHV-6 is also detected in lesions of Langerhans cell histiocytosis in the syndrome of Langerhans cell histiocytosis (Leahy et al., 1993; Csire et al., 2007a).

2.5.2 Clinical manifestations

Asymptomatic HHV-6 reactivation is common after allogeneic bone marrow transplantation (Cone et al.,1999), but reactivation has also been linked to bone marrow suppression, encephalitis, gastroduodenitis, colitis, pneumonitis, rash, and acute graft-versus-host disease, all of which have been reviewed by others (De Bolle et al., 2005). Liver dysfunction is also associated with HHV-6 infection; although usually mild, it can be fatal hepatitis and chronic hepatitis. Primary HHV-6 infection has also been associated with cases of idiopathic thrombocytopenic purpura. Further, human herpesvirus 6 infection has also been associated with pneumonitis, with the infected cells being primarily intraalveolar macrophages, plus some lymphocytes.

Concentrations of HHV-6 genomes in lung tissue and their relation to changes in serologic titers support an association between HHV-6 infection and idiopathic pneumonitis in immunocompromised hosts. HHV-6 reactivates early after HSCT and is found in the blood in about half of all allo-HSCT recipients, making it difficult to make disease association. Two viral variants of HHV-6 have been identified (A and B), but the HHV-6B is most frequently associated with disease among immuncompromised patients. Longitudinal studies in HSCT recipients found the viral reactivation to occur at a median of 20 days after transplantation, and that viral shedding for some patients was prolonged, and correlated poorly with clinical improvement (Zerr et al., 2005). A clinical syndrome consisting of central nervous system dysfunction, impaired memory, secondary hypothyroidism, and delayed platelet engrafment are common disease manifestations. HHV-6 viraemia among allogenic transplant recipients is associated with the increase in all-cause mortality, and viraemia appears to be increased when patients are transplanted for disease other than first remission, when donor and recipient are sex mismatched, and among younger patients.

2.5.3 Laboratory diagnosis

HHV-6 virus isolation is easily recovered from peripheral blood mononuclear cells of patients with exanthema subitum during the acute phase. Cytopathic effect (CPE) develops within 7 to 10 days. The refractile giant cells usually contain one or two nuclei and, after the occurrence of the CPE, lytic degeneration of the cells takes place. The rate of virus isolation from mononuclear cells was 100% on days 0 to 2 (just before appearance of skin rash), 82% on day 3, and 20% on day 4.

Numerous HHV-6 serologic assays have been described, including IFA, ELISA, neutralization, and immunoblot. IFA is the most commonly applied method, with HHV-6 infected cells being used as the antigens. For detection of IgM, separation of serum IgM from IgG and IgA significantly increases the specificity.

Antigenemia tests: such tests have been used for the diagnosis of HHV-6 infection in blood, but there is limited experience as their use has not been widespread.

HHV-6 DNA can be detected via PCR techniques (sPCR, n-PCR) from blood, cerebrospinal fluid (CSF), tissue samples, and other samples in view of the differing natural histories of variants A and B. Quantitative PCR (Q-PCR or real-time PCR) analysis on blood and CSF is the method of choice for diagnosis.

Possibile techniques include *in situ* hybridization and immunohistochemistry, but these are not generally available.

2.5.4 Prevention

Antiviral prophylaxis against HHV-6: foscarnet, ganciclovir and cidofovir have been shown to inhibit HHV-6 replication. Data from two small non-randomized studies of HSCT recipients suggest that prophylactic gancyclovir can prevent recurrent HHV-6 infection (Tokimasa et al., 2002, Rapaport et al., 2002).

2.5.5 Therapy

Foscarnet and gancyclovir, alone or in combination, have been used as treatment for HHV-6 infection. For treatment of HHV-6 encephalitis foscarnet or ganciclovir are recommended as first-line therapies after HSCT. Cidofovir is recommended as a second-line therapy.

2.6 Human herpesvirus 7 (HHV-7)

Human herpesvirus 7 (HHV-7) belongs to the *Roseolovirus* genus of the *Betaherpesvirinae* subfamily of the *Herpesviridae family*. HHV-7 was first described in 1990 (Frenkel et al., 1990). HHV-7 was isolated in 1990 from a healthy individual whose cells were stimulated with antibody against CD3 and then incubated with interleukin-2. The virus is one of the causative agents of exanthema subitum (Tanaka et al., 1994) and has been associated with febrile convulsions in young children (Ward et al., 2005). After primary infection of CD 4+T lymphocytes, HHV-7 infects (similar to HHV-6) epithelial cells of salivary glands and various organs (lungs, skin, mammary gland, liver, kidney and tonsils). HHV-7 could be reactivated from lately infected peripheral blood mononuclear cells by T-cell activation. Thus, HHV-7 can provide transacting functions, mediating HHV-6 reactivation from latency (Tanaka-Taya et al., 2000).

2.6.1 Epidemiology
HHV-7 infection appears to occur slightly later than HHV-6. As for HHV-6, seroprevalence declines over the first 5 to 6 months, as maternal antibody wanes, then increases fairly rapidly up to 4 years of age. HHV-7 is ubiquitous, with more than 44%-91% of adults having antibody to virus.

2.6.2 Clinical manifestations
Although the frequency of clinical illness is lower, primary infection with HHV-7 causes illness similar to that of HHV-6, including exanthem subitum, high fever, and neurologic symptoms (e.g., febrile convulsions).

In 1997, Drago et al. reported the association of pityriasis rosea with HHV-7 infection and proposed that it is a clinical presentation of HHV-7 reactivation. Peripheral blood mononuclear cell (PBMC) from patients with pityriasis rosea showed ballooning cells and syncytia after 7 days in culture, whereas PBMC from controls and patients recovered from pityriasis rosea did not. PCR identified HHV-7 DNA in PBMC, plasma, and skin from all patients with active pityriasis rosea, and only in the PBMC 10 to 14 months later. HHV-7 detection after HSCT is relatively infrequent, and there are only a handful of cases in which HHV-7 is associated with central nervous system disease (Yoshikawa et al., 2003).

2.6.3 Laboratory diagnosis
HHV-7 is sometimes isolated from peripheral blood of patients with exanthema subitum, and can be readily isolated from saliva by using methods as described above for HHV-6. Isolation of HHV-6 from saliva is uncommon, although its DNA is often detectable there. HHV-7 serology techniques are immunoblot, IFA, and ELISA assays for HHV-7 antibodies. The ELISA was the most sensitive, whereas the immunoblot was the most specific. As mentioned, antibody avidity assays enable identification of recent primary infections (Ward 2005). PCR techniques (sPCR, n-PCR, Q-PCR or RT-PCR) can be used to detect HHV-7 DNA of blood, cerebrospinal fluid (CSF), tissue, or other samples.

2.6.4 Prevention
In view of the limited data, no recommendations can be made regarding HHV-7 as a potential pathogen in leukemia patients or after HSCT.

2.6.5 Therapy
The majority of conditions due to infection do not require antiviral medication, but the severe complications may be treated with ganciclovir and its derivates or foscarnet and cidofovir.

2.7 Human herpesvirus 8 (HHV-8) [Kaposi's sarcoma associated herpesvirus (KSHV)]
Kaposi's sarcoma associated herpesvirus (KSHV; human herpesvirus 8, HHV-8) is the most recently discovered human herpesvirus (Chang et al., 1994). Kaposi's sarcoma (KS) is a complex, angioproliferative and inflammatory lesion that was first described by Kaposi in the late 19th century (Kaposi, 1872). HHV-8 belongs to the *Rhadinovirus* genus of the *Gammaherpesvirinae* subfamily of the *Herpesviridae family*. HHV-8 is the ethiologic agent of Kaposi's sarcoma, and has been implicated in other B-cell lymphoproliferative disorders including primary effusion lymphoma and a subset of multricentric Castleman disease. HHV-8 has been implicated in the pathogenesis of several other diseases, including multiple

myeloma, Waldenstörm macroglobulinaemia, and monoclonal gammopathy with unknown significance (Mikala et al., 1999).

2.7.1 Epidemiology

The prevalence of HHV-8 infection is very high in older children and adults in Africa and the Amazon basin (50-100%), medium in the Mediterranean (5-25%), and low in North America, North and West Europe (2-5%). Transmission of the virus is sexual; in homosexual and bisexual persons, seroprevalence rates are substantially lower among women than men. Transmission is possible via saliva in areas of high epidemicity. HHV-8 may be transmitted by blood transfusion and solid organ transplantation (Hladik et al., 2006).

2.7.2 Clinical manifestations

Transplant patients may acquire HHV-8 from the allograft, blood products, caregivers, or from family members. Cutaneuous or visceral Kaposi's sarcomas develop with a reported incidence of 0.5-5.0% in solid organ recipients (Jenkins et al., 2002).

2.7.3 Laboratory diagnosis

The first successful cultivation of HHV-8 used PEL cell lines explanted from patients with advanced AIDS (Renne et al., 1996). HHV-8 diagnostic serology techniques may include immunoblot, IFA, and ELISA assays for HHV-8 antibodies (Sarmati 2001; Juhasz et al., 2001). These are useful for donors and recipients in at risk population, but wherever available, are of variable sensitivity and specificity (Sergerie et al., 2004).

HHV-8 DNA can be detected via PCR techniques (sPCR, n-PCR, Q-PCR or RT-PCR) from the whole blood, plasma or serum, cerebrospinal fluid (CSF), tissue or other samples. Possible techniques may include *in situ* hybridization and immunohistochemistry, but these are not generally available.

2.7.4 Prevention

In view of the limited data, no recommendations can be made regarding HHV-8 as a potential pathogen in leukemia patients or after HSCT.

2.7.5 Therapy

Antiviral agents that target herpesvirus DNA synthesis, such as ganciclovir, foscarnet and cidofovir, inhibit HHV-8 lytic replication and can prevent Kaposi sarcoma (Cohen & Powderly 2004). Several HIV protease inhibitors may interfere with tumor growth and angiogenesis, and one protease inhibitor, nelfinavir, directly inhibits HHV-8 replication *in vitro* (Gantt & Casper, 2011).

3. Conclusion

The spectrum of viral infections for patients with haematological diseases is expanding and diagnosis has increased because of new molecular diagnostic techniques. The group of human herpesviruses consists of eight members. Primary and reactivation infections are characteristic of these pathogens. Viral latency can be predicted by serological screening and it is useful for disease management. Antiviral therapy is now routinely used for prevention and therapy. Viral immunization remains investigational, except for the VZV vaccination (Cheuk et al., 2011).

Human herpesviruses are a major cause of related morbidity and mortality in hematologic diseases. This chapter focuses on the epidemiology and prevention strategies for human herpesviruses in this population (see Table 1.).

Virus	Disease -------------------- Population	Surveillance ---------------- (Monitoring)	Recommended antiviral agent	Preventative measure	Timing and Duration
HHV-1 & HHV-2 (HSV-1 & HSV-2)	Reactivation, rare first infection Mucositis Esophagitis Pneumonitis or hepatitis	Baseline serologies Prophylaxis if seropositive ---------------- (No)	ACV GCV VACV VGCV FAM	Prophylaxis: IV ACV 5mg/kg BID oral ACV 200mg TID oral VACV 500mg BID	Initiate prophylaxis with start of chemotherapy Continue for 3-5 weeks post-chemotherapy
	HSCT			ACV 250mg per meter-squared IV q12h or oral ACV 200mg TID oral VACV 500mg BID FAM 750 mg po q24h or 500mg BID or 250mg TID	at least 30 days post-tranplantation
	Leukemia				during neutropenia
	Alemtuzumab therapy				2 months after therapy or until CD4> 100 cells/ul
HHV-3 (VZV)	Primary infection varicella, reactivation herpes zoster	Baseline serologies preventative therapy if seronegative	ACV GCV VACV VGCV FAM	post-exposure prophylaxis ACV 800mg QID, VACV 1g TID post-exposure passive immunization VZIG (0.2-1ml/kg IV) or IVIG (300-500 mg/kg IV	antiviral agents are until 21 days post-exposure passive immunization within 96 hours of exposure
		Monitor if seropositive		herpes zoster treatment with antivirals	
HHV-4 (EBV)	HSCT	Baseline serologies	GCV foscarnet cidofovir	No evidence for the use of prophylactic therapy	

Virus	Disease -------------------- Population	Surveillance ---------------- (Monitoring)	Recommended antiviral agent	Preventative measure	Timing and Duration
HHV-5 (CMV)	Reactivation CMV viraemia CMV syndrome Organ Disease (CNS, pneumonitis, GI)	Baseline serologies, weekly CMV PCR or pp65 antigenemia	GCV foscarnet cidofovir VGCV	Pre-emptive IV GCV 5mg/kg BID oral VGCV 900mg BID	
	HSCT	weekly CMV PCR or pp65 antigenemia			chemotherapy to 2-6 months, post therapy treatment for at least 1 week or until CMV PCR is negative and patient asymptomatic
	Alemtuzumab therapy				
HHV-6		Baseline serologies ?	foscarnet GCV	No evidence for the use of prophylactic therapy	
HHV-7		Baseline serologies ?	GCV foscarnet cidofovir	No evidence for the use of prophylactic therapy	
HHV-8 (KSHV)		Baseline serologies ?	GCV foscarnet cidofovir nelfinavir	No evidence for the use of prophylactic therapy	

Abbreviations: ACV-acyclovir, GCV-ganciclovir, VACV-valacyclovir, VGCV-valganciclovir, HSCT-hematopoietic stem cell transplantation, GVHD-graft-versus-host disease, IV-intavenous, BID-two times per day, TID-three times per day, QID-four times per day, VZIG-Varicella-zoster immunoglobulin, IVIG-intravenous immunoglobulin, FAM-Famciclovir, CNS-central nervous system, GI-gastrointestinal

Table 1. Recommendations for Surveillance and Prophylaxis in Patients with Hematologic Diseases

Viral infections remain a common complication in patients with hematologic diseases, especially in those receiving intensive chemotherapy. Fortunately, there are effective prophylactic and preventative mesures available to help control these infections.

Human herpesviruses have been implicated in the pathogenesis of several diseases. An increasing number of malignancies are being associated with EBV (e.g. LPD, non-Hodgkin's lymphoma, Hodgkin's diseases, Burkitts's lymphoma, NK-cell leukemia). HHV-8 has been suggested as a possible etiologic agent of several diseases. These include multiple myeloma, Waldenstörm's macroglobulinaemia, and monoclonal gammopathy with unknown significance. Multiple myeloma is a genetically and clinically heterogeneous disease. Recently, (at least) 5 prognostically and biologically different subgroups have been described based on karyotype and type of cyclin expression (Gertz & Greipp 2004). HHV-8 infection may play a role in the disease process of only one or more subgroups of myeloma patients while not in others. In the history of HHV-8 research, it has been exceedingly difficult to obtain lymphoid cell lines (e.g. effusion lymphoma) devoid of EBV genome (Renne et al. 1996).

This brings up the point of possible interaction between these two lymphotropic herpesviruses, at least in diseases of the lymphoid system. A similar interaction of HHV-6 and 8 has been described *in vitro*. EBV-seronegative patients may be prone to HHV-8 reactivation, the possible interaction of EBV early proteins with the activation of latently harbored HHV-8 genomes. This might occur also in such cases when the two viruses are not replicating in the same cell, but viral membrane proteins i.e. ZEBRA or interleukin-like molecules shed (IL10) by the EBV producing B-cells might interact with B cells or bone marrow cells carrying latent HHV-8 mini-chromosomes.

It may be possible that the continuously replicating myeloma cells release both EBV and HHV-8, since latent virus infected cells are usually blocked in the G0-G1 phases of the cell cycle. When myeloma cells enter the S-phase, the availability of DNA replication machinery may activate the DNA viruses persisting in a small proportion of cells. The absence of CMV reactivation can be understood, since the sites of latency are the CD34+ progenitor cells of monocytes. The main site of replication is the B lymphocytes and many other cells in the human body. In conclusion, the data also indicate that in addition to HHV-8, the transitional reactivation of EBV may also play a role in the pathogenesis of MM (Csire et al. 2007b).

Prospective studies are needed to clarify the spectrum of viral infections and risk factors for disease better, and to define effective prevention and treatment strategies. Fortunately, clinicians and virologists are increasingly aware of the most appropriate therapeutic options based on improved monitoring and characteriziation of the antiviral therapy.

4. Acknowledgment

The authors would like to thank György Berencsi for helpful discussions, and Borbála Stubán, Zsuzsanna Zlinszky and Margit Zolyómi for their helpful assistance.

5. References

Ablashi, D. V.; Devin C. L.; Yoshikawa, T.; Lautenschlager, I.; Luppi, M. , Kuhl U. & Komaroff, A. L. (2010). Human herpesvirus-6 in multiple non-neurological diseases. *J. Med. Virol.*, Vol. 82, No.11, (November 2010), pp. 1903–1910, ISSN1096-9071

Almeida, J. D.; Howatson, A. F. & Williams, M. G. (1962). Morphology of varicella (chickenpox) virus. *Virology*, Vol.16, (March, 1962), pp. 353-355, ISSN 0042-6822

Ambinder R. F. (2007). Epstein-barr virus and hodgkin lymphoma. *Hematology Am Soc Hematol Educ Program*, Vol. 1, (2007) pp.204-209, ISSN 1520-4391

Anaisse, E. J.; Kontoyiannis, D. P.; O'Brien, S.; Kantarjian, H.; Robertson, L.; Lerner, S. & Keating, M. J. (1998). Infections in patients with chronic lymphotic leukemia treated with fludarabine. *Ann Intern Med,* Vol.129, No.7, (1998), pp. 559-566, ISSN 0003-4819

Angarone, M. & Ison, M. G. (2008). Prevention and early treatment of opportunistic viral infections in patients with leukemia and allogeneic stem cell transplantation recipients. *J Natl Compr Canc Netw,* Vol.6, No.2, (Ferbruary 2008), pp. 191-201, ISSN 1540-1405

Angarone, M. (2011). Epidemiology and prevention of viral infections in patients with hematologic malignancies. *Infect Disord Drug Targets,* Vol.11, No.1, (February 2011), pp. 27-33, ISSN 1871-5265

Arbuckle, J. H. & Medveczky, P. G. (2011). The molecular biology of human herpesvirus-6 latency and telomere integration. *Microbes Infect*, Vol.13, No.8-9, (August 2011), pp: 731-741, ISSN 1286-4579

Arbuckle, J.H.; Medveczky, M. M.; Luka, J.; Hadley, S. H.; Luegmayr, A.; Ablashi, D.; Lund T. C.; Tolar, J.; De Meirleir, K.; Montoya, J. G.; Komaroff, A. L.; Ambros, P. F. & Medveczky, P. G. (2010). The latent human herpesvirus-6A genome specifically integrates in telomeres of human chromosomes in vivo and in vitro, *Proc Natl Acad Sci U S A,* Vol.107, No.12, (March 2010), pp: 5563-5568, ISSN 0027-8424

Boeckh, M.; Kim, H. W.; Flowers, M. E.; Meyers, J. D. & Bowden, R. A. (2006). Long-term acyclovir for prevention of varicella zoster virus disease after allogeneic hematopoietic cell transplantation-randomized double-blind placebo-controlled study. *Blood,* Vol.107, No5, (March 2006), pp. 1800-1805, ISSN 0006-4971

Chang, Y.; Cesarman, E.; Pessin, M. S.; Lee, F.; Culpepper, J.; Knowles, D. M. & Moore, P. S. (1994). Identification of herpesvirus-like DNA sequences in AIDS-associated Kaposi's sarcoma. *Science,* Vol.266, No.5192, (December 1994), pp. 1865-1869, ISSN 0036-8075

Chayavichitsilp, P.; Buckwalter, J. V.; Krakowski, A. C. & Friedlander, S. F. (2009). Herpes simplex. *Pediatrics in Review,* Vol.30, No.4, (April 2009), pp.119-129, ISSN 0191-9601

Cheuk, D. K.; Chiang, A. K.; Lee, T. L.; Chan, G. C. & Ha, S. Y. (2011). Vaccines for prophylaxis of viral infections in patients with hematological malignancies. *Cochrane Database Syst Rev,* Vol.3, (March 2011), CD006505.

Cohen, J. & Powderly, W. G. (2004). *Infectious Diseases (Second edition)* Elsevier Limited ISBN 978-0-323-04579-7

Cone, R. W.; Huang, M. L.; Corey, L. ;Zeh, J.; Ashley, R. & Bowden, R. (1999). Human herpesvirus 6 infections after bone marrow transplantation: clinical and virologic manifestations. *J. Infect. Dis.,* Vol.179, No.2, (February 1999), pp. 311–318. ISSN 0022-1899

Corey, L. & Handsfield, H. (2000). Genital herpes and public health: addressing a global problem. *JAMA*, Vol.283, No.6, (February 2000), pp. 791–794, ISSN 0098-7484

Csire, M.; Mikala, G.; Jákó, J.; Masszi, T.; Jánosi, J.; Dolgos, J.; Füle, T.; Tordai, A.; Berencsi, G. & Vályi-Nagy, I. (2007a) Persistent long-term human herpesvirus 6 (HHV-6) infection in a patient with langerhans cell histiocytosis. *Pathol Oncol Res,* Vol.13, No.2, (July 2007), pp. 157-160, ISSN 1219-4956

Csire, M.; Mikala, G; Peto, M.; Jánosi, J.; Juhász, A.; Tordai, A.; Jákó, J.; Domján, G.; Dolgos, J.; Berencsi, G. & Vályi-Nagy, I. (2007b). Detection of four lymphotropic herpesviruses in Hungarian patients with multiple myeloma and lymphoma. *FEMS Immunol Med Microbiol.* Vol.49, No.1, (February 2007), pp.62-67, ISSN 0928-8244

Davison, A. J. (2002). Evolution of the herpesviruses. *Veterinary Microbiology,* Vol.86, No.1-2,(April 2002), pp. 69-88, ISSN 0378-1135

De Bolle, L.; Naesens, L. & De Clercq, E. (2005). Update on human herpesvirus 6 biology, clinical features, and therapy. *Clin. Microbiol. Rev,* Vol.18, No.1, (January 2005), pp. 217–245, ISSN 0893-8512

Delecluse, H. J.; Feederle, R.; O'Sullivan, B. & Taniere, P. (2007). Epstein Barr virus-associated tumours: an update for the attention of the working pathologist. *J Clin Pathol* Vol.60, No12, (December 2007), pp. 1358-1364, ISSN 0021-9746

Drago, F.; Ranieri, E.; Malaguti, F.; Losi, E. & Rebora, A. (1997) Human herpesvirus 7 in pityriasis rosea. *Lancet,* Vol.349, No.9062, (May 1997), pp. 1367-1368, ISSN0140-6736

Epstein, M.; Achong, B. & Barr, Y. (1964). Virus particles in cultured lymphoblasts from Burkitt's lymphoma. *Lancet,* Vol.1, No.7335, (March 1964), pp. 702-703, ISSN 0140-6736

Fatahzadeh, M. & Schwartz, R. A. (2007). Human herpes simplex virus infections: epidemiology, pathogenesis, symptomatology, diagnosis, and management. *J. Am. Acad. Dermatol.* Vol. 57, No.5, (November 2007), pp.737-763, ISSN 0190-9622

Fellay, J.; Venetz, J. P.; Pascual, M.; Aubert, J. D.; Seudoux, C. & Meylan, P. R. (2005). Treatment of cytomegalovirus infection or disease in solid organ transplant recipients with valganciclovir. *Am J Transplant,* Vol.5, No7, (July 2005), pp. 1781-1782, ISSN 1600-6135

Fleming, D. T.; McQuillan, G. M.; Johnson, R. E.; Nahmias, A. J.; Aral, S. O.; Lee, F. K. & St Louis, M. E. (1997) Herpes simplex virus type 2 in the United States, 1976-1994. *N Engl J Med,* Vol.337, No. 16, (October 1997), pp. 1105–1111, ISSN 0028-4793

Frenkel, N.; Schirmer, E. C.; Wyatt, L. S.; Katsafanas, G.; Roffman, E.; Danovich, R. M. & June, C. H. (1990). Isolation of a new herpesvirus from CD4+ T cells. *Proc Natl Acad Sci U S A,* Vol.87, No.2, (January 1990), pp. 748-752, ISSN 0027-8424

Gantt, S. & Casper, C. (2011). Human herpesvirus 8-associated neoplasms: the roles of viral replication and antiviral treatment. *Curr Opin Infect Dis.* Vol.24, No.4, (August 2011), pp. 295-301, ISSN 0951-7375

Gershon, A. A.; Steinberg, S. P. & Schmidt, N. J. (1999). Varicella-zoster virus. In: *Manual of Clinical Microbiology.* Balows, A.; Hauseler, W. J.; Herrman, K. L. et al. eds. Washington DC: American Society for Microbiology; (1999) 7th edition, pp. 900-911, ISBN1-55581-126-4, Washington, USA

Gertz, M. A. & Greipp, P. R. (2004). *Multiple Myeloma and Related Plasma Cell Diorders, Springer-Verlag,* ISBN 3-540-00811-X, Berlin Heidelberg New York

Gilbert, N. D.; Moellering, R. C.; Eliopoulos, G. M.; Chambers, H. F. & Saag, M. S. (2010) *The Stanford Guide to Antimicrobial Therapy 2010,* Pocket Editions, ISBN 978-1-930808-59-1, Sperryville, Virginia, USA

Gnann, J. (2003). *Herpes Simplex and Varicella Zoster Virus Infections After Hemopetic Stem Cell or Solid Organ Transplantation* (2 edition), Lippincott Williams & Wilkins, ISBN 9781562558202, Philadelphia, Pennsylvania, USA

Gross, G.; Schöfer, H.; Wassilew, S.; Friese, K.; Timm, A.; Guthoff, R.; Pau, H. W.; Malin, J. P.; Wutzler, P. & Doerr, H. W. (2003). Herpes zoster guideline of the German

Dermatology Society (DDG). *J Clin Virol*, Vol.26, No.3, (April 2003), pp. 277-289, ISSN 1986-6532

Gu, S.Y.; Huang, T. M.; Ruan, L.; Miao, Y. H.; Lu, H.; Chu, C.M.; Motz, M. & Wolf H. (1995). First EBV vaccine trial in humans using recombinant vaccinia virus expressing the major membrane antigen. *Dev Biol Stand*, Vol.84, (1995), pp. 171-177, ISSN 0301-5149

Hata, A.; Asanuma, H.; Rinki, M.; Sharp, M.; Wong, R. M.; Blume, K. & Arvin, A. M. (2002). Use of an inactivated varicella vaccine in recipients of hematopoietic-cell Transplants. *N Engl J Med*, Vol.347, No.1, (July 2002), pp. 26-34, ISSN 0028-4793

Hettmann, A.; Gerle, B.; Barcsay, E.; Csiszár, C. & Takács, M. (2008). Seroprevalence of HSV-2 in Hungary and comparison of the HSV-2 prevalence of pregnant and infertile women. *Acta Microbiol Immunol Hung*, Vol.55, No.4, (December 2008), pp. 429-436, ISSN 1217-8950

Hladik, W., Dollard, S. C.; Mermin, J.; Fowlkes, A. L.; Downing, R.; Amin, M. M.; Banage, F.; Nzaro, E.; Kataaha, P.; Dondero, T. J.; Pellett, P. E. & Lackritz, E. M. (2006). Transmission of human herpesvirus 8 by blood transfusion. *N Engl J Med*, Vol.355, No.13, (September 2006), pp. 1331-1338, ISSN 0028-4793

Ho, M. (1991). *Cytomegalovirus: Biology and Infection*, 2nd ed. Plenum Publishing, ISBN 10 030643654X, New York, USA

Islam, M. S.; Anoop, P.; Gordon-Smith, E. C.; Rice, P.; Datta-Nemdharry, P. & Marsh, J. C. (2010). Epstein-Barr virus infections after allogeneic stem cell transplantation: a comparison between non-malignant and malignant hematological disorders. *Hematology*, Vol.15, No.5, (October 2010), pp.344-350, ISSN 1466-4860

Jancel, T. & Penzak, S. R. (2009). Antiviral therapy in patients with hematologic malignancies, transplantation, and aplastic anemia. *Semin Hematol*. Vol.46, No.3, (July 2009), pp. 230-247. ISSN 0037-1963

Jenkins, F. J.; Hoffman, L. J. & Liegey-Dougall, A. (2002). Reactivation of and primary infection with human herpesvirus 8 among solid-organ transplant recipients. *J. Infect. Dis.*, Vol.185, No.9, (May 2002), pp.1238-1243, ISSN 0022-1899

Jones, C. A. & Cunningham, A. L. (2004). Vaccination Strategies to Prevent Genital Herpes and Neonatal Herpes Simplex Virus (HSV) Disease. *Herpes*, Vol.11, No.1, (2004), pp. 12-17. ISSN 0969-7667

Juhasz, A.; Konya, J.; Beck, Z.; Remenyik, E.; Veress, G.; Begany, A.; Medgyessy, I.; Hunyadi J. & Gergely, L. (2001). HHV-8 ELISA based on a one step affinity capture of biotinylated K8.1. antigen. *Journal of Medical Virology*, Vol.94, No.1-2, (May 2001), pp.163–172, ISSN 0146-6615

Kalpoe, J. S.; Kroes, A. C.; Verkerk, S.; Claas, E. C.; Barge, R. M. & Beersma, M. F. (2006). Clinical relevance of quantitative varicella-zoster virus (VZV) DNA detection in plasma after stem cell transplantation. *Bone Marrow Transplant*, Vol.38, No.1, (July 2006), pp. 41-46, ISSN 0268-3369

Kaposi, M. (1872). Idiopathisches multiples pigmentsarkom her haut. *Arch Dermatol Shypilol*, Vol.4, (1872), pp. 265-273, DOI: 10.1007/BF01830024

Kaufman, B.; Gandhi, S. A.; Louie, E.; Rizzi, R.; Illei, P. (1997) Herpes simplex virus hepatitis: case report and review, *Clin Infect Dis*, Vol.24, No.5, (May 1997), pp. 334-338, ISSN 1058-4838

Knipe, D. M. & Howley, P.M. (2007) *Fields Virology (Fifth Edition)*, Lippincott Williams & Wilkins, ISBN-13: 978-0-7817-6060-7, ISBN-10:07817-6060-7 Philadelphia, Pennsylvania, USA

Kurata T., Iwasaki T., Sata T., Wakabayashi, T.; Yamaguchi, K.; Okuno, T.; Yamanishi, K. & Takei, Y. (1990). Viral pathology of human herpesvirus 6 infection. *Adv. Exp. Med. Biol*, Vol.278, (1990), pp. 39–47, ISSN 0065-2598

Leahy, M. A.; Krejci, S. M.; Friednash, M.; Stockert, S. S.; Wilson, H.; Huff, J. C.; Wetson , W. & Brice, S.L. (1993). Human herpesvirus 6 is present in lesions of Langerhans cell histiocytosis. *J. Invest. Dermatol*, Vol.101, No.5, (November 1993), pp. 642–645, ISSN 0022-202X

Levine, P. H.; Jahan, N.; Murari, P.; Manak, M. & Jaffe, E. S. (1992). Detection of human herpesvirus 6 in tissues involved by sinus histiocytosis with massive lymphadenopathy (Rosai–Dorfman disease). *J. Infect. Dis*, Vol.166, No.2, (August 1992), pp. 291–295, ISSN 0022-1899

Ljungman, P.; de la Camara, R.; Cordonnier, C.; Einsele, H.; Engelhard, D.; Reusser, P.; Styczynski, J. & Ward, K. (2008). European Conference on Infections in Leukemia, (2008) Management of CMV, HHV-6, HHV-7 and Kaposi-sarcoma herpesvirus (HHV-8) infections in patients with hematological malignancies and after SCT. *Bone Marrow Transplant*, Vol.42, No.4, (August 2008), pp. 227-240, ISSN 0268-3369

Locksley, R. M., Flournoy, N.; Sullivan, K. M. & Meyers, J. D. (1985). Infection with varicella-zoster virus after marrow transplantation. *J Infect Dis*, Vol.152, No.6, (December 1985), pp. 1172-1181, ISSN 0022-1899

Lowenstein, A. (1919). Aetiologische untersuchungen uber den fieberhaften, herpes, *Munch Med Wochenschr* Vol.66, pp. 769-770, ISSN 0027-2973

Lundgren, G.; Wilczek, H.; Lönnqvist, B.; Lindholm, A.; Wahren, B. & Ringdén, O. (1985). Acyclovir prophylaxis in bone marrow transplant recipients. *Scand J Infect Dis Suppl*, (1985) Vol.47, No. pp 137-44, ISSN 0036-5548

McMillan, J. A.; Weiner, L. B.; Higgins, A. M. & Lamparella V. J.(1993). Pharyngitis associated with herpes simplex virus in college students. *Pediatr Infect Dis J*, Vol.12, No.4, (April 1993), pp 280-284, ISSN 08913668

Mikala, G.; Xie, J.; Berencsi, G.; Kiss, C.; Márton, I.; Domján, G. & Vályi-Nagy, I. (1999). Human herpesvirus 8 in hematologic diseases. *Pathol Oncol Res*, Vol.5, No.1, (January 1999), pp. 73-79, ISSN 1219-4956

Minarovits, J.; Gonczol, E. & Valyi-Nagy, T. (2007). *Latency Strategies of Herpesviruses*, Springer, ISBN-10: 0-378-32464-X ISBN-13:978-0387-32464-7, New York, NY, USA

Ng, A. P.; Worth, L.; Chen, L.; Seymour, J. F.; Prince, H. M.; Slavin, M. & Thursky, K. (2005). Cytomegalovirus DNAemia and disease: incidence, natural history and management in settings other than allogeneic stem cell transplantation. *Haematologica*, Vol.90, No.12, (December 2005), pp. 1672-1679, ISSN 0390-6078

Oxman, M. N. (2010). Zoster vaccine: current status and future prospects. *Clin Infect Dis*, Vol.51, No.2, (July 2010), pp. 197-213, ISSN 1058-4838

Rapaport, D.; Engelhard, D.; Tagger, G.; Or, R. & Frenkel, N. (2002). Antiviral prophylaxis may prevent human herpesvirus-6 reactivation in bone marrow transplant recipients. *Transpl Infect Dis*, Vol.4, No.1, (March 2002), pp. 10-16, ISSN 1399-3062

Renne, R.; Zhong, W.; Herndier, B.; Kedes, D.; McGrath, M. & Ganem, D. (1996). Lytic growth of Kaposi's sarcoma-associated herpesvirus (human herpesvirus 8) in B cell lymphoma cells in culture. *Nature Med.* Vol.2, No.3, (March 1996), pp. 342-346, ISSN 1078-8956

Reusser, P. (2002). Management of viral infections in immunocompromised cancer patients. *Swiss Med Wkly*,Vol.132, No.27-28, (July 2002), pp. 374-378, ISSN 1424-7860

Ribes, J.; Steele, A.; Seabolt J. & Baker, D. (2001). Six-year study of the incidence of herpes in genital and nongenital cultures in a central Kentucky medical center patient population. *J Clin Microbiol*, Vol.39, No.9, (September 2001), pp. 3321–3325, ISSN 0095-1137

Salahuddin, S. Z.; Ablashi, D. V.; Markham, P. D.; Josephs, S. F.; Sturzenegger, S.; Kaplan, M.; Halligan, G.; Biberfeld, P.; Wong-Staal, F.; Kramarsky, B. et al.(1986). Isolation of a new virus, HBLV, in patients with lymphoproliferative disorders. *Science*, Vol.234, No.4776, (October 1986), pp 596-601, ISSN 0036-8075

Sandherr, M.; Einsele, H.; Hebart, H.; Kahl, C.; Kern, W.; Kiehl, M.; Massenkeil, G.; Penack, O.; Schiel, X.; Schuettrumpf, S.; Ullmann, A. J. & Cornely, O. A. (2006). Antiviral profilaxis in patients with hematological malignancies and solid tumors:Guidlines of the Infectious Diseqse Working Party (AGIHO) of the German Society of Hematology and Oncology (DGHO), *Ann Oncol.* Vol.17, No.7, (July 2006), pp. 1051-1059, ISSN 0923-7534

Sarmati, L. (2001). Serological testing for human herpesvirus 8. *Herpes*, Vol.8, No.3, (November 2001), pp. 76-79, ISSN 0969-7667

Sawyer, M. H.; Chamberlin, C. J.; Wu, Y. N.; Aintablian, N. & Wallace, M. R. (1994). Detection of varicella-zoster virus DNA in air samples from hospital rooms. *J Infect Dis*, Vol.169, No 1, (January 1994), pp. 91-94, ISSN0022-1899

Schneweiss, K. E. (1962). Serological studies on the type differentiation of Herpesvirus hominis (Article in German; Serologische Untersuchungen zur Typendifferenzierung des Herpesvirus hominis). *Z Immun Exp Ther*, Vol.124, (September 1962), pp 24-28, ISSN 7864-6374

Sergerie, Y.; Abed, Y.; Roy, J. & Boivin, G. (2004). Comparative evaluation of three serological methods for detection of human herpesvirus 8-specific antibodies in Canadian allogeneic stem cell transplant recipients. *J Clin Microbiol*, Vol.42, No.6, (June, 2004), pp. 2663-2667, ISSN 0095-1137

Stanberry, L. R. (2004) Clinical trials of prophylactic and therapeutic herpes simplex virus vaccines. *Herpes*, Vol.11, Suppl 3, (August 2004), pp.161-169, ISSN 0969-7667

Steinberg, S. P. & Gershon, A. A. (1991). Measurement of antibodies to varicella-zoster virus by using a latex agglutination test. *J Clin Microbiol*, Vol.29, No7, (July 1991), pp. 1527-1529, ISSN 0095-1137

Styczynski, J.; Reusser, P.; Einsele, H.; de la Camara, R.; Cordonnier, C.; Ward, K. N.; Ljungman, P. & Engelhard, D. (2009), Second European Conference on Infections in Leukemia. Management of HSV, VZV and EBV infections in patients with haematological malignancies and after SCT: guidelines from the Second European Conference on Infections in Leukemia. *Bone Marrow Transplant*, Vol.43, No.10, (May 2009), pp. 757-770, ISSN 0268-3369

Sung, H. & Schleiss, M.R. (2010) Update on the current status of cytomegalovirus vaccines. *Expert Rev Vaccines,* Vol.9, No.11, (November 2010), pp. 1303-1314, ISSN 1476-0584

Takahashi, M.; Otsuka, T.; Okuno, Y.; Asano, Y. & Yazaki, T. (1974). Live vaccine used to prevent the spread of varicella in children in hospital. *Lancet,* Vol.2, No.7892, (November 1974), pp. 1288-90, ISSN0140-6736

Tanaka, K.; Kondo, T.; Torigoe, S.; Okada, S.; Mukai, T. & Yamanishi, K. (1994). Human herpesvirus 7: another causal agent for roseola (exanthem subitum). *J Pediatr,* Vol.125, No.1, (July 1994), pp. 1-5, ISSN0022-3476

Tanaka-Taya, K.; Kondo, T.; Nakagawa, N.; Inagi, R.; Miyoshi, H.; Sunagawa, T.; Okada, S. & Yamanishi, K. (2000). Reactivation of human herpesvirus 6 by infection of human herpesvirus 7. *J Med Virol,* Vol.60, No.3, (March 2000), pp. 284-289, ISSN ISSN1096-9071

Tokimasa, S.; Hara, J.; Osugi, Y.; Ohta, H.; Matsuda, Y.; Fujisaki, H.; Sawada, A.; Kim, J. Y.; Sashihara, J.; Amou, K.; Miyagawa, H.; Tanaka-Taya, K.; Yamanishi, K. & Okada, S. (2002). Ganciclovir is effective for prophylaxis and treatment of human herpesvirus-6 in allogeneic stem cell transplantation. *Bone Marrow Transplant,* Vol.29, No.7, (April 2002), pp. 595-598, ISSN 0268-336

Tzanck, A. & Aron-Brunietiere, R. (1949). Cytodiagnostic immediate des dermatoses bullenses. *Gaz Med Port,* Vol.2, No.3, (1949) pp. 667-675, NLM ID 17040250R

Vickrey, E.; Allen, S.; Mehta, J. & Singhal, S. (2009). Acyclovir to prevent reactivation of varicella zoster virus (herpes zoster) in multiple myeloma patients receiving bortezomib therapy. *Cancer,* Vol.115, No.1, (January 2009), pp. 229-232, ISSN 0008-543X

von Bokay, J. (1909). Uber den etiologischen zusammenhang der Varizellen mit gewissen Fallen von Herpes Zoster. *Wien Klin Wochenschr,* Vol.22, (1909), pp.1323-1326, ISSN 0043-5325

Wade, J. C. (2006). Viral infections in patients with hematological malignancies. *Hematology Am Soc Hematol Educ Program,* (2006) pp. 368-374, ISSN 1520-4391

Ward, K. N. (2005). The natural history and laboratory diagnosis of human herpesviruses-6 and -7 infections in the immunocompetent. *J Clin Virol,* Vol.32, No.3, (March 2005), pp. 183-193, ISSN 1386-6532

Ward, K. N.; Andrews, N. J.; Verity, C. M. Miller, E. & Ross, E. M. (2005). Human herpesviruses-6 and -7 each cause significant neurological morbidity in Britain and Ireland. *Arch Dis Child,* Vol.90, No.6, (June 2005), pp. 619-623, ISSN 0003-9888

Weinstock, D. M.; Boeckh, M.; Boulad, F.; Eagan, J. A.; Fraser, V. J.; Henderson, D. K.; Perl, T. M.; Yokoe, D. & Sepkowitz, K. A. (2004). Postexposure prophylaxis against varicella-zoster virus infection among recipients of hematopoietic stem cell transplant: unresolved issues. *Infect Control Hosp Epidemiol,* Vol.25, No.7, (July 2004), pp. 603-608, ISSN 0899-823X

Weller, T. H. (1953). Serial propagation in vitro of agents producing inclusion bodies derived from varicella and herpes zoster. *Proceedings of the Society for Experimental Biology and Medicine,* Vol.83, No.2, (June 1953), pp. 340-346, ISSN 0037-9737

Wilson, J. B. & May, G. H. W. (2001). *Epstein-Barr Virus Protocols (Methods in Molecular Biology; 174),* Humana Press Inc., ISBN 0-89603-690-1, Totowa, New Jersey, USA

Yamanishi,K.; T. Okuno, K.; Shiraki, M.; Takahashi, T.; Kondo, Y.; Asano & T. Kurata (1988). Identification of human herpesvirus-6 as a causal agent for exanthem subitum, *Lancet,* Vol.1, No.8594, (May 1988), pp. 1065–1067, ISSN 0140-6736

Yoshikawa, T.; Yoshida, J.; Hamaguchi, M.; Kubota, T.; Akimoto, S.; Ihira, M.; Nishiyama, Y. & Asano Y. (2003). Human herpesvirus 7-associated meningitis and optic neuritis in a patient after allogeneic stem cell transplantation. *J Med Virol*, Vol.70, No.3, (July 2003), pp. 440-443, ISSN 1096-9071

Zerr, D. M.; Corey, L.; Kim, H. W.; Huang, M. L.; Nguy, L. & Boeckh, M. (2005). Clinical outcomes of human herpesvirus 6 reactivation after hematopoietic stem cell transplantation. *Clin Infect Dis,* Vol.40, No.7, (April 2005), pp. 932-940, ISSN 1058-4838

Zhou, W.; Longmate, J.; Lacey, S.F.; Palmer, J. M.; Gallez-Hawkins, G.; Thao, L.; Spielberger, R.; Nakamura, R.; Forman, S. J.; Zaia, J. A. & Diamond, D. J. (2009). Impact of donor CMV status on viral infection and reconstitution of multifunction CMV-specific T cells in CMV-positive transplant recipients. *Blood,* Vol.113, No.25, (June 2009), pp. 6465–6476, ISSN 0006-4971

7

Zoster-Associated Pain and Post Herpetic Neuralgia

Tamara Ursini[1], Monica Tontodonati[1], Ennio Polilli[2], Lucio Pippa[3] and Giustino Parruti[2]
[1]*Infectious Disease Clinic, G. d'Annunzio University, School of Medicine, Chieti, Italy*
[2]*Infectious Diseases Unit, Pescara General Hospital, Pescara,*
[3]*FondazioneOnlus Camillo de Lellis per l'Innovazione e la Ricerca in Medicina, Pescara, Italy*

1. Introduction

Herpes zoster (HZ, shingles) is a disease characterized by monolateral vesicular rash and pain, due to reactivation of VZV in the context of a waning specific anti-VZV cell-mediated immunity. Reactivation of VZV produces a new wave of viral replication within the dorsal root ganglia where latency was established after primary infection and its spread downwards to peripheral metameric fibers through the skin, all sensorial manifestations being the expression of VZV-related inflammatory response in sensory ganglia and nerve fibers. Systemic symptoms (fever, headache, malaise) are rare, being observed in some 20% of patients. Other manifestations as facial palsy can be observed in peculiar localizations as zoster oticus, or in particular categories of patients, such as vesicular dissemination in severely immunodepressed patients (Dworkin et al., 2007).

2. Epidemiology

HZ is a common disease, and HZ incidence was estimated in up to 1 million new cases every year in the United States (Schmader et al., 2008). The average lifetime risk was estimated as high as 30% in the general population; as a consequence, it affects almost half of the population aged over 65 during lifetime (Insinga et al., 2005; Yawn et al., 2007; Dworkin et al., 2007). Incidence all around the world was estimated in several studies, being calculated as 1.2-5.2 cases/person-years (Hope-Simpson, 1965; di Luzio Paparatti et al., 1999; Chidiac et al., 2001; Insinga et al., 2005; Yawn et al., 2007; Gauthier et al., 2009). Most of these studies were retrospective, based on health research or insurance databases. This may have possibly introduced selection biases, as some HZ cases, such as mild cases not ever seeking medical care, may have not been recorded or may have been incorrectly coded under the CDC ICD-9 or similar coding systems (Joesoef et al., 2011). Detailed information about pain, clinical aspects and therapy are not usually present in such databases, even though these studies usually include larger number of patients in comparison with prospective collections. In at least two cases, however, prospective evaluation of the incidence of HZ has been attempted in recent years (Oxman et al., 2005; Parruti et al., 2010). The Shingles

Prevention Study (Oxman et al., 2005) was a randomized double-blind placebo-controlled trial set up to demonstrate that vaccination against VZV can decrease the incidence and severity of HZ and post herpetic neuralgia (PHN), its more frequent complication. In this study 38,546 healthy subjects aged >60 years were randomly assigned to receive either a mock vaccine or an investigational live-attenuated VZV vaccine. In the large placebo arm (19,276 subjects) the incidence of HZ was 11.12 cases/1000 person-years (Oxman et al., 2005). An Italian cohort (Parruti et al., 2010) prospectively enrolled HZ patients of any age (mean age was 58 years, with 46% of patients aged <60 years) presenting to general practitioners, pediatricians or hospital specialists (dermatology, infectious diseases, pain management center) in a Local Health District. Incidence of HZ was prospectively calculated in a subset of that study, that is considering only cases consecutively enrolled by general practitioners, whose reference population is known. HZ incidence was 3.99 cases/person-years, over a total reference population of nearly 35,000 persons (Tontodonati, unpublished personal data). These data are largely congruent with those reported using different experimental models (di Luzio Paparatti et al., 1999; Chidiac et al., 2001; Insinga et al., 2005; Yawn et al., 2007; Gauthier et al., 2009). It is widely accepted that HZ incidence increases with age: even though HZ is not rare among young people, median age at presentation is around 64 years (Dworkin et al., 2007). Some decades ago, Hope-Simpson (Hope-Simpson, 1965) conducted a longitudinal study among his own outpatients, being a general practitioner, and estimated an increasing incidence of HZ from pediatric to older age: he estimated an incidence of 0.74 cases/person-years in children aged ≤10 years, 2.5 in patients aged 20-45 years, up to 7.8 cases/person-years in patients aged ≥65. HZ estimates in different countries (Iceland, France, Netherlands, United Kingdom, USA) and with different methodologies confirmed that HZ incidence rises with age (Hegalsson et al., 2000; Chidiac et al., 2001; Opstelten et al., 2002; Insinga et al., 2005; Yawn et al., 2007; Gauthier et al., 2009; Oxman et al., 2005). HZ incidence is known to increase in immunodepression, being more frequent and aggressive in transplant recipients, cancer patients, HIV-infected people, and in patients with autoimmune diseases (rheumatoid arthritis and lupus erythematosus sistemicus among others), diabetes, hypertension, renal failure and chronic obstructive pulmonary disease (Hata et al., 2011; Yi et al., 2010; Yang et al., 2011; Schmader et al., 2008). Notwithstanding this evidence, HZ can be considered a disease involving immunocompetent subjects in the vast majority of cases (Hegalsson et al., 2000; Oxman et al., 2005; Yawn et al., 2007; Parruti et al., 2010; Drolet et al., 2010). Contacts with patients with Varicella, more frequent for some professionals as pediatricians and teachers, turned out to be protective (Thomas et al., 2004), in line with the biological assumption that exposure to VZV may boost and strengthen natural cell-mediated immunity (Vossen et al., 2004). Recent studies investigated the role of Varicella vaccination programs in the epidemiology of HZ. Pediatric Varicella vaccination with a live attenuated vaccine was first introduced in the United States in 1995 and in many other countries in the following years. Universal Varicella vaccination programs will decrease the number of wild type Varicella cases (Jumaan et al., 2005; Schmader et al., 2008,; Reynolds et al., 2008). As contacts with patients with Varicella may be protective for HZ (Thomas & Hall, 2004), the decrease of Varicella in the general population will likely produce an increase in the incidence of HZ in the absence of parallel plans of population-wide HZ vaccination (Reynolds et al., 2008; van Hoek et al., 2011; n Schmader et al., 2008). Some other factors have been associated with an increased incidence of HZ. Trauma and surgical interventions have been suggested in several case reports, case series and a single case-control study (Foye et al., 2000; Levy & Smyth, 2002; Evans & Lee, 2004; Thomas et al., 2004; Godfrey et al., 2006). Psychological stress was also associated with an increasing incidence of HZ (Thomas & Hall, 2004). Finally it is unclear whether a real difference exist in the incidence of HZ between sexes, female sex purportedly representing a predisposing factor in some studies (Thomas & Hall, 2004).

Post Herpetic Neuralgia (PHN) is the most common complication of HZ, ensuing in 10 to 20% of patients on average. Its prevalence has been estimated to range from 500,000 up to 1 million cases in United States (Schmader et al., 2008). Its incidence has been calculated in several studies in parallel with the incidence of HZ (Hope-Simpson, 1975; Hegalsson et al., 2000; Opstelten et al., 2002; Scott et al., 2003; Parruti et al, 2010). The first study deserving quotation is again by Hope-Simpson in 1975 (Hope-Simpson, 1975). Among his outpatients, he observed HZ and kept note of PHN during a period of over 25 years: he calculated the incidence of PHN as 14.3% and he observed an increase in PHN in older patients, with incidence raising up to 34.4% in patients aged >80. This observation was later confirmed in several studies. A large prospective population-based study was conducted in Iceland some years ago on local residents (Hegalsson et al., 2000). Lost to follow up were really few, and the study period was extraordinary long. They found a relatively low incidence of PHN in 421 HZ patients (6.95% in subjects aged >60), followed up to 7.6 years and gave formal evidence that PHN may last for as long as 5 to 7 years in a small proportion of patients (Hegalsson et al., 2000). A Dutch study estimated an incidence of 6.5% or 2.6% according to different definitions of PHN used (pain persisting at 1 and 3 months after HZ rash onset, respectively) (Opstelten et al., 2002). A significantly higher proportion of incident cases was reported in an English study, whereby PHN incidence was calculated in a prospective sample of patients referring to general practitioners in East London (Scott et al., 2003). The authors observed a 38% incidence at 6 weeks and 27% at 3 months after rash onset. Such differences may partly be due to different definitions of PHN (as discussed below), to a proactive search for pain persistence in some prospective studies, and to the lack of data on pain severity in most studies. All these methodological issues may have well hampered reporting of cases with less intense pain persistence, making comparisons difficult, as well as a meta-analytic evaluation of the incidence of PHN hardly obtainable. Finally, a wide array of factors influencing the incidence of PHN has been described in recent years (see below). A significant variation in the distribution of such factors in different populations may well contribute to the variability in the incidence of PHN in different studies.

3. Prodromal and acute pain in herpes zoster

Moving from the epidemiological to the clinical perspective, pain in HZ is the main element as it severely impacts patients' life in the acute phase, as well as within prodromic phases and possibly during persistence after rash healing. As the predominant HZ clinical feature, pain has been described as prodromal, acute and post herpetic; more recently, some authors proposed a new classification (Jung et al., 2004) as acute, subacute and post herpetic neuralgia (120 days after rash healing). More comprehensively, however, pain can be considered as a continuum from its prodromal phase to its latest presence in post herpetic neuralgia. The definition of post herpetic neuralgia has been questioned until recently, the most important matter of discussion being the time threshold to define its onset. Pain often begins in the same area as cutaneous lesions, even before rash appearance, being the only clue possibly leading to the early diagnosis of HZ until rash appears: in this phase it is referred to as **prodromal pain**. Its characteristics are similar to that of acute pain during rash: it is described as sharping, burning, lancinating, shooting or throbbing, with a variable duration from 1-2 days up to one week (Volpi et al., 2007; Benbernou et al., 2011). It has been extensively investigated because of its important role in the diagnosis and of its predictive value for HZ severity and complications (see discussion below). A recent study (Benbernou et al., 2011) investigated prodromal pain and its burden of illness in a prospective sample of HZ patients referring to general practitioners and specialists: prodromal pain was common, occurring in almost 75% of patients aged ≥50 years, its mean duration before rash onset being 5 days and nearly half of patients rating their pain as severe. The authors clearly showed that the intensity of prodromal pain was related to the number of cutaneous lesions, as well as to the intensity of acute HZ pain. Prodromal pain is probably the clinical expression of the beginning of VZV reactivation and subsequent inflammatory responses in latently infected ganglia (Garry et al., 2005): its duration is likely to reflect the time necessary to VZV to replicate, run downwards along sensory nerve fibers, replicate in the skin and produce inflammatory damage and necrosis that is expressed in the appearance of the rash. Prodromal pain has also been associated with the risk of PHN: the higher its intensity and the longer its duration, the higher gets the probability that PHN may ensue after rash healing (Decroix et al., 2000; Jung et al., 2004; Katz et al., 2005; Volpi et al., 2008). This association may suggest that in patients destined to establish PHN replication of VZV in the ganglia and nerve fibers may be more long-lasting (Kleischmidt-Demasters & Gilden, 2001; Gilden et al., 2000). Pain accompanies the typical rash from onset to resolution. Typically, HZ appears as a monolateral dermatomeric papulo-vesicular rash, spreading proximal to distal in the involved regions (*see Figure 1*). First erythematous at its onset, rash rapidly evolves into papules and then vesicles, usually within 12-24 hours; vesicles tend to be confluent, clusters appearing more often where nerve fibers reach on skin surface (e.g. parasternal, median axillary, paravertebral; *see Figure 1.A*). They finally develop into ulcers and crusts. New waves of vesicles can ensue up to 3-7 days after rash onset in immunocompetent patients, so that lesions in different evolutive stages can be observed at the same time. Crusts detach in the following 3-4 weeks, leaving long-lasting scars and dischromic alterations in few cases. Pain has been reported as more intense when HZ is localized in the cranial dermatomes, that are involved in approximately 10 to 15 % of cases, whereas thoracic dermatomes are involved in over one half of cases (Dworkin et al., 2007). Pain can worsen into the rash phase, or it can appear for the first time in patients not experiencing prodromal pain. It has the same features as prodromal pain and may be accompanied by pruritus. The **acute phase** is dominated by a typical neuropathic pain, sharply confined along the involved dermatome(s) in the immunocompetent patient. Pain is often associated with neighboring allodynia and hyperalgesia, with an area of hypoalgesia surrounding all the involved areas. Patients often report that even a slight contact with clothes or with sheets can produce profound discomfort. Indeed in HZ this is the major cause of sleep disturbances and loss of working days. In a small proportion of patients, VZV-related pain can appear in the complete absence of cutaneous lesions, being then referred to as "zoster sine herpete": this entity has been supported by serological and molecular evidence of VZV reactivation in some acute pain syndromes, clinically very similar to HZ (Nagel et al., 2007; Dworkin et al., 2007).

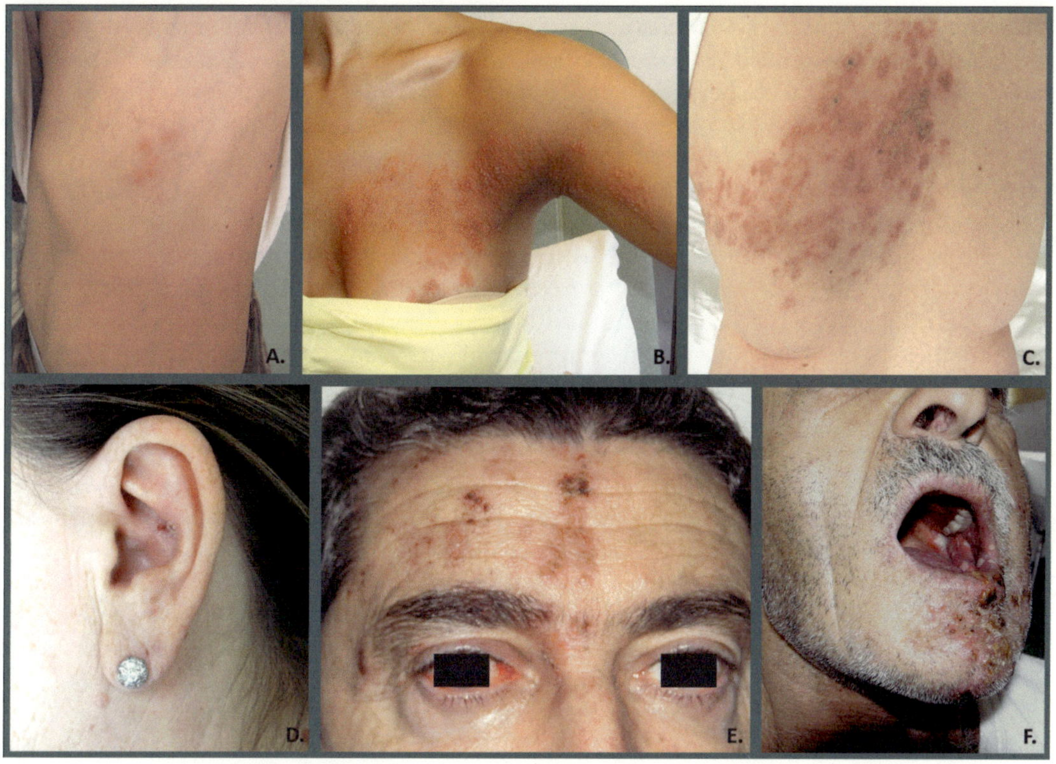

Fig. 1. Different clinical manifestations and localization of HZ rash. **A.** Minimally expressive rash, expressing in only few papules in the median axillary region. **B.** Typical dermatomeric rash, with a high number of lesions in the vesicular phase. Note that HZ rash never crosses the median line. **C.** Multidermatomeric rash, highly skin-destructing with a large number of lesions expressing in purulent vesicles; typical in immunodepressed patients. **D.** HZ oticus, vesicle within the ear. **E.** HZ ophtalmicus, involving the first branch of trigeminal nerve and the eye. **F.** Devastating maxillary HZ, involving with vesicles, crusts and ulcers the skin surface, the internal mucosa of the mouth and the tongue surface until the median line. Personal clinical experience.

4. Post herpetic neuralgia

HZ is usually a self limiting disease, with pain quenching at the end of vesicular eruptions. In a significant proportion of patients, however, it can persist or relapse months to years after rash healing, being then referred to as PHN. Pain in PHN is described as burning, throbbing or lancinating, similarly to that in acute HZ, or electric-shock-like, intermittent or continuous, sometimes associated with allodynia or hyperesthesia; it spreads along the interested dermatome(s) in the same way as during HZ. PHN has been variously defined as pain persisting or resuming 4, 6, 8, 12 weeks, and up to 6 months after rash healing. At the end of the 90's, Dworkin and Portenoy proposed a definition that was widely accepted: they set the time point for the diagnosis of PHN at 3 months after rash healing (Dworkin & Portenoy, 1996), referring to pain persisting at earlier time points as *Zoster-Associated Pain* (ZAP). More recently this definition has been revised, with a further distinction (Arani et al.,

2001; Jung et al., 2004, Niv & Maltsman-Tseikhin, 2005): pain present within 30 days from the onset of rash is defined as acute herpetic neuralgia; pain present between 30 and 120 days is defined as subacute herpetic neuralgia; pain persisting after 120 days from the onset of HZ is defined as PHN. Moreover other authors introduced the concept that only clinically relevant pain should be defined as PHN, to avoid overestimation of the problem: they proposed PHN to be defined as pain ≥3 on a 10-point VAS scale persisting 120 days after rash healing (Coplan et al., 2004; Oxman et a., 2005; Thyregod et al., 2007). All these definitions, however, introduce purely arbitrary partitions of an entity that is a continuum, from prodromal to post herpetic pain. According to this more comprehensive view, in recent years PHN has been considered and valued differently. Some authors proposed to measure its total burden with a single comprehensive parameter. Coplan et al. used an area-under-the-curve (AUC) method to combine measures of HZ pain intensity and duration (Coplan et al., 2004). The AUC was calculated by multiplying the average of two consecutive worst pain scores by the number of days between the scores. AUC highly correlated with other pain, quality-of-life and activities-of-daily-living validated questionnaires, showing its efficacy to take into account the total burden of HZ pain. This approach was developed and validated to assess and quantify HZ burden of illness (HZBOI) in the Shingles Prevention Study (Oxman et al., 2005). The prospective Italian study already quoted had a very similar approach, using verbal rating pain scores instead of worst pain scores in the calculation of AUC (Parruti et al., 2010). A recent study (Drolet et al., 2010) used a slightly different measure (HZ severity of illness, HZSOI) in which scores below 3 on a 0-to-10 scale were considered as zero, as they have been demonstrated not to affect relevantly quality of life and activities of daily living (Thyregod et al., 2007). The predictive role of HZSOI for greater acute and post herpetic pain burden was assessed in 261 HZ patients enrolled within 14 days of rash onset, strictly followed with different pain questionnaires up to 6 months (Drolet et al., 2010). Greater acute burden was significantly associated with higher pain intensity at presentation, higher number of cutaneous lesions, lower income and conditions of immunodepression. Higher acute pain severity, lower income, being immunocompromised, older age and not receiving antivirals were also predictors of greater post herpetic burden. All these attempts introduced a potentially relevant tool to better estimate the impact of HZ and PHN in real life and to thoroughly assess the cost-efficacy of preventive extensive vaccination for HZ. In this approach to ZAP and PHN, structured tools for pain assessment have been valued. Verbal rating scales, asking to the patient to define his pain as no pain, mild, moderate, intense or very intense, are easy to handle in real clinical life, but don't allow to stratify and better characterize pain. Visual Analogue Scales (VAS) have been extensively investigated and used in various settings of pain clinical management (Hao et al., 1994; Thyregod et al., 2007), allowing a more precise identification of the single patient's pain level, and being easily understood by patients. Other structured tools have been defined in recent years: McGill Pain Questionnaire and its Short Form (Melzack 2005) are widely used for pain evaluation in a consistent part of more recent studies (Melzack & Togerson, 1971; Thyregod et al., 2007; Ursini et al., 2010) as they allow to evaluate different pain dimensions (sensory, affective and mixed features). Zoster Brief Pain Inventory (ZBPI) is the more specific tool designed on-purpose for HZ pain (Coplan et al., 2004): it includes discomfort other than pain, such as itch, occurring in the same area as HZ rash. It measures the severity of pain (current, least and worst) in the last 24 hours on an 0-to-10 scale, together with HZ pain interference with various activities of daily life. This tool was shown to have a good validity in the context of ZAP and PHN (Coplan et al., 2004; Oxman et al., 2005). Both HZ and PHN have a considerable impact on patients' quality of life and daily life activities. A few studies investigated this impact, especially in recent years, in order to assess the total burden of these conditions and possibly to establish the cost-effectiveness of HZ vaccination. Poorer physical, role and social functioning and greater emotional distress was reported in a sample of 110 patients with intense acute pain in HZ (Katz et al., 2004), using a composite measure of overall pain burden in the first 30 days after rash onset. In this sample, patients experienced average pain of moderate intensity most of the time. In a multicenter prospective study enrolling 261 HZ patients followed up to 6 months, HZ had a major impact on the quality of life, especially on sleep (64%), enjoyment of life (58%) and general activities (53%). In the same study, PHN mostly affected enjoyment of life, mood and sleep (Drolet et al., 2010). An interesting study with a different methodology was conducted in Germany, enrolling patients by means of telephone interviews (Weinke et al., 2010). More than 11,000 subjects were contacted and 280 were enrolled, having experienced HZ in the previous 5 years. They were asked about ZAP and its characteristics and impact on quality of life. Both HZ and PHN had substantial impact on daily activities, mobility, work, sleep, social relationships and overall quality of life. Authors agreed that more attention should be paid to this aspect of HZ and PHN in designing research studies and health and prevention policies, as it is certainly the most important element from the patient's perspective.

The understanding of the pathophysiological mechanisms underlying the onset of chronic pain typical of PHN is still an open challenge. The initial viral replication causes direct damage by neuritic inflammation on the rear dorsal root, resulting in the involvement of the corresponding nerve and of spinal cord metamers. Necrosis of neural and scaffolding cells in the posterior root ganglia occurring during the acute phase of HZ is followed by fibrosis and destruction of nerve tissue at all levels of pain transmission, from peripheral afferent fibers to the spinal cord (Johnson, 2003; Bartley, 2009). Several studies have documented atrophy of the posterior horn in the spinal cord, fibrosis of the posterior root ganglia and loss of cutaneous innervation, with pathological degeneration of cell bodies and axons of primary afferent neurons (Dworkin et al., 2007). Therefore, patients with PHN often experience hypoesthesia (mainly as a result of peripheral denervation) and pallestesia (mainly for non-uniform loss of the various nerve fibers resulting in impaired sensory discrimination) in association with pain. Anyway, the precise mechanisms at the basis of typical pain in PHN remains still unclear and attempts to explain this by a single unifying theory elusive. The pathophysiology of PHN may involve both peripheral and central mechanisms. According to the gate control theory, a sensory input reduction from peripheral nerves starting from Aβ fibers causes an increase of Aδ and C fibers firing onto the posterior horn of the spinal cord: this last event, in turn, "opens the gate" to pain "from deafferentation". PHN, then, could be viewed as a chronic pain syndrome due to deafferentation (Oaklander et al., 2001). Other authors have tried to clarify the central mechanisms underlying the genesis and persistence of pain in PHN. Sensitized C fibers would not be responsible for hyperalgesia in PHN, but the mechanism involved would stand in the strengthening of existing synaptic connections between the central pain pathways and peripheral Aβ fibers (Baron & Saguez, 1993). The traditional theories of pain in PHN, as exposed above, have mainly focused on anatomical and functional changes of nerve cells and pain pathways. However, several studies revealed interesting aspects about CNS support cells and structures. It is known that glia (astrocytes and oligodendrocytes) and their receptors produce factors influencing neuronal functioning. A study in 2001 showed that persistent inflammation in glial cells is involved in the induction and maintenance of various conditions characterized by chronic pain (Watkins et al., 2001). At the level of the peripheral nervous system, Schwann cells and satellite cells in dorsal root ganglia of the posterior roots constitute together the peripheral glia, with many similarities with oligodendrocytes and astrocytes (Sorkin et al ., 2007). Damage of myelinated fibers would activate Schwann cells and satellite cells, releasing in turn neuro-excitatory mediators such as TNF-α (Hanani et al., 2005). According to this hypothesis, these substances would act as the mediators of neuronal damage (Oaklander et al., 1998). Other support structures putatively involved in the pathogenesis of chronic pain are *vasa nervorum* and *nervi nervorum,* which are responsible for vascular and nervous support, respectively, of the nervous system itself. All the layers of a nerve are "innervated" and have a subtle but important complex of nociceptors: *nervi nervorum* are potentially able to induce a neurogenic inflammatory reaction (Sauer et al., 1999; Bove et al. 2008), through the release of substance P, calcitonin gene-related peptide and nitric oxide, increasing permeability of *vasa nervorum* of the neighboring blood vessels (Zochodne et al., 1997; Bove et al., 2008). The hypothesis that the activation of trophic (*vasa nervorum* and *nervi nervorum*) and support structures (Schwann and satellite cells) of the peripheral nerve would play an important pathogenic role in PHN may have important therapeutic implications (Bartley, 2009). In recent years, another interesting hypothesis has been worked out. In 2003, Gilden et al. reported the case of a patient with PHN followed for 11 year (Gilden et al., 2003). In the initial phase, the detection of VZV DNA in blood mononuclear cells in 2 consecutive occasions suggested the use of antivirals in an attempt to quenching pain. In random blood assays following treatment with famciclovir, VZV DNA was not detected. The patient, however, discontinued treatment for 5 five times: on all these occasions, the VZV genome was again detectable in blood mononuclear cells and pain resumed. Considering the recurrence of VZV DNA after discontinuation of treatment in parallel with the presence of segments of the VZV genome in blood mononuclear cells, the increase of cell-mediated response to VZV and the positive clinical response to the resumption of antiviral therapy induced the authors to speculate that PHN could be supported by chronic ganglionitis induced by VZV. Although this hypothesis was based on the persistence of VZV DNA in blood mononuclear cells, the mechanisms involved in the development of this syndrome are still unknown. To this end, several studies in recent years attempted to evaluate the role of the immune system in the pathogenesis of PHN. A Chinese work published in 2009 analyzed the relationship between the trigger pro-inflammatory cytokine produced by T lymphocytes in the acute phase of HZ and the development of PHN. The 74 subjects enrolled in the study were divided into 3 groups: a first group of patients who developed PHN, a second group with HZ in the acute phase and a control group. All subjects underwent clinical evaluation of pain (by VAS) and determination of serum levels of T-lymphocyte-derived cytokines. This study showed that patients with PHN had IL-6 serum levels higher than subjects with HZ. The levels of other cytokines (TNF-α, IL-1β, IL-8) were, however, similar between the two groups. These findings would indicate that these cytokines are implicated in the pathogenesis of HZ but not in that of PHN. However IL-6, a pro-inflammatory cytokine considered an early tissue damage marker, would play an important role in the pathophysiological mechanisms underlying the development of chronic pain in PHN, as demonstrated by the correlation between serum levels of this cytokine and the VAS scores obtained in patients with PHN (Zhu et al., 2009).

The different hypotheses so far postulated are not mutually exclusive, so that the factors involved in the pathophysiology of chronic pain in PHN may well be multifactorial. Therefore, further studies are needed to link all these findings together, to allow a more comprehensive view of this severe and disrupting condition and to develop targeted therapies for PHN.

Beyond PHN, other complications of HZ have been described, although much rarer that PHN (Dworkin et al., 2007, Gilden et al., 2000,; Nagel & Gilden, 2007). All of these are related to the endothelial and vascular involvement that relapsing bursts of VZV replication in HZ may cause, having been exploratory described both in vivo and in vitro (Gilden et al., 2009). They include stroke in its extreme manifestation, that is when endothelial damage lead to large vessel occlusion(s) (Kang et al., 2009). Other neurological syndromes with a vascular genesis have been related to VZV, including large vessel granulomatous arteritis, causing multifocal encephalitis in the immunocompetent host, and small-vessel encephalitis, relatively more frequent in the immunocompromised hosts (Gilden et al., 2000, Nagel & Gilden, 2007). Transverse myelitis is another fortunately rare but invalidating expression of small vessel involvement in the spinal cord (Gilden et al., 2000). Finally, retinal necrosis may occur in a small proportion of patients (Nagel & Gilden, 2007).

In summary, the updated epidemiology and clinical appraisal of HZ manifestations generate a renewed picture of a frequent disease that has per se a very relevant impact on the quality of life and social functioning of the affected patients. Adding to that the invalidating impact of PHN, still poorly treatable and ultimately incurable, as well as the major impact of the rarer but even more serious vascular and neurological complications of HZ, the questions as to whether HZ and its complications can be predicted and prevented become of the highest clinical interest.

5. Can ZAP and PHN be predicted?

Predictors of PHN in the acute phase of HZ have been extensively investigated in order to point out patients who are at higher risk of developing this painful syndrome and need to be monitored more carefully during follow-up. ZAP gained due attention only recently, even though pain at presentation was assessed in most of trials and cohorts on HZ and PHN (Dworkin et al., 1998; Chidiac et al., 2001; Dworkin et al., 2001). Acute pain at HZ presentation is rated as severe in a consistent proportion of patients (25%, 41%, 70%, ...) and has been addressed for its impact on quality of life (Chidiac et al., 2001; Dworkin et al., 2001). Recently, an Italian study on 519 HZ patients showed that female patients who were older, present or past smokers, with a history of trauma or surgery at the site of HZ were more likely to have moderate-severe pain at HZ presentation (Parruti et al., 2010). In another Italian study on 533 HZ patients, the intensity of pain at presentation was associated with the extent of rash, presence of prodromal pain, dysesthesia, education level and depression, but not with gender, anxiety or quality of life (Volpi et al., 2007). In a Dutch study on 598 patients, female gender, younger age, severity of rash, shorter duration of rash prior to inclusion, longer duration of prodromal pain, and an anxious character were independently associated with higher intensity of acute zoster pain (Opstelten et al., 2007). Pain severity at presentation has not been investigated in other settings and more attention should be given to this element that dominates HZ clinics. More recently, acute HZ pain has been considered as a continuum and not only as a single point measure, and acute pain burden has been evaluated in a prospective study conducted across Canada (Drolet et al., 2010): greater acute burden was associated with greater pain intensity at presentation, greater number of lesions, lower income and being immunocompromised. Further studies on acute pain in different settings could be similarly useful. PHN, on the other hand, has been extensively investigated in different settings and a great deal of information is now available. PHN has been repeatedly associated with **older age** (Dworkin & Portenoy, 1996; Choo et al., 1997,; Dworkin et al., 1998; Decroix et al., 2000; Opstelten et al., 2002; Kurokawa et al., 2002; Scott et al., 2003; Jung et al., 2004; Opstelten et al., 2007; Volpi et al., 2008; Parruti et al., 2010; Drolet et al., 2010). Some decades ago, Hope-Simpson already envisaged this association observing his own HZ outpatients (Hope-Simpson, 1975), and in the following years older age has been one of the factors more frequently associated in almost all studies where it was investigated. Indeed several cohort studies (Choo et al., 1997, Dworkin et al., 1998; Decroix et al., 2000; Opstelten et al., 2002; Kurokawa et al., 2002; Scott et al., 2003; Jung et al., 2004; Opstelten et al., 2007; Volpi et al., 2008; Parruti et al., 2010; Drolet et al., 2010) found significantly older age in patients developing PHN, in samples up to 1,900 patients. The SPS placebo arm, as well, provided evidence as to the predictive role of older age: enrolled subjects were stratified in two subgroups (60-69 years and ≥70 years), and PHN incidence in the 19,247 subjects was 0.74 cases/1,000 person-years in the first subgroup and 2.13 cases/1,000 person-years in the older (Oxman et al., 2005). Central and peripheral nervous systems in the elderly may probably tolerate less efficiently the damage associated to VZV reactivation and the consequent burst of immune response (Baron et al., 1997). **Pain at presentation**, together with older age, is the other best-established risk factor for PHN (*see Figure 2 and 3*): the more severe pain is at presentation, the more frequent PHN will be. It has to be considered that there are some difficulties in lumping up data from studies using different definitions and designs: trials have larger number of patients compared to cohort studies, but cohorts allow to search for a larger number of variables, even though not all planned at the beginning of the study. Some years ago, trials on antiviral therapy for HZ suggested the importance of pain intensity at presentation in predicting PHN (Dworkin et al., 1998; Whitley et al., 1999); several cohort studies confirmed these data in real life (Decroix et al., 2000; Scott et al., 2003; Jung et al., 2004; Katz et al., 2005; Opstelten et al., 2007; Volpi et al., 2008; Parruti et al., 2010) (*see Figure 2 and 3*). The pathogenesis of this correlation is still unclear: the intensity of acute pain may reflect central structural and functional processes, such as excitotoxic damage in the dorsal horn, and damage to primary afferent nociceptors (Bennett , 1994).

Other factors have been proposed as possible predictors of PHN. **Severity of rash**, assessed as the number of lesions appearing on the patients' skin at presentation, has been significantly associated with PHN in several studies (*see Figure 3*) (Dworkin et al., 1998; Whitley et al., 1999; Nagasako et al., 2002; Kurokawa et al., 2002; Jung et al., 2004; Opstelten et al., 2007; Volpi et al., 2008). HZ patients with greater rash severity at presentation have a greater risk of PHN, suggesting a relationship between the extent of neural damage and the development of PHN; this interesting and comprehensive hypothesis, however, has not been yet demonstrated (Nagasako et al., 2002). In a recent survey, rash severity was correlated with age and immunodepression but not with use of steroids and diabetes (Tontodonati, unpublished personal data). The presence of **prodromal symptoms** (pain, dysesthesia, allodynia, …) and their duration before the appearance of rash had a negative predictive value for PHN of 95% (Jung et al., 2004; Volpi et al., 2007; Decroix et al., 2000; Katz et al., 2005): this association may reflect a more intense involvement of nerve fibers by

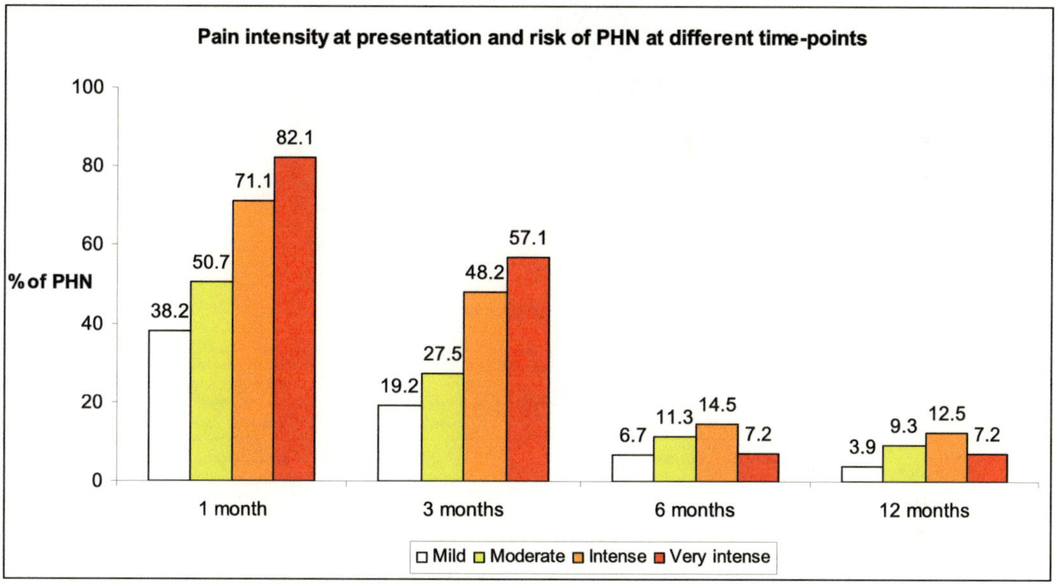

Fig. 2. Pain intensity at presentation and risk of PHN at different time-points. Pain at presentation predicts PHN: the higher pain at HZ presentation is, the higher risk of developing PHN will be (Parruti et al., 2010, with permission).

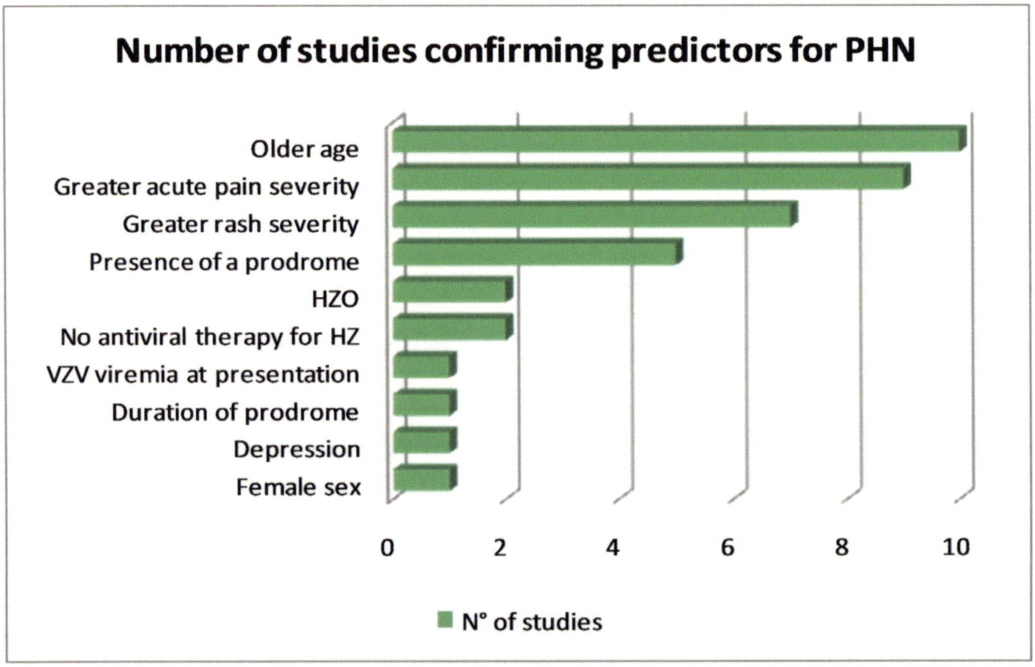

Authors	Patients	Design	PHN definition
Choo 1997	821 HZ – PHN n.d.	Retrospective	Pain persisting 1m and 2m after rash onset
Dworkin 1998	419 HZ – 129 (n.d.) PHN	Famciclovir trial	Pain following rash healing, 1 (and 3) m after HZ diagnosis
Whitley 1999	n.d.	Acyclovir and prednisone trial	Time to cessation of acute neuritis (Cox)
Decroix 2000	1897 HZ – PHN n.d	Open-label valacyclovir trial	Time to cessation of ZAP (Cox)
Opstelten 2002	837 HZ – 54 PHN	Retrospective	Pain 1m after HZ diagnosis
Nagasako 2002	1778 HZ – PHN n.d.	4 famciclovir trials	Pain present 3m after rash onset
Kurokawa 2002	263 HZ – PHN n.d	Prospective	Pain persisting >3m-6m after HZ diagnosis
Scott 2003	278 HZ – 42 (78) PHN	Prospective	Pain present at 6w (and 3m) after HZ diagnosis
Jung 2004	965 HZ – 114 PHN	2 famciclovir trials	Pain persisting 120d after rash onset
Katz 2005	129 HZ – 20 PHN	Prospective	Pain persisting 120d after rash onset
Opstelten 2007	598 HZ – 46 PHN	Prospective (in the PINE study)	Pain ≥30/100 VAS 3m after HZ diagnosis
Volpi 2008	219 HZ – 70 PHN	Prospective	Pain present 6m after HZ diagnosis
Parruti 2010	519 HZ – 226 (130) PHN	Prospective	Pain persisting / relapsing 1 (and 3) m after HZ diagnosis

Fig. 3. Evidence confirming predictors of PHN. Several studies with different size and designs have investigated predictors of PHN. Older age and greater pain at presentation are the best well-established risk factors, emerging in most studies with no regards to different designs.

Viral reactivation in the early phases of HZ, leading to extended damage and PHN (Watson et al., 1991). Uncertainties still remain about **antiviral therapy** for preventing the occurrence of PHN in ordinary clinical settings. Most data come from clinical trials where antivirals were administered ≤72 hours from the onset of rash: this could have been a bias as most patients in real practice seek for medical attention after 72 hours (Volpi et al., 2008), antivirals being anyhow prescribed usually in the first 7 days from rash onset. As a consequence, the preventive role of antiviral therapy has been questioned until recently: a recent meta-analysis including most of these trials concluded that the role of therapy in preventing PHN is still uncertain (Li et al., 2009). However, different data came from different study designs. Conflicting results emerged even in trials on antivirals (Gnann, 2007): in a famciclovir trial (Dworkin et al., 1998), treatment of acute HZ significantly reduced both the incidence and the duration of PHN, whatever defined. A recent cohort prospective study (Parruti et al., 2010) collected all the incident cases of HZ in a specifically created network of General Practitioners and Hospital Centers in a local health service in Central Italy, resuming data from 519 cases on an estimated reference population of nearly 35,000 persons. In multivariate analyses for both PHN and the total pain burden due to HZ and PHN, PHN appeared to be significantly more frequent in patients who did not receive antiviral therapy and total ZAP was much higher in this small proportion of patients. Indeed, antiviral therapy is now largely prescribed for its documented positive effect in reducing viral shedding, new vesicular eruptions and pain intensity in the acute phase of HZ; these results suggest that antiviral therapy may be useful even in reducing the incidence of PHN and total ZAP. Further studies are needed, however, as the best way to assess this point would be an on purpose designed RCT. **Localization of HZ** has been associated with PHN, being more frequent in ophthalmic and thoracic zoster (Volpi et al., 2008). Serological and laboratory findings have been investigated, in order to identify novel predictors among elements easily accessible in a blood sample, as specific antibodies or VZV viremia. A prospective observational cohort study collecting HZ cases occurring among a network of General Practitioners in East London (Scott et al., 2003) suggested that higher levels of VZV DNA at HZ presentation may be a strong independent predictor of pain persistence (*see Figure 3*). **Surgical interventions** and **mechanical trauma** have been suggested as predictors of VZV reactivation, but their possible role in predicting PHN has been poorly investigated. In a recent prospective survey on 519 HZ patients (Parruti et al., 2010), trauma and surgical interventions were associated with higher pain intensity at presentation, only trauma being associated with a higher risk of PHN. Furthermore **cigarette smoking** has been scantly evaluated as a possible risk factor for pain intensity at presentation or PHN. In the same survey (Parruti et al., 2010), it was associated with both higher pain at presentation and higher risk of PHN, probably due to the prospective and proactive nature of the investigation. Indeed, smoking has not been searched for PHN prediction in other studies, in spite of data suggesting a possible role in chronic pain syndromes (Weingarten et al., 2008), subclinical peripheral neuropathy (Agrawal et al., 2007) and smoke-induced impairment of cell-mediated immunity (Sopori & Zozak, 1998). Further studies are needed to confirm these interesting and novel predictors. **Psychosocial factors** have been proposed to be associated both with a higher ZAP burden and higher risk of PHN. Depression, together with the severity of HZ disease at presentation, was associated with higher pain intensity and ZAP burden (Volpi et al., 2007). In a small prospective study (Dworkin et al., 1992), greater anxiety, greater depression, lower life satisfaction and greater disease conviction were predictors at baseline for chronic zoster pain. In a large prospective sample of HZ patients in the Netherlands (Opstelten et al., 2007), investigating different psychological predictors for PHN, only trust in healthcare was associated with PHN risk, that is patients who expect that others will find remedies to their own pain could have a higher incidence of chronic pain. Hence, psychological factors may be useful in evaluating patients with HZ, even though further studies are needed. Finally, **female sex** has been proposed as a predictor of PHN, not yet reaching, however, a convincing level of evidence so far (Jung et al., 2004; Volpi et al., 2008; Parruti et al., 2010).

6. What is the best therapy for acute HZ to control ZAP and PHN?

6.1 Antiviral therapy

HZ is a self limiting disease, as patient's immune response usually contains viral replication. Treatment of the acute phase with antiviral drugs is widely recommended at present to contain vesicular eruption and diffusion and to reduce acute pain and malaise in the affected patients. The FDA approved acyclovir, valacyclovir (prodrug of acyclovir), famcyclovir (prodrug of penciclovir) and brivudin for HZ therapy. All these molecules are nucleoside analogues needing phosphorylation from viral thymidin-kinase. Their triphosphate forms inhibit viral DNA synthesis by competing as a substrate for viral DNA polymerase (Gnann, 2007). There have been no serious adverse reactions to these drugs, nausea and headache being the most common side effects in 10-20% of patients (Gnann, 2007). Dosage reduction is required in patients with renal insufficiency according to creatinine serum levels because of their renal excretion. Clinical trials did not find any difference in their cutaneous and analgesic effect. In clinical practice, however, some factors should be considered in the choice of HZ antiviral therapy. Acyclovir is the cheapest antiviral, with 5 doses of 800 mg per day necessary to achieve adequate serum levels. Therapy with acyclovir should last for 7-10 days. Furthermore acyclovir is the only one available in parenteral formulation. Valacyclovir has a higher bio-availability, allowing 3 doses of 1,000 mg per day for 7 days. Famcyclovir recommended schedule for HZ is 500 mg 3 times daily for 7 days. Brivudin can be prescribed once daily, 125 mg for 7 days. Valacyclovir, famcyclovir and brivudin have been shown to achieve higher blood concentration, compared with acyclovir. This may be relevant, due to physiological barriers hampering antiviral penetration in VZV-infected tissues (nervous tissue, CNS) and to relatively poor sensitivity of VZV to these drugs. Pharmacokinetic differences among drugs may be relevant as to their impact on patient's compliance to therapy, always related to final efficacy. Oral antiviral therapy for HZ is widely recommended for all immunocompetent patients aged ≥50 years, with moderate to severe pain intensity at presentation, as they have been shown to have higher risk of complications. However, given the safety profile of antivirals, and the persistent risk of complications even in patients with no demonstrated risk factors, antiviral therapy is recommended at present for every patient with HZ onset to reduce the duration of viral shedding, promote resolution of skin lesions, and limit the duration of pain (Gnann, 2007). Most trials in the literature considered antivirals as worth prescribing only <72 hours from rash onset. This time-points, however, do not necessarily reflect the end of viral replication in the skin. In clinical practice nearly half of patients get to medical observation and start antiviral therapy within this time-point, the others starting in general within the first 7 days from rash onset (Volpi et al., 2007; Parruti et al., 2010). A recent trial on 156 HZ patients, investigating the effect of antiviral therapy started

before and after 72 hours from rash onset, showed no significant difference in pain reduction, healing of lesions and PHN incidence (Rasi et al., 2010), thus providing valuable evidence for prescription of antivirals even beyond the 72-hour threshold. In immunocompromised patients with a higher incidence of HZ per se, antiviral therapy reduces dissemination, severity of disease and mortality. Acyclovir is the first choice in its intravenous formulation, 10-15 mg/kg every 8 hours, to administer up to 7 days after the ending of new vesicular eruptions or until healing is complete (Gnann, 2007). Valacyclovir in immunocompromised patients has been valued in a small trial (Arora et al., 2008). Its use needs further evidence, acyclovir remaining the best recommended drug in such patients.
The end of viral replication is the main aim of antiviral therapy in acute HZ: this objective should be pursued in parallel with the attempt to reduce the pain perceived, which mainly influences patient's quality of life. The classes of drugs currently available for this purpose are the following: corticosteroids, tricyclic antidepressants, anticonvulsants, opioid analgesics.

6.2 Corticosteroids

Although corticosteroids have limited effectiveness in reducing chronic pain, they may have some beneficial effect on acute pain: a number of studies in the literature have shown their positive action in association with antiviral therapy. The addition of prednisolone to the treatment with acyclovir was effective in reducing pain, in accelerating the regression of skin lesions and facilitating the return of the patient to normal daily activities (Whitley et al., 1996). Dworkin et al. (Dworkin et al., 2007) have shown that the use of corticosteroids in combination with antiviral therapy reduced the time to return to a restful sleep and normal activities of daily life and the use of analgesics. The German Society of Dermatology recommended the use of corticosteroids in acute herpetic pain, based on the results of two large prospective studies that showed the efficacy of high-dose corticosteroids is association with antiviral therapy both in alleviating Zoster - related pain and in accelerating rash healing (Gross et al., 2003). No study has, however, showed a preventive role of corticosteroids for PHN.

6.3 Tricyclic antidepressants (TCAs)

Tricyclic antidepressants (amitriptyline, nortriptyline) have a documented effect in the treatment of neuropathic pain syndromes, but their use in the acute phase of HZ has not yet been adequately investigated. In fact, although TCAs reduce pain by inhibiting reuptake of serotonin and norepinephrine (Stankus et al., 2000), they require at least 3 months to exert positive effects. In a randomized trial of patients older than 60 years, it was observed that 25 mg amiptriptyline, administered within 48 hours of rash onset and continued for 90 days, yielded a 50% reduction in pain at 6 months compared to placebo (Bowsher, 1997). In this context, it is important to emphasize that such drugs should be used with extreme caution, taking into account the severe anticholinergic side effects associated with their use, as they may precipitate an acute confusional state and may cause cardiac arrhythmias up to sudden cardiac death, especially in elderly patients (Wareham & Breuer, 2007).

6.4 Opioids

Opioid analgesics, such as oxycodone, morphine and tramadol are widely used in acute herpetic pain, often in combination with acetaminophen (paracetamol) or other nonsteroidal anti-inflammatory drugs (NSAIDs). However, among these drugs, only oxycodone and tramadol have been the subject of studies specifically designed for acute herpetic pain. Oxycodone reduces acute pain, but there is yet no evidence of a possible role of this drug in the prevention of PHN. A recent randomized placebo-controlled trial compared the effectiveness of oxycodone and gabapentin in reducing acute pain, showing that oxycodone provided a greater pain relief (Dworkin et al., 2009). Tramadol, however, is effective in the treatment of PHN, but its efficacy in the treatment of acute herpetic pain has not been evaluated (Boureau et al., 2003).

6.5 Antiepileptics

Among the antiepileptic drugs, pregabalin and gabapentin have a demonstrated effect on chronic neuropathic pain, documented in several clinical studies and lack of significant side effects or drug interactions. Based on these data and considering the effectiveness of these drugs in other conditions of acute pain, gabapentinoids are also used for acute herpetic pain. Berry et al. showed that gabapentin reduced acute HZ pain (Berry et al., 2005). Preliminary evidences suggest a similar efficiency of pregabalin, in conjunction with an even better tolerability profile (Jensen-Dahm et al., 2011). Further prospective and on purpose designed evaluations, however, appear opportune before their use for acute herpetic pain may be widely recommended.

6.6 Nerve blocks

Use of nerve block injections is another option in the conventional medical armamentary for acute herpetic pain. Local anaesthetics may be injected around the affected nerves, providing immediate pain relief, typically lasting 12-24 hours (Roxas, 2005). Location of the nerve block is dependent on the involved dermatome. If head, neck or arms are affected, a stellate ganglion block is performed, with injections placed at the base of the neck, just above the collarbone. Dermatomal patterns involving chest, trunk or lower extremities are addressed via epidural blocks. Long term relief can be accomplished by repeating the procedure 2-3 times within a two-week period, provided it is administered at an early stages of the disease (Roxas, 2005). Although epidural, intrathecal, and sympathetic nerve blocks have all been used in the treatment of pain caused by HZ and PHN, the effectiveness of nerve blocks in reducing or preventing PHN is still somewhat controversial (Johnson, 1997). However, there are a few controlled randomized trials of nerve blocks in the prevention of PHN. Yanagida et al. reported no prophylactic effect of early sympathetic blockade on PHN (Yanagida et al., 1987). Two randomized trials have been performed for the prevention of PHN by single or repetitive epidural injections of anesthetics and steroids in the acute HZ (van Wijck et al., 2006; Pasqualucci et al., 2000). Van Wijck et al. showed no significant effect of epidural injections in reducing the incidence of PHN; Pasqualucci et al. reported that repetitive epidural administration of bupivacaine and methylprednisolone was significantly more effective in preventing PHN at 12 months compared with acyclovir and prednisolone. More recently, Genlin and colleagues examined the effectiveness of repetitive paravertebral injections with local anaesthetics and steroids for the prevention of PHN in patients with acute HZ. The findings of this randomized study show that repetitive paravertebral injections with bupivacaine and methylprednisolone in acute herpetic phase within 7 days of rash onset reduce the incidence of PHN more effectively than standard treatments (oral administration of acyclovir and analgesics) (Genlin et al., 2009). This preliminary evidence, in conclusion, would suggest that the repetition of the blockade procedure may be crucial to the long-term efficacy of ZAP control. Further data, however, are auspicable.

6.7 Other treatment options

In addition to the use of the above mentioned medications, alternative medical practices have been recently investigated for controlling acute herpetic pain (Ursini et al, 2011; Fleckenstein et al., 2009). Acupuncture, an ancient form of medicine that originated in China several thousand years ago, has been used by Canadian physicians since the 1970s. Research on the neurophysiology of acupuncture analgesia supports the theory that it is primarily mediated via the selective release of neuropeptides in the central nervous system. Furthermore, evidence is rapidly accumulating on the immunomodulating actions of acupuncture, as well as on its effects on neuroendocrine regulation, muscle and cardiovascular tone and the psycho-emotional sphere (Rapson et al., 2008). Acupuncture has long been regarded as an effective therapy for pain management in different conditions. Although several reports documented its use in HZ and PHN (Coghlan, 1992; He et al., 2007), sizes in investigated samples were generally very small. A recent three-armed, partially blinded trial, known as ACUZoster, which is still ongoing and whose study protocol was recently published, represents the first randomized, controlled study attempting to directly compare acupuncture and standard analgesia (gabapentin) for acute herpetic pain (Fleckenstein et al., 2009). The first evidence of a potential role of acupuncture in the treatment of acute herpetic pain was provided by a randomized, controlled, open-label trial (Ursini et al., 2011). Patients with intense or very intense pain at presentation of HZ were randomized to receive acupuncture or standard pharmacological treatment. Despite the limited dimensions of the study populations (105 patients randomized, 66 patients treated), no significant differences in pain reduction after 4 weeks of treatment between the two study arms were evidenced Furthermore, under the assumption that acupuncture may have an immune-modulating activity (Quirico et al., 1996; Yan et al., 1991), evaluation of the incidence of PHN at 3, 6 and 12 months after rash onset, as well as of the total pain burden during follow-up, might have revealed an ability of this medical tool to influence the rate of pain persistence and relapses. However, the incidence of PHN at 3, 6 and 12 months, as well as the mean pain burden during follow-up, were overlapping in the 2 arms. Given that patients treated with acupuncture carry a lower risk of cumulative drug toxicity, should these findings be confirmed by the ensuing ACUZoster trial and/or by other investigations, acupuncture might be appropriately considered among the available therapeutic options for the control of severe acute HZ related pain.

6.8 Synthetic approach to acute herpetic pain

Under a practical point of view, the approach to the patient can be summarized as follows (Dworkin et al., 2007): in patients with mild to moderate pain, pain therapy may be based on the use of paracetamol or other NSAIDs, possibly associated with mild opioids as codeine; antiviral therapy should be added whatever the time interval between pain onset and patient's presentation (Dworkin et al., 2007; Parruti et al., 2010). In patients with moderate to severe pain, pain therapy should consider fist-line opioid analgesics (oxycodone), which can be administered in combination with gabapentin or pregabalin, nortriptyline or corticosteroids, associated in various possible combinations for those patients who do not respond promptly to single agent therapy. Only in severe pain, uncontrolled by antiviral and analgesic combinations, the use of nerve blocks may be taken into account, and better practised repeatedly (Dworkin et al., 2007). The acquisition of a growing body of evidence in favour of the effectiveness of acupuncture may make the management of acute herpetic pain (and PHN, as described below) even more complex, allowing the patient suffering with VZV-related painful conditions to be eligible for acupuncture, in addition to conventional therapy *(see Figure 4)*.

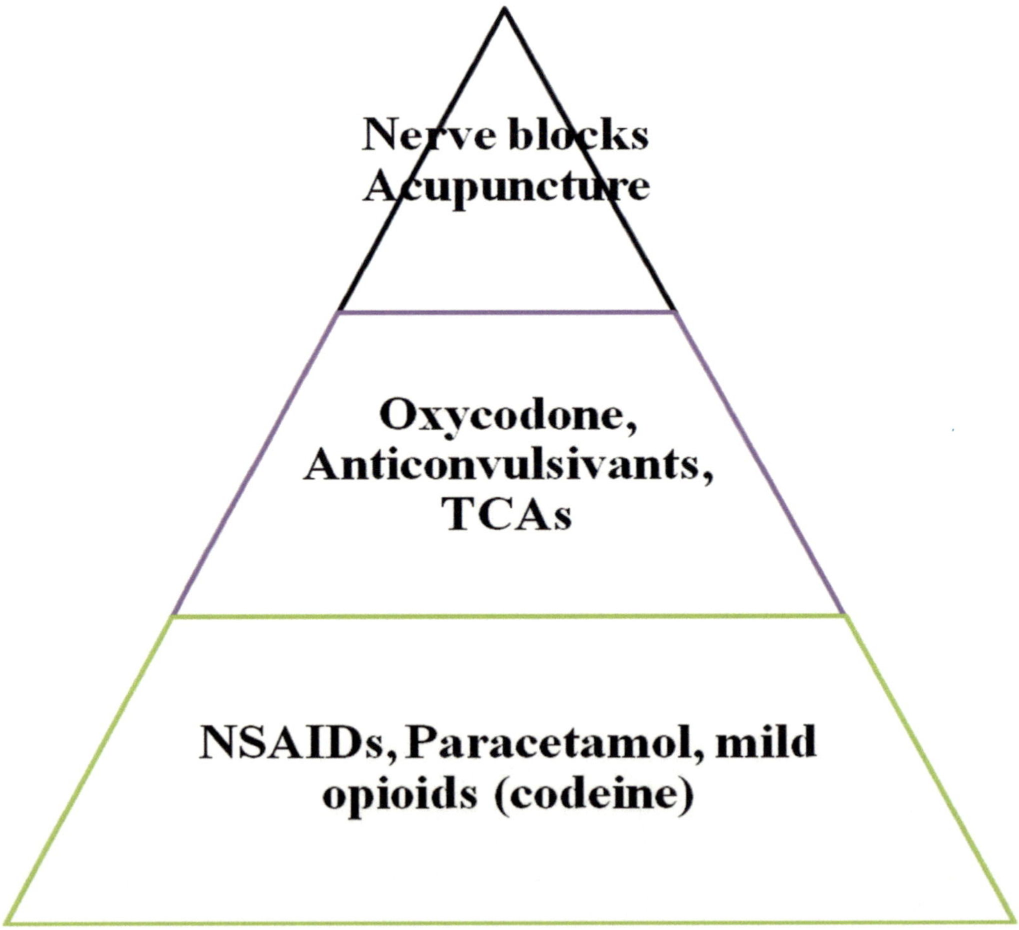

Fig. 4. Step-by-step strategy for management of acute herpetic pain.

Finally, it is important to underline that antiviral therapy can now be regarded as a cornerstone in the treatment of ZAP, according to recent acquired data on the genesis of pain and its persistence (Dworkin et al., 2007; Parruti et al., 2010).

7. What is the best therapy for PHN?

A large body of evidence indicates that some pharmacologic agents, including opioids, TCAs, antiepileptic drugs and lidocaine patches, may result in at least partial pain relief for a significant but limited proportion of patients with PHN, and that some of these patients may find the adverse effects of the above medications outweighing their benefits (Hempenstall et al., 2005; Wu & Raja, 2008). Therefore, the most formidable challenge in the framework of HZ is the treatment of PHN. The lack of fully effective treatments stands in the nature of PHN, whose exact patho-physiological mechanisms are still elusive. Consequently, it is difficult to establish specifically targeted therapies, a task calling for further research efforts. Indeed, as this condition does not adequately respond in many cases to none of the conventional agents tested, many efforts are ongoing even in the field of alternative therapeutic options. The management of PHN, however, is and will be complex, requiring a multidisciplinary approach, including drug therapy and non-pharmacological adjunctive therapies.

7.1 Antidepressants

Several systematic reviews indicate that TCAs are effective in neuropathic pain and PHN (Attal et al., 2010; Hempenstall et al., 2005; Niv & Maltsman-Tseikhin, 2005), being superior to Selective Serotonin Reuptake Inhibitors (SSRI) (Attal et al., 2006; Saarto & Wiffen, 2010). No studies assessed the use of Serotonin-Noradrenalin Reuptake Inhibitors (SNRI) for this condition. It is believed that TCAs have an analgesic action by blocking the re-uptake of serotonin and norepinephrine, a blockade enhancing the inhibition of spinal cord neurons involved in pain perception (Basmaum & Fields, 1978). Among this class, the most commonly used compounds are amitriptyline, nortriptyline and desipramine. Amitriptyline led to a reduction in pain in 47-66% of patients, desipramine and nortriptyline in 55% to 63% (Schamder, 2001; Watson et al., 1998). Nortriptyline and desipramine are generally preferred to amitriptyline because of lower incidence of anticholinergic side effects such as sedation, orthostatic hypotension, cognitive decline, and constipation (Watson et al., 1998). Furthermore, despite amitriptyline is probably the most widely studied TCA for the treatment of PHN, nortriptyline and desipramine have recently been shown to be equally effective (Watson & Oaklander, 2002; Hempenstall et al., 2005; Rowbotham et al., 2005). A limiting factor in the clinical use of TCAs is represented by their side effects, including dry mouth, fatigue, dizziness, sedation, constipation, urinary retention, and palpitations. Other side effects include orthostatic hypotension, weight gain, blurred vision, and QT prolongation. Such side effects may be of particular concern in the elderly population and in patients with a history of cardiac arrhythmia or ischemic heart disease. Although there is no standard guidance for ECG screening prior to their administration, TCAs may cause ECG changes (prolonged QT) and it may be prudent to obtain a baseline ECG in patients with cardiac disease (Sansone et al., 2002; Vieweg et al., 2003; Dworkin & Schmader, 2003).

7.2 Antiepileptics

Among anticonvulsants, gabapentin and pregabalin have established efficacy in PHN, several trials showing the non inferiority of gabapentin versus nortriptyline (Gilron et al., 2009; Hempenstall et al., 2005). Although the precise mechanism of analgesia of gabapentin is uncertain, it is believed that gabapentin may act at the $\alpha 2\delta$ subunits of voltage-dependent channels to decrease calcium influx, which in turn inhibits the release of neurotransmitters (such as glutamate) from the central terminals of primary afferent fibers in the spinal cord (Fink et al., 2002). Several randomized controlled trials (RCTs) and a few meta-analyses have established the analgesic efficacy of gabapentin for the treatment of pain in PHN. RCTs have shown that a daily dose of 1800-3600 mg given for 1-2 weeks, is effective in reducing pain and improving sleep, mood and patients' quality of life (Rowbotham et al., 1998; Rice et al., 2001; Johnson, 2003). More recent studies have shown that a dose of 3600 mg daily can reduce pain by 43% (Niv & Maltsman-Tseikhin, 2005). The main reported side effects are drowsiness, dizziness, ataxia, mild peripheral edema, and a worsening of cognitive impairment in elderly patients. To reduce adverse events and increase compliance, gabapentin should be initially used at lower doses (100-300 mg in a single dose at bedtime) and then continued at a dose of 100-300 mg three times a day (Mustafa et al., 2009), titring the analgesic effect and the occurrence of side effects (Dworkin & Schmader, 2003). Adjustment of its dose on the basis of renal function tests is also recommended, since the drug is excreted unchanged in urine (Johnson, 2003). Among gabapentinoids, both gabapentin and pregabalin are likely to provide analgesia by a similar mechanism of action. Although there are no meta-analyses examining the analgesic efficacy of pregabalin in PHN, there are a few RCTs in support. In 2004, the use of pregabalin for the treatment of diabetic neuropathy and PHN was approved in Europe and the United States. A randomized controlled trial in 2004 showed the effectiveness of this drug in the treatment of PHN: pregabalin was superior to placebo in reducing pain and improving mood, pain interference with sleep and patients' quality of life (Sabatowski et al., 2004). Pregabalin was well tolerated even by elderly patients. The commonly reported side effects were drowsiness, dizziness and mild peripheral edema. Studies conducted to date have shown an analgesic efficacy and good tolerability profile at doses of 150/600 mg, administered in 2 or 3 daily doses. The optimal dose to be administered, however, has not yet been thoroughly assessed. Other recently studied antiepileptic drugs are sodium divalproate and oxcarbazepine, which demonstrated a significant efficacy in reducing pain and improving patients' quality of life (Criscuolo et al., 2005; Kochar et al., 2005). Both of them have shown a good safety profile, with few side effects (dizziness and nausea, in particular). The use of other anticonvulsants such as phenytoin, carbamazepine, lamotrigine and sodium valproate for PHN is not adequately supported by the literature.

7.3 Opioids

Although opioid analgesics are accepted as a cornerstone for the treatment of nociceptive and cancer pain, their role in the management of chronic neuropathic pain such as that of PHN has been debated, as some clinicians consider neuropathic pain to be resistant to the analgesic effects of opioids. The controversy over their efficacy in relieving neuropathic pain reflects the use of multiple definitions and pain assessment methodologies for neuropathic pain in experimental trials and interindividual differences in opioid responsiveness (Wu & Raja, 2008). In addition, many other factors, such as opioid-related side effects, development of tolerance, exaggerated fear of addiction, and differences in governmental health policies contribute to such controversy (Wu & Raja, 2008). In spite of that, opioids may be considered as part of a comprehensive plan for the treatment of PHN (Cohen et al., 2006; Niv & Maltsman-Tseikhin, 2005; Johnson, 2003; Dworkin & Schmader, 2003), when pain is moderate to severe, with significant impact on quality of life after proven inefficacy of first-line agents. Among the investigated formulations, oxycodone, morphine, fentanyl, buprenorphine, methadone, and weaker opioids such as dihydrocodeine and tramadol were found to be effective. Treatment should be started with a short-acting opioid, replaced after 1-2 weeks with a long-acting formulation (controlled-release morphine, controlled-release oxycodone, methadone, transdermal fentanyl) when the first was not fully effective. Constipation, nausea, and sedation are common adverse effects associated with opioid use for chronic neuropathic pain. Tramadol has a unique pharmacological profile, which makes it one of the most effective drug of its class in controlling neuropathic pain. It is a synthetic derivative of codeine with a dual mechanism of action: one of the opioid type (is a weak μ receptors agonist), and the other similar to that of TCAs (inhibition of norepinephrine and serotonin reuptake). An additional way of action of this compound consists in activating post-synaptic α2 adrenergic receptors. Such an activation results in a block of transmission of nociceptive stimuli to the central level. Several studies have shown the effectiveness of tramadol in reducing neuropathic pain, particularly PHN and diabetic neuropathy (Hempenstall et al., 2005; Boreau et al., 2003; Harati et al., 1998). As side effects, tramadol may causes nausea, vomiting, dizziness, constipation, drowsiness and headache; it also increases the risk of serotonin syndrome in patients using antidepressants such as SSRIs, TCAs or inhibitors of mono-amino oxidase in combination (Christo et al., 2007) *(see Table 1).*

DRUG	INITIAL DOSAGE	TITRATION	ADVERSE EFFECTS
TCAs	10 mg every evening	Increase by 10 mg every 7 days to 50 mg, then to 100 mg and then to 150 mg nightly	Sedation, xerostomia, confusion, weight gain, dizziness
GABAPENTIN	100 mg three times daily	100-300 mg increases every 5 days to total dose of 1800-3600 mg/day	Somnolence, dizziness, ataxia, fatigue
PREGABALIN	75 mg twice daily	Increase to 150 mg twice daily within 1 week	Somnolence, dizziness
OXICODONE sustained-release	10 mg every 12 hours	As needed for pain while balancing analgesia and adverse effects	Nausea, constipation, sedation, cognitive dysfunction, hormonal changes
Transdermal FENTANYL	12 μg/hour, changed every 3 days	As needed for pain while balancing analgesia and adverse effects	Nausea, constipation, sedation, cognitive dysfunction, skin irritation, hormonal changes
Transdermal BUPRENORPHINE	35 μg/hour, changed every 3 days	As needed for pain while balancing analgesia and adverse effects	Nausea, constipation, sedation, cognitive dysfunction, skin irritation, hormonal changes
Immediate-release TRAMADOL	50 mg/day	Increase by 50 mg every 3-4 days to total dose between 100-400 mg/day divided dose	Nausea, emesis, dizziness, vertigo, somnolence, headache, constipation

Table 1. Summary of effective systemic drugs for PHN. Initial dosage, titration and adverse effects are reported.

7.4 Topical therapies

Local anesthetics may provide analgesia in neuropathic pain states, where an accumulation of neuronal-specific sodium channels may contribute to pain, including that of PHN (Mao & Chen, 2000). Topical treatments including lidocaine patches and capsaicin cream/patches have been studied for the treatment of PHN (Niv & Maltsman-Tseikhin, 2005). Topical adhesive patches containing 5% lidocaine (700 mg) have been used for the treatment of PHN with benefit (Comer & Lamb, 2000). Although there are few studies on their efficacy, the available clinical trials in patients with allodynia suggest that lidocaine is effective in providing pain relief with minimal systemic absorption and few side effects, the most frequent being mild skin irritation at the side of application (Khaliq et al., 2007; Binder et al., 2009; Hans et al., 2009). Furthermore, patients may respond well to topical lidocaine even if the skin is completely deprived of nociceptors (Wasner et al., 2005).

Capsaicin, the pungent ingredient in hot chili pepper, results in excitation of nociceptive afferents when applied topically. However, repeated application of capsaicin results in desensitization of unmyelinated epidermal nerve fibers and hypoalgesia (Nolano et al., 1999; Knotkova et al., 2008). Low-concentration (0.025% or 0.075) capsaicin creams have demonstrated efficacy in the topical treatment of PHN and neuropathic pain conditions (Knotkova et al., 2008). Recently, a high-concentration (8%) synthetic capsaicin dermal patch has been developed with the aim of providing more rapid and long-lasting pain relief after a single application. Banckonja et al. (Backonja et al., 2009) evidenced that a one-off application of high concentration (8%) of capsaicin patch for 60 minutes was more effective than a low concentration patch over 12 weeks. Adverse events reported were local reactions at the application site (pain, erythema). Therefore, as evidenced by a Cochrane review, capsaicin either as repeated application of a low dose (0.075%) cream, or even a single application of a high dose (8%) patch may provide a good degree of pain relief to some patients with painful neuropathic conditions (Derry et al., 2009). Capsaicin dermal patches have been approved in the EU for the treatment of peripheral neuropathic pain in non-diabetic adults either alone or in combination with other pain medications. Capsaicin dermal patches are also approved in the US only for management of neuropathic pain associated with PHN (McCormack, 2010).

7.5 Interventional management

A wide variety of interventional options, such as sympathetic and other nerve block, intrathecal injections and spinal cord stimulations have been analyzed as potential treatments for PHN. Interventional options are part of a comprehensive (invasive e non invasive) strategy for the treatment of PHN (*see Figure 5*). Selective sympathetic nerve blocks have been one of the more common interventional strategies used for pain relief for both acute HZ and PHN. Although the precise mechanisms by which the sympathetic nervous system contributes to neuropathic pain are unclear, experimental data indicate that abnormal activation of the α-adrenergic receptors in primary afferent neurons, direct interactions between primary afferent neurons and efferent sympathetic nerves resulting from neuronal regeneration and sprouting after nerve injury and tissue trauma may all contribute to sympathetically mediated pain (Janig et al., 1996; Wu et al., 2000). The incidence of severe complications from sympathetic nerve blocks is extremely low and, depending on the location of the nerve block, may consist of local anesthetic toxicity (such as seizures), pneumothorax, intraspinal/neuraxial injection, or neurologic injury (van Wijck et al., 2010; Wu & Raja, 2008). Some data suggest a link between sympathetic activity and pain in PHN, as patients with PHN demonstrate increased levels of pain and worsening of their allodynia after local administration of adrenergic agonists (Choi et al., 1997). Thus, administration of sympathetic nerve blocks may theoretically interrupt the sympathetic-sensory interactions contributing to pain of HZ and PHN. Sympathetic nerve blocks for the treatment of PHN were evaluated mainly in retrospective studies. In a few of them, a reduction in pain was initially noted, but this effect was not maintained in the long run. Therefore, there is inadequate evidence for a long-term effect of sympathetic nerve blocks in PHN (van Wijck et al., 2010; Wu & Raja, 2008; Wu et al., 2000).

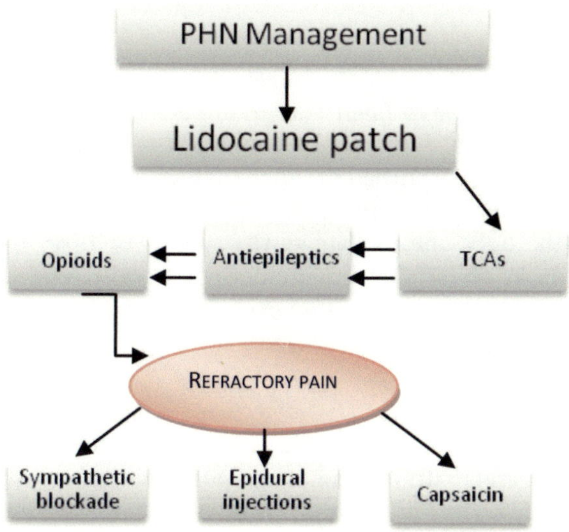

Fig. 5. Strategy for management of PHN.

Use of epidural blocks (through injections of corticosteroids with or without local anesthetics) has been reported for the treatment of acute HZ (Ahn et al., 2001) as an effective treatment shortening the total duration and reducing the severity of pain in combination with antiviral agent. A single epidural injection of steroids and local anesthetics in the acute phase of HZ may have a modest effect in reducing zoster-associated pain for 1 month after injection and is not effective for prevention of PHN. Furthermore, the value of epidural injections for the treatment of existing PHN has not been evaluated (van Wijck et al., 2010).

Continuous infusions of analgesic agents (typically an opioid or local anesthetic) via an externalized intrathecal catheter or internalized intrathecal pump may also be used for the treatment of PHN, although no controlled trials examining the analgesic efficacy of these modalities are available (Angel et al., 1998; Nitescu et al., 1998).

In extreme cases, refractory to all treatment options, other interventional strategies were described in the literature. Although there are limitations in the quality and quantity of available data, current evidence suggests that Spinal Cord Stimulation be effective in the management of severe neuropathic pain (Grabow et al., 2003).

The effect of subcutaneous injections, transcutaneous nerve stimulations, percutaneous nerve stimulations, and radiofrequency on HZ and PHN has not been established. There is minor anecdotal evidence for the efficacy of these techniques, and the risk for complications, such as exacerbation of pain, is unknown. There are no controlled studies for any of these interventional procedures (van Wijck et al., 2010).

Reported surgical options for PHN include trigeminal or spinal peripheral neurectomy, deep brain stimulation, dorsal root entry zone lesions, cordotomy, and mesencephalotomy. Microsurgical DREZotomy or dorsal root entry zone lesions may interrupt small nociceptive fibers and neurons in the dorsal horn of the spinal cord. General indications for this procedure include well-localized pain, neuropathic pain including PHN, and excessive spasticity associated with severe pain The role of these invasive surgical treatments in the management of PHN is uncertain, as there are no controlled studies to date (Wu & Raja, 2008).

7.6 Other therapies

A number of other therapies have been explored, such as NMDA receptor antagonists, topical NSAIDs and TCAs, vincristine iontophoresis, botox, minocycline and cryoanalgesia. There is, however, little evidence that justifies evaluation of the efficacy of these therapeutic options. Acupuncture is another option to treat PHN. A clinical report (Lewith et al., 1983), the only one to date retrievable in English, on the possible role of acupuncture in PHN, lacks of sufficient methodological consistency to be quoted in terms of efficacy. A current Cochrane project, however, is due in the near future on this topic (Wang et al., 2009).

7.7 Psychological interventions

Neuropathic pain reduces quality of life, including mood, physical and social functioning. Depression and pain coping strategies, such as catastrophizing and social support, predict pain severity in chronic pain states. Therefore, the importance of psychosocial support and long-term follow- up for severe cases should, however, not be overlooked as sometimes it is the final tool to resort on for otherwise intractable cases (Wu & Raja, 2008).

7.8 Recommendations and combination therapies

Recent guidelines on evidence-based management of neuropathic pain and PHN provide distinct recommendations for first, second, and third line treatment, including possible drug combinations for each step. European Federation of Neurological Societies (EFNS) guidelines recommend TCA or gabapentin/pregabalin as first line treatment in PHN (level A). Topical lidocaine (level A, less consistent results), with its excellent tolerability, may be considered first line in the elderly, especially if there are concerns regarding the CNS side effects of oral medications. In such cases, a trial of 2–4 weeks is justified. Strong opioids (level A) and capsaicin creams are recommended as a second choice. Capsaicin patches are promising (level A), but the long-term effects of repeated applications are not clarified, particularly on sensation. (Attal et al., 2010) *(see Table 2).*

Although drugs and drug classes have been discussed individually for the purpose of this chapter, combination therapy associating more than 1 drug class may be useful in providing additive if not synergistic analgesia. The benefits of combination therapies are supported by a recent study, indicating that the combination of gabapentin and morphine achieved better analgesia at lower doses of each drug than either of the 2 drugs as a single agent in patients with PHN and diabetic neuropathy (Gilron et al.,2009).

Level A rating for efficacy	Level B rating for efficacy	Level A/B rating for inefficacy or discrepant results	Recommendations for first line	Recommendations for second line
Capsaicin 8% patch Gabapentin Lidocaine plasters Opioids Pregabalin TCA	Capsaicin cream Valproate	Benzydamide topical Dextromethorphan Memantine Lorazepam Mexiletine COX-2 inhibitor Tramadol	Gabapentin Pregabalin TCA Lidocaine plasters	Capsacin Opioids

Table 2. Classification of evidence for drug treatment in PHN and recommendations for use (adapted from EFNS guidelines, 2010).

8. Can PHN be prevented?

PHN is the most frequent complication of HZ, it hardly affects patients' life and it is often refractory to current combination treatments, pain persisting in spite of any therapy nearly in half of patients. Several approaches have been investigated for PHN prevention. Prevention clearly appears so far the most interesting path to face with this condition. Antivirals have been addressed for their potential role in prevention as the stop on viral replication in acute phase was hypothesized to reduce pathological damage to nerve fibers and the subsequent onset of PHN. As their role in accelerating rash healing and acute pain resolution is widely recognized, results on their role in PHN prevention are still controversial: a recent Cochrane review (Li et al., 2009) raises some doubts about their efficacy, concluding that there is insufficient evidence from RCTs to support their use with this peculiar aim. In spite of that, studies with different designs suggest some opposite results. Another review (Vander Straten et al., 2001) suggested that antivirals in the acute phase of HZ appear to be effective in reducing PHN severity and duration, but not its incidence. Dworkin et al. (Dworkin et al., 1998) found that patients receiving antiviral therapy (famciclovir *versus* placebo) had a significant lower prevalence of PHN in a cohort study of 419 HZ patients. Parruti et al. (Parruti et al., 2010) showed that HZ patients not prescribed antivirals in the acute phase have a significantly higher risk of developing PHN, in a prospective cohort of 519 HZ unselected patients addressing a real-life clinical setting. The role of antivirals in preventing PHN is still a matter of debate. Corticosteroids prescribed in the acute phase of HZ have been shown to be uneffective in preventing PHN onset in several trials and in a recent review (Chen et al., 2010), as well as antidepressants (Saarto & Wiffen, 2010). As greater acute pain severity predispose to higher risk of PHN onset, pain relief in acute HZ has been investigated as to its possible preventive role. Interventional techniques, such as topical local anesthetics, subcutaneous local anesthetics and corticosteroids, percutaneous electrical nerve stimulation, sympathetic and epidural blocks, have been proposed as prevention: they can produce an effective short-term pain relief in the acute phase, thus reducing the important burden of pain in this time frame, but their effect in reducing PHN incidence remains unclear (Opstelten et al., 2004).

In 1995, vaccination for varicella with a wild-type VZV Oka-strain was introduced under an FDA recommendation and at present a universal coverage vaccination program is ongoing in the USA and several other countries. Varicella vaccine at higher dosage (at least 14 times) than that used in Varicella vaccination was suggested to be protective for the development of HZ. The Shingles Prevention Study (Oxman et al. 2005) was a randomized double-blind placebo-controlled trial designed to demonstrate that vaccination against VZV can decrease the incidence and severity of HZ and PHN. 38,546 healthy subjects aged over than 60 years were recruited and randomly assigned to receive a mock vaccine or an investigational anti-VZV vaccine. They were trained to recognize early HZ sings and to refer quickly to study sites in the evenience of HZ. After vaccination, they were followed for 3.13 years on average. The incidence of HZ was significantly reduced, from 11.12 per 1,000 person-years in the placebo arm to 5.42 per 1,000 person-years in the vaccine arm (Oxman et al. 2005). The incidence of PHN, defined as pain ≥30/100 at 90 days from the onset of rash, was markedly reduced in the vaccine arm, from 1.38 to 0.46 per 1,000 person-years. Moreover, vaccinated subjects developing HZ and PHN had significantly less pain and discomfort, with the burden of illness due to HZ, calculated as described by Coplan et al. (Coplan et al., 2004), being reduced by 61.1%. Zoster vaccination reduced overall HZ and PHN incidence by 51.3% and 66.5%, respectively (*see Figure 6*) (Oxman et al., 2005), giving evidence for a major protective role. This cornerstone study, however, had some limitations, as it included only subjects aged >60 and excluded subjects with relevant and frequent comorbidities such as diabetes, chronic obstructive pulmonary diseases, cancer, HIV and other cases of immunodepression. For these reasons, it does not allow to draw conclusions as to safety and efficacy of HZ vaccine in these subsets of subjects that are relevant in real practice and that a priori would largely benefit from vaccine administration, having a higher risk to develop HZ and PHN and a heavier total burden of illness. Further studies are needed to better define these elements.

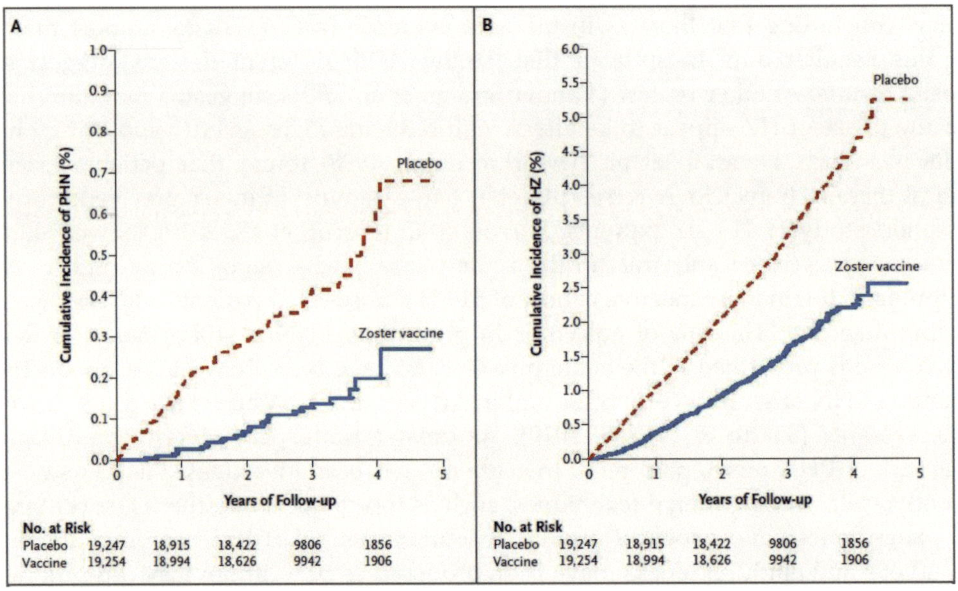

Fig. 6. Kaplan-Meier estimates of the effect of HZ vaccine on HZ (A) and PHN incidence (B). HZ and PHN incidence were significantly lower in the vaccine group compared to the placebo group (waiting for permission from Oxman et al., 2005).

Since 2006, when HZ vaccine was approved by FDA and recommended for adults aged >60 in the United States, the real cost-effectiveness of HZ vaccination for the general population has been widely investigated. Several studies assessed the economic burden of HZ and PHN, showing that they are frequent and costly conditions, also in terms of impact on quality of life, as discussed above (Scott et al., 2006; Stein et al.,2009; Gil et al., 2009; Gialloreti et al., 2010; Aunhachoke et al., 2011; Hornberger & Robertus, 2006). For instance, in Italy a recent study estimated that total annual costs for HZ and PHN were €41.2 Million, including both direct and indirect costs (Gialloreti et al., 2010). Vaccine cost-effectiveness was determined by decision models in multiple large countries (Canada, England and Wales, Italy), suggesting that immunization would increase quality-adjusted life-years (QALYs) (Najafzadeh et al., 2009; van Hoek et al., 2009; Gialloreti et al., 2011). In general, studies evaluating vaccine cost-effectiveness agree on its relevance in the elderly population (Hornberger & Robertus, 2006; Pellissier et al., 2007; Rothberg et al., 2007; van Hoek et al., 2011; Annemans et al., 2010; Gilden, 2011). Furthermore it has been supposed that vaccination could be equally cost-effective also in younger people, aged <50, as about 19% of HZ cases occur between 50 and 59 years of age. Further studies are once more needed to assess this point.

9. References

Agrawal, D.; Vohra, R., Gupta, PP. & Sood S. (2007). Subclinical peripheral neuropathy in stable middle-aged patients with chronic obstructive pulmonary disease. *Singapore Med J.* 48:887-94.

Ahn, HJ.; Lim, HK.; Lee, YB.; Hwang, SM.; Lee, WS.; Ahn, SK. & Choi EH. (2007). The effects of famciclovir and epidural block in the treatment of herpes zoster. *J Dermatol.* 28:208-216.

Angel, IF.; Gould, HJ. Jr & Carey ME. (1998) Intrathecal morphine pump as a treatment option in chronic pain of nonmalignant origin. *Surg Neurol.* 49:92-98.

Annemans, L.; Bresse, X.; Gobbo, C. & Papageorgiou M. (2010) Health economic evaluation of a vaccine for the prevention of herpes zoster (shingles) and post-herpetic neuralgia in adults in Belgium. *J Med Econ.* 13(3):537-51.

Arani, RB.; Soong, SJ.; Weiss, HL.; Wood, MJ.; Fiddian, PA.; Gnann, JW. & Whitley R. (2001). Phase specific analysis of herpes zoster associated pain data: a new statistical approach. *Stat Med.* 30;20(16):2429-39.

Arora, A.; Mendoza, N.; Brantley, J.; Yates, B.; Dix, L. & Tyring S. (2008). Double-blind study comparing 2 dosages of valacyclovir hydrochloride for the treatment of uncomplicated herpes zoster in immunocompromised patients 18 years of age and older. *J Infect Dis.* 1;197(9):1289-95.

Attal, N.; Cruccu, G.; Haanpää, M.; Hansson, P.; Jensen, TS.; Nurmikko, T.; Sampaio, C.; Sindrup, S.; Wiffen P; EFNS Task Force. (2006). EFNS guidelines on pharmacological treatment of neuropathic pain. *Eur J Neurol.* 13(11):1153-69.

Attal, N.; Cruccu, G.; Baron R.; Haanpää, M.; Hansson, P.; Jensen, TS.; Nurmikko, T.; European Federation of Neurological Societies. (2010). EFNS guidelines on the pharmacological treatment of neuropathic pain: 2010 revision *Eur J Neurol.* 17(9):1113-e88.

Aunhachoke, K.; Bussaratid, V.; Chirachanakul, P.; Chua-Intra, B.; Dhitavat, J.; Jaisathaporn, K.;, Kaewkungwal, J.; Kampirapap, K.; Khuhaprema, T.; Pairayayutakul, K.;

Pitisuttithum, P.; Sindhvananda, J.; Thaipisuttikul, Y. & Thai Herpes Zoster Study Group. (2011). Measuring herpes zoster, zoster-associated pain, post-herpetic neuralgia-associated loss of quality of life, and healthcare utilization and costs in Thailand. *Int J Dermatol.* 50(4):428-35.

Backonja, M.; Wallace, MS.; Blonsky, ER.; Cutler, BJ.; Malan P. Jr.; Rauck, R.; Tobias, J.; NGX-4010 C116 Study Group. (2008). NGX-4010, a high-concentration capsaicin patch, for the treatment of postherpetic neuralgia: a randomised, double-blind study. *Lancet Neurol.* 7(12):1106-12.

Baron, R. & Saguez, M. (1993). Postherpetic neuralgia. Are C-nociceptors involved in signalling and maintenance of tactile allodynia? *Brain.* 116: 1477-1496.

Baron, R.; Haendler, G. & Schulte, H. (1997). Afferent large fiber polyneuropathy predicts the development of postherpetic neuralgia. *Pain.* 73(2):231-8.

Bartley, J. (2009). Post herpetic neuralgia, schwann cell activation and vitamin D. *Medical Hypothesis.* 73: 927-929.

Basbaum, AI. & Fields HL. (1978). Endogenous pain control mechanisms: review and hypothesis. *Ann Neurol.* 4(5):451-62.

Benbernou, A.; Drolet, M.; Levin, MJ.; Schmader, KE.; Oxman, MN.; Johnson, R.; Patrick, D.; Camden, S.; Mansi, JA. & Brisson M. (2011). Association between prodromal pain and the severity of acute herpes zoster and utilization of health care resources. *Eur J Pain.* [Epub ahead of print].

Bennett, GJ. (1994). Hypotheses on the pathogenesis of herpes zoster-associated pain. *Ann Neurol.* 35 Suppl:S38-41.

Berry, JD. & Petersen, KL. (2005). A single dose of gabapentin reduces acute pain and allodynia in patients with herpes zoster. *Neurology.* 65(3):444-7.

Binder, A.; Bruxelle, J.; Rogers, P.; Hans, G.; Boster, I. & Baron, R. (2009). Topical 5% lidocaine (lignocaine) medicated plaster treatment for post-herpetic neuralgia. *Clin Drug Investig.* 29: 393–408.

Boureau, F.; Legallicier, P. & Kabir-Ahmadi, M. (2003). Tramadol in post-herpetic neuralgia: a randomized, double blind, placebo-controlled trial. *Pain.* 104: 323-31.

Bove, GM (2008). Epi-perineurial anatomy, innervation, and axonal nociceptive mechanisms. *J Bodyw Mov Ter.* 9: S19-30.

Bowsher, D. (1997). The effects of pre-emptive treatment of post-herpetic neuralgia with amitriptyline: a randomized, double-blind, placebo-controlled trial. *J Pain Symptom Manage.* 13: 327-31.

Chen, N.; Yang, M.; He, L.; Zhang, D.; Zhou, M. & Zhu C. (2010). Corticosteroids for preventing postherpetic neuralgia. *Cochrane Database Syst Rev.* 8;(12):CD005582.

Chidiac, C.; Bruxelle, J.; Daures, JP.; Hoang-Xuan, T.; Morel, P.; Leplège, A.; El Hasnaoui, A. & de Labareyre, C. (2001). Characteristics of patients with herpes zoster on presentation to practitioners in France. *Clin Infect Dis.* 1;33(1):62-9.

Choi, B. & Rowbotham, MC. (1997). Effect of adrenergic receptor activation on post-herpetic neuralgia pain and sensory disturbances. 69:55-63.

Choo, PW.; Galil, K.; Donahue, JG.; Walker, AM.; Spiegelman, D. & Platt R. (1997). Risk factors for postherpetic neuralgia. *Arch Intern Med.* 9;157(11):1217-24.

Christo, PJ.; Hobelmann, G. & Maine, DN. (2007) Post-herpetic neuralgia in older adults: evidence-based approaches to clinical management. *Drugs Aging.* 24 (1): 1-19.

Coghlan, CJ. (1992). Herpes zoster treated by acupuncture. *Cent Afr J Med.* 38:466-467.

Cohen, SP. & Raja, SN. (2006). The middle way: a practical approach to prescribing opioids for chronic pain. *Nat Clin Pract Neurol.* 2(11):580-1.

Comer, AM. & Lamb, HM. (2000). Lidocaine patch 5%. *Drugs* 59:245-249, 2000.

Coplan, PM.; Schmader, K.; Nikas A.; Chan, IS.; Choo, P.; Levin, MJ.; Johnson, G.; Bauer, M.; Williams, HM.; Kaplan, KM. et al. (2004). Development of a measure of the burden of pain due to herpes zoster and postherpetic neuralgia for prevention trials: adaptation of the brief pain inventory. *J Pain.* 5(6):344-56.

Criscuolo, S.; Auletta, C.; Lippi, S.; Brogi, F. & Brogi, A. (2005). Oxcarbazepine monotherapy in postherpetic neuralgia unresponsive to carbamazepine and gabapentin. *Acta Neurol Scand.* 111: 229-32.

Decroix, J.; Partsch, H.; Gonzalez, R.; Mobacken, H.; Goh, CL.; Walsh, JB. et al. (2000). Factors influencing pain outcome in herpes zoster: an observational study with valaciclovir. Valaciclovir International Zoster Assessment Group (VIZA). *J Eur Acad Dermatol Venereol.* 14(1):23-33.

Derry, S.; Lloyd, R.; Moore RA. & McQuay, HJ. (2009). Topical capsaicin for chronic neuropathic pain in adults *Cochrane Database Syst Rev.* 7;(4):CD007393.

di Luzio Paparatti, U.; Arpinelli, F. & Visonà, G. (1999). Herpes zoster and its complications in Italy: an observational survey. *J Infect.* 38(2):116-20.

Drolet, M.; Brisson, M.; Levin, MJ.; Schmader, KE.; Oxman, MN.; Johnson, RW.; Camden, S. & Mansi, JA. (2010 Oct). A prospective study of the herpes zoster severity of illness. *Clin J Pain.* 2010 Oct;26(8):656-66.

Drolet, M.; Brisson, M.; Schmader, K.; Levin, M.; Johnson, R.; Oxman, M.; Patrick D.; Camden, S. & Mansi, JA. (2010 Nov) Predictors of postherpetic neuralgia among patients with herpes zoster: a prospective study. *J Pain.* 11(11):1211-21.

Drolet, M.; Brisson, M.; Schmader, KE.; Levin, MJ.; Johnson, R.; Oxman, MN.; Patrick, D.; Blanchette, C. & Mansi, JA. (2010 Nov). The impact of herpes zoster and postherpetic neuralgia on health-related quality of life: a prospective study. *C M A J.* 9;182(16):1731-6.

Dworkin, RH.; Hartstein, G.; Rosner, HL.; Walther, RR.; Sweeney, EW. & Brand, L. (1992). A high-risk method for studying psychosocial antecedents of chronic pain: the prospective investigation of herpes zoster. *J Abnorm Psychol.* 101(1):200-5.

Dworkin, RH. & Portenoy, RK. (1996). Pain and its persistence in herpes zoster. *Pain.* 67(2-3):241-51.

Dworkin, RH.; Boon, RJ.; Griffin, DR. & Phung, D. (1998). Postherpetic neuralgia: impact of famciclovir, age, rash severity, and acute pain in herpes zoster patients. *J Infect Dis.* 178 Suppl 1:S76-80.

Dworkin, RH.; Nagasako, EM.; Johnson, RW.; Griffin, DR. (2001) Acute pain in herpes zoster: the famciclovir database project. *Pain.* 94(1):113-9.

Dworkin, RH. & Schmader, KE. (2003). Treatment and prevention of postherpetic neuralgia. *CID.* 36: 877-82.

Dworkin, RH.; Johnson, RW.; Breuer, J.; Gnann, JW.; Levin, MJ.; Backonja, M. et al. (2007). Recommendations for the management of herpes zoster. *Clin Infect Dis.* 1;44 Suppl 1:S1-26.

Dworkin, RH.; Barbano, RL.; Tyring, SK.; Betts, RF.; McDermott, MP.; Pennella-Vaughan, J.; Bennett, GJ.; Berber, E.; Gnann, JW.; Irvine, C.; Kamp, C.; Kieburtz, K.; Max, MB. &

Schmader, KE. (2009). A randomized placebo-controlled trial of oxycodone and og gabapentin for acute pain in herpes zoster. *Pain,* 142(3):209-17.

Evans, RW. & Lee AG. (2004). Herpes zoster ophthalmicus, ophthalmoplegia, and trauma. *Headache.* 2004. 44(3):286-8.

Fink, K.; Dooley, DJ. & Meder, WP. (2002). Inhibition of neuronal Ca2+ influx by gabapentin and pregabalin in the human neocortex. *Neuropharmacology.* 42: 229-36.

Fleckenstein, J.; Kramer, S.; Hoffrogge, P.; Thoma, S.; Lang, PM.; Lehmeyer, L.; Schober, GM.; Pfab, F.; Ring, J.; Weisenseel, P.; Schotten, KJ.; Mansmann, U. & Irnich D. (2009). Acupuncture in acute herpes zoster pain therapy (ACUZoster) - design and protocol of a randomised controlled trial. *BMC Complement Altern Med.* 12;9:31.

Foye, PM.; Stitik, TP.; Nadler, SF. & Chen B. (2000). A study of post-traumatic shingles as a work related injury. *Am J Ind Med.* 38(1):108-11.

Garry, EM.; Delaney, A.; Anderson, HA.; Sirinathsinghji, EC.; Clapp, RH.; Martin, WJ.; Kinchington, PR.; Krah, DL.; Abbadie, C.& Fleetwood-Walker, SM. (2005). Varicella zoster virus induces neuropathic changes in rat dorsal root ganglia and behavioral reflex sensitisation that is attenuated by gabapentin or sodium channel blocking drugs. *Pain.* 118(1-2):97-111.

Gialloreti, LE.; Merito, M.; Pezzotti, P.; Naldi, L.; Gatti, A.; Beillat, M.; Serradell, L.; di Marzo, R. & Volpi A. (2010). Epidemiology and economic burden of herpes zoster and post-herpetic neuralgia in Italy: a retrospective, population-based study. *BMC Infect Dis.* 3;10:230.

Gil, A.; Gil, R.; Alvaro, A.; San Martín, M. & González A. (2009). Burden of herpes zoster requiring hospitalization in Spain during a seven-year period (1998-2004). *BMC Infect Dis.* 7;9:55.

Gilden, DH.; Kleinschmidt-DeMasters, BK.; LaGuardia, JJ.; Mahalingam, R. & Cohrs RJ. (2000). Neurologic complications of the reactivation of varicella-zoster virus. *N Engl J Med.* 2;342(9):635-45.

Gilden, DH.; Cohrs, RJ.; Hayward, AR.; Wellish, M. & Mahalingam R. (2003) Chronic varicella-zoster virus ganglionitis-a possible cause of postherpetic neuralgia. *J Neurovirol.* 9(3):404-7.

Gilden, D.; Cohrs, RJ.; Mahalingam, R. & Nagel, MA. (2009). Varicella zoster virus vasculopathies: diverse clinical manifestations, laboratory features, pathogenesis, and treatment. *Lancet Neurol.* 8(8):731-40.

Gilden, D. (2011). Efficacy of live zoster vaccine in preventing zoster and postherpetic neuralgia. *J Intern Med.*269(5):496-506.

Gilron, I.; Bailey, JM.; Tu, D.; Holden, RR.; Jackson, AC. & Houlden, RL. (2009). Nortriptyline and gabapentin, alone and in combination for neuropathic pain: a double-blind, randomised controlled crossover trial. *Lancet.* 10;374(9697):1252-61.

Gnann, Jr. JW. (2007). Antiviral therapy of varicella-zoster virus infections. In: Arvin A, Campadelli-Fiume G, Mocarski E, Moore PS, Roizman B, Whitley R, Yamanishi K, editors. Human Herpesviruses: Biology, Therapy, and Immunoprophylaxis. Cambridge: Cambridge University Press; 2007. Chapter 65.

Godfrey, EK.; Brown, C. & Stambough, JL. (2006). Herpes zoster--varicella complicating anterior thoracic surgery: 2 case reports. *J Spinal Disord Tech.* 19(4):299-301.

Grabow, TS.; Tella, PK. & Raja SN. (2003). Spinal cord stimulation for complex regional pain syndrome: An evidence-based medicine review of the literature. *Clin J Pain.* 19:371-383.

Gross, G.; Schofer, H. & Wassilew, S. (2003). Herpes zoster guidelines of the German Dematology Society. *J Clin VIrol.* 26 (3): 277-89.

Hanani M. (2005). Satellite glial cells in sensory ganglia: from form to function. *Brain.* 48:457-76.

Hans, G.; Sabatowski, R.; Binder, A.; Boesl, I.; Rogers, P. & Baron R. (2009). Efficacy and tolerability of a 5% lidocaine medicated plaster for the topical treatment of post-herpetic neuralgia: results of a long-term study. *Curr Med Res Opin.* 25: 1295–1305.

Hao, S.; Tian, B. & Wang L. (1994). A primary evaluation of VAS for use in clinical experimentral pain assessment. *Zhongguo Yi Xue Ke Yuan Xue Bao.* 16:397-399.

Harati, Y.; Gooch, C. & Swenson, M. (1998). Double-blind randomized trial of tramadol for the treatment of the pain of diabetic neuropathy. *Neurology.* 50 (6):1842-6.

Hata, A.; Kuniyoshi, M. & Ohkusa Y. (2011). Risk of Herpes zoster in patients with underlying diseases: a retrospective hospital-based cohort study. *Infection.* Jul 29.

He, Y. & Fang, R. (2007). Treatment of 60 cases of senile herpes zoster by encircled acupuncture plus valaciclovir. *J Acupunct Tuina Sci.* 5:171-173.

Hegalsson, S.; Petursson, G..; Gudmundsson, S. & Sigurdsson, JA. (2000). Prevalence of postherpetic neuralgia after a single episode of herpes zoster: prospective study with a long-term follow up. *BMJ.* 321:1-4

Hempenstall, K.; Nurmikko, TJ.; Johnson, RW.; A'Hern, RP. & Rice AS. (2005). Analgesic therapy in postherpetic neuralgia: a quantitative systematic review. *PLoS Med.* 2(7):e164.

Hope-Simpson, RE. (1965). The Nature of Herpes Zoster: a long-term study and a new hypothesis. *Proc R Soc Med.* 58:9-20.

Hope-Simpson, RE. (1975). Postherpetic neuralgia. *J R Coll Gen Pract.* 25(157):571-5.

Hornberger, J. & Robertus, K. (2006). Cost-effectiveness of a vaccine to prevent herpes zoster and postherpetic neuralgia in older adults. *Ann Intern Med.* 5;145(5):317-25.

Insinga, RP.; Itzler, RF.; Pellissier, JM.; Saddier, P. & Nikas, AA. (2005). The incidence of herpes zoster in a United States administrative database. *J Gen Intern Med.* 20(8):748-53.

Janig, W.; Levine, JD. & Michaelis, M. (1996). Interactions of sympathetic and primary afferent neurons following nerve injury and tissue trauma. *Prog Brain Res.* 113:161-184.

Jensen-Dahm, C.; Rowbotham, MC.; Reda, H. & Petersen KL. (2011). Effect of a single dose of pregabalin on herpes zoster pain. *Trial.,* 28;12:55.

Ji, G. ; Niu, J. ; Shi, Y. ; Hou, L. ; Lu, Y. & Xiong L. (2009). The effectiveness of repetitive paravertebral injections with local anesthetics and steroids for the prevention of postherpetic neuralgia in patients with acute herpes zoster. *Anesth Analg.* 109(5):1651-5.

Joesoef, MR.; Leung, J.; Harpaz, R. & Bialek SR. (2011). Potential coding error of herpes zoster (HZ) vaccination and HZ diagnosis in administrative data. *Vaccine.* 3;29(11):2008-9.

Johnson, RW. (1997). Herpes zoster and postherpetic neuralgia. Optimal treatment. *Drugs Aging.* 10:80-94.

Johnson, R. (2003). Herpes Zoster in the immunocompetent patient: management of Post-herpetic Neuralgia. *Herpes.* 10: 2: 38-45.

Jumaan, AO.; Yu, O.; Jackson, LA.; Bohlke, K.; Galil, K. & Seward JF. (2005). Incidence of herpes zoster, before and after varicella-vaccination-associated decreases in the incidence of varicella, 1992-2002. *J Infect Dis.* 15;191(12):2002-7.

Jung, BF.; Johnson, RW.; Griffin, DR. & Dworkin, RH. (2004). Risk factors for postherpetic neuralgia in patients with herpes zoster. *Neurology.* 11;62(9):1545-51.

Kang, JH.; Ho, JD.; Chen, YH. & Lin, HC. (2009). Increased risk of stroke after a herpes zoster attack: a population-based follow-up study. *Stroke.* 40(11):3443-8.

Katz, J.; Cooper, EM.; Walther, RR.; Sweeney, EW. & Dworkin, RH. (2004). Acute pain in herpes zoster and its impact on health-related quality of life. *Clin Infect Dis.* 1;39(3):342-8.

Katz, J.; McDermott, MP.; Cooper, EM.; Walther, RR.; Sweeney, EW. & Dworkin RH. (2005). Psychosocial risk factors for postherpetic neuralgia: a prospective study of patients with herpes zoster. *J Pain.* 6(12):782-90.

Khaliq, W; Alam, S. & Puri, N. (2007). Topical lidocaine for the treatment of postherpetic neuralgia. *Cochrane Database Syst Rev.* 18;(2):CD004846.

Kleinschmidt-DeMasters, BK. & Gilden DH. (2001). Varicella-Zoster virus infections of the nervous system: clinical and pathologic correlates. *Arch Pathol Lab Med.* 125(6):770-80.

Knotkova, H.; Pappagallo, M. & Szallasi A. (2008) Capsaicin (TRPV1 Agonist) therapy for pain relief: farewell or revival? *Clin J Pain.* 24(2):142-54.

Kochar, DK.ù; Garg, P. & Bumb, RA. (2005). Divalproex sodium in the management of post-herpetic neuralgia: a randomized double-blind placebo-controlled study. *Q J M.* 98:29-34.

Kurokawa, I. ; Kumano, K. & Murakawa, K.; Hyogo Prefectural PHN Study Group. (2002). Clinical correlates of prolonged pain in Japanese patients with acute herpes zoster. *J Int Med Res.* 30(1):56-65.

Levy, JM. & Smyth SH. (2002). Reactivation of herpes zoster after liver biopsy. *J Vasc Interv Radiol.* 2002. 13(2 Pt 1):209-10.

Lewith, GT.; Field J. & Machin D. (1983). Acupuncture compared with placebo in post-herpetic pain. *Pain* . 17:361-368.

Li, Q.; Chen, N.; Yang, J.; Zhou, M.; Zhou, D.; Zhang, Q. & He L. (2009). Antiviral treatment for preventing postherpetic neuralgia. *Cochrane Database Syst Rev.* 15;(2):CD006866.

Mao, J. & Chen LL. (2000). Gabapentin in pain management. *Anesth Analg.* 91(3):680-7.

McCormack, PL. (2010). Capsaicin dermal patch: in non-diabetic peripheral neuropathic pain. *Drugs.* 1;70(14):1831-42.

Melzack, R. & Torgerson, WS. (1971). On the language of pain. *Anesthesiology.* 34:50-59.

Melzack, R. (2005). The McGill pain questionnaire: from description to measurement. *Anesthesiology.* 103(1):199-202.

Nagasako, EM.; Johnson, RW.; Griffin, DR. & Dworkin, RH(2002). Rash severity in herpes zoster: correlates and relationship to postherpetic neuralgia. *J Am Acad Dermatol.* 46(6):834-9.

Nagel, MA. & Gilden, DH. (2007). The protean neurologic manifestations of varicella-zoster virus infection. *Cleve Clin J Med.* 74(7):489-94, 496, 498-9.

Najafzadeh, M.; Marra, CA.; Galanis, E. & Patrick, DM. (2009). Cost effectiveness of herpes zoster vaccine in Canada. *Pharmacoeconomics*. 27(12):991-1004.

Nitescu, P.; Dahm, P.; Appelgren, L. & Curelaru I. (1998). Continuous infusion of opioid and bupivacaine by externalized intrathecal catheters in long-term treatment of "refractory" nonmalignant pain. *Clin J Pain*. 14:17-28.

Niv, D. & Maltsman-Tseikhin, A. (2005). Postherpetic neuralgia: the never-ending challenge. *Pain Pract*. 5(4):327-40.

Nolano, M.; Simone, DA.; Wendelschafer-Crabb, G.; Johnson, T.; Hazen, E. & Kennedy, WR. (1999) Topical capsaicin in humans: Parallel loss of epidermal nerve fibers and pain sensation. *Pain* 81:135-145.

Oaklander, AL.; Romans, K.; Horasek, S.; Stocks, A.; Hauer, P. & Meyer, RA. (1998). Unilateral postherpetic neuralgia is associated with bilateral sensory neuron damage. *Ann Neurol*. 44: 789-95.

Oaklander, AL. (2001). The density of remaining nerve endings in human skin with and without postherpetic neuralgia after shingles. *Pain* , 92: 139-45.

Opstelten, W.; Mauritz, JW.; de Wit, NJ.; van Wijck, AJ.; Stalman, WA. & van Essen GA. (2002). Herpes zoster and postherpetic neuralgia: incidence and risk indicators using a general practice research database. *Fam Pract*. 19(5):471-5.

Opstelten, W.; van Wijck, AJ. & Stolker, RJ. (2004). Interventions to prevent postherpetic neuralgia: cutaneous and percutaneous techniques. *Pain*. 107(3):202-6.

Opstelten, W.; van Loon, AM.; van Wijck, AJ. & Moons, KG. (2007). Correlates of acute pain in herpes zoster. *J Clin Virol*. 39(3):238-9.

Opstelten, W.; Zuithoff, NP.; van Essen, GA. et al. (2007). Predicting postherpetic neuralgia in elderly primary care patients with herpes zoster: prospective prognostic study. *Pain*. 132 Suppl 1:S52-9.

Oxman, MN.; Levin, MJ.; Johnson, GR. et al. (2005). A vaccine to prevent herpes zoster and postherpetic neuralgia in older adults. *N Engl J Med*. 2;352(22):2271-84.

Parruti, G.; Tontodonati, M.; Rebuzzi, C.; Polilli, E.; Sozio, F.; Consorte, A.; Agostinone, A.; Di Masi, F.; Congedo, G.; D'Antonio, D.; Granchelli, C.; D'Amario, C.; Carunchio, C.; Pippa, L.; Manzoli, L.; Volpi, A. & VZV Pain Study Group. (2010). Predictors of pain intensity and persistence in a prospective Italian cohort of patients with herpes zoster: relevance of smoking, trauma and antiviral therapy. *BMC Med*. 11;8:58.

Pasqualucci, A.; Pasqualucci, V.; Galla, F.; De Angelis, V.; Marzocchi, V.; Colussi, R.; Paoletti, F.; Girardis, M.; Lugano, M. & Del Sindaco F. (2000). Prevention of post-herpetic neuralgia: acyclovir and prednisolone versus epidural local anesthetic and methylprednisolone. *Acta Anaesthesiol Scand*. 44(8):910-8.

Pellissier, JM.; Brisson, M. & Levin, MJ. (2007). Evaluation of the cost-effectiveness in the United States of a vaccine to prevent herpes zoster and postherpetic neuralgia in older adults. *Vaccine*. 28;25(49):8326-37.

Quirico, PE. LG. & Allais G. (1996). L'effetto immunomodulatore dell'agopuntura. *G Ital Riflessot Agopunt*. 8:175-179.

Rapson, LM. & Banner, R. (2008). Acupuncture for pain management. *Geriatric Aging*. 11(2):93-97.

Rasi, A.; Heshmatzade Behzadi, A.; Rabet, M.; Hassanloo, J.; Honarbakhsh, Y.; Dehghan, N. & Kamrava SK. (2010). The efficacy of time-based short-course acyclovir therapy in treatment of post-herpetic pain. *J Infect Dev Ctries*. 24;4(11):754-60.

Reynolds, MA.; Chaves, SS.; Harpaz, R.; Lopez, AS. & Seward, JF. (2008). The impact of the varicella vaccination program on herpes zoster epidemiology in the United States: a review. *J Infect Dis* 1;197 Suppl 2:S224-7.

Rice, AS. & Maton, S. (2001). Gabapentin in postherpetic neuralgia: a randomized, double-blind, placebo controlled study. *Pain.* 94: 215-24.

Rothberg, MB.; Virapongse, A. & Smith KJ. (2007). Cost-effectiveness of a vaccine to prevent herpes zoster and postherpetic neuralgia in older adults. *Clin Infect Dis.* 15;44(10):1280-8.

Rowbotham, MC.; Reisner, LA.; Davies, PS. & Fields, HL. (2005). Treatment response in antidepressant-naïve postherpetic neuralgia patients: double-blind, randomized trial. *J Pain..* 6(11):741-6.

Rowbotham, M.; Harden, N. ,Stacey, B. ,Bernstein, P. & Magnus-Muller, L. (1998). Gabapentin for the treatment of postherpetic neuralgia: a randomized controlled trial. *J A M A.* 280:837-42.

Roxas, M. (2006). Herpes zoster and post-herpetic neuralgia: diagnosis and therapeutic considerations. *Altern Med Rev.* 11(2):102-113.

Saarto, T. & Wiffen, PJ. (2010). Antidepressants for neuropathic pain: a Cochrane review. *J Neurol Neurosurg Psychiatry.* 81(12):1372-3.

Sabatowski, R.; Galvez, R. & Cherry, DA. (2004). Pregabalin reduces pain and improves sleep and mood disturbances in patients with post-herpetic neuralgia: results of a randomized, placebo-controlled clinical trial. *Pain.* 109:26-35.

Sansone, RA.; Todd, T. & Meier, BP. (2002). Pretreatment ECGs and the prescription of amitriptyline in an internal medicine clinic. *Psychosomatics.* 43(3):250-1.

Sauer, SK.; Bove, GM.; Averbeck, B. & Reeh, PW. (1999). Rat peripheral nerve components release calcitonin gene-related peptide and prostaglandin E2 in response to noxious stimuli: evidence that nervi nervorum are nociceptors. *Neuroscience.* 92:319-25.

Schmader, K. (2001). Herpes zoster in older adults. *CID.* 32: 1481-6.

Schmader, K.; Gnann JW. Jr. & Watson, CP. (2008). The epidemiological, clinical, and pathological rationale for the herpes zoster vaccine. *J Infect Dis.* 1;197 Suppl 2:S207-15.

Scott, FT.; Leedham-Green, ME.; Barrett-Muir, WY. et al. (2003). A study of shingles and the development of postherpetic neuralgia in East London. *J Med Virol.* 70 Suppl 1:S24-30.

Scott, FT.; Johnson, RW.; Leedham-Green, M.; Davies, E.; Edmunds, WJ. & Breuer, J. (2006). The burden of Herpes Zoster: a prospective population based study. *Vaccine.* 27;24(9):1308-14.

Sopori, ML. & Kozak, W. (1998). Immunomodulatory effects of cigarette smoke. *J Neuroimmunol.* 83:148-56.

Sorkin, LA. & Schafers, M. (2007). Immune cells in peripheral nerve. In: De Leo, JA.; Sorkin, LA. ; Watkins, LR. Immune and glial regulation of pain, IASP Press;2007. p. 1-19.

Stankus, SJ.; Dlugopolski, M. & Packer D. (2000) Management of herpes zoster (shingles) and posteherpetic neuralgia. *Am Fam Physician.* 61(8):2437-44, 2447-8.

Stein, AN.; Britt, H.; Harrison, C.; Conway, EL.; Cunningham, A.& Macintyre, CR. (2009). Herpes zoster burden of illness and health care resource utilization in the Australian population aged 50 years and older. *Vaccine.* 22;27(4):520-9.

Thomas, SL. & Hall, AJ. (2004). What does epidemiology tell us about risk factors for herpes zoster? *Lancet Infect Dis.* 4(1):26-33.

Thomas, SL.; Wheeler, JG. & Hall, AJ. (2004). Case-control study of the effect of mechanical trauma on the risk of herpes zoster. *BMJ.* 21;328(7437):439.

Thyregod, HG.; Rowbotham, MC.; Peters, M.; Possehn, J. ;Berro, M. & Petersen KL. (2007). Natural history of pain following herpes zoster. *Pain.* 128(1-2):148-56.

Ursini, T.; Tontodonati, M.; Manzoli, L.; Polilli, E.; Rebuzzi, C.; Congedo, G.; Di Profio, S.; Marani Toro, P.;, Consorte, A.; Placido, G.; Laganà, S.; D'Amario, C.; Granchelli, C., Parruti G.; Pippa, L; & the VZV Pain Study Group. (2011). Acupuncture for the treatment of severe acute pain in Herpes Zoster: results of a nested, open-label, randomized trial in the VZV Pain Study. *BMC Complement Altern Me.,* 5;11(1):46.

van Hoek, AJ.; Gay, N.; Melegaro, A.; Opstelten, W. & Edmunds, WJ. (2009). Estimating the cost-effectiveness of vaccination against herpes zoster in England and Wales. *Vaccine.* 25;27(9):1454-67.

van Hoek, AJ.; Melegaro, A.; Zagheni, E.; Edmunds, WJ. % Gay, N. (2011). Modelling the impact of a combined varicella and zoster vaccination programme on the epidemiology of varicella zoster virus in England. *Vaccine.* 16;29(13):2411-20.

van Wijck, AJ.; Opstelten, W.; Moons, KG.; van Essen, GA.; Stolker, RJ.; Kalkman, CJ. & Verheij, TJ. (2006). The PINE study of epidural steroids and local anaesthetics to prevent postherpetic neuralgia: a randomised controlled trial. *Lancet.* 21;367(9506):219-24.

van Wijck ,AJ.; Wallace, M.; Mekhail, N. & van Kleef, M. (2011). Evidence-based interventional pain medicine according to clinical diagnoses. 17. Herpes zoster and post-herpetic neuralgia *Pain Pract.* 11(1):88-97

Vander Straten, M.; Carrasco, D.; Lee, P. & Tyring, SK. (2001). Reduction of postherpetic neuralgia in herpes zoster. *J Cutan Med Surg.* 5(5):409-16.

Vieweg, WV. & Wood, MA. (2004). Tricyclic antidepressants, QT interval prolongation, and torsade de pointes. *Psychosomatics.* 45(5):371-7.

Volpi, A.; Gatti, A.; Serafini, G.; Costa, B.; Suligoi, B.; Pica, F.; Marsella, LT.; Sabato, E. & Sabato, AF. (2007). Clinical and psychosocial correlates of acute pain in herpes zoster. *J Clin Virol.* 38(4):275-9.

Volpi, A.; Gatti, A.; Pica, F.; Bellino, S.; Marsella, LT. & Sabato, AF. (2008). Clinical and psychosocial correlates of post-herpetic neuralgia. *J Med Virol.* 80(9):1646-52.

Vossen, MT.; Gent, MR.; Weel, JF.; de Jong, MD.; van Lier, RA. & Kuijpers, TW. (2004). Development of virus-specific CD4+ T cells on reexposure to Varicella-Zoster virus. *J Infect Dis.* 1;190(1):72-82.

Wang, P.; Zhao, J. & Wu T. (2009). Acupuncture for postherpetic neuralgia (Protocol). *Cochrane Database of Systematic Reviews* 2009, Issue 2. Art. No.: CD007793. DOI: 10.1002/14651858.CD007793.

Wareham, DW. & Breuer, J. (2007). Herpes zoster. *BMJ.* 334(7605):1211-5.

Wasner, G.; Kleinert, A.; Binder, A.; Schattschneider, J. & Baron, R. (2005). Postherpetic neuralgia: Topical lidocaine is effective in nociceptor-deprived skin. *J Neurol.* 252:677-686.

Watkins, LR.; Milligan, ED. & Maier, SF. (2001). Glial attivation: a driving force for the pathological pain. *Trends Neurosci.* 24:450-5.

Watson, CP.; Deck, JH.; Morshead, C.; Van der Kooy, D. & Evans, RJ. (1991). Post-herpetic neuralgia: further post-mortem studies of cases with and without pain. *Pain.* 44(2):105-17.

Watson, CP.; Vernich, L.; Chipman, M. & Reed, K. (1998) Nortriptyline versus amitriptyline in postherpetic neuralgia: a randomized trial. *Neurology.* 51:1166-71.

Watson, CP. & Oaklander, AL. (2002). Postherpetic neuralgia. *Pain Practice* . 2(4):295-307.

Weingarten, TN.; Moeschler, SM.; Ptaszynski, AE.; Hooten, WM.; Beebe, TJ. & Warner, DO. (2008). An assessment of the association between smoking status, pain intensity, and functional interference in patients with chronic pain. *Pain Physician.* 11:643-53.

Weinke, T.; Edte, A.; Schmitt, S. & Lukas K. (2010). Impact of herpes zoster and post-herpetic neuralgia on patients' quality of life: a patient-reported outcomes survey. *Z Gesundh Wiss.* 18(4):367-374.

Whitley, RJ.; Weiss, H. &, Gnann JW. (1996). Acyclovir with and without prednisone for the treatment of herpes zoster. A randomized, placebo-controlled trial. The national institute of allergy and infectious diseases collaborative antiviral study group. *Ann Intern Med.* 125: 376-83.

Whitley, RJ.; Weiss, HL.; Soong, SJ. & Gnann, JW. (1999). Herpes zoster: risk categories for persistent pain. *J Infect Dis.* 179(1):9-15.

Wu, CL.; Marsh, A. & Dworkin, RH(2000). The role of sympathetic nerve blocks in herpes zoster and postherpetic neuralgia. *Pain.* 87:121-129.

Wu, CL. & Raja, SN. (2008). An update on the treatment of postherpetic neuralgia. *J Pain.* 9(1 Suppl 1):S19-30.

Yan, WK.; Wang, JH. & Chang, QQ. (1991). Effect of leu-enkephalin in striatum on modulating cellular immune during electropuncture. *Sheng Li Xue Bao.* 43:451-456.

Yanagida, H.; Suwa, K. & Corssen G. (1987). No prophylactic effect of early sympathetic blockade on postherpetic neuralgia. *Anestesiology.* 66:73-6.

Yang, YW.; Chen, YH.; Wang, KH.; Wang, CY. & Lin, HW. (2011). Risk of herpes zoster among patients with chronic obstructive pulmonary disease: a population-based study. *CMAJ.* 22;183(5):E275-80.

Yawn, BP.; Saddier, P.; Wollan, PC.; St Sauver, JL.; Kurland, MJ. & Sy, S. (2007). A population-based study of the incidence and complication rates of herpes zoster before zoster vaccine introduction. *Mayo Clin Proc.* 2007. 82(11):1341-9.

Yi, YS.; Chung, JS.; Song, MK. et al. (2010). The risk factors for herpes zoster in bortezomib treatment in patients with multiple myeloma. *Korean J Hematol.* 45(3):188-92.

Zhu, SM.; Liu, YM.; An, ED. & Chen, QI (2009). Influence of systemic immune and cytokine responses during the acute phase of zoster on the development of postherpetic neuralgia. *J Zhejiang Univ Sci B.* 10 (8): 625-630.

Zochodne, DW. (1997). Local events within the injured and regenerating peripheral nerve trunk: the role of the microenvironment and microcirculation. *Biomed Rev.* 8: 37-54.

8

Varicella Zoster Virus Infection in Pregnancy

Irena Narkeviciute[1] and Jolanta Bernatoniene[2]
[1]*Vilnius University Clinic of Children's Diseases,*
[2]*Bristol Royal Hospital for Children,*
[1]*Lithuania*
[2]*UK*

1. Introduction

Varicella-zoster virus (VZV) is one of the eight herpesviruses that infect humans. The virus causes two diseases: the primary infection, varicella (chickenpox), and secondary or clinical manifestation of latent infection, herpes zoster (shingles). Though VZV infection rarely occurs during pregnancy, the disease is likely to be associated with significant complications for both mother and fetus: pregnant women are several times more likely to develop fatal varicella than non-pregnant patients, the fetus is at high risk of congenital varicella syndrome (CVS), and the neonate is at high risk of a severe or fatal form of varicella.

1.1 Varicella

Ninety percent of varicella cases occur in children between the age of 1 and 14 years. Varicella is a highly contagious disease and affects nearly all susceptible children with an attack rate approaching 90% following a household exposure to the illness. Transmission occurs mainly via direct contact and through respiratory droplets that contain the virus, making the disease highly contagious even before the first onset of rash. Varicella is generally regarded as a mild, self-limited viral illness with occasional complications in healthy children, and it is usually characterized by fever, malaise, and vesicular rash on the trunk, face, scalp, extremities, and oropharynx. The incubation period is usually 14-16 days, but can range from 10 to 21 days. The incubation period may be prolonged to 28 days if varicella zoster immunoglobulin (VZIG) has been administered. Transplacental transmission from mother to fetus occurs during maternal viraemia, and the incubation period for neonatal infection is 11 days (range 9-15 days) from the onset of maternal disease. The period of infectivity begins 1-2 days before the appearance of rash until the lesions crust over, usually 4 to 5 days after the onset of the rash (Centers for Disease Control and Prevention [CDC], 1996; Riley, 1998). Initially, the lesions appear as macules which tend to progress to vesicules which may erupt every 1-2 days. Once ruptured, these vesicules crust over. The lesions may be at various stages in the same area of skin and the rash is characteristically pruritic. The illness normally evolves over about 5 days.

Seroepidemiological studies performed between 1973 and 2000 in different industrial countries revealed that up to 26% of women of reproductive age do not possess VZV-specific IgG class antibodies (Sauerbrei & Wutzler, 2005). Currently, most pregnant women living in the US and Europe are not susceptible to the development of varicella, because

more than 90% of women of childbearing age are protected by virus-specific IgG class antibodies. The average incidence of varicella in pregnant women has been calculated as 2-3 per 1,000 pregnancies (Enders & Miller, 2000). The epidemiology of varicella differs between countries with temperate climates and those with tropical climates. VZV is acquired at less frequency and at older ages in tropical and subtropical geographical zones. The rate of susceptibility to VZV is 16% (CDC, 1996). The latest seroepidemiological study carried out in 7980 pregnant women from various regions of the word demonstrated a prevalence of VZV antibodies of 93.1% in women born in Western European countries and 80.3% in women born in Central and Eastern Europe, Asia and Africa (Knowles et al., 2004).
Although the clinical course of varicella in children is usually mild, it may be severe or fatal in pregnant women. Varicella is estimated to be 25 times more likely to be severe in adults than in children. There is thought to be an even greater risk associated with pregnancy, particularly during the third trimester. Presumably, this is caused by maternal immunosuppression, which is most intense during this period (Gershon, 2001).

1.2 Herpes zoster

Herpes zoster (HZ) is caused by reactivation of latent VZV infection in sensory nerve root ganglia, which resulted during the attack of primary varicella infection. It usually occurs in about 15% of people over their lifetime, most commonly in elderly and immunocompromised populations. People with herpes zoster are capable of transmitting VZV to varicella susceptible individuals, although the patients with zoster infection are thought to be less infectious than the patients suffering with the primary varicella. Herpes zoster or shingles is characterized by a painful, unilateral vesicular rash that is usually restricted to unilateral dermatomal distribution and can occur on the trunk or face, although the rash may involve an extremity. The lesions, full of infectious virus, tend to coalesce. The individual is considered contagious to varicella susceptible until the skin lesions have dried. Most lesions may be present for days to weeks in immunocompromised patients. Pain is often a major complaint rather than itching. Zoster seems to increase in severity with increasing age; young people rarely have a severe form of the illness. Zoster is essentially not a fatal illness in otherwise healthy individuals. There is little information on the risk of developing zoster during pregnancy. Fortunately, herpes zoster during pregnancy and during the perinatal period is not associated with any known birth defect and problems for newborns, unless the women are immunocompromised (Enders et al., 1994; Miller et al., 1989; Sauerbrei & Wutzler, 2000).

2. Varicella in pregnancy

If the pregnant women give a history of contact with varicella or shingles, a careful history including previous vaccinations must be taken to confirm the significance of the exposure and the susceptibility of the patient. The women should have a blood test to assess the presence or absence of the immunity to varicella. The algorithm for the assessment and management of varicella exposure during pregnancy is demonstrated in figure 1.
Varicella is much less common in adults than in children; however, it is associated with greater morbidity and mortality. Varicella results in the death of 25 people/year in England and Wales and 75% of these deaths occur in adults (Rawson et al., 2001). The data suggest that 5-14% of adults with varicella develop pulmonary involvement, which

may vary in severity from a subclinical form, only detected on X-ray or lung function tests, to a severe and potentially fatal illness (Nathwani et al., 1998). The disease usually develops within 3-5 days of the rash and is associated with cough, dyspnea, fever, and tachypnea. Additionally, cyanosis, pleuritic pain in the chest, and hemoptysis can occur and secondary bacterial infections are frequent. The chest X-ray findings include a diffuse or nodular infiltrative pattern often seen in peribronchial distribution involving both lungs. The X-ray findings may be more severe than the clinical appearance (Daley et al., 2008; Haake et al., 1990).

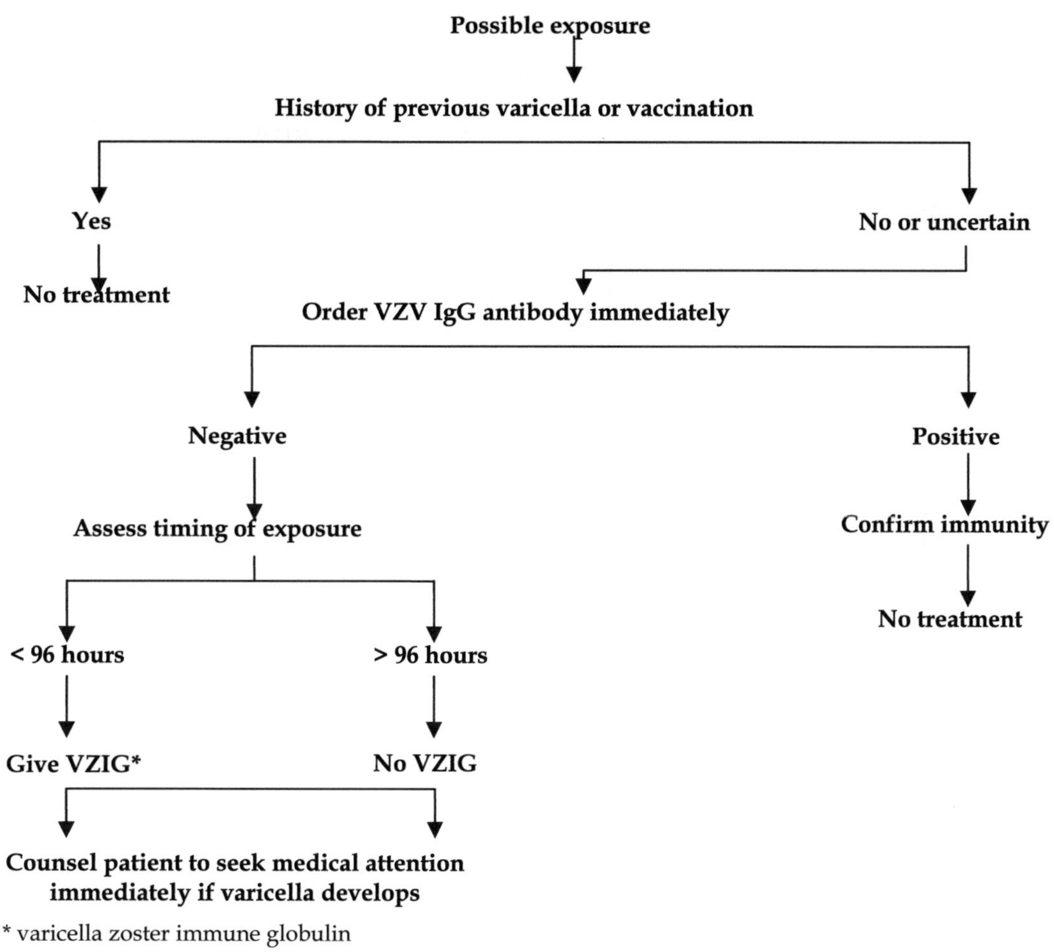

Fig. 1. Management of exposure to varicella during pregnancy (Gardella & Brown, 2007, as cited in Heuchan & Isaacs, 2001)

Pregnant women appear no more likely than other adults to develop pneumonia (Royal College of Obstetricians and Gynaecologists [RCOG], 2001) which can occur in up to 10% of pregnant women suffering with varicella (Harger et al., 2002); however, varicella pneumonia may be more severe in pregnant compared to non-pregnant women. The severity of this complication seems to increase in later gestation (Tan & Koren, 2005). Smoking and the occurrence of at least 100 skin lesions are well known risk factors for the development of VZV pneumonia (Harger et al., 2002). The mortality rate in untreated pregnant women is as high as 40% (Haake et al., 1990), therefore varicella pneumonia in pregnancy is considered a medical emergency. However, more recent studies suggest that the mortality has decreased to 10-11% for both non-pregnant and pregnant patients, most likely due to the effective antiviral therapy and better respiratory management (Chandra et al., 1998).

Encephalitis causing acute cerebellar ataxia can occur up to 21 days after the onset of the varicella rash (Sissons, 2003). Fortunately, more severe forms of encephalitis are uncommon (0.1–0.2% of cases of varicella), but they have a mortality of around 5–20% (Sissons, 2003).

Possible haemorrhagic complications of chickenpox include acute thrombocytopenia, or purpura fulminans associated with arterial thrombosis and haemorrhagic gangrene (Sissons, 2003). Although encephalitis and haemorrhagic complications are rare, their development may severely complicate pregnancy. Multiorgan involvement including hepatitis, myocarditis, and pericarditis is associated with a high mortality. Fetal loss may result from maternal sepsis, fever and hypoxia (Daley et al., 2008).

There is no evidence that uncomplicated chickenpox in the mother significantly increases the likelihood of spontaneous abortion during the first 20 weeks of pregnancy (3.0% in one study) or intrauterine death after the 20th week (0.7%) (Enders et al., 1994; Hinshaw & Fayyad, 2000; Office for National UK Statistics, 2005).

3. Management of the pregnant woman who develops varicella or herpes zoster

Most pregnant women who develop varicella illness do not require hospitalization; they can be reassured and sent home for daily or more frequent reviews if clinically indicated (Morgan-Capner et al., 2002). Indications for referral to hospital include the development of respiratory or/and neurological symptoms, a wide-spreading haemorrhagic rash or bleeding, a dense rash with or without mucosal lesions, the appearance of new lesions after 6 days, and a history of significant immunosuppression. Also, the women close to term should be considered for hospitalization because of the risk of developing haemorrhagic complications or varicella of the newborn (RCOG, 2001). Furthermore, if the woman smokes cigarettes, has chronic lung disease, is taking corticosteroids, or is in the latter half of pregnancy, a hospital assessment should be considered, even in the absence of complications (Heuchan & Isaacs, 2001; RCOG, 2001).

If the pregnant woman develops the first signs of chickenpox illness, an appropriate treatment should be decided in consultation with a multidisciplinary team: obstetrician or fetal medicine specialist, virologist, and neonatologist. Depending on the severity of the maternal condition, a respiratory physician, intensive care specialist, and infectious disease specialist may also be involved. Timing and mode of delivery must be individualized (Morgan-Capner et al., 2002; RCOG, 2001).

As the only safe therapeutic agent, acyclovir is indicated for pregnant women with varicella. The studies suggest that acyclovir administered in a dosage of 800mg five times a day for 7 days reduces the duration of fever and symptomatology of varicella in immunocompetent patients if commenced within 24 hours of developing the rash when compared with placebo (Wallace et al. 1992). This randomized controlled trial did not have sufficient power to comment on the impact of early oral acyclovir on the serious complications of varicella. Data suggest that there is no increase in the risk of fetal malformation with acyclovir in pregnancy, although the theoretical risk of teratogenesis persists in the first trimester (Ratanajamit et al., 2003; Stone et al., 2004). Intravenous acyclovir (10mg/kg three times daily for at least 5 days (7-10)) is indicated for pregnant women with severe illness, complications and/or risk factors (Kempf et al., 2007; Morgan-Capner et al., 2002). VZIG has no therapeutic benefit once varicella has developed (Nathwani et al., 1998).

The woman may also need symptomatic relief with paracetamol and/or ibuprofen, although ibuprofen should be avoided after 30 weeks of gestation because it may cause premature closure of the ductus arteriosus (Prodigy, 2005). Systemic antihistamines should also be avoided during the first trimester and breast-feeding (Prodigy, 2005; Drug and Therapeutics Bulletin [DTB], 2002).

Delivery during the viraemic period may be extremely hazardous. There are significant maternal risks associated with bleeding, thrombocytopenia, disseminated intravascular coagulopathy, and hepatitis. Also, there is a high risk of varicella of the newborn with significant morbidity and mortality (Meyers, 1974; Miller et al., 1989). Therefore, where relevant and practical, the delivery should be delayed until 5 days after the onset of maternal illness to allow for passive transfer of antibodies that could protect the baby from the infection (RCOG, 2001). Supportive treatment and intravenous acyclovir is therefore desirable, allowing resolution of the rash, immune recovery, and transfer of protective antibodies from the mother to the fetus. Delivery may be required in women to facilitate assisted ventilation in cases where varicella pneumonia is complicated by respiratory failure (RCOG, 2001).

There is no evidence available to us to inform decisions about the optimum method of anaesthesia for women requiring delivery by caesarean section. General anaesthesia may exacerbate varicella pneumonia. There is a theoretical risk of transmitting the VZV from skin lesions to the central nervous system via spinal anaesthesia. This results in advice that epidural anaesthesia may be safer than spinal anaesthesia, because the dura is not penetrated. A site free of cutaneous lesions should be chosen for needle placement (Brown et al., 2003).

Women hospitalized with varicella should be nursed in isolation from babies or potentially susceptible pregnant women or non-immune staff (RCOG, 2001).

Treatment of herpes zoster in imunocompetent pregnant women should be symptomatic; topical or systemic antiviral therapy is not recommended (Kempf et al., 2007).

4. Consequences of varicella in pregnancy

Varicella acquired during pregnancy may have serious consequences for fetus and neonate. Maternal varicella associated with viraemia can transmit the virus to the fetus by either transplacental route or by ascending infection from the lesions in the birth canal. The possible outcomes of VZV infection during pregnancy depends on the time of the disease and includes spontaneous abortion, fetal malformation, premature delivery, fetal growth restriction, or postnatal infection. In infancy, herpes zoster may be the first clinical manifestation of VZV infection after the primary infection *in utero* (Table 1).

Maternal disease	Timing during pregnancy	Consequences for mother, fetus, term neonate
Varicella	At any stage	Intrauterine death, neonatal or infantile zoster
	5-24th weeks	Congenital varicella sindrome (risk: 2%, mortality: 30%)
	At any stage, especially in the third trimester	Maternal pneumonia (risk: 10-20%, mortality: 10-45%)
	Near term: ≥5 days before delivery	Neonatal varicella at ages 10 (-12) days (risk: 20-50%, mortality: 0%)
	Near term: ≤4-5 days before to 2 days after delivery	Neonatal varicella 0-4 days after birth (risk: 20-50%, mortality: 0-3%); neonatal varicella 5-10 (-12) days after birth (risk: 20-50%, mortality: 20-25%)
Normal zoster	At any stage	No risk for severe maternal, fetal or neonatal infections

Table 1. Potential consequences of varicella-zoster virus infections during pregnancy (Sauerbrei, 2010)

4.1 Congenital varicella syndrome

Since the first report in 1947 (Laforet & Lynch, 1947) more than 130 cases of congenital varicella syndrome have been described in the English and German literature (Sauerbrei & Wutzler, 2005). CVS can occur in about 12% of infected fetuses (Prober et al., 1990). Prospective studies in Europe and North America demonstrated that the incidence of congenital anomalies after maternal varicella in the first 20 weeks of pregnancy is about 1-2% (Enders et al., 1994; Pastuszak et al., 1994). Before the 5th and after the 24th gestational weeks, the probability of CVS is extremely low (Sauerbrei, 2010). Overall the incidence of CVS in nine reported cohort studies was 0.55% in the first trimester, 1.4% in the second trimester, and 0% in the third trimester (Tan & Koren, 2006).

Although a few cases of fetal abnormalities have been reported after maternal herpes zoster, clinical evidence suggests that herpes zoster infection during pregnancy does not cause the congenital varicella syndrome or neonatal varicella. This is because the fetus passively acquires, and is protected by, the mother's varicella antibodies produced in response to the initial varicella infection (RCOG, 2001).

Congenital varicella syndrome is usually characterized by unusual cutaneous defects with cicatricial skin scars in dermatomal distribution, neurological defects secondary to probable intrauterine VZV encephalitis (cortical atrophy, spinal cord atrophy, limb paresis, seizures, microcephaly, Horner's syndrome, encephalitis, mental retardation), eye disease (microphthalmia, enophthalmia, chorioretinitis, cataract, nystagmus, anisocoria, optic atrophy), limb hypoplasia or diminished limb growth, and other skeletal anomalies. Less frequent abnormalities include muscle hypoplasia and affections of the internal organs as well as gastrointestinal, genitourinary, and cardiovascular manifestations (Sauerbrei, 2010).

It is not known whether VZIG reduces the risk of CVS. A prospective study was carried out in 108 women who developed varicella infection despite VZIG prophylaxis. Eighty percent of these women received VZIG in the first and second trimester and there were no cases of

CVS or infants with IgM antibodies at birth reported (Enders & Miller, 2000). However, no conclusion can be drawn from this, given the rarity of CVS. Criteria for diagnosis of CVS listed in Table 2.

- **Appearance of maternal varicella during pregnancy**
- **Neonate or fetus with**
  - congenital skin lesions in dermatomal distribution and/or
  - neurological defects,
  - eye diseases,
  - limb hypoplasia

- **Proof of intrauterine VZV infection by**
  - detection of viral DNA using polymerase chain reaction and/or
  - presence of specific IgM/persistence of IgG beyond 7 months of age
  - appearance of zoster during early infancy

Table 2. Criteria used for diagnosis of congenital varicella syndrome (Sauerbrei, 2010)

Prenatal diagnosis of CVS is possible using detailed fetal ultrasonography and/or fetal magnetic resonance imaging and can be useful to look for limb anomalies or other morphological abnormalities caused by intrauterine varicella. VZV DNA can be detected by PCR in fetal blood, amniotic fluid, or placental villi. VZV IgM in fetal blood can be detected. No cases of CVS occurred when the amniotic fluid obtained during amniocentesis was negative for VZV DNA. If the amniotic fluid is PCR positive for VZV and the ultrasound is normal at 17-21 weeks, the risk of CVS is still low. If the repeat ultrasound is normal at 23-24 weeks the risk of CVS is remote. However, the risk of CVS increases significantly if the ultrasound scan reveals features compatible with CVS and the DNA is found in the amniotic fluid. (Mouly et al., 1997). A negative PCR for VZV in amniotic fluid, and a normal ultrasound scan results from 23 weeks onwards, suggest a low risk of intrauterine infection (Table 3).

Weeks of gestation	PCR	High level ultrasound	Risk for CVS with severe malformation
Initial			
17-21	(+) Amniocentesis	Normal	Uncertain
Repeat			
23-24	(+) Amniocentesis	Normal	Unlikely
22-24	(+) Amniocentesis (±) cord blood	Abnormal	High
18-22/>23	(-)Amniocentesis	Normal	Low

Table 3. Prenatal diagnosis using ultrasound and PCR for risk of CVS (Enders & Miller, 2000)

The prognosis of infants born with CVS is poor, with death in infancy resulting from intractable gastroesophageal reflux, severe recurrent aspiration pneumonia, and respiratory failure due to dysfunction of the autonomic nervous system (Smith & Arvin, 2009). Nearly 30% of neonates born with CVS died during the first months of life. A follow-up report in the literature showed that in spite of initially poor prognosis, a good long-term outcome can occur in patients with CVS (Schulze & Dietzsch, 2000).

4.2 Neonatal varicella

If maternal varicella occurs 1–4 weeks before delivery, up to 50% of babies may be infected. Approximately 23% of these develop clinical varicella despite high titers of passively acquired maternal antibodies (Miller et al., 1989). When the mother's rash appeared 7–3 days before delivery, progressively fewer infants had antibodies.

Infection may occur by transplacental viraemia, ascending infection from the birth canal, or through direct contact with infectious lesions during and after delivery. Varicella occurring in the first 12 days of life is described as intrauterine-acquired neonatal varicella infection. If the infection is diagnosed after the 12th day of the neonatal period, VZV is most likely acquired postnatally. (Enders & Miller, 2000). The severity of intrauterine-acquired neonatal varicella is closely related to the time of onset of the maternal infection, as transplacentally transmitted antibodies may reduce the severity of symptoms in the neonate (Table 1). Generalized neonatal varicella can be fatal if mothers develop varicella rash between 4-5 days before and 2 days after delivery since these neonates are not protected from severe disease by the maternal antibodies. A fatal outcome is more likely if the neonatal disease occurs between 5 and 10 days after delivery. Infants born to mothers with varicella within this high risk period are usually initially well-appearing. Varicella presents with the classical skin lesions, but can disseminate with pneumonia, hepatitis, encephalitis, and severe coagulopathy resulting from liver failure and thrombocytopenia (Prober & Arvin, 1987). Before VZV immunoglobulin was available, the risk of death among neonates born to mothers with the onset of rash up to four days before delivery was 31% (Meyers, 1974). The rate decreased to 7% when the use of VZIG was introduced and neonatal intensive care improved (Miller et al., 1989). Neonatal varicella within the first 4 days after birth has usually been found to be mild (Sauerbrei & Wutzler, 2001).

When the history of maternal varicella is in the few weeks preceding delivery, the infants may be asymptomatic or may have cutaneous lesions at birth or developing shortly thereafter, but are at low risk of dissemination of varicella disease or complications (Smith & Arvin, 2008).

Premature neonates younger than 28 weeks gestation must be considered to have an increased risk for severe neonatal varicella during the first 6 weeks after birth (Advisory Committee on Immunization Practices [ACIP], 1996; Deutsche Gesellschaft für Pädiatrische Infektologie [DGPI], 2003). They are unlikely to have protecting maternal antibodies due to the reduced gestation period and the lack the transplacental transfer of maternal IgG to VZV.

The diagnosis of neonatal varicella is usually based on typical clinical picture. The clinical findings may be confirmed by serological methods, detection of VZV DNA in skin swabs or biopsies, or liquor and tissue samples using PCR (Sauerbrei, 2010). When varicella pneumonia is suspected, broncho-alveolar lavage may be obtained for the VZV DNA detection.

We report three clinical cases of neonatal varicella: two transmitted in utero and one acquired postnatally.

4.2.1 Case report 1

A 6-day-old baby boy was hospitalized on the first day of his illness with a history of a maculovesicular skin rash noticed on his face and back. On admission, he had normal temperature and he weighed 3960 g. The next day, he was noticed to have haemorrhagic fluid in some of the vesicles, and subsequently he developed pustules with infiltration as well as necrosis of the surrounding tissues on the 5th day of the illness. He spiked temperatures up to 38°C on day 4 and a few days later (day 6) his condition deteriorated even further. He was spiking fevers up to 39°C; he had poor appetite and dropped his weight to 3440g. Peripheral blood analysis performed on the 1st, 5th and 11th day of his illness was within normal limits. His chest was clear on auscultation with no evidence of any obvious respiratory compromise. However, on day 7 a chest x-ray demonstrated fine bilateral foci with a minor reaction of interlobular pleura on the right side which was very suggestive of varicella pneumonitis. The patient received 2 ml (50 IU) of intravenous human varicella zoster immunoglobuline (VZIG; Varitect, Germany) on the 2nd day of the admission. He was also given a course of second generation cephalosporin between the day 5 and 9 of his illness. The patient's condition was significantly improved and he was discharged home on the 12th day of his illness.

Of note, the mother had varicella infection 5 days before the delivery. The incubation period for the newborn was 11 days (Figure 2).

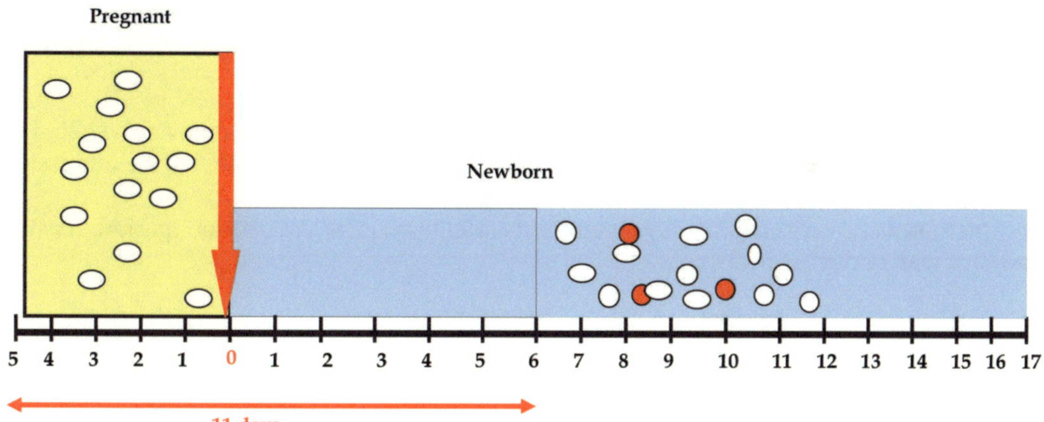

Fig. 2. Newborn varicella aquired from the mother in prenatal period. Varicella of the pregnant woman started at 5 days before delivery; severe varicella of newborn, at 6 days of age. The incubation period of varicella for the newborn was 11days.

4.2.2 Case report 2

A 2-day-old newborn presented with a widespread maculovesicular skin rash and was hospitalized on the first day of his illness (Figure 3).

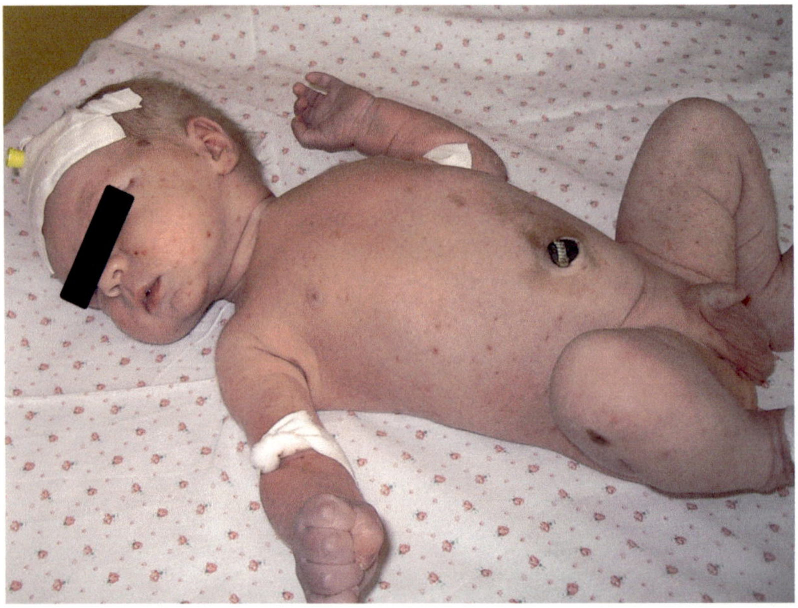

Fig. 3. Male neonate with intrauterine acquired varicella, day 3 of the illness. There was a history of maternal varicella 12 days before the delivery.

On physical examination, the newborn was afebrile and generally appeared well. His peripheral blood analysis was entirely normal. He remained very well during the admission and he was discharged from the hospital on day 4.

The mother had varicella 12 days before the delivery. The incubation period for the newborn was 14 day (Figure 4).

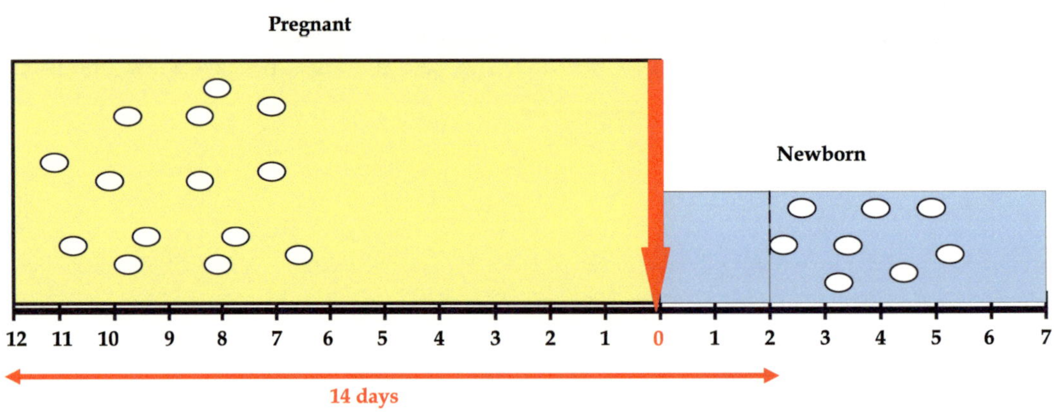

Fig. 4. Prenatally acquired newborn varicella. The mother developed varicella 12 days before the delivery. Mild varicella illness of newborn was diagnosed at 2 days of age. The incubation period of varicella for the neonate was 14 days.

4.2.3 Case report 3

We report a 22-day-old baby boy who at the age of 3 days was in a close contact with his 10-year old sister who had clinically unrecognized varicella. Her serological investigation confirmed the diagnosis of varicella by detecting VZV- IgM class antibodies (ELISA, Enzygnost; Dade Behring, Germany). Serum VZV-IgM concentration was raised to 0.939 (pos. > 0.200 OD) on the 9th day of his illness. Varicella of the neonate started after 14 days of the incubation period. A clinical course of the varicella illness was mild (Figure 5).

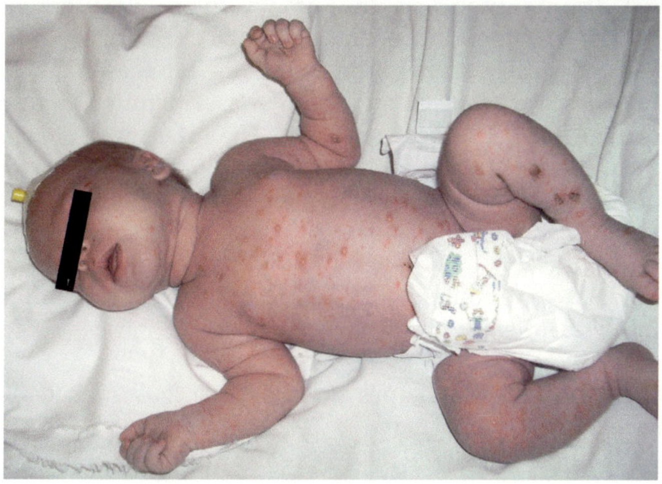

Fig. 5. A 22 day old newborn with postnatally acquired varicella, day 5 of the illness. The index case was a 10 year old sister.

Three days after the delivery, the mother was in direct contact with her daughter who was ill with varicella. As a result, the mother developed varicella thirteen days later, but fortunately the illness was mild (Figure 6).

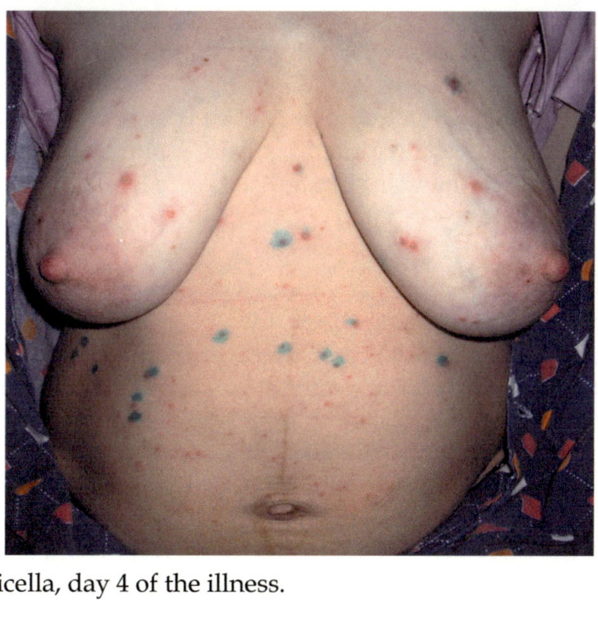

Fig. 6. Maternal varicella, day 4 of the illness.

4.3 Herpes zoster in young infants

Nearly 20% of infants with intrauterine-acquired VZV primary infection develop herpes zoster in the first or second year of life, usually with uncomplicated course (Sauerbrei & Wutzler, 2003). The observed risk of zoster when maternal infection occurs before 24 weeks was 0.8%, compared to a 1.7% observed risk if maternal varicella was after 25 weeks (Enders et al., 1994). The risk of postnatal herpes zoster infection in infancy was 3.8% in cases when maternal amniotic fluid had been positive for VZV DNA by PCR (Mouly et al., 1997). The symptoms are the same as in adults, although the skin lesions are less prominent and the symptoms of acute neuritis are mild or absent. Unlike adults, children do not suffer with post-herpetic neuralgia (Helgason et al., 2000). Serious complications have been reported in only one case of a four-month-old infant whose mother had had varicella at 17 weeks' gestation. The infant was born full term without complications; however, aged three months, he developed herpes zoster associated with generalized seizures. The clinical picture and VZV DNA detected in his cerebrospinal fluid by PCR were consistent with central nervous system infection (Sauerbrei et al., 2003).

Herpes zoster in infants who acquired VZV in utero has been self-limited. If the zoster is extensive and painful, treatment with acyclovir (initially by intravenous, followed by oral) for seven to 10 days is recommended.

We report two patients with typical herpes zoster, whose mothers had varicella during the second-third trimester of their pregnancy.

4.3.1 Case report 4

A thirteen and a half month old girl was hospitalized on the 7th day of her illness because of ongoing restlessness, disturbed sleep, and a rash, which she had developed on day 4 of her restlessness. On examination, she had a right-sided vesicular skin rash along T10-12, L1-2 dermatomes (Picture 2). Otherwise, she appeared generally well. Her peripheral blood analysis was completely normal. The patient received symptomatic treatment and was discharged home 4 days later. VZV-IgG and IgM class antibodies (ELISA, Enzygnost; Dade Behring, Germany) were detected in the blood serum on the 9th and 29th days of the illness. VZV-IgG concentration was 0.135 and 2.142; VZV-IgM was 0.038 and 0.704, respectively (pos. > 0.200 OD). Of note, she was born prematurely at week 36 of gestation via Caesarean section. Initially she required intubation and ventilation for her backbone injury identified at birth. The mother suffered with moderate varicella during the 26th week of her pregnancy.

4.3.2 Case report 5

A 10 month old girl was hospitalized on the 6th day of her illness due to her ongoing restlessness, fever, and a rash noticed on the right side of her chest. On the 5th day she developed a maculovesicular rash and started spiking temperatures up to 38.5°C. On physical examination, she had vesicular skin lesions observed on the right side of her chest along T6-7 dermatomes. Otherwise, the girl appeared generally well. Peripheral blood analysis was entirely normal. Varicella immune status was established on the 8th and 22nd day of the illness. Her VZV-IgG concentrations were 0.200 and 2.462, and VZV-IgM levels were 0.122 and 0.412, respectively (pos. > 0.200 OD). The patient received symptomatic treatment for 6 days and was discharged in good health thereafter.

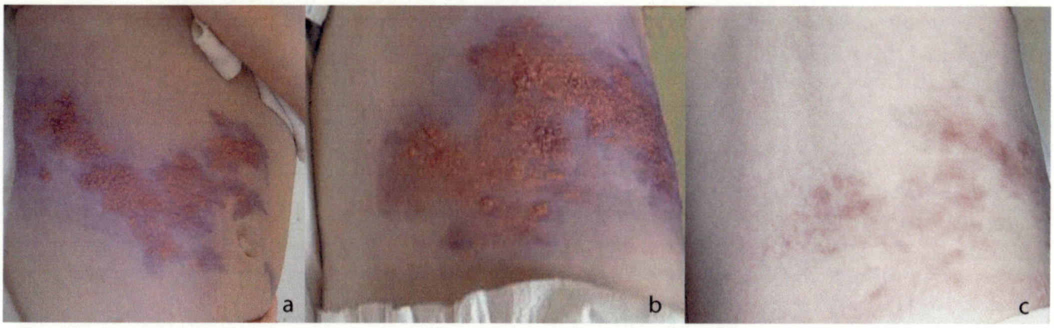

Fig. 7. The patient with herpes zoster following maternal varicella acquired during pregnancy. Day 7 of the illness. a) A typical anterior vesicular skin rash along the T10-12 and L1-2 dermatomes on the right side. b) A typical posterior vesicular skin rash along the T10-12 and L1-2 dermatomes on the right side. c) Post inflammatory skin hyperpigmentation following zoster, day 29 of the illness.

Early manifestation of herpes zoster may be explained by the immature cell-mediated immune response in young children and/or the decrease of maternally derived antibodies (Sauerbrei & Wutzler, 2000). The hypothesis was confirmed by our two clinical cases. Neither of them had detectable VZV-IgG antibodies at the beginning of the illness. High titers of serum VZV-IgG and IgM antibodies were discovered only 3–4 weeks later.

5. Management of neonatal varicella

Varicella zoster immunoglobulin, administered to the infants whose mothers developed varicella (but not herpes zoster) at around term, may attenuate infection and significantly reduce the risk of life-threatening neonatal varicella (Enders, 1985; Miller et al., 1989). VZIG should be given at birth to neonates who meet any of the following criteria (Sauerbrei, 2010):

- their mothers develop rash between 7 days before and 7 days after birth;
- they were born within the last 7 days, the mother is seronegative and they have had significant non-maternal post-natal exposure (e.g. from a sibling);
- they have been exposed to varicella and are at risk because of potentially inadequate transfer of maternal antibodies. This includes neonates born before 28 weeks gestation; or weighing less than 1,000g; or who have had repeated blood sampling with replacement by packed red cell infusion; or those requiring intensive or prolonged special care nursing. VZIG can be issued without antibody testing but, where possible, such infants should be tested.

Other infants whose mothers have a positive history of varicella and/or a positive VZV antibody result will usually have maternal antibody and do not require VZIG. Severe neonatal varicella can occur despite VZIG administration (Reynolds et al., 1999). Neonatal varicella should be treated promptly with acyclovir (Table 4, Figure 8).

Postnatally, the mother and neonate should be isolated from other mothers and babies on the ward, but not from each other. Breast-feeding of neonates exposed to maternal varicella should be encouraged. If the mother has varicella lesions close to the nipple, milk should be expressed until the lesions have crusted (Morgan-Capner et al., 2002). Where other members of the family have varicella at home and the mother is seronegative, discharge should be delayed until the baby is at least 7 days old (Morgan-Capner et al., 2002).

VZIG after intrauterine exposure to VZV		
Neonates whose mothers develop varicella within 5 days before and 2 days after delivery	Intravenously: 1 ml/kg or intramuscularly: 125 U or 0.5 mg/kg	Immediately after birth or onset of maternal rash
VZIG after postnatal exposure		
Premature neonates with negative maternal varicella history	Intravenously: 1 ml/kg or intramuscularly: 125 U or 0.5 mg/kg	Within 96 hours after exposure
Premature neonates <28 weeks gestation or <1,000 g birth weight independent of maternal varicella history	Intravenously: 1 ml/kg or intramuscularly: 125 U or 0.5 mg/kg	Within 96 hours after exposure
Antiviral treatment of neonatal varicella		
Suspected neonatal varicella	Acyclovir intravenously: 3 x 10-15 mg/kg	Length of therapy: 5-7 days

Table 4. Administration of VZIG and acyclovir in neonates to prevent neonatal varicella (Sauerbrei, 2010; ACIP, 1996; DGPI, 2003)

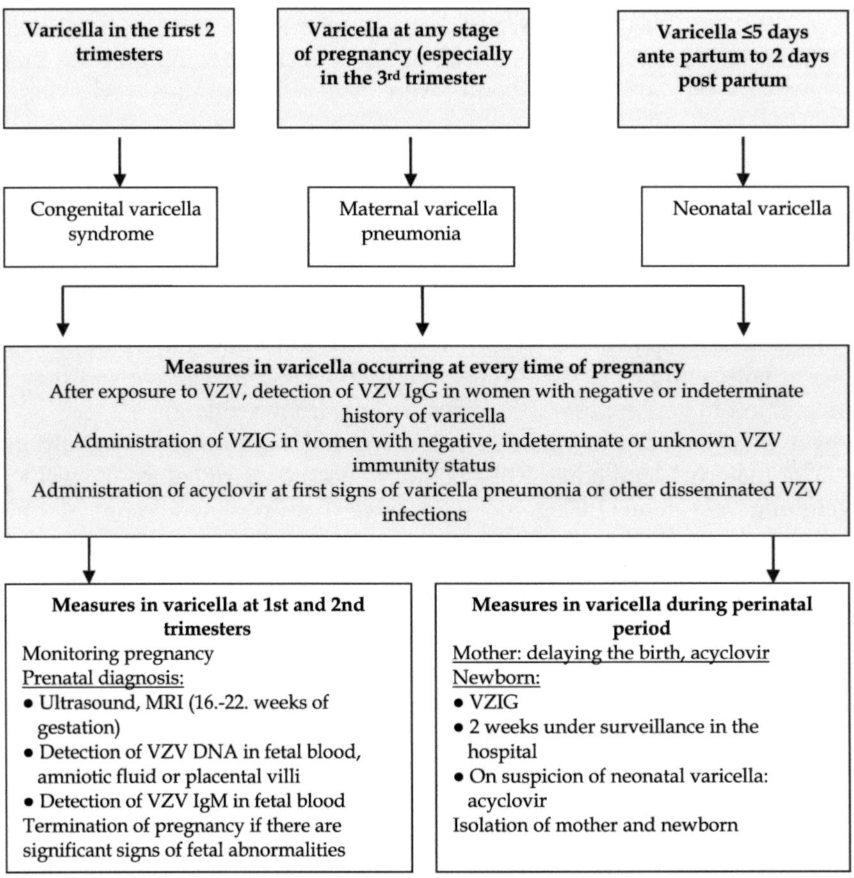

Fig. 8. Measures in case of varicella during pregnancy depending on the point of time of infection (Sauerbrei , 2010)

All neonates with maternal or other exposure must be followed up for 14–16 days (by the GP, midwife, health visitor or in hospital) and acyclovir should be given if there is any evidence of infection (RCOG, 2001).

6. Varicella prevention

The aim of varicella immunisation is to protect from exposure those who are at the most risk of serious illness. Varicella vaccination prepregancy or postpartum is an effective prophylaxis of chickenpox in pregnant women and neonates, and should be considered for seronegative women before pregnancy or in the postpartum period. Live-attenuated varicella vaccine, made from the OKA strain, was licensed in the United States in 1995 and is currently recommended for universal administration in early childhood. Following its introduction, the incidence of primary varicella infection has fallen by 90% and the mortality related to the condition has decreased by two-thirds (Ngyuen et al., 2005). The vaccine has also been shown to be safe and effective in preventing chickenpox in adults (Gershon et al., 1990). The two-dose varicella vaccine schedule administered to suseptible adolescents and adults provides about 75% protection, and the single-dose schedule in children about 95% protection against clinical varicella (Annunziato & Gershon, 2000). In both age groups, most of the breakthrough infections are modified, and vaccinated individuals who contract varicella develop fewer lesions and less systemic illness than unvaccinated individuals (Immunisation against infections disease, Varicella, online, updated 2011). Currently, a two-dose regimen of varicella vaccine, given four to eight weeks apart, is recommended to susceptible individuals (Gardella & Brown, 2007; Department of Health, 2004). In the UK, varicella immunisation is only offered to specific individuals who are in regular or close contact with those at risk (Department of Health, 2004).

Women who are pregnant should not receive varicella vaccine and pregnancy should be avoided for three months following the last dose (Department of Health, 2004). Studies have shown that the vaccine virus is not transferred to the infant through breast milk (Bohlke et al., 2003) and therefore breast feeding women can be vaccinated if necessary.

Inadvert exposures to the vaccine in pregnancy have been reported to a register. No cases of congenital varicella have been reported so far. Furthermore, the rate of occurrence of congenital anomalies was similar to that reported in the general population (Merck Pregnancy Registry Program, 2003).

The varicella immune status of women planning a pregnancy can be determined by obtaining a past history of primary varicella infection or by checking the serum for varicella antibodies in those who have no history or uncertain history of previous infection. A previous history of varicella infection is 97-99% predictive of the presence of serum varicella antibodies (CDC, 1996). Routine serologic testing is not recommended for pregnant women who received 2 doses of varicella vaccine, since seroconvertion rate after the second dose of varicella immunization is as high as 99% (Kuter et al., 1995). Non-immune pregnant women should be advised to avoid exposure to chickenpox or shingles and to immediately inform healthcare workers of a potential exposure. The US Advisory Committee on Immunization Practices recommends that postpartum women without evidence of immunity be given the first dose of vaccine before discharge from the hospital, and the second dose of vaccine at the follow-up postpartum visit six to eight weeks after delivery (Marin et al., 2007).

If the pregnant woman has had a significant exposure to varicella infection or shingles, a careful history must be taken to confirm the significance of the contact, any past history of chickenpox or shingles, vaccination, and the susceptibility of the patient. Significant contact is defined as contact in the same room for 15 minutes or more, face-to-face contact and contact in the setting of a large open ward. The UK Advisory Group on Chickenpox considers any close contact during the period of infectiousness to be significant (Nathwani et al., 1998). If the woman's immunity to chickenpox is unknown and if there is any doubt about previous infection, or if there is no previous history of chickenpox or shingles, serum should be tested for VZV IgG. At least 80–90% of women tested will have VZ IgG and can be reassured (McGregor et al., 1987).

If the woman has a past history of chickenpox or shingles or two doses of a varicella containing vaccine, and is not immunosuppressed, protection can be assumed and reassurance given.

If the pregnant woman is VZV negative, has indeterminate or unknown serologic status, she should be given VZIG as soon as possible (Figure 1), preferably within 72-96 h after the exposure (Smith & Arvin, 2009). VZIG is effective when given up to 10 days after contact (RCOG, 2001). VZIG recommended intramuscularly at a concentration of 125 U/10 kg of body weight, up to a maximum of 625 U (ACIP, 1996) or 0.5 ml/kg of body weight (DGPI, 2003). A dosage of 1 ml/kg of body weight can be administered intravenously as alternative (DGPI, 2003). The primary reason for VZIG prophylaxis in pregnant women is to reduce severity of maternal disease and reduce the risk of fetal infection for women contracting varicella in the first 20 weeks of pregnancy. The risk of fatal varicella is estimated to be about five times higher in pregnant than non-pregnant adults, with fatal cases concentrated late in the second or early in the third trimester (Enders & Miller, 2000). One study showed a significant reduction in the risk of congenital VZV infection in women who developed varicella after VZIG prophylaxis compared with women who developed varicella without VZIG prophylaxis; however, the study was too small to assess whether the risk of CVS was reduced (Enders et al., 1994). A case of CVS has been reported in the infant of a woman exposed at the eleventh week of gestation and who developed clinical varicella despite post-exposure prophylaxis with VZIG (Pastuszak et al., 1994). About 50% of susceptible pregnant women given VZIG after a household exposure to chickenpox will develop clinical varicella, although the disease may be attenuated; the clinical attack rates are similar whether VZIG is given within 72 hours or four to ten days after contact (Enders & Miller, 2000; Miller et al., 1993). A further quarter will be infected sub-clinically (Miller et al., 1993). Severe maternal varicella may still occur despite VZIG prophylaxis. Prompt treatment with acyclovir is indicated in such cases. Women who have had exposure to chickenpox or shingles (regardless of whether or not they have received VZIG) should be asked to notify their doctor or midwife early if a rash develops (Nathwani et al., 1998).

Neither immunoglobulin nor acyclovir treatment have been shown to prevent vertical transmission or CVS (McKendrick et al., 2007).

If there is another exposure to chickenpox or shingles three weeks or more after the first use of VZIG, the need for VZIG needs to be reassessed. If more than six weeks have elapsed since first issue, antibody testing should be performed using a new (recent) sample ((Health Protection Agency [HPA], 2011).

As VZIG does not always prevent chickenpox, the woman should be managed as being possibly infectious 8–28 days after VZIG, and should be asked to contact her family doctor if she develops a rash. Up to 50% may develop a modified form of disease. Maternal pneumonia associated with chickenpox infection has been reported despite the timely VZIG administration (HPA, 2001).

7. References

Advisory Committee on Immunization Practices (ACIP). (1996). Prevention of varicella. *Morbidity and Mortality Weekly Report*, Vol.45, pp. 1-36

Annunziato, P.W. & Gershon, A.A. (2000). Primary vaccination against varicella, In: *Varicella-zoster virus*, A.M. Arvin & A.A. Gershon (Eds), pp. ??? Cambridge, Cambridge University Press

Bohlke, K.; Galil, K.; Jackson, L.A.; Schmid, D.S.; Starkovich, P.; Loparev, V.N. & Seward, J.F. (2003). Postpartum varicella vaccination: is the vaccine virus excreted in breast milk? *Obstetrics & Gynecology*. Vol.102 (5 Pt 1), pp. 970-977

Brown, N.W.; Parsons, A.P. & Kam, P.C. (2003). Anaesthetic considerations in a parturient with varicella presenting for Caesarean section. *Anaesthesia*, Vol.58, No.11, pp. 1092-1095

Centers for Disease Control and Prevention (CDC). (1996). Prevention of varicella: Recommendations of the Advisory Committee on Immunization (ACIP). *Morbidity and Mortality Weekly Report*, Vol.45 (RR-11), pp. 1-25

Chandra, P.C.; Patel, H., Schiavello, H.J. & Briggs, S.L. (1998). Successful pregnancy outcomeafter complicated varicella pneumonia. *Obstetrics & Gynecology*, Vol.92, (4 Pt 2), pp. 680-682

Chickenpox, pregnancy and the newborn. (2005). *Drug and Therapeutics Bulletin*, Vol.43, No.9, pp. 69-72 [Downloaded from dtb.bmj.com on May 16, 2011 - Published by group.bmj.com]

Daley, A.J.; Thorpe, S. & Garland, S.M. (2008). Varicella and the pregnant woman:prevention and management. *Australian and New Zealand J of Obstetrics and Gynaecology*, Vol.48, No.1 (Feb), pp. 26-33 Department of Health. (2004). Varicella [online]. Available: http://www.dh.gov.uk/assetRoot/04/07/31/40/04073140.pdf [Accessed 18 August 2005]

Deutsche Gesellschaft für Pädiatrische Infektiologie. (2003). *Handbuch 2003: Infektionen im Kindesalter*, pp. 732-739, Futuramed, München

Enders, G. & Miller, E. (2000). Varicella and herpes zoster in pregnancy and the newborn. In: *Varicella-zoster virus. Virology and Clinical Management*, A.M. Arvin & A.A. Gershon (Eds.), pp. 317-347, University Press, Cambridge

Enders, G.; Miller, E.; Cradock-Watson, J.; Bolley, I. & Ridehalgh, M. (1994). Consequences of varicella and herpes zoster in pregnancy: prospective study of 1739 cases. *Lancet*, Vol.343, No.8912 (Jun 18), pp. 1548-1551

Enders, G. (1985). Management of varicella-zoster contact and infection in pregnancy using a standartized varicella-zoster ELISA test. *Postgraduate Medical Journal*, Vol.61, (Suppl 4), pp. 23-30

Gardella, C. & Brown, Z.A. Managing varicella zoster infection in pregnancy. (2007). *Cleveland Clinic Journal of Medicine*, Vol.74, No.4 (Apr), pp. 290-296

Gershon, A.A. & Steinberg, S.P. (1990). Live attenuated varicella vaccine: protection in healthy adults compared with leukemic children. National Institute of Allergy and Infectious Diseases Varicella Vaccine Collaborative Study Group. *Journal of Infectious Diseases*, Vol.161, No.4, pp. 661-666

Gershon, A.A. (2001). Chickenpox, measles, and mumps. In: *Infections of the Fetus and Newborn Infant, 5th ed.*, J. Remington, J. Klein, (Eds.), pp. 683-732, Saunders, Philadelphia

Haake, D.A.; Zakowski, P.C.; Haake, D.L. & Bryson, X.J. (1990). Early treatment with acyclovir for varicella pneumonia in otherwise healthy adults: retrospective controlled study and review. *Reviews of Infectious Diseases*, Vol.12, No.5 (Sep-Oct), pp. 788-798

Harger, J.H.; Ernest, J.M.; Thurnau, G.R.; Moawad, A.; Momirova, V.; Landon, M.B.; Paul, R.; Miodovnik, M.; Dombrowski, M.; Sibai, B. & Van Dorsten P. (2002). Risk factors and outcome of varicella-zoster virus pneumonia in pregnant women. *Journal of Infectious Diseases*, Vol. 185, No.4, (Jan 17), pp. 422-427 Health Protection Agency, UK (2011). Guidance on viral rash in pregnancy [online]. Available: http://www.hpa.org.uk/web/HPAweb&HPAwebStandard/HPAweb_C/1195733745858

Helgason, S; Petursson, G.; Gudmundsson, S. & Sigurdsson, J.A. (2000). Prevalence of postherpetic neuralgija after a first episode of herpes zoster: prospective study with long term follow up. *British Medical Journal*, Vol.321, No.7264 (Sep 30), pp. 794-796

Petursson, G. & Sigurdsson, J.A. (2000). Prevalence of postherpetic neuralgia after a first episode of herpes zoster: prospective study with long term follow up. *British Medical Journal*, Vol.321, No.7264, pp. 794-796

Heuchan, A.M. & Isaacs, D. (2001). The management of varicella-zoster virus exposure and infection in pregnancy and the newborn period. *The Medical Journal of Australia*, Vol.174, No.6, pp. 288-292

Hinshaw, K. & Fayyad, A. (2000). The management of early pregnancy loss – (25) Oct 2000 [online]. Available: http://www.rcog.org.uk/printindex.asp?PageID=515 [Accessed 18 August 2005]

Department of Health. (2006). Varicella, In: Immunisation against infectious disease - The Green Book, D. Salisbury, M. Ramsy, K. Noakes, (Eds), pp.421-442, TSO, UK (updated 2011). [online]. Available: http://www.dh.gov.uk/prod_consum_dh/groups/dh_digitalassets/@dh/@en/documents/digitalasset/dh_128074.pdf.

Kempf, W.; Meylan, P.; Gerber, S.; Aebi, C.; Agosti, R.; Büchner, S.; Coradi, B.; Garweg, J.;Hirsch, H.H.; Kind, C.; Lauper, U.; Lautenschlager, S.; Russer, P.; Ruef, C.;Wunderli, W. & Nadal, D. (2007). Swiss recommendations for the management of

varicella zoster virus infections. *Swiss Medical Weekly*, Vol.137, No.17-18 (May 5), pp. 239-251

Knowles, S.J.; Grindy, K.; Cahill, I. & Cafferkey M.T. (2004). Susceptibility to infection rash illness in pregnant women from diverse geographical regions. *Communicable Disease and Public Health*, Vol.7, No.4, pp. 344-348

Kuter, B.J.; Ngai, A.; Patterson, C.M.; Staehle, B.O.; Cho, I.; Matthews, H.; Provost, P.J. & White, C.J. (1995). Safety, tolerability, and immunogenicity of two regimens of Oka/Merck varicella vaccine (Varivax) in healthy adolescents and adults. *Vaccine*, Vol.13, No.11, pp. 967-972

Laforet, E.G. & Lynch, C.L. Jr. (1947). Multiple congenital defects following maternal varicella. *New England Journal of Medicine*, Vol.236, No.15 (April 10), pp. 534-537

McGregor, J.A.; Mark, S.; Crawford, G.P. & Levin, M.J. (1987). Varicella zoster antibody testing in the care of pregnant women exposed to varicella. *American Journal of Obstetrics and Gynecology*, Vol.157, No.2, pp.281–284

Marin, M.; Guris, D.; Chaves, S.S.; Schmid, S. & Seward, J.F. (2007). Prevention of varicella: recommendations of the Advisory Committee on Immunization Practices (ACIP).

Morbidity and Mortality Weekly Report. Recommendations and Reports, Vol.56 (RR-4), pp. 1-40

McKendrick, M.W.; Lau, J.; Alston, S. & Bremner, J. (2007). VZV infection in pregnancy: a retrospective review over 5 years in Sheffield and discussion on the potential utilization of varicella vaccine in prevention. *Journal of Infection*, Vol.55, No.1, pp.64-67

Merck Pregnancy Registry Program (2003). *Merck/CDC pregnancy registry for Varivax*, the eight annual report

Meyers, J.D. (1974). Congenital varicella in term infants: risk reconsidered. *Journal of Infectious Diseases*, Vol.129, No.2 (Feb), pp. 215-217

Miller, E.; Cradock-Watson, J.E. & Ridehalgh, M.K. (1989). Outcome in newborn babies given anti-varicella zoster immunoglobulin after perinatal maternal infection with varicella zoster virus. *Lancet*, Vol.2, No.8659 (Aug 12), pp. 371-373

Miller, E.; Marshall, R. & Vurdien, J.E. (1993). Epidemiology, outcome and control of varicella-zoster infection. *Reviews of Medical Microbiology*, Vol.4, pp. 222-230

Morgan-Capner, P. & Crowcroft, N.S. (2002). Guidelines on the management of, and exposure to, rash illness in pregnancy (including consideration of relevant antibody screening programmes in pregnancy). *Communicable Disease and Public Health*, Vol.5, No.1 (Mar), pp. 59-71

Mouly, F.; Mirlesse, V.; Meritel, J.F.; Rozenberg, F.; Poissonier, M.H.; Lebon, P. & Daffos, F. (1997). Prenatal diagnosis of fetal varicella-zoster virus infection with polymerase chain reaction of amniotic fluids in 107 cases. *American Journal of Obstetrics and Gynecology*, Vol. 177, No.4 (Oct), pp. 894-898

Nathwani, D.; Maclean, A.; Conway, S. & Carrington, D. (1998). Varicella infections in pregnancy and the newborn. *Journal of Infection*, Vol.36, (Suppl 1), pp. 59-71

Nguyen, H.Q.; Jumaan, A.O. & Seward, J.F. (2005). Decline in mortality due to varicella after implementation of varicella vaccination in the United States. *New England Journal of Medicine*, Vol.352, No.5 (Feb 3), pp. 450-458

Office for National Statistics (2005). Deaths 2001: Childhood, infant and perinatal mortality: stillbirths, infant deaths and childhood deaths under 15 (rates) [online]. Available: http://www.statistics.gov.uk/STATBASE/xsdataset.asp?%20%20%20More=Y&vlnk=6667&All=Y&B2.x=24&B2.y=11 [Accessed 18 August 2005]

Oral antihistamines for allergic disorders. (2002). *Drug and Therapeutics Bulletin*, Vol.40, pp. 59-62

Pastuszak, A.L.; Levy, M.; Schick, B.; Zuber, C.; Feldkamp, M.; Gladstone, J.; Bar-Levy, F.; Jackson, E, Donnenfeld, A.; Meschino, W. & Koren, G. (1994). Outcome after maternal varicella infection in the first 20 weeks of pregnancy. *New England Journal of Medicine*, Vol.330, No.13 (Mar 31), pp. 901-905

Prober, C.G. & Arvin, A.M. (1987). Perinatal viral infections. *European Journal of Clinical Microbiology*, Vol.6, No.3 (Jun), pp. 245-261

Prober, C.G.; Gershon, A.A.; Grose, C.; McCracken, G.H. Jr.& Nelson, J.D. (1990). Consensus: varicella-zoster infections in pregnancy and the perinatal period. *Pediatric Infectious Disease Journal*, Vol.9, No.12 (Dec), pp. 865-869 Prodigy. (2004). Chickenpox [online]. Available from:
www.prodigy.nhs.uk/guidance.asp?gt= Chickenpox [Accessed 18 August 2005]

Ratanjamit, C.; Vinther Skriver, M.; Jepsen, P.; Chongsuvivatwong, V.; Ober, J. & Sorensen, H.T. (2003). Adverse pregnancy outcome in women exposed to acyclovir during pregnancy: a population based observational study. *Scandinavian Journal of Infectious Diseases*, Vol.35, No.4, pp. 255-259

Rawson, H.; Crampin, A. & Noah, N. (2001). Deaths from chickenpox in England and Wales.1995-7: analysis of routine mortality data. *Britsh Medical Journal*, Vol.323, pp. 1091-1093

Reynolds, L.; Struik, S. & Nadel, S. Neonatal varicella: varicella zoster immunoglobulin (VZIG) does not prevent disease. (1999). *Archives of Disease in Childhood. Fetal and Neonatal Ed*, Vol.81, No.1 (Jul), F69-70

Riley, L. (1998). Varicella-zoster virus infection in pregnancy. Available from: *UptoDate*, 34 Washington St., Suite 100, Wellesley, MA 02481, on CD-ROM and by subscription at www.uptodate.com

Royal College of Obstetricians and Gynaecologists. (2001). Chickenpox in pregnancy [online]. Available:
http://www.rcog.org.uk/resourses/Public/pdf/Chickenpox_No13.pdf

[Accessed 18 August 2005]

Sauerbrei, A. & Wutzler, P. (2000). The congenital varicella sindrome. *Journal of Perinatology*, Vol.20 (8 Pt 1), pp. 548-554

Sauerbrei, A. & Wutzler, P. (2003). Das fetale Varizellensyndrom. *Monatsschrift fur Kinderheilkunde*, Vol.151, pp. 209-213

Sauerbrei, A,; Pawlak, J.; Luger, C. & Wutzler, P. (2003). Intracerebral varicella-zoster virus reactivation in congenital varicella sindrome. *Development Medicine and Child Neurology*, Vol.45, No.12 (Dec), pp. 837-840

Sauerbrei, A. & Wutzler, P. (2005). Varicella-zoster virus infections during pregnancy: Epidemiology, clinical symptoms, diagnosis, preventon and therapy. *Current Pediatric Reviews*, Vol.1, pp. 205-216

Sauerbrei, A. & Wutzler, P. (2001). Neonatal varicella. *Journal of Perinatology*, Vol.21, No.8 (Dec), pp. 545-549

Sauerbrei, A. (2010). Review of varicella-zoster virus infections in pregnant women and neonates. *Health*, Vol.2, No.2, pp. 143-152

Schulze, A. & Dietzsch, H.J. (2000). The natural history of varicella embryopathy: A 25-year follow-up. *Journal of Pediatrics*, Vol.137, No.6 (Dec), pp. 871-874

Sissons, J.G. (2003). Herpesviruses (ecluding Epstein-Barr virus). In: *Oxford Textbook of Medicine*, D.A. Warrell et al. (Eds.), Fourth Editon, Vol.1, Sections 1-10, Oxford University press, Oxford

Smith, C.K. & Arvin, M.A. (2009). Varicella in the fetus and newborn. *Seminars in Fetal & Neonatal Medicine*, Vol.14, No.4 (Aug), pp. 209-217

Stone, K.M.; Reiff-Eldridge, R.; White, A.D.; Cordero, J.F.; Brown, Z.; Alexander, E.R. & Andrews, E.B. (2004). Pregnancy outcomes following systemic prenatal acyclovir exposure: conclusions from the International acyclovir pregnancy registry, 1984-1999. *Birth Defects Research.Part A, Clinical and Molecular Teratology*, Vol.70, No.4 (Apr), pp. 201-207.

Tan, M.P. & Koren, G. (2006). Chickenpox in pregnancy: revisited. *Reproductive Toxicology*, Vol.21, No.4 (May), pp. 410-420

Wallace, M.R.; Bowler, W.A.; Murray, N.B.; Brodine, S.K. & Oldfield, E.C. (1992). Treatment of adult varicella with oral acyclovir. A randomized, placebo-controlled trial. *Annals of Internal Medicine*, Vol.117, No.5 (Sep 1), pp. 358-363

9

KSHV Paracrine Effects on Tumorigenesis

Ramona Jochmann[1], Peter Lorenz[3], Priya Chudasama[1], Christian Zietz[2], Michael Stürzl[1] and Andreas Konrad[1]
[1]*Division of Molecular and Experimental Surgery, Department of Surgery, University Medical Centre Erlangen, Erlangen,*
[2]*Institute for Pathology, University Medical Centre Carl Gustav Carus, Dresden,*
[3]*Gefäßzentrum Münchner Freiheit, Munich,*
Germany

1. Introduction

In 1994, Chang and colleagues isolated two viral DNA fragments from Kaposi's sarcoma (KS) patients which showed homologies to, but were distinct from, genes coding for capsid and tegument proteins of two herpesviruses - namely, Epstein-Barr virus and Herpesvirus saimiri (Y. Chang et al., 1994). These new herpesvirus-like sequences led to the definition of a new human herpesvirus, namely, Kaposi's sarcoma-associated herpesvirus (KSHV, or human herpesvirus type-8, HHV-8). Shortly afterwards it was shown that KSHV is closely associated with KS tumours (Dupin et al., 1995; Huang et al., 1995; Moore & Chang, 1995), indicating that KSHV is the etiologic agent of KS.

KSHV infection can be detected in several different cell types, including B-cells (Monini et al., 1999), T-cells (Harrington et al., 1996; Sirianni et al., 1997b), monocytes (Blasig et al., 1997), macrophages (Sirianni et al., 1997a), endothelial cells (Boshoff et al., 1995), and dendritic cells (Rettig et al., 1997). Apart from KS, infection with KSHV leads to the development of two other tumour diseases: primary effusion lymphoma (PEL), and a subset of multicentric Castleman's disease (MCD) (Cesarman et al., 1995; Soulier et al., 1995). While PEL and MCD are primary disorders of the B-cell lineage, KS originates from endothelium-derived cells. KS is classified into four different epidemiological forms: classic KS, iatrogenic KS, African endemic KS, and AIDS-associated epidemic KS. All forms have the same histological features, but reveal different progression rates and risk factors, and evolve in different populations (Friedman-Kien & Saltzman, 1990).

The classic KS primarily affects elderly men of Eastern European or Mediterranean origin and usually proceeds very slowly. Patients receiving immunosuppressive therapy (e.g. after solid-organ transplantation) are at increased risk for iatrogenic KS. This rare form of KS is more aggressive than classic KS (Stickler & Friedman-Kien, 1991). The interruption or modulation of the immunosuppressive therapy is usually sufficient for the regression of iatrogenic KS (Stallone et al., 2005; Wijnveen et al., 1987). The African endemic KS is much more aggressive and affects adults as well as children, predominantly in Sub-Saharan Africa (Stickler & Friedman-Kien, 1991). In the endemic regions, KS accounts for up to 13% of all malignancies (Parkin et al., 2008). The most clinically aggressive form of KS is the AIDS-associated epidemic KS (AKS). This entity is the most common cancer in patients infected with the human immunodeficiency virus type-1 (HIV-1). HIV-1-positive homosexual men are predominantly affected (J.N. Martin et al., 1998). The fact that co-infection with HIV-1 acts as co-factor for AKS development is specifically supported by the significant decline of AKS incidence after the introduction of highly active anti-retroviral therapy (HAART) for treatment of HIV-1 infection (J. Gill et al., 2002; Ledergerber et al., 1999). Nevertheless, KS is still among the most commonly observed tumours in certain regions of central Africa, and is a clinical threat for organ transplant recipients (Parkin et al., 2008; Trattner et al., 1993).

In 1996, the complete genome sequence of KSHV was made available, indicating that KSHV encodes more than 86 genes (Neipel et al., 1997; Russo et al., 1996). The large KSHV genome provides innumerable possibilities to interfere with cellular signalling cascades in the course of the viral life cycle and thereby induce tumorigenesis. It is still an unsolved question how KSHV may initiate and/or perpetuate KS development. Research on KS tumorigenesis was hampered for long time by the fact that an efficient *in vitro* culture system for KSHV infection and replication in endothelial derived cells was lacking. Moreover, an appropriate animal model system in which KSHV transmission causes KS is missing. Sporadic observations of KS development in common marmosets (New World primates) require still further confirmation (H. Chang et al., 2009). In this chapter, we will review the histopathology of KS and the oncogenic potential of KSHV.

2. KS histogenesis and the biology of the KS spindle cells

KS was first described by Moritz Kaposi in 1872 as an idiopathic multiple pigment sarcoma of the skin (Kaposi, 1872). KS is a multifocal, highly vascularised tumour of endothelial origin with a complex histology. Apart from KSHV-positivity, KS lesions contain three further hallmarks – (1) a pronounced inflammatory infiltrate composed of monocytes, macrophages, T-cells and dendritic cells, (2) neovascular spaces, which are incomplete or dilated vessel-like structures, often associated with extravasated erythrocytes and oedema, and (3) predominantly in later stages of tumour development, bundles of spindle shaped cells, which are called the KS spindle cells and are considered to be the tumour cells of KS (Gottlieb & Ackerman, 1988; Grayson & Pantanowitz, 2008; Stickler & Friedman-Kien, 1991). The tumour occurs at onset predominantly in the skin, visceral organs, and lymph nodes, while in progressed late stages, all organs can be affected (Pantanowitz & Dezube, 2008). KS evolves over time from the early patch stage to the intermediate plaque stage and manifests later on into a nodular stage. The patch stage is characterized by pinpoint macules on the skin with proliferating endothelial cells, which form the slit-like neovascular structures. These neovascular channels are only partially lined with KSHV-positive cells (Dupin et al., 1999), lack coating by pericytes or smooth muscle cells, and are prone to leakage and rupture (McNutt et al., 1983). Early-stage lesions are further characterized by the presence of infiltrating inflammatory cells such as macrophages, monocytes, dendritic cells, and B- and T-cells (Gottlieb & Ackerman, 1988). Productive KSHV infection of B-cells, monocytes, and macrophages within KS lesions has been described (Ascherl et al., 1999a; Blasig et al., 1997; Stürzl et al., 2001), indicating that these cells may represent the viral replication reservoirs. In the plaque stage, flat macules and patches start to enlarge vertically to slightly elevated lesions termed papules or plaques. In this stage, the typical KS spindle cells appear. In the nodular stage, the KS spindle cells become the predominant cell type. Up to 80% of these cells are infected by KSHV, wherein the virus resides mainly in the latent stage of the viral life cycle (Staskus et al., 1997; Stürzl et al., 1997). These cells were initially considered as the main proliferating element of KS.

The nature of the KS spindle cells has been debated for many years. Nowadays, it is commonly accepted that the spindle cells are of endothelial origin, as most of them express markers of both lymphatic and blood vessel derived endothelial cells (Boshoff et al., 1995; Stürzl et al., 1992a). However, whether these cells originate from lymph or blood vessel endothelial cells (LECs and BECs respectively) is still not unequivocally proven. Initial *in vivo* studies of AIDS- and classic KS showed that the KS spindle cells are of endothelial origin (CD31-positive), and related to, or even derived from, LECs. The KS spindle cells stained positive for the typical lymph endothelial markers vascular endothelial growth factor receptor (VEGFR)-3 and podoplanin (Dupin et al., 1999; Skobe et al., 1999; Weninger et al., 1999), but were negative for BEC marker (Beckstead et al., 1985; Roth et al., 1992), excluding their origin from blood vessel or hematopoietic cells.

However, several further studies showed that KSHV does not only infect LECs, but also BECs (Carroll et al., 2004; Moses et al., 1999; Poole et al., 2002). Microarray analyses revealed that infection with KSHV seems to induce a cellular reprogramming of each cell type towards the gene expression profile of the other, driving these cells away from their terminally differentiated state towards the opposing lineage (Hong et al., 2004; Petrova et al., 2002; H.W. Wang et al., 2004). This was supported by observations that KSHV-infection of BECs led to increased expression of LEC markers such as VEGFR-3, podoplanin, LYVE-1, PROX1, VEGF-A and VEGF-C (Carroll et al., 2004; Sivakumar et al., 2008), while in parallel, KSHV infection of LECs led to increased expression of BEC markers (H.W. Wang et al., 2004). Thus, the resulting infected LECs or BECs are more similar to one another than their uninfected counterparts. This is in agreement with the observation that KS spindle cells do not represent the typical transcriptional profile of LECs nor of BECs, but instead are poorly differentiated, expressing markers of both lymphatic and blood vessel endothelium (Cornelissen et al., 2003; Lagos et al., 2007; Pyakurel et al., 2006b; H.W. Wang et al., 2004).

Currently, two hypotheses describe the origin of the KS spindle cells: the first hypothesis suggests that KSHV infects both BECs and LECs, and induces a transcriptional dedifferentiation towards the gene expression profile of an endothelial precursor cell (EPC) (R. Liu et al., 2010). This hypothesis is supported by the studies of Chang et al., where a high-throughput approach was employed to study the genome-wide alternative splicing events in LECs and $CD34^{+}$ EPCs (T.Y. Chang et al., 2011). The authors found a significant difference in the exon usage between LECs and $CD34^{+}$ EPCs, and observed that KSHV infection of LECs resulted in a LEC-to-precursor dedifferentiation-like reprogramming. Moreover, it seems that KSHV prefers LECs, as (1) mature endothelial cells surrounding normal vascular blood vessels within a KS lesion are only very rarely infected with KSHV (Dupin et al., 1999; Lorenz, 2007) and (2) LECs exhibit an increased number of viral genome copies per cell compared to BECs, indicating that the virus replicates more efficiently in LECs than in BECs (H.W. Wang et al., 2004). The second hypothesis suggests that KSHV productively infects and replicates in $CD34^{+}$ EPCs, which might serve as the KSHV reservoir (Della Bella et al., 2008; Henry et al., 1999; Pellet et al., 2006; Wu et al., 2006). This is in accordance with the observation that $CD34^{+}$ circulating endothelial cells are increased in classic KS patients (Taddeo et al., 2008) and that KSHV-infected $CD34^{+}$ hematopoietic progenitor cells are transmitted through the graft during transplantation (Barozzi et al., 2003). KSHV infection of circulating EPCs might drive their gene expression profile towards a more lymphatic genotype. This would explain the simultaneous expression of marker proteins for lymphatic endothelial cells, blood vessel endothelial cells, and pericytes, which originate all from $CD34^{+}$ EPCs.

3. KS tumorigenesis

As detailed above, KS lesions display a remarkable diversity of cell types, dominated by endothelial-derived KS spindle cells (Regezi et al., 1993; Stürzl et al., 1992a). While the infiltrating inflammatory cells appear already during the early patch stage, the KS spindle cells start to appear in the intermediate plaque stage and are present in increased numbers in late nodular stages. In the late stages of KS, nearly all spindle cells are infected (Dupin et al., 1999; Katano et al., 2000; Staskus et al., 1997; Stürzl et al., 1997), indicating that the spindle cells constitute the main tumour mass of KS. The abundance of spindle cells in late stage lesions is thought to derive from the growth and/or survival advantages of infected over uninfected cells due to oncoviral transformation by KSHV.

3.1 KS: Reactive hyperplasia rather than true malignancy?

Among the oncoviruses, especially throughout the herpesviruses, virus-induced transformation of cells occurs mostly due to the continuous expression of viral proteins in the host cell. For example, among the closest relatives of KSHV, the herpesvirus saimiri (HVS) transforms T-cells by expressing the saimiri transformation-associated protein (Stp) and in the HVS subgroup C additionally the tyrosine kinase-interacting protein (Tip) (Biesinger et al., 1995; Duboise et al., 1998; Murthy et al., 1989), while the Epstein-Barr virus (the only other known member of the human pathogenic gamma-herpesviruses) transforms resting primary human B-cells by continuously expressing the latent membrane protein-1 (LMP-1) (D. Wang et al., 1985). In contrast, it is still unclear whether KSHV-infection results in full tumorigenic cell transformation, and the underlying mechanisms of KS tumorigenesis are unknown. Several studies have tried to address these questions, but the mechanisms of cell alteration used by KSHV differ from that of other oncogenic viruses.

One crucial question is whether KS represents a hyperplastic proliferation or a clonal neoplastic growth. Several features indicate a neoplastic transformation of the KS spindle cells, such as anchorage independent growth and prolonged survival due to increased telomerase activity (Chen et al., 2001; Flore et al., 1998; Moses et al., 1999), protection from apoptosis (Mori et al., 1996; Morris et al., 1996; Stürzl et al., 1999; Thurau et al., 2009), increased angiogenesis, inflammation, invasion and metastasis (Gottlieb & Ackerman, 1988), genomic instability (Cuomo et al., 2008; Pan et al., 2004; Pyakurel et al., 2006a; Si & Robertson, 2006), and immune evasion strategies (Means et al., 2002), as well as the ability to reprogram the cellular metabolism (Karki et al., 2011; Montaner, 2007). Moreover, two studies indicated monoclonal expansion of KS. In the first study, KS clonality has been assessed by determining the methylation pattern of the X-linked androgen receptor gene (HUMARA) (Rabkin et al., 1997). The authors proved concordance among the methylation pattern of the HUMARA alleles in several different KS tumours from a given patient (in total, 8 female patients), indicating that multiple KS lesions in the same patient arise from a single clone of cells (Rabkin et al., 1997). The second study examined the clonal loss of the Y-chromosome in 20 of 23 male KS biopsies, as analysed by comparative genomic hybridisation (CGH) analysis (Pyakurel et al., 2006a). However, this study did not clarify if KSHV preferentially infects endothelial precursor cells that have sporadically lost their Y-chromosome or whether KSHV infection triggers the loss of the Y chromosome.

In contrast, a considerable amount of evidence is supporting a hyperplastic process of tumour development. First, KS spindle cells seem to be incompletely immortalised. This is indicated by the fact that (1) explanted KS cells are strongly dependent on external cytokines and growth factors for the growth *in vitro* (Ensoli et al., 1989; Roth et al., 1989) and for the induction of tumours in immunodeficient mice (Salahuddin et al., 1988) and (2) KS spindle cells loose their ability to proliferate *ad infinitum* after explantation (Gao et al., 2003; Grossmann et al., 2006; Roth et al., 1989).

Second, KSHV-infected spindle cells do not exhibit enhanced proliferation in KS lesions, but on the contrary, show significantly reduced proliferation rates as compared to uninfected cells (Kaaya et al., 2000; Kaaya et al., 1995; Köster et al., 1996). In this context, Pyakurel and colleagues showed that only a small fraction (up to 5%) of all latency-associated nuclear antigen (LANA)-1-positive KS spindle cells proliferate in KS lesions (Pyakurel et al., 2004). Our data confirmed these findings (Lorenz, 2007). KS lesions were stained for LANA-1 as a marker for infected cells (Fig. 1C, brown staining) and for Ki67 as a marker for proliferating cells (Fig. 1C, blue staining). Using double staining procedure of KS lesions, we could demonstrate that KSHV-infected cells were only rarely proliferating, while the main proliferating population was composed of uninfected cells (Fig. 1C). By contrast, in body cavity based lymphoma cells, most of the infected cells (Fig. 1A, LANA-1, brown staining) are also proliferating (Fig. 1B, Ki67, brown staining). Thus, in KS lesions, the KSHV-infected cells do not represent the major proliferative element.

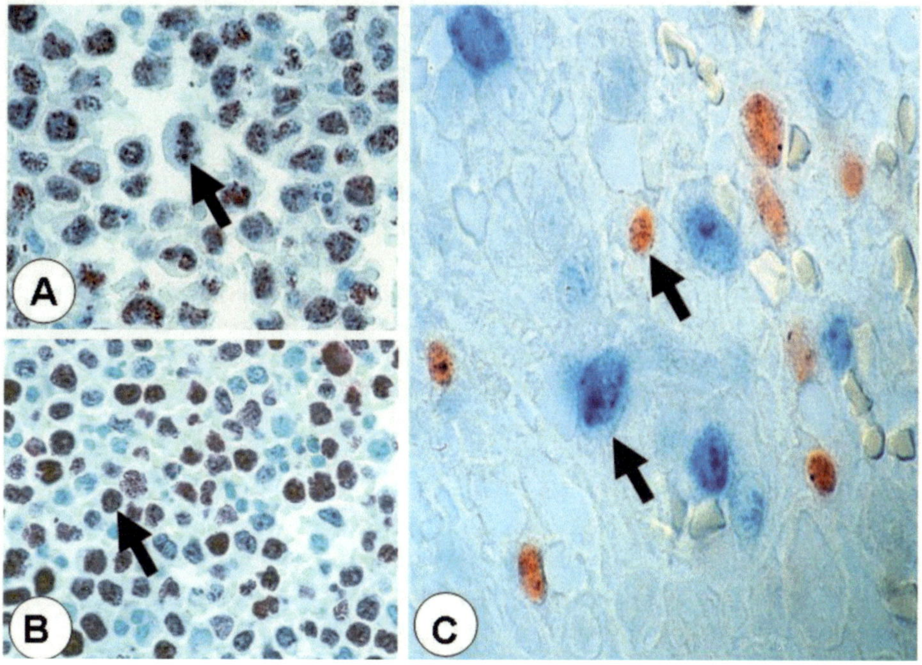

Fig. 1. KSHV infection and cell proliferation in body cavity-based lymphomas (A, B) and KS (C). Immunohistochemical detection of KSHV-LANA-1 (A) and of the proliferation-associated antigen Ki67 (B) in body cavity-based lymphoma cells shows that almost every infected cell is proliferating. Immunohistochemical double staining procedure of KSHV-LANA-1 (C, brown staining) and of the proliferation-associated antigen Ki67 (C, blue staining) in KS tissue shows that KSHV-infected cells are only rarely proliferating and that the major proliferative activity is observed in non-infected cells. Examples of positively stained cells are indicated by arrows.

Third, several studies provided evidence that KS expansion is polyclonal. The largest study was performed in 2007 on 62 biopsies. In order to investigate the cellular clonality of KS lesions, the authors determined the size heterogeneity of the KSHV-fused terminal repeat region (Duprez et al., 2007). The authors revealed in 59 cases a clonal pattern. Of those, 11 KS lesions were monoclonal, while 48 were oligoclonal expansions. Other studies sustain these findings, although performed with a smaller number of biopsies (Delabesse et al., 1997; P.S. Gill et al., 1998; Judde et al., 2000).
Fourth, KS lesions show a substantial rate of spontaneous remission, observed after the introduction of HAART (J. Gill et al., 2002; Ledergerber et al., 1999), cessation of immunosuppression (Kondo et al., 2000; Nagy et al., 2000), or treatment with ganciclovir or foscarnet, which selectively inhibits lytic KSHV replication (Glesby et al., 1996; Mocroft et al., 1996). Together, these features imply that KS is not a true malignancy, but rather a polyclonal reactive hyperplasia.

3.2 Contribution of latency and lytic replication to KS tumorigenesis

As typical for herpesviruses, KSHV establishes a latent state of infection after entering the cell. During latency, only a few viral genes are expressed, among them are the LANA-1, viral cyclin, viral FLICE-inhibitory protein (vFLIP), Kaposin, and the viral-encoded microRNAs. All of the latently expressed proteins have been shown to have individual transforming potential by driving cell proliferation and preventing apoptosis (Friborg et al., 1999; Muralidhar et al., 1998; Radkov et al., 2000; Stürzl et al., 1999; Stürzl et al., 2001; Sun et al., 2003; Verschuren et al., 2002). Therefore, it was long assumed that latently expressed proteins are involved in KS tumorigenesis and that latently infected cells contribute significantly to the development of KS. The fact that most of the KS spindle cells are latently infected is in line with the herpesviral persuasion that the latency program drives tumorigenesis.
Nevertheless, several lines of evidence suggest that latent replication is not sufficient to induce KS. First, KS is typically observed in patients with higher circulating KSHV loads, indicating that lytic expression is necessary for the recruitment and *de novo* infection of cells (Campbell et al., 2000; Whitby et al., 1995). Second, ganciclovir and foscarnet have been shown to mediate the long-term remission of KS (Glesby et al., 1996; Mocroft et al., 1996), again indicating that ongoing lytic replication is necessary for lesion formation. Third, immunosuppression favours KS development, and this is connected with KSHV reactivation and lytic replication (Bourboulia et al., 2004; D.F. Martin et al., 1999). Fourth, cells expressing only latent genes are unable to induce tumour formation in nude mice, unless cells expressing viral G protein-coupled receptor (vGPCR), a lytic cycle protein, are co-injected (Montaner et al., 2006). A contribution of lytic replication to the development of KS is further sustained by the fact that a minority of cells within KS lesions do express lytic viral proteins and produce virions (Orenstein et al., 1997; Staskus et al., 1997).
By now, the crucial question arises concerning the way lytically infected cells might contribute to KS tumour development, albeit (1) only up to 2% of the infected cells within KS lesions replicate lytically and (2) all lytically infected cells die after virus release. The common hypothesis is based on the fact that KSHV encodes many viral lytic genes whose products are secreted factors homologous to cellular chemokines, cytokines, and growth factors, such as the viral interleukin (IL)-6 and the three viral chemokines (vCCL-1, -2, and -3, or alternatively named viral macrophage inflammatory protein, vMIP-I, -II, and III)

(Nicholas, 2003). The vIL-6 is produced and released by infected cells during lytic infection and activates cell proliferation (Meads & Medveczky, 2004) and local angiogenesis (Aoki et al., 1999), while the viral MIPs are agonists for cellular chemokine receptors and exhibit angiogenic properties (Boshoff et al., 1997; Endres et al., 1999; C. Liu et al., 2001; Stine et al., 2000). The vMIP-I was shown to induce the migration of endothelial cells, which suggests that uninfected endothelial cells are recruited to the KS lesion as a target for infection (Haque et al., 2001) and vMIP-II was demonstrated to be a selective chemoattractant for Th2 cells and monocytes (Sozzani et al., 1998). Furthermore, two KSHV transmembrane proteins - K1, an immunoreceptor tyrosine-based activation motif (ITAM) containing receptor, and vOX2, a glycosylated cell surface protein belonging to the immunoglobulin superfamily homologous to the cellular OX2 protein - are suggested to be important for secretion of cellular inflammatory cytokines and growth factors. K1 induces the expression of VEGF and matrix metalloproteinase-9 (MMP-9) in endothelial cells (L. Wang et al., 2004), indicating its role in proliferation and migration of these cells. Solubilised vOX2 stimulates monocytes, macrophages, and dendritic cells to produce the inflammatory cytokines IL-1β, IL-6, monocyte chemoattractant protein 1 (MCP-1), and tumour necrosis factor α (TNF-α) (Chung et al., 2002). Thus, lytically infected cells are thought to produce or activate signalling molecules which promote inflammation and angiogenesis in the KS lesions in a paracrine manner.

In addition, KSHV encodes a vGPCR, a homologue of the cellular IL-8 receptor CXCR2, which has a mutation within the highly conserved DRY sequence, rendering the receptor constitutively active. Therefore, the vGPCR was long thought to play a key role in the initiation of KS. This was further enforced in 2003, when Montaner and colleagues succeeded in engineering a novel transgenic mouse that allowed endothelial cell-specific retroviral transduction. With that technique, they expressed several single KSHV genes that were assumed to have oncogenic properties in mouse endothelial cells. The authors showed that the vGPCR was the only gene that was able and sufficient to induce angioproliferative tumours that resembled human KS (Montaner et al., 2003). Thus, lytically expressed vGPCR may contribute to KS pathogenesis. As vGPCR is a protein produced only during the lytic replication of KSHV, its expression should correlate with the rate of lytically replicating cells in KS lesions. Concordantly, in all KS mouse models, expression of vGPCR is restricted to a small subset of cells within the lesions, which is similar to the part of lytically replicating cells in human KS. This supports the hypothesis that vGPCR influences tumour growth by paracrine mechanisms promoted by the cytokines, chemokines, and growth factors secreted by vGPCR-expressing cells (Jham & Montaner, 2010). However, it remains to be proven if the vGPCR alone (together with latently infected cells) is sufficient to trigger KS tumorigenesis or additional factors are necessary.

3.3 Interplay between inflammatory cytokines and angiogenic factors in KS tumorigenesis

KS tumorigenesis is characterized by the interplay between three processes: proliferation, inflammation and angiogenesis. These processes are connected by paracrine signalling pathways driven by the interplay between viral gene products, inflammatory cytokines, and growth factors released not only by infected cells, but also by chemoattracted infiltrating inflammatory cells. KSHV-infected cells secrete factors, such as MCP-1 or granulocyte-macrophage-colony-stimulating factor (GM-CSF), to recruit and activate inflammatory cells (especially CD8^{+}-T-cells, plasma cells, monocytes and macrophages) to the site of infection (Barillari et al., 1992; Ensoli & Stürzl, 1998; Sciacca et al., 1994). To further enhance the infiltration and binding of immune cells within the lesions, KS spindle cells express additionally high levels of adhesion molecules, such as intercellular adhesion molecule 1 (ICAM-1), vascular cell adhesion molecule 1 (VCAM-1), and E-selectin (Fiorelli et al., 1995; Galea et al., 1998). The recruited and activated infiltrating inflammatory cells in turn release inflammatory cytokines (IC), such as IFN-γ, IL-1β, TNF-α, and IL-6, which are essential for the activation and proliferation of cells comprised in the KS lesions. Interestingly, these cytokines can induce uninfected endothelial cells to acquire the phenotypic and functional features of KS spindle cells (Fiorelli et al., 1998; Monini et al., 1999; Qin et al., 2010; Samaniego et al., 1995; Sirianni et al., 1998; Stürzl et al., 1995). In accordance, these cytokines are also detected *in vivo* at increased concentrations in the serum of patients with all forms of KS and of individuals at high risk for KS (Emilie et al., 1990; Ensoli et al., 1992; Fuchs et al., 1989; Hober et al., 1989).

The presence of an inflammatory milieu is further supported by several studies that have been performed to analyse the impact of KSHV infection on the transcriptome or proteome of endothelial cells. KSHV-infection is associated with a strong IFN-related cell response. Up-regulation of several interferon-inducible proteins, interferon-induced transmembrane protein 1 (IFI9-27), myxovirus resistance protein 1 (MxA), CXCL11, and members of the guanylate binding protein (GBP) family were observed (Chandriani & Ganem, 2007; Lagos et al., 2007; Moses et al., 2002; Naranatt et al., 2004; Poole et al., 2002; Stürzl et al., 2009). Of these factors, especially GBP-1 has been shown to have antiangiogenic effects in endothelial cells *in vitro* and *in vivo* (Guenzi et al., 2001; Guenzi et al., 2003; Hammon et al., 2011; Lubeseder-Martellato et al., 2002; Naschberger et al., 2008), which might explain the observed reduced proliferation rate in infected spindle cells within KS lesions.

Additionally to the IC, the infiltrating inflammatory cells release the angiogenic growth factors basic fibroblast growth factor (bFGF) and VEGF, which are known to induce angiogenesis, vascular permeability, and oedema, the typical histological features of KS (Barillari et al., 1992; Barillari et al., 1999; Samaniego et al., 1998). These angiogenic growth factors were detected at increased concentrations in the serum of HIV-1 infected patients, supporting their important role in KS pathogenesis (Ascherl et al., 1999b). Furthermore, another growth factor, namely PDGF-B, was shown to be an important paracrine mitogen in KS lesions. *In vitro*, PDGF-B activates the proliferation and migration of KS spindle cells. *In vivo* gene expression analysis revealed that PDGF-B, as well as the PDGF-receptor, is present in KS lesions (Köster et al., 1996; Stürzl et al., 1995; Stürzl et al., 1992b). Accordingly, treatment of AIDS-related KS patients with imatinib, an inhibitor of the PDGF-receptor, induced clinical regression of KS in five out of ten patients within four weeks of therapy. Imatinib is also active against c-kit, another receptor tyrosine kinase that has been implicated in KS formation. Thus, further molecular studies and clinical trials are necessary to better elucidate the significance of PDGF-receptor and c-kit expression in KS and the therapeutic role of imatinib (Koon et al., 2005; Rossi et al., 2009).

The angiogenic environment in the KS lesions is further promoted by numerous paracrine or juxtacrine active proteins expressed by KSHV-infected cells. For example, increased expression of Angiopoeitin-2 (Ang-2), angiopoietin-related protein 4, angiopoietin-like polypeptide, ephrins A1 and B2, endothelin convertase, serpin B2 (plasminogen activator inhibitor 2), VEGF-A and -C, thrombomodulin, members of the matrix metalloproteinases

(MMP-1 and -9), urokinase-type plasminogen activator receptor, CXCR7, and MCP-1 has been observed upon KSHV infection (Chandriani & Ganem, 2007; Cornali et al., 1996; Moses et al., 2002; Naranatt et al., 2004; Poole et al., 2002; Thewes et al., 2000; Vart et al., 2007). Of those, Ang-2 is thought to destabilise endothelial cells interaction and to prime endothelial cells to respond to angiogenic stimuli, such as VEGF (Gale et al., 2002). It also plays an important function in lymphangiogenesis (Gale et al., 2002) and regulates the expression of inflammatory proteins in endothelial cells (Fiedler et al., 2006).

Moreover, lytically replicating KSHV-infected cells express a vGPCR, which has the ability to up-regulate the activity of numerous transcription factors, such as hypoxia inducible factor-1α (HIF-1α), nuclear factor-kappaB (NF-κB), activator protein-1 (AP-1), cAMP response element-binding protein (CREB) and nuclear factor of activated T cells (NFAT), and thereby mediates the secretion of paracrine factors promoting endothelial cell survival, proliferation and angiogenesis. Among the paracrine-acting factors are angiogenic growth factors such as VEGF, bFGF, and VEGFR-2, pro-inflammatory chemokines and cytokines such as IL-1β, IL-2, IL-4, IL-6, IL-8, MIP-1, and TNF-α, and adhesion molecules such as ICAM-1, VCAM-1, and E-selectin (Arvanitakis et al., 1997; Bais et al., 1998; Grisotto et al., 2006; D. Martin et al., 2008; Montaner et al., 2004; Schwarz & Murphy, 2001; Sodhi et al., 2000; Yang et al., 2000).

In summary, viral proteins and virus-induced cellular proteins are secreted by infected cells and act in autocrine and paracrine loops to recruit inflammatory cells into the lesions, which in turn secrete inflammatory cytokines, chemokines, and angiogenic growth factors. The fact that KSHV-infection leads to up-regulation of angiogenesis-related and interferon-inducible genes in endothelial cells highlights the importance of an inflammatory-angiogenic milieu during KS tumorigenesis. This is further sustained by the observation that these genes are strongly transcribed, although KSHV encodes a DNA exonuclease SOX/orf37, which mediates the shut-off of host transcription during the lytic cycle of KSHV (Chandriani & Ganem, 2007). All these secreted proteins appear to cooperate in the activation of endothelial cells and are important for tumour neovascularisation and KS development (Ensoli et al., 1992; Ensoli et al., 1989; Ganem, 1995; Safai et al., 1985).

3.4 Paracrine model of KS tumorigenesis

The presence of paracrine-acting factors in KS lesions and the transcriptome analyses of infected endothelial cells (see above) argue for a paracrine stimulation of proliferation in the KS lesions. The current theory is that the paracrine-driven cell proliferation is promoted by the concerted action of latent and lytic gene products inducing a specific "tumorigenic" environment of growth factors and cytokines. In this scenario, KSHV-infected cells may stimulate the proliferation of uninfected endothelial cells in the vicinity and/or recruit endothelial cells in a paracrine manner, and thereby increase the number of target cells for *de novo* infection with virus particles released from lytic replicating cells. Accordingly, proliferation might be driven by latently, and a few lytically, infected cells, and the initial tumour mass might be predominantly formed by uninfected endothelial cells (in early lesions). The abnormal cell proliferation of uninfected endothelial cells may contribute to the increased formation of dilated vessels with abnormal structure and the formation of spindle cells observed in the course of KS development. Subsequent KSHV infection of these cells may predominantly result in a survival advantage of these cells with reduced proliferation rate, overall resulting in the stabilisation of KS lesions. This is supported by several data.

First, KS spindle cells exhibit up-regulation of the VEGFR and increased response to growth factors (Brown et al., 1996; Flore et al., 1998; Sivakumar et al., 2008). Second, KS spindle cells show increased protection against apoptosis, mainly through activation of the NF-κB signal transduction pathway (Keller et al., 2000; Konrad et al., 2009; Stürzl et al., 1999; Thurau et al., 2009). Third, in KS spindle cells, the prosurvival phosphatidylinositol 3-kinase/Akt signal transduction pathway is activated (Montaner et al., 2001; L. Wang & Damania, 2008). Finally, infection of endothelial cells with KSHV increases telomerase activity (Flore et al., 1998), causing prolonged growth and survival of the infected cells beyond their natural lifespan. Thus, during the progression of KS, more and more endothelial cells might be attracted to the lesions and become infected with KSHV, thereby resulting in the histological presentation observed above (Fig. 1): a high number of latently infected spindle cells with a low proliferation rate.

4. Acknowledgements

This work was supported by grants of the Deutsche Forschungsgemeinschaft (DFG-GK1071, STU317/2-1), the German Federal Ministry of Education and Research (BMBF, Polyprobe-Study) and the German Cancer Aid to M.S., and of the Interdisciplinary Centre for Clinical Research (IZKF) of the University Medical Centre Erlangen to M.S. and to R.J., and of the Erlangen's fund for performance-based start-up funding and promotion of young researchers (ELAN) of the University Medical Centre Erlangen to A.K. and R.J..

5. References

Aoki, Y., Jaffe, E.S., Chang, Y., Jones, K., Teruya-Feldstein, J., Moore, P.S. & Tosato, G. (1999). Angiogenesis and hematopoiesis induced by Kaposi's sarcoma-associated herpesvirus-encoded interleukin-6, *Blood* 93(12): 4034-4043.

Arvanitakis, L., Geras-Raaka, E., Varma, A., Gershengorn, M.C. & Cesarman, E. (1997). Human herpesvirus KSHV encodes a constitutively active G-protein-coupled receptor linked to cell proliferation, *Nature* 385(6614): 347-350.

Ascherl, G., Hohenadl, C., Monini, P., Zietz, C., Browning, P.J., Ensoli, B. & Sturzl, M. (1999a). Expression of human herpesvirus-8 (HHV-8) encoded pathogenic genes in Kaposi's sarcoma (KS) primary lesions, *Adv Enzyme Regul* 39: 331-339.

Ascherl, G., Hohenadl, C., Schatz, O., Shumay, E., Bogner, J., Eckhart, L., Tschachler, E., Monini, P., Ensoli, B. & Stürzl, M. (1999b). Infection with human immunodeficiency virus-1 increases expression of vascular endothelial cell growth factor in T cells: implications for acquired immunodeficiency syndrome-associated vasculopathy, *Blood* 93(12): 4232-4241.

Bais, C., Santomasso, B., Coso, O., Arvanitakis, L., Raaka, E.G., Gutkind, J.S., Asch, A.S., Cesarman, E., Gershengorn, M.C. & Mesri, E.A. (1998). G-protein-coupled receptor of Kaposi's sarcoma-associated herpesvirus is a viral oncogene and angiogenesis activator, *Nature* 391(6662): 86-89.

Barillari, G., Buonaguro, L., Fiorelli, V., Hoffman, J., Michaels, F., Gallo, R.C. & Ensoli, B. (1992). Effects of cytokines from activated immune cells on vascular cell growth and HIV-1 gene expression. Implications for AIDS-Kaposi's sarcoma pathogenesis, *J Immunol* 149(11): 3727-3734.

Barillari, G., Sgadari, C., Palladino, C., Gendelman, R., Caputo, A., Morris, C.B., Nair, B.C., Markham, P., Nel, A., Stürzl, M. & Ensoli, B. (1999). Inflammatory cytokines synergize with the HIV-1 Tat protein to promote angiogenesis and Kaposi's sarcoma via induction of basic fibroblast growth factor and the alpha v beta 3 integrin, *J Immunol* 163(4): 1929-1935.

Barozzi, P., Luppi, M., Facchetti, F., Mecucci, C., Alu, M., Sarid, R., Rasini, V., Ravazzini, L., Rossi, E., Festa, S., Crescenzi, B., Wolf, D.G., Schulz, T.F. & Torelli, G. (2003). Post-transplant Kaposi sarcoma originates from the seeding of donor-derived progenitors, *Nat Med* 9(5): 554-561.

Beckstead, J.H., Wood, G.S. & Fletcher, V. (1985). Evidence for the origin of Kaposi's sarcoma from lymphatic endothelium, *Am J Pathol* 119(2): 294-300.

Biesinger, B., Tsygankov, A.Y., Fickenscher, H., Emmrich, F., Fleckenstein, B., Bolen, J.B. & Broker, B.M. (1995). The product of the Herpesvirus saimiri open reading frame 1 (tip) interacts with T cell-specific kinase p56lck in transformed cells, *J Biol Chem* 270(9): 4729-4734.

Blasig, C., Zietz, C., Haar, B., Neipel, F., Esser, S., Brockmeyer, N.H., Tschachler, E., Colombini, S., Ensoli, B. & Stürzl, M. (1997). Monocytes in Kaposi's sarcoma lesions are productively infected by human herpesvirus 8, *J Virol* 71(10): 7963-7968.

Boshoff, C., Endo, Y., Collins, P.D., Takeuchi, Y., Reeves, J.D., Schweickart, V.L., Siani, M.A., Sasaki, T., Williams, T.J., Gray, P.W., Moore, P.S., Chang, Y. & Weiss, R.A. (1997). Angiogenic and HIV-inhibitory functions of KSHV-encoded chemokines, *Science* 278(5336): 290-294.

Boshoff, C., Schulz, T.F., Kennedy, M.M., Graham, A.K., Fisher, C., Thomas, A., McGee, J.O., Weiss, R.A. & O'Leary, J.J. (1995). Kaposi's sarcoma-associated herpesvirus infects endothelial and spindle cells, *Nat Med* 1(12): 1274-1278.

Bourboulia, D., Aldam, D., Lagos, D., Allen, E., Williams, I., Cornforth, D., Copas, A. & Boshoff, C. (2004). Short- and long-term effects of highly active antiretroviral therapy on Kaposi sarcoma-associated herpesvirus immune responses and viraemia, *AIDS* 18(3): 485-493.

Brown, L.F., Tognazzi, K., Dvorak, H.F. & Harrist, T.J. (1996). Strong expression of kinase insert domain-containing receptor, a vascular permeability factor/vascular endothelial growth factor receptor in AIDS-associated Kaposi's sarcoma and cutaneous angiosarcoma, *Am J Pathol* 148(4): 1065-1074.

Campbell, T.B., Borok, M., Gwanzura, L., MaWhinney, S., White, I.E., Ndemera, B., Gudza, I., Fitzpatrick, L. & Schooley, R.T. (2000). Relationship of human herpesvirus 8 peripheral blood virus load and Kaposi's sarcoma clinical stage, *AIDS* 14(14): 2109-2116.

Carroll, P.A., Brazeau, E. & Lagunoff, M. (2004). Kaposi's sarcoma-associated herpesvirus infection of blood endothelial cells induces lymphatic differentiation, *Virology* 328(1): 7-18.

Cesarman, E., Chang, Y., Moore, P.S., Said, J.W. & Knowles, D.M. (1995). Kaposi's sarcoma-associated herpesvirus-like DNA sequences in AIDS-related body-cavity-based lymphomas, *N Engl J Med* 332(18): 1186-1191.

Chandriani, S. & Ganem, D. (2007). Host transcript accumulation during lytic KSHV infection reveals several classes of host responses, *PLoS One* 2(8): e811.

Chang, H., Wachtman, L.M., Pearson, C.B., Lee, J.S., Lee, H.R., Lee, S.H., Vieira, J., Mansfield, K.G. & Jung, J.U. (2009). Non-human primate model of Kaposi's sarcoma-associated herpesvirus infection, *PLoS Pathog* 5(10): e1000606.

Chang, T.Y., Wu, Y.H., Cheng, C.C. & Wang, H.W. (2011). Differentially regulated splice variants and systems biology analysis of Kaposi's sarcoma-associated herpesvirus-infected lymphatic endothelial cells, *Nucleic Acids Res*.

Chang, Y., Cesarman, E., Pessin, M.S., Lee, F., Culpepper, J., Knowles, D.M. & Moore, P.S. (1994). Identification of herpesvirus-like DNA sequences in AIDS-associated Kaposi's sarcoma, *Science* 266(5192): 1865-1869.

Chen, Z., Smith, K.J., Skelton, H.G., 3rd, Barrett, T.L., Greenway, H.T., Jr. & Lo, S.C. (2001). Telomerase activity in Kaposi's sarcoma, squamous cell carcinoma, and basal cell carcinoma, *Exp Biol Med (Maywood)* 226(8): 753-757.

Chung, Y.H., Means, R.E., Choi, J.K., Lee, B.S. & Jung, J.U. (2002). Kaposi's sarcoma-associated herpesvirus OX2 glycoprotein activates myeloid-lineage cells to induce inflammatory cytokine production, *J Virol* 76(10): 4688-4698.

Cornali, E., Zietz, C., Benelli, R., Weninger, W., Masiello, L., Breier, G., Tschachler, E., Albini, A. & Stürzl, M. (1996). Vascular endothelial growth factor regulates angiogenesis and vascular permeability in Kaposi's sarcoma, *Am J Pathol* 149(6): 1851-1869.

Cornelissen, M., van der Kuyl, A.C., van den Burg, R., Zorgdrager, F., van Noesel, C.J. & Goudsmit, J. (2003). Gene expression profile of AIDS-related Kaposi's sarcoma, *BMC Cancer* 3: 7.

Cuomo, M.E., Knebel, A., Morrice, N., Paterson, H., Cohen, P. & Mittnacht, S. (2008). p53-Driven apoptosis limits centrosome amplification and genomic instability downstream of NPM1 phosphorylation, *Nat Cell Biol* 10(6): 723-730.

Delabesse, E., Oksenhendler, E., Lebbe, C., Verola, O., Varet, B. & Turhan, A.G. (1997). Molecular analysis of clonality in Kaposi's sarcoma, *J Clin Pathol* 50(8): 664-668.

Della Bella, S., Taddeo, A., Calabro, M.L., Brambilla, L., Bellinvia, M., Bergamo, E., Clerici, M. & Villa, M.L. (2008). Peripheral blood endothelial progenitors as potential reservoirs of Kaposi's sarcoma-associated herpesvirus, *PLoS One* 3(1): e1520.

Duboise, S.M., Guo, J., Czajak, S., Desrosiers, R.C. & Jung, J.U. (1998). STP and Tip are essential for herpesvirus saimiri oncogenicity, *J Virol* 72(2): 1308-1313.

Dupin, N., Fisher, C., Kellam, P., Ariad, S., Tulliez, M., Franck, N., van Marck, E., Salmon, D., Gorin, I., Escande, J.P., Weiss, R.A., Alitalo, K. & Boshoff, C. (1999). Distribution of human herpesvirus-8 latently infected cells in Kaposi's sarcoma, multicentric Castleman's disease, and primary effusion lymphoma, *Proc Natl Acad Sci U S A* 96(8): 4546-4551.

Dupin, N., Grandadam, M., Calvez, V., Gorin, I., Aubin, J.T., Havard, S., Lamy, F., Leibowitch, M., Huraux, J.M., Escande, J.P. & et al. (1995). Herpesvirus-like DNA sequences in patients with Mediterranean Kaposi's sarcoma, *Lancet* 345(8952): 761-762.

Duprez, R., Lacoste, V., Briere, J., Couppie, P., Frances, C., Sainte-Marie, D., Kassa-Kelembho, E., Lando, M.J., Essame Oyono, J.L., Nkegoum, B., Hbid, O., Mahe, A., Lebbe, C., Tortevoye, P., Huerre, M. & Gessain, A. (2007). Evidence for a multiclonal origin of multicentric advanced lesions of Kaposi sarcoma, *J Natl Cancer Inst* 99(14): 1086-1094.

Emilie, D., Peuchmaur, M., Maillot, M.C., Crevon, M.C., Brousse, N., Delfraissy, J.F., Dormont, J. & Galanaud, P. (1990). Production of interleukins in human immunodeficiency virus-1-replicating lymph nodes, *J Clin Invest* 86(1): 148-159.

Endres, M.J., Garlisi, C.G., Xiao, H., Shan, L. & Hedrick, J.A. (1999). The Kaposi's sarcoma-related herpesvirus (KSHV)-encoded chemokine vMIP-I is a specific agonist for the CC chemokine receptor (CCR)8, *J Exp Med* 189(12): 1993-1998.

Ensoli, B., Barillari, G. & Gallo, R.C. (1992). Cytokines and growth factors in the pathogenesis of AIDS-associated Kaposi's sarcoma, *Immunol Rev* 127: 147-155.

Ensoli, B., Nakamura, S., Salahuddin, S.Z., Biberfeld, P., Larsson, L., Beaver, B., Wong-Staal, F. & Gallo, R.C. (1989). AIDS-Kaposi's sarcoma-derived cells express cytokines with autocrine and paracrine growth effects, *Science* 243(4888): 223-226.

Ensoli, B. & Stürzl, M. (1998). Kaposi's sarcoma: a result of the interplay among inflammatory cytokines, angiogenic factors and viral agents, *Cytokine Growth Factor Rev* 9(1): 63-83.

Fiedler, U., Reiss, Y., Scharpfenecker, M., Grunow, V., Koidl, S., Thurston, G., Gale, N.W., Witzenrath, M., Rosseau, S., Suttorp, N., Sobke, A., Herrmann, M., Preissner, K.T., Vajkoczy, P. & Augustin, H.G. (2006). Angiopoietin-2 sensitizes endothelial cells to TNF-alpha and has a crucial role in the induction of inflammation, *Nat Med* 12(2): 235-239.

Fiorelli, V., Gendelman, R., Samaniego, F., Markham, P.D. & Ensoli, B. (1995). Cytokines from activated T cells induce normal endothelial cells to acquire the phenotypic and functional features of AIDS-Kaposi's sarcoma spindle cells, *J Clin Invest* 95(4): 1723-1734.

Fiorelli, V., Gendelman, R., Sirianni, M.C., Chang, H.K., Colombini, S., Markham, P.D., Monini, P., Sonnabend, J., Pintus, A., Gallo, R.C. & Ensoli, B. (1998). gamma-Interferon produced by CD8+ T cells infiltrating Kaposi's sarcoma induces spindle cells with angiogenic phenotype and synergy with human immunodeficiency virus-1 Tat protein: an immune response to human herpesvirus-8 infection?, *Blood* 91(3): 956-967.

Flore, O., Rafii, S., Ely, S., O'Leary, J.J., Hyjek, E.M. & Cesarman, E. (1998). Transformation of primary human endothelial cells by Kaposi's sarcoma-associated herpesvirus, *Nature* 394(6693): 588-592.

Friborg, J., Jr., Kong, W., Hottiger, M.O. & Nabel, G.J. (1999). p53 inhibition by the LANA protein of KSHV protects against cell death, *Nature* 402(6764): 889-894.

Friedman-Kien, A.E. & Saltzman, B.R. (1990). Clinical manifestations of classical, endemic African, and epidemic AIDS-associated Kaposi's sarcoma, *J Am Acad Dermatol* 22(6 Pt 2): 1237-1250.

Fuchs, D., Reibnegger, G., Dierich, M.P. & Wachter, H. (1989). Cytokines and acquired immunodeficiency syndrome, *Am J Med* 86(4): 509.

Gale, N.W., Thurston, G., Hackett, S.F., Renard, R., Wang, Q., McClain, J., Martin, C., Witte, C., Witte, M.H., Jackson, D., Suri, C., Campochiaro, P.A., Wiegand, S.J. & Yancopoulos, G.D. (2002). Angiopoietin-2 is required for postnatal angiogenesis and lymphatic patterning, and only the latter role is rescued by Angiopoietin-1, *Dev Cell* 3(3): 411-423.

Galea, P., Frances, V., Dou-Dameche, L., Sampol, J. & Chermann, J.C. (1998). Role of Kaposi's sarcoma cells in recruitment of circulating leukocytes: implications in pathogenesis, *J Hum Virol* 1(4): 273-281.

Ganem, D. (1995). AIDS. Viruses, cytokines and Kaposi's sarcoma, *Curr Biol* 5(5): 469-471.

Gao, S.J., Deng, J.H. & Zhou, F.C. (2003). Productive lytic replication of a recombinant Kaposi's sarcoma-associated herpesvirus in efficient primary infection of primary human endothelial cells, *J Virol* 77(18): 9738-9749.

Gill, J., Bourboulia, D., Wilkinson, J., Hayes, P., Cope, A., Marcelin, A.G., Calvez, V., Gotch, F., Boshoff, C. & Gazzard, B. (2002). Prospective study of the effects of antiretroviral therapy on Kaposi sarcoma--associated herpesvirus infection in patients with and without Kaposi sarcoma, *J Acquir Immune Defic Syndr* 31(4): 384-390.

Gill, P.S., Tsai, Y.C., Rao, A.P., Spruck, C.H., 3rd, Zheng, T., Harrington, W.A., Jr., Cheung, T., Nathwani, B. & Jones, P.A. (1998). Evidence for multiclonality in multicentric Kaposi's sarcoma, *Proc Natl Acad Sci U S A* 95(14): 8257-8261.

Glesby, M.J., Hoover, D.R., Weng, S., Graham, N.M., Phair, J.P., Detels, R., Ho, M. & Saah, A.J. (1996). Use of antiherpes drugs and the risk of Kaposi's sarcoma: data from the Multicenter AIDS Cohort Study, *J Infect Dis* 173(6): 1477-1480.

Gottlieb, G.J. & Ackerman, A.B. (1988). In: Kaposi's sarcoma: A Text and Atlas *eds., Philadelphia: Lea & Febiger.*

Grayson, W. & Pantanowitz, L. (2008). Histological variants of cutaneous Kaposi sarcoma, *Diagn Pathol* 3: 31.

Grisotto, M.G., Garin, A., Martin, A.P., Jensen, K.K., Chan, P., Sealfon, S.C. & Lira, S.A. (2006). The human herpesvirus 8 chemokine receptor vGPCR triggers autonomous proliferation of endothelial cells, *J Clin Invest* 116(5): 1264-1273.

Grossmann, C., Podgrabinska, S., Skobe, M. & Ganem, D. (2006). Activation of NF-kappaB by the latent vFLIP gene of Kaposi's sarcoma-associated herpesvirus is required for the spindle shape of virus-infected endothelial cells and contributes to their proinflammatory phenotype, *J Virol* 80(14): 7179-7185.

Guenzi, E., Töpolt, K., Cornali, E., Lubeseder-Martellato, C., Jorg, A., Matzen, K., Zietz, C., Kremmer, E., Nappi, F., Schwemmle, M., Hohenadl, C., Barillari, G., Tschachler, E., Monini, P., Ensoli, B. & Stürzl, M. (2001). The helical domain of GBP-1 mediates the inhibition of endothelial cell proliferation by inflammatory cytokines, *Embo J* 20(20): 5568-5577.

Guenzi, E., Töpolt, K., Lubeseder-Martellato, C., Jörg, A., Naschberger, E., Benelli, R., Albini, A. & Stürzl, M. (2003). The guanylate binding protein-1 GTPase controls the invasive and angiogenic capability of endothelial cells through inhibition of MMP-1 expression, *Embo J* 22(15): 3772-3782.

Hammon, M., Herrmann, M., Bleiziffer, O., Pryymachuk, G., Andreoli, L., Munoz, L.E., Amann, K.U., Mondini, M., Gariglio, M., Airo, P., Schellerer, V.S., Hatzopoulos, A.K., Horch, R.E., Kneser, U., Sturzl, M. & Naschberger, E. (2011). Role of guanylate binding protein-1 in vascular defects associated with chronic inflammatory diseases, *J Cell Mol Med* 15(7): 1582-1592.

Haque, N.S., Fallon, J.T., Taubman, M.B. & Harpel, P.C. (2001). The chemokine receptor CCR8 mediates human endothelial cell chemotaxis induced by I-309 and Kaposi sarcoma herpesvirus-encoded vMIP-I and by lipoprotein(a)-stimulated endothelial cell conditioned medium, *Blood* 97(1): 39-45.

Harrington, W.J., Jr., Bagasra, O., Sosa, C.E., Bobroski, L.E., Baum, M., Wen, X.L., Cabral, L., Byrne, G.E., Pomerantz, R.J. & Wood, C. (1996). Human herpesvirus type 8 DNA sequences in cell-free plasma and mononuclear cells of Kaposi's sarcoma patients, *J Infect Dis* 174(5): 1101-1105.

Henry, M., Uthman, A., Geusau, A., Rieger, A., Furci, L., Lazzarin, A., Lusso, P. & Tschachler, E. (1999). Infection of circulating CD34+ cells by HHV-8 in patients with Kaposi's sarcoma, *J Invest Dermatol* 113(4): 613-616.

Hober, D., Haque, A., Wattre, P., Beaucaire, G., Mouton, Y. & Capron, A. (1989). Production of tumour necrosis factor-alpha (TNF-alpha) and interleukin-1 (IL-1) in patients with AIDS. Enhanced level of TNF-alpha is related to a higher cytotoxic activity, *Clin Exp Immunol* 78(3): 329-333.

Hong, Y.K., Foreman, K., Shin, J.W., Hirakawa, S., Curry, C.L., Sage, D.R., Libermann, T., Dezube, B.J., Fingeroth, J.D. & Detmar, M. (2004). Lymphatic reprogramming of blood vascular endothelium by Kaposi sarcoma-associated herpesvirus, *Nat Genet* 36(7): 683-685.

Huang, Y.Q., Li, J.J., Kaplan, M.H., Poiesz, B., Katabira, E., Zhang, W.C., Feiner, D. & Friedman-Kien, A.E. (1995). Human herpesvirus-like nucleic acid in various forms of Kaposi's sarcoma, *Lancet* 345(8952): 759-761.

Jham, B.C. & Montaner, S. (2010). The Kaposi's sarcoma-associated herpesvirus G protein-coupled receptor: Lessons on dysregulated angiogenesis from a viral oncogene, *J Cell Biochem* 110(1): 1-9.

Judde, J.G., Lacoste, V., Briere, J., Kassa-Kelembho, E., Clyti, E., Couppie, P., Buchrieser, C., Tulliez, M., Morvan, J. & Gessain, A. (2000). Monoclonality or oligoclonality of human herpesvirus 8 terminal repeat sequences in Kaposi's sarcoma and other diseases, *J Natl Cancer Inst* 92(9): 729-736.

Kaaya, E., Castanos-Velez, E., Heiden, T., Ekman, M., Catrina, A.I., Kitinya, J., Andersson, L. & Biberfeld, P. (2000). Proliferation and apoptosis in the evolution of endemic and acquired immunodeficiency syndrome-related Kaposi's sarcoma, *Med Oncol* 17(4): 325-332.

Kaaya, E., Parravicini, C., Ordonez, C., Gendelman, R., Berti, E., Gallo, R.C. & Biberfeld, P. (1995). Heterogeneity of spindle cells in Kaposi's sarcoma: comparison of cells in lesions and in culture, *J Acquir Immune Defic Syndr Hum Retrovirol* 10(3): 295-305.

Kaposi (1872). Idiopathisches multiples Pigmentsarkom der Haut, *Archives of Dermatological Research* 4(2): 265-273.

Karki, R., Lang, S.M. & Means, R.E. (2011). The MARCH family E3 ubiquitin ligase K5 alters monocyte metabolism and proliferation through receptor tyrosine kinase modulation, *PLoS Pathog* 7(4): e1001331.

Katano, H., Sato, Y., Kurata, T., Mori, S. & Sata, T. (2000). Expression and localization of human herpesvirus 8-encoded proteins in primary effusion lymphoma, Kaposi's sarcoma, and multicentric Castleman's disease, *Virology* 269(2): 335-344.

Keller, S.A., Schattner, E.J. & Cesarman, E. (2000). Inhibition of NF-kappaB induces apoptosis of KSHV-infected primary effusion lymphoma cells, *Blood* 96(7): 2537-2542.

Kondo, Y., Izumi, T., Yanagawa, T., Kanda, H., Katano, H. & Sata, T. (2000). Spontaneously regressed Kaposi's sarcoma and human herpesvirus 8 infection in a human immunodeficiency virus-negative patient, *Pathol Int* 50(4): 340-346.

Konrad, A., Wies, E., Thurau, M., Marquardt, G., Naschberger, E., Hentschel, S., Jochmann, R., Schulz, T.F., Erfle, H., Brors, B., Lausen, B., Neipel, F. & Stürzl, M. (2009). A systems biology approach to identify the combination effects of human herpesvirus 8 genes on NF-kappaB activation, *J Virol* 83(6): 2563-2574.

Koon, H.B., Bubley, G.J., Pantanowitz, L., Masiello, D., Smith, B., Crosby, K., Proper, J., Weeden, W., Miller, T.E., Chatis, P., Egorin, M.J., Tahan, S.R. & Dezube, B.J. (2005). Imatinib-induced regression of AIDS-related Kaposi's sarcoma, *J Clin Oncol* 23(5): 982-989.

Köster, R., Blatt, L.M., Streubert, M., Zietz, C., Hermeking, H., Brysch, W. & Stürzl, M. (1996). Consensus-interferon and platelet-derived growth factor adversely regulate proliferation and migration of Kaposi's sarcoma cells by control of c-myc expression, *Am J Pathol* 149(6): 1871-1885.

Lagos, D., Trotter, M.W., Vart, R.J., Wang, H.W., Matthews, N.C., Hansen, A., Flore, O., Gotch, F. & Boshoff, C. (2007). Kaposi sarcoma herpesvirus-encoded vFLIP and vIRF1 regulate antigen presentation in lymphatic endothelial cells, *Blood* 109(4): 1550-1558.

Ledergerber, B., Telenti, A. & Egger, M. (1999). Risk of HIV related Kaposi's sarcoma and non-Hodgkin's lymphoma with potent antiretroviral therapy: prospective cohort study. Swiss HIV Cohort Study, *BMJ* 319(7201): 23-24.

Liu, C., Okruzhnov, Y., Li, H. & Nicholas, J. (2001). Human herpesvirus 8 (HHV-8)-encoded cytokines induce expression of and autocrine signaling by vascular endothelial growth factor (VEGF) in HHV-8-infected primary-effusion lymphoma cell lines and mediate VEGF-independent antiapoptotic effects, *J Virol* 75(22): 10933-10940.

Liu, R., Li, X., Tulpule, A., Zhou, Y., Scehnet, J.S., Zhang, S., Lee, J.S., Chaudhary, P.M., Jung, J. & Gill, P.S. (2010). KSHV-induced notch components render endothelial and mural cell characteristics and cell survival, *Blood* 115(4): 887-895.

Lorenz, P. (2007). Latenz-assoziiertes-nukleäres-Antigen (LANA) des Humanen-Herpesvirus 8 (HHV 8) im AIDS-assoziierten Kaposi-Sarkom, In: *PhD thesis/dissertation, LMU Munich, Germany*, 06/14/2007, Available from: http://edoc.ub.uni-muenchen.de/7109/

Lubeseder-Martellato, C., Guenzi, E., Jörg, A., Töpolt, K., Naschberger, E., Kremmer, E., Zietz, C., Tschachler, E., Hutzler, P., Schwemmle, M., Matzen, K., Grimm, T., Ensoli, B. & Stürzl, M. (2002). Guanylate-binding protein-1 expression is selectively induced by inflammatory cytokines and is an activation marker of endothelial cells during inflammatory diseases, *Am J Pathol* 161(5): 1749-1759.

Martin, D., Galisteo, R., Ji, Y., Montaner, S. & Gutkind, J.S. (2008). An NF-kappaB gene expression signature contributes to Kaposi's sarcoma virus vGPCR-induced direct and paracrine neoplasia, *Oncogene* 27(13): 1844-1852.

Martin, D.F., Kuppermann, B.D., Wolitz, R.A., Palestine, A.G., Li, H. & Robinson, C.A. (1999). Oral ganciclovir for patients with cytomegalovirus retinitis treated with a ganciclovir implant. Roche Ganciclovir Study Group, *N Engl J Med* 340(14): 1063-1070.

Martin, J.N., Ganem, D.E., Osmond, D.H., Page-Shafer, K.A., Macrae, D. & Kedes, D.H. (1998). Sexual transmission and the natural history of human herpesvirus 8 infection, *N Engl J Med* 338(14): 948-954.

McNutt, N.S., Fletcher, V. & Conant, M.A. (1983). Early lesions of Kaposi's sarcoma in homosexual men. An ultrastructural comparison with other vascular proliferations in skin, *Am J Pathol* 111(1): 62-77.

Meads, M.B. & Medveczky, P.G. (2004). Kaposi's sarcoma-associated herpesvirus-encoded viral interleukin-6 is secreted and modified differently than human interleukin-6: evidence for a unique autocrine signaling mechanism, *J Biol Chem* 279(50): 51793-51803.

Means, R.E., Lang, S.M., Chung, Y.H. & Jung, J.U. (2002). Kaposi's sarcoma associated herpesvirus immune evasion strategies, *Front Biosci* 7: e185-203.

Mocroft, A., Youle, M., Gazzard, B., Morcinek, J., Halai, R. & Phillips, A.N. (1996). Anti-herpesvirus treatment and risk of Kaposi's sarcoma in HIV infection. Royal Free/Chelsea and Westminster Hospitals Collaborative Group, *AIDS* 10(10): 1101-1105.

Monini, P., Colombini, S., Stürzl, M., Goletti, D., Cafaro, A., Sgadari, C., Butto, S., Franco, M., Leone, P., Fais, S., Melucci-Vigo, G., Chiozzini, C., Carlini, F., Ascherl, G., Cornali,

E., Zietz, C., Ramazzotti, E., Ensoli, F., Andreoni, M., Pezzotti, P., Rezza, G., Yarchoan, R., Gallo, R.C. & Ensoli, B. (1999). Reactivation and persistence of human herpesvirus-8 infection in B cells and monocytes by Th-1 cytokines increased in Kaposi's sarcoma, *Blood* 93(12): 4044-4058.

Montaner, S. (2007). Akt/TSC/mTOR activation by the KSHV G protein-coupled receptor: emerging insights into the molecular oncogenesis and treatment of Kaposi's sarcoma, *Cell Cycle* 6(4): 438-443.

Montaner, S., Sodhi, A., Molinolo, A., Bugge, T.H., Sawai, E.T., He, Y., Li, Y., Ray, P.E. & Gutkind, J.S. (2003). Endothelial infection with KSHV genes in vivo reveals that vGPCR initiates Kaposi's sarcomagenesis and can promote the tumorigenic potential of viral latent genes, *Cancer Cell* 3(1): 23-36.

Montaner, S., Sodhi, A., Pece, S., Mesri, E.A. & Gutkind, J.S. (2001). The Kaposi's sarcoma-associated herpesvirus G protein-coupled receptor promotes endothelial cell survival through the activation of Akt/protein kinase B, *Cancer Res* 61(6): 2641-2648.

Montaner, S., Sodhi, A., Ramsdell, A.K., Martin, D., Hu, J., Sawai, E.T. & Gutkind, J.S. (2006). The Kaposi's sarcoma-associated herpesvirus G protein-coupled receptor as a therapeutic target for the treatment of Kaposi's sarcoma, *Cancer Res* 66(1): 168-174.

Montaner, S., Sodhi, A., Servitja, J.M., Ramsdell, A.K., Barac, A., Sawai, E.T. & Gutkind, J.S. (2004). The small GTPase Rac1 links the Kaposi sarcoma-associated herpesvirus vGPCR to cytokine secretion and paracrine neoplasia, *Blood* 104(9): 2903-2911.

Moore, P.S. & Chang, Y. (1995). Detection of herpesvirus-like DNA sequences in Kaposi's sarcoma in patients with and without HIV infection, *N Engl J Med* 332(18): 1181-1185.

Mori, S., Murakami-Mori, K., Jewett, A., Nakamura, S. & Bonavida, B. (1996). Resistance of AIDS-associated Kaposi's sarcoma cells to Fas-mediated apoptosis, *Cancer Res* 56(8): 1874-1879.

Morris, C.B., Gendelman, R., Marrogi, A.J., Lu, M., Lockyer, J.M., Alperin-Lea, W. & Ensoli, B. (1996). Immunihistochemical detection of Bcl-2 in AIDS-associated and classical Kaposi's sarcoma, *Am J Pathol* 148(4): 1055-1063.

Moses, A.V., Fish, K.N., Ruhl, R., Smith, P.P., Strussenberg, J.G., Zhu, L., Chandran, B. & Nelson, J.A. (1999). Long-term infection and transformation of dermal microvascular endothelial cells by human herpesvirus 8, *J Virol* 73(8): 6892-6902.

Moses, A.V., Jarvis, M.A., Raggo, C., Bell, Y.C., Ruhl, R., Luukkonen, B.G., Griffith, D.J., Wait, C.L., Druker, B.J., Heinrich, M.C., Nelson, J.A. & Fruh, K. (2002). Kaposi's sarcoma-associated herpesvirus-induced upregulation of the c-kit proto-oncogene, as identified by gene expression profiling, is essential for the transformation of endothelial cells, *J Virol* 76(16): 8383-8399.

Muralidhar, S., Pumfery, A.M., Hassani, M., Sadaie, M.R., Kishishita, M., Brady, J.N., Doniger, J., Medveczky, P. & Rosenthal, L.J. (1998). Identification of kaposin (open reading frame K12) as a human herpesvirus 8 (Kaposi's sarcoma-associated herpesvirus) transforming gene, *J Virol* 72(6): 4980-4988.

Murthy, S.C., Trimble, J.J. & Desrosiers, R.C. (1989). Deletion mutants of herpesvirus saimiri define an open reading frame necessary for transformation, *J Virol* 63(8): 3307-3314.

Nagy, S., Gyulai, R., Kemeny, L., Szenohradszky, P. & Dobozy, A. (2000). Iatrogenic Kaposi's sarcoma: HHV8 positivity persists but the tumors regress almost completely without immunosuppressive therapy, *Transplantation* 69(10): 2230-2231.

Naranatt, P.P., Krishnan, H.H., Svojanovsky, S.R., Bloomer, C., Mathur, S. & Chandran, B. (2004). Host gene induction and transcriptional reprogramming in Kaposi's sarcoma-associated herpesvirus (KSHV/HHV-8)-infected endothelial, fibroblast, and B cells: insights into modulation events early during infection, *Cancer Res* 64(1): 72-84.

Naschberger, E., Croner, R.S., Merkel, S., Dimmler, A., Tripal, P., Amann, K.U., Kremmer, E., Brueckl, W.M., Papadopoulos, T., Hohenadl, C., Hohenberger, W. & Sturzl, M. (2008). Angiostatic immune reaction in colorectal carcinoma: Impact on survival and perspectives for antiangiogenic therapy, *Int J Cancer* 123(9): 2120-2129.

Neipel, F., Albrecht, J.C. & Fleckenstein, B. (1997). Cell-homologous genes in the Kaposi's sarcoma-associated rhadinovirus human herpesvirus 8: determinants of its pathogenicity?, *J Virol* 71(6): 4187-4192.

Nicholas, J. (2003). Human herpesvirus-8-encoded signalling ligands and receptors, *J Biomed Sci* 10(5): 475-489.

Orenstein, J.M., Alkan, S., Blauvelt, A., Jeang, K.T., Weinstein, M.D., Ganem, D. & Herndier, B. (1997). Visualization of human herpesvirus type 8 in Kaposi's sarcoma by light and transmission electron microscopy, *AIDS* 11(5): F35-45.

Pan, H., Zhou, F. & Gao, S.J. (2004). Kaposi's sarcoma-associated herpesvirus induction of chromosome instability in primary human endothelial cells, *Cancer Res* 64(12): 4064-4068.

Pantanowitz, L. & Dezube, B.J. (2008). Kaposi sarcoma in unusual locations, *BMC Cancer* 8: 190.

Parkin, D.M., Sitas, F., Chirenje, M., Stein, L., Abratt, R. & Wabinga, H. (2008). Part I: Cancer in Indigenous Africans--burden, distribution, and trends, *Lancet Oncol* 9(7): 683-692.

Pellet, C., Kerob, D., Dupuy, A., Carmagnat, M.V., Mourah, S., Podgorniak, M.P., Toledano, C., Morel, P., Verola, O., Dosquet, C., Hamel, Y., Calvo, F., Rabian, C. & Lebbe, C. (2006). Kaposi's sarcoma-associated herpesvirus viremia is associated with the progression of classic and endemic Kaposi's sarcoma, *J Invest Dermatol* 126(3): 621-627.

Petrova, T.V., Makinen, T., Makela, T.P., Saarela, J., Virtanen, I., Ferrell, R.E., Finegold, D.N., Kerjaschki, D., Yla-Herttuala, S. & Alitalo, K. (2002). Lymphatic endothelial reprogramming of vascular endothelial cells by the Prox-1 homeobox transcription factor, *EMBO J* 21(17): 4593-4599.

Poole, L.J., Yu, Y., Kim, P.S., Zheng, Q.Z., Pevsner, J. & Hayward, G.S. (2002). Altered patterns of cellular gene expression in dermal microvascular endothelial cells infected with Kaposi's sarcoma-associated herpesvirus, *J Virol* 76(7): 3395-3420.

Pyakurel, P., Massambu, C., Castanos-Velez, E., Ericsson, S., Kaaya, E., Biberfeld, P. & Heiden, T. (2004). Human herpesvirus 8/Kaposi sarcoma herpesvirus cell association during evolution of Kaposi sarcoma, *J Acquir Immune Defic Syndr* 36(2): 678-683.

Pyakurel, P., Montag, U., Castanos-Velez, E., Kaaya, E., Christensson, B., Tonnies, H., Biberfeld, P. & Heiden, T. (2006a). CGH of microdissected Kaposi's sarcoma lesions reveals recurrent loss of chromosome Y in early and additional chromosomal changes in late tumour stages, *AIDS* 20(14): 1805-1812.

Pyakurel, P., Pak, F., Mwakigonja, A.R., Kaaya, E., Heiden, T. & Biberfeld, P. (2006b). Lymphatic and vascular origin of Kaposi's sarcoma spindle cells during tumor development, *Int J Cancer* 119(6): 1262-1267.

Qin, Z., Kearney, P., Plaisance, K. & Parsons, C.H. (2010). Pivotal advance: Kaposi's sarcoma-associated herpesvirus (KSHV)-encoded microRNA specifically induce IL-6 and IL-10 secretion by macrophages and monocytes, *J Leukoc Biol* 87(1): 25-34.

Rabkin, C.S., Janz, S., Lash, A., Coleman, A.E., Musaba, E., Liotta, L., Biggar, R.J. & Zhuang, Z. (1997). Monoclonal origin of multicentric Kaposi's sarcoma lesions, *N Engl J Med* 336(14): 988-993.

Radkov, S.A., Kellam, P. & Boshoff, C. (2000). The latent nuclear antigen of Kaposi sarcoma-associated herpesvirus targets the retinoblastoma-E2F pathway and with the oncogene Hras transforms primary rat cells, *Nat Med* 6(10): 1121-1127.

Regezi, J.A., MacPhail, L.A., Daniels, T.E., DeSouza, Y.G., Greenspan, J.S. & Greenspan, D. (1993). Human immunodeficiency virus-associated oral Kaposi's sarcoma. A heterogeneous cell population dominated by spindle-shaped endothelial cells, *Am J Pathol* 143(1): 240-249.

Rettig, M.B., Ma, H.J., Vescio, R.A., Pold, M., Schiller, G., Belson, D., Savage, A., Nishikubo, C., Wu, C., Fraser, J., Said, J.W. & Berenson, J.R. (1997). Kaposi's sarcoma-associated herpesvirus infection of bone marrow dendritic cells from multiple myeloma patients, *Science* 276(5320): 1851-1854.

Rossi, G., Sartori, G., Rusev, B.C. & Sgambato, A. (2009). Expression and molecular analysis of c-kit and PDGFRs in Kaposi's sarcoma of different stages and epidemiological settings, *Histopathology* 54(5): 619-622.

Roth, W.K., Brandstetter, H. & Stürzl, M. (1992). Cellular and molecular features of HIV-associated Kaposi's sarcoma, *AIDS* 6(9): 895-913.

Roth, W.K., Werner, S., Schirren, C.G. & Hofschneider, P.H. (1989). Depletion of PDGF from serum inhibits growth of AIDS-related and sporadic Kaposi's sarcoma cells in culture, *Oncogene* 4(4): 483-487.

Russo, J.J., Bohenzky, R.A., Chien, M.C., Chen, J., Yan, M., Maddalena, D., Parry, J.P., Peruzzi, D., Edelman, I.S., Chang, Y. & Moore, P.S. (1996). Nucleotide sequence of the Kaposi sarcoma-associated herpesvirus (HHV8), *Proc Natl Acad Sci U S A* 93(25): 14862-14867.

Safai, B., Johnson, K.G., Myskowski, P.L., Koziner, B., Yang, S.Y., Cunningham-Rundles, S., Godbold, J.H. & Dupont, B. (1985). The natural history of Kaposi's sarcoma in the acquired immunodeficiency syndrome, *Ann Intern Med* 103(5): 744-750.

Salahuddin, S.Z., Nakamura, S., Biberfeld, P., Kaplan, M.H., Markham, P.D., Larsson, L. & Gallo, R.C. (1988). Angiogenic properties of Kaposi's sarcoma-derived cells after long-term culture in vitro, *Science* 242(4877): 430-433.

Samaniego, F., Markham, P.D., Gallo, R.C. & Ensoli, B. (1995). Inflammatory cytokines induce AIDS-Kaposi's sarcoma-derived spindle cells to produce and release basic fibroblast growth factor and enhance Kaposi's sarcoma-like lesion formation in nude mice, *J Immunol* 154(7): 3582-3592.

Samaniego, F., Markham, P.D., Gendelman, R., Watanabe, Y., Kao, V., Kowalski, K., Sonnabend, J.A., Pintus, A., Gallo, R.C. & Ensoli, B. (1998). Vascular endothelial growth factor and basic fibroblast growth factor present in Kaposi's sarcoma (KS) are induced by inflammatory cytokines and synergize to promote vascular permeability and KS lesion development, *Am J Pathol* 152(6): 1433-1443.

Schwarz, M. & Murphy, P.M. (2001). Kaposi's sarcoma-associated herpesvirus G protein-coupled receptor constitutively activates NF-kappa B and induces proinflammatory cytokine and chemokine production via a C-terminal signaling determinant, *J Immunol* 167(1): 505-513.

Sciacca, F.L., Stürzl, M., Bussolino, F., Sironi, M., Brandstetter, H., Zietz, C., Zhou, D., Matteucci, C., Peri, G., Sozzani, S. & et al. (1994). Expression of adhesion molecules, platelet-activating factor, and chemokines by Kaposi's sarcoma cells, *J Immunol* 153(10): 4816-4825.

Si, H. & Robertson, E.S. (2006). Kaposi's sarcoma-associated herpesvirus-encoded latency-associated nuclear antigen induces chromosomal instability through inhibition of p53 function, *J Virol* 80(2): 697-709.

Sirianni, M.C., Uccini, S., Angeloni, A., Faggioni, A., Cottoni, F. & Ensoli, B. (1997a). Circulating spindle cells: correlation with human herpesvirus-8 (HHV-8) infection and Kaposi's sarcoma, *Lancet* 349(9047): 255.

Sirianni, M.C., Vincenzi, L., Fiorelli, V., Topino, S., Scala, E., Uccini, S., Angeloni, A., Faggioni, A., Cerimele, D., Cottoni, F., Aiuti, F. & Ensoli, B. (1998). gamma-Interferon production in peripheral blood mononuclear cells and tumor infiltrating lymphocytes from Kaposi's sarcoma patients: correlation with the presence of human herpesvirus-8 in peripheral blood mononuclear cells and lesional macrophages, *Blood* 91(3): 968-976.

Sirianni, M.C., Vincenzi, L., Topino, S., Scala, E., Angeloni, A., Gonnella, R., Uccini, S. & Faggioni, A. (1997b). Human herpesvirus 8 DNA sequences in CD8+ T cells, *J Infect Dis* 176(2): 541.

Sivakumar, R., Sharma-Walia, N., Raghu, H., Veettil, M.V., Sadagopan, S., Bottero, V., Varga, L., Levine, R. & Chandran, B. (2008). Kaposi's sarcoma-associated herpesvirus induces sustained levels of vascular endothelial growth factors A and C early during in vitro infection of human microvascular dermal endothelial cells: biological implications, *J Virol* 82(4): 1759-1776.

Skobe, M., Brown, L.F., Tognazzi, K., Ganju, R.K., Dezube, B.J., Alitalo, K. & Detmar, M. (1999). Vascular endothelial growth factor-C (VEGF-C) and its receptors KDR and flt-4 are expressed in AIDS-associated Kaposi's sarcoma, *J Invest Dermatol* 113(6): 1047-1053.

Sodhi, A., Montaner, S., Patel, V., Zohar, M., Bais, C., Mesri, E.A. & Gutkind, J.S. (2000). The Kaposi's sarcoma-associated herpes virus G protein-coupled receptor up-regulates vascular endothelial growth factor expression and secretion through mitogen-activated protein kinase and p38 pathways acting on hypoxia-inducible factor 1alpha, *Cancer Res* 60(17): 4873-4880.

Soulier, J., Grollet, L., Oksenhendler, E., Cacoub, P., Cazals-Hatem, D., Babinet, P., d'Agay, M.F., Clauvel, J.P., Raphael, M., Degos, L. & et al. (1995). Kaposi's sarcoma-associated herpesvirus-like DNA sequences in multicentric Castleman's disease, *Blood* 86(4): 1276-1280.

Sozzani, S., Luini, W., Bianchi, G., Allavena, P., Wells, T.N., Napolitano, M., Bernardini, G., Vecchi, A., D'Ambrosio, D., Mazzeo, D., Sinigaglia, F., Santoni, A., Maggi, E., Romagnani, S. & Mantovani, A. (1998). The viral chemokine macrophage inflammatory protein-II is a selective Th2 chemoattractant, *Blood* 92(11): 4036-4039.

Stallone, G., Schena, A., Infante, B., Di Paolo, S., Loverre, A., Maggio, G., Ranieri, E., Gesualdo, L., Schena, F.P. & Grandaliano, G. (2005). Sirolimus for Kaposi's sarcoma in renal-transplant recipients, *N Engl J Med* 352(13): 1317-1323.

Staskus, K.A., Zhong, W., Gebhard, K., Herndier, B., Wang, H., Renne, R., Beneke, J., Pudney, J., Anderson, D.J., Ganem, D. & Haase, A.T. (1997). Kaposi's sarcoma-associated herpesvirus gene expression in endothelial (spindle) tumor cells, *J Virol* 71(1): 715-719.

Stickler, M.C. & Friedman-Kien, A.E. (1991). Kaposi's sarcoma, *Clin Dermatol* 9(1): 39-47.

Stine, J.T., Wood, C., Hill, M., Epp, A., Raport, C.J., Schweickart, V.L., Endo, Y., Sasaki, T., Simmons, G., Boshoff, C., Clapham, P., Chang, Y., Moore, P., Gray, P.W. & Chantry, D. (2000). KSHV-encoded CC chemokine vMIP-III is a CCR4 agonist, stimulates angiogenesis, and selectively chemoattracts TH2 cells, *Blood* 95(4): 1151-1157.

Stürzl, M., Blasig, C., Schreier, A., Neipel, F., Hohenadl, C., Cornali, E., Ascherl, G., Esser, S., Brockmeyer, N.H., Ekman, M., Kaaya, E.E., Tschachler, E. & Biberfeld, P. (1997). Expression of HHV-8 latency-associated T0.7 RNA in spindle cells and endothelial cells of AIDS-associated, classical and African Kaposi's sarcoma, *Int J Cancer* 72(1): 68-71.

Stürzl, M., Brandstetter, H. & Roth, W.K. (1992a). Kaposi's sarcoma: a review of gene expression and ultrastructure of KS spindle cells in vivo, *AIDS Res Hum Retroviruses* 8(10): 1753-1763.

Stürzl, M., Brandstetter, H., Zietz, C., Eisenburg, B., Raivich, G., Gearing, D.P., Brockmeyer, N.H. & Hofschneider, P.H. (1995). Identification of interleukin-1 and platelet-derived growth factor-B as major mitogens for the spindle cells of Kaposi's sarcoma: a combined in vitro and in vivo analysis, *Oncogene* 10(10): 2007-2016.

Stürzl, M., Hohenadl, C., Zietz, C., Castanos-Velez, E., Wunderlich, A., Ascherl, G., Biberfeld, P., Monini, P., Browning, P.J. & Ensoli, B. (1999). Expression of K13/v-FLIP gene of human herpesvirus 8 and apoptosis in Kaposi's sarcoma spindle cells, *J Natl Cancer Inst* 91(20): 1725-1733.

Stürzl, M., Konrad, A., Alkharsah, K.R., Jochmann, R., Thurau, M., Marquardt, G. & Schulz, T.F. (2009). The contribution of systems biology and reverse genetics to the understanding of Kaposi's sarcoma-associated herpesvirus pathogenesis in endothelial cells, *Thromb Haemost* 102(6): 1117-1134.

Stürzl, M., Roth, W.K., Brockmeyer, N.H., Zietz, C., Speiser, B. & Hofschneider, P.H. (1992b). Expression of platelet-derived growth factor and its receptor in AIDS-related Kaposi sarcoma in vivo suggests paracrine and autocrine mechanisms of tumor maintenance, *Proc Natl Acad Sci U S A* 89(15): 7046-7050.

Stürzl, M., Zietz, C., Monini, P. & Ensoli, B. (2001). Human herpesvirus-8 and Kaposi's sarcoma: relationship with the multistep concept of tumorigenesis, *Adv Cancer Res* 81: 125-159.

Sun, Q., Zachariah, S. & Chaudhary, P.M. (2003). The human herpes virus 8-encoded viral FLICE-inhibitory protein induces cellular transformation via NF-kappaB activation, *J Biol Chem* 278(52): 52437-52445.

Taddeo, A., Presicce, P., Brambilla, L., Bellinvia, M., Villa, M.L. & Della Bella, S. (2008). Circulating endothelial progenitor cells are increased in patients with classic Kaposi's sarcoma, *J Invest Dermatol* 128(8): 2125-2128.

Thewes, M., Elsner, E., Wessner, D., Engst, R. & Ring, J. (2000). The urokinase plasminogen activator system in angiosarcoma, Kaposi's sarcoma, granuloma pyogenicum, and angioma: an immunohistochemical study, *Int J Dermatol* 39(3): 188-191.

Thurau, M., Marquardt, G., Gonin-Laurent, N., Weinländer, K., Naschberger, E., Jochmann, R., Alkharsah, K.R., Schulz, T.F., Thome, M., Neipel, F. & Stürzl, M. (2009). Viral inhibitor of apoptosis vFLIP/K13 protects endothelial cells against superoxide-induced cell death, *J Virol* 83(2): 598-611.

Trattner, A., Hodak, E., David, M. & Sandbank, M. (1993). The appearance of Kaposi sarcoma during corticosteroid therapy, *Cancer* 72(5): 1779-1783.

Vart, R.J., Nikitenko, L.L., Lagos, D., Trotter, M.W., Cannon, M., Bourboulia, D., Gratrix, F., Takeuchi, Y. & Boshoff, C. (2007). Kaposi's sarcoma-associated herpesvirus-encoded interleukin-6 and G-protein-coupled receptor regulate angiopoietin-2 expression in lymphatic endothelial cells, *Cancer Res* 67(9): 4042-4051.

Verschuren, E.W., Klefstrom, J., Evan, G.I. & Jones, N. (2002). The oncogenic potential of Kaposi's sarcoma-associated herpesvirus cyclin is exposed by p53 loss in vitro and in vivo, *Cancer Cell* 2(3): 229-241.

Wang, D., Liebowitz, D. & Kieff, E. (1985). An EBV membrane protein expressed in immortalized lymphocytes transforms established rodent cells, *Cell* 43(3 Pt 2): 831-840.

Wang, H.W., Trotter, M.W., Lagos, D., Bourboulia, D., Henderson, S., Makinen, T., Elliman, S., Flanagan, A.M., Alitalo, K. & Boshoff, C. (2004). Kaposi sarcoma herpesvirus-induced cellular reprogramming contributes to the lymphatic endothelial gene expression in Kaposi sarcoma, *Nat Genet* 36(7): 687-693.

Wang, L. & Damania, B. (2008). Kaposi's sarcoma-associated herpesvirus confers a survival advantage to endothelial cells, *Cancer Res* 68(12): 4640-4648.

Wang, L., Wakisaka, N., Tomlinson, C.C., DeWire, S.M., Krall, S., Pagano, J.S. & Damania, B. (2004). The Kaposi's sarcoma-associated herpesvirus (KSHV/HHV-8) K1 protein induces expression of angiogenic and invasion factors, *Cancer Res* 64(8): 2774-2781.

Weninger, W., Partanen, T.A., Breiteneder-Geleff, S., Mayer, C., Kowalski, H., Mildner, M., Pammer, J., Stürzl, M., Kerjaschki, D., Alitalo, K. & Tschachler, E. (1999). Expression of vascular endothelial growth factor receptor-3 and podoplanin suggests a lymphatic endothelial cell origin of Kaposi's sarcoma tumor cells, *Lab Invest* 79(2): 243-251.

Whitby, D., Howard, M.R., Tenant-Flowers, M., Brink, N.S., Copas, A., Boshoff, C., Hatzioannou, T., Suggett, F.E., Aldam, D.M., Denton, A.S. & et al. (1995). Detection of Kaposi sarcoma associated herpesvirus in peripheral blood of HIV-infected individuals and progression to Kaposi's sarcoma, *Lancet* 346(8978): 799-802.

Wijnveen, A.C., Persson, H., Bjorck, S. & Blohme, I. (1987). Disseminated Kaposi's sarcoma--full regression after withdrawal of immunosuppressive therapy: report of a case, *Transplant Proc* 19(5): 3735-3736.

Wu, W., Vieira, J., Fiore, N., Banerjee, P., Sieburg, M., Rochford, R., Harrington, W., Jr. & Feuer, G. (2006). KSHV/HHV-8 infection of human hematopoietic progenitor (CD34+) cells: persistence of infection during hematopoiesis in vitro and in vivo, *Blood* 108(1): 141-151.

Yang, T.Y., Chen, S.C., Leach, M.W., Manfra, D., Homey, B., Wiekowski, M., Sullivan, L., Jenh, C.H., Narula, S.K., Chensue, S.W. & Lira, S.A. (2000). Transgenic expression of the chemokine receptor encoded by human herpesvirus 8 induces an angioproliferative disease resembling Kaposi's sarcoma, *J Exp Med* 191(3): 445-454.

Part 3

Infection in Animals

10

Herpesviruses of Fish, Amphibians and Invertebrates

Steven van Beurden and Marc Engelsma
Central Veterinary Institute, part of Wageningen UR
Faculty of Veterinary Medicine, Utrecht University
The Netherlands

1. Introduction

Herpesviruses are large and complex DNA viruses which infect a wide range of vertebrates and invertebrates, including humans and domestic animals (Davison et al., 2005a). Severe infections are usually only observed in foetuses and very young or immunocompromised individuals, but economic consequences for livestock can be significant. Certain herpesviruses may also cause serious disease in non-reservoir host species - for example, Bovine malignant catharral fever. Prevention and treatment are complicated due to the ability of herpesviruses to persist as a latent infection.

In general, the occurrence of herpesviruses is host-specific (Davison, 2002). Most herpesviruses have evolved with their hosts over long periods of time and are well adapted to them. This view is supported by molecular phylogenetic data, and consistent with the generally modest pathogenicity of these viruses. In order to understand the evolutionary origin and consequences of herpesviruses infecting higher vertebrates, a profound understanding of the taxonomy of lower vertebrate and invertebrate herpesviruses is needed.

In many of the major aquaculture species, such as carp, salmon, catfish, eel, sturgeon and oyster, herpesviruses have been identified (Table 1). These herpesviruses merely represent the focus of current fish disease research, and it is expected that many other herpesviruses of lower vertebrates exist. The herpesviruses infecting fish, amphibians, and invertebrates make up two families, which are only distantly related to the well-known family of herpesviruses of mammals, birds, and reptiles (Davison et al., 2009).

In the last decades several mass mortality outbreaks in fish and oysters were found to be associated with herpesvirus infections. Management strategies are taken at fish farms to reduce the production losses due to these viruses. Several less-pathogenic fish herpesviruses are known to induce skin tumours and tumour-like proliferations (Anders & Yoshimizu, 1994), and one amphibian herpesvirus causes renal adenocarcinoma (McKinnell & Carlson, 1997). Experimental studies on these spontaneously-occurring viral tumours may serve as a model for viral carcinogenesis in humans. Interestingly, the course of infection of both the high pathogenic and tumour-inducing alloherpesviruses seems to be dependent on host age and ambient water temperature.

Genus	Virus name	Common name	Natural host(s)	Key reference for taxonomy
Batrachovirus	*Ranid herpesvirus 1*	Lucké tumour herpesvirus	Leopard frog (*R. pipiens*)	(Davison et al., 2006)
	Ranid herpesvirus 2	Frog virus 4	Leopard frog (*R. pipiens*)	(Davison et al., 2006)
Cyprinivirus	*Cyprinid herpesvirus 1*	Carp pox	Common carp (*C. carpio*)	(Waltzek et al., 2005)
	Cyprinid herpesvirus 2	Goldfish hematopoietic necrosis virus	Goldfish (*C. auratus*)	(Waltzek et al., 2005)
	Cyprinid herpesvirus 3	Koi herpesvirus	Common carp (*C. carpio carpio*) & Koi (*C. carpio koi*)	(Waltzek et al., 2005)
Ictalurivirus	*Acipenserid herpesvirus 2*	White sturgeon herpesvirus 2	White sturgeon (*A. ransmontatus*)	(Kurobe et al., 2008)
	Ictalurid herpesvirus 1	Channel catfish virus	Channel catfish (*I. punctatus*)	(Davison, 1992)
	Ictalurid herpesvirus 2	Ictalurus melas herpesvirus	Black bullhead (*A. melas*) & Channel catfish (*I. punctatus*)	(Doszpoly et al., 2008)
Salmonivirus	*Salmonid herpesvirus 1*	Herpesvirus salmonis	Rainbow trout (*O. mykiss*)	(Waltzek et al., 2009)
	Salmonid herpesvirus 2	Coho salmon herpesvirus	Salmon spp. (*Oncorhynchus* spp.)	(Waltzek et al., 2009)
	Salmonid herpesvirus 3	Epizootic epitheliotrophic disease virus	Lake trout (*S. namaycush*)	(Waltzek et al., 2009)
Unclassified alloherpesviruses	*Acipenserid herpesvirus 1*	White sturgeon herpesvirus 1	Sturgeon spp. (*Acipenser* spp.)	(Kurobe et al., 2008)
	Anguillid herpesvirus 1	Eel herpesvirus	European eel (*A. anguilla*) & Japanese eel (*A. japonica*)	(van Beurden et al., 2010)
	-	Pilchard herpesvirus	Pacific sardine (*S. sagax*)	(Doszpoly et al., 2011a)
Uncharacterized alloherpesviruses	Esocid herpesvirus 1	Blue spot disease virus	Northern pike (*E. Lucius*) & muskellunge (*E. masquinongy*)	-
	Percid herpesvirus 1	Herpesvirus vitreum	Walleye (*S. vitreum*)	-
	Pleuronectid herpesvirus 1	Herpesvirus scopthalami	Turbot (*S. maximua*)	-
		Atlantic salmon papillomatosis virus	Atlantic salmon (*S. salar*)	-
		Herpesvirus of osmerus eperlanus 1	European smelt (*O. eperlanus*) & rainbow smelt (*O. mordax*)	-
		Tilapia larvae encephalitis virus	Tilapia (*Oreochromis* spp.)	-
		Viral epidermal hyperplasia/necrosis	Japanese flounder (*P. esus*)	-
		-	Angelfish (*P. altum*)	-
		-	Golden ide (*L. ide*)	-
		-	Red striped rockfish (*S. proriger*)	-
		-	Smooth dogfish (*M. canis*)	-
Ostreavirus	*Ostreid herpesvirus 1*	Oyster herpesvirus	Japanese oyster (*C. gigas*) & other bivalves	(Davison et al., 2005b)
Unclassified malacoherpesvirus	*Abalone herpesvirus 1*	Abalone herpesvirus	Abalone (*H. diversicolor supertexta*)	(Savin et al., 2010)

Table 1. Classified, characterized and uncharacterized fish and amphibian herpesviruses of the family *Alloherpesviridae*, and invertebrate herpesviruses of the family *Malacoherpesviridae*

Herpesviruses of fish, amphibians and invertebrates form an important and potentially large group of many yet-undiscovered pathogens. Although the fundamental characteristics of herpesviruses of humans and several other mammals have been thoroughly studied, there is still little knowledge of the herpesviruses of lower vertebrates and invertebrates. This lack of knowledge hampers the development of therapeutic and preventive strategies.

This book chapter describes the fundamentals of herpesviruses infecting fish, amphibians and invertebrates, including their biology, classification and taxonomy, capsid structure and structural proteins, and genome organization and gene conservation. Where possible, a comparison with herpesviruses infecting higher vertebrates is made. An overview of the current knowledge on gene expression, latency and virulence factors of alloherpesviruses, as well as the characterization of specific genes and the development of vaccines, is given at the end of this chapter.

2. Biology of fish, amphibian and invertebrate herpesviruses

2.1 Frog herpesviruses

The North American leopard frog (*Rana pipiens*) is occasionally affected with a renal adenocarcinoma known as the Lucké tumour. A viral aetiology was proposed based on the presence of acidophilic inclusions in tumour cell nuclei, and transmission experiments (Lucké, 1934; 1938). Viral particles were observed by electron microscopy (EM) about 20 years later (Fawcett, 1956). Yet another decade later, the virus was characterized as a herpes-type virus (Lunger, 1964), later designated *Ranid herpesvirus 1* (RaHV-1). Tumour formation could be induced by injection with purified RaHV-1 (Mizell et al., 1969), and Koch-Henle's postulates were fulfilled (Naegele et al., 1974). Virus replication is promoted by low temperature (Granoff, 1999), whereas induction of metastasis is promoted by high temperature (Lucké & Schlumberger, 1949; McKinnell & Tarin, 1984). Although RaHV-1 cannot be cultured in cell lines, it was the first amphibian herpesvirus subjected to extensive genomic studies (Davison et al., 1999).

During an attempt to isolate the causative agent of the Lucké tumour from pooled urine of tumour-bearing frogs, another virus - designated frog virus 4 - was isolated using a frog embryo cell line (Rafferty, 1965). The virus was shown to possess the morphological characteristics of a herpesvirus (Gravell et al., 1968), but appeared to be clearly distinctive from the Lucké tumour herpesvirus with regard to the possibility of *in vitro* propagation and genomic properties (Gravell, 1971). In addition, frog virus 4 has no oncogenic potential, although it infects leopard frog embryos and larvae effectively (Granoff, 1999). Frog virus 4 was later designated *Ranid herpesvirus 2* (RaHV-2).

2.2 Catfish herpesviruses

In the United States, during the rapid expansion of the pond-cultured channel catfish (*Ictalurus punctatus*) industry in the late 1960s, high mortalities were reported in fingerlings and fry shortly after transfer from the hatchery to the fry ponds (Wolf, 1988). Moribund fish showed behavioural changes (swimming in spirals and hanging vertically with the head at the water surface), exophthalmus, pale or haemorrhagic gills, external and internal haemorrhages, and distension of abdomen (ascites and oedema) and stomach (Fijan et al., 1971). In 1968 a virus was isolated from various fish farms, designated channel catfish virus. A year later the virus was shown to be a herpesvirus which replicated best at 25-33 °C (Wolf

& Darlington, 1971), later designated *Ictalurid herpesvirus 1* (IcHV-1). Although mortality among young channel catfish may be very high, the effects of the disease can be minimized through management practices (Wolf, 1988). IcHV-1 has been studied extensively ever since (Kucuktas & Brady, 1999), starting with the biological properties (including pathogenicity and diagnostic possibilities), followed by molecular and structural studies, as well as vaccine development. IcHV-1 was the first fish herpesvirus for which the genome sequence became available (Davison, 1992), which had a significant impact on herpesvirus taxonomy.
In the summer of 1994 another catfish herpesvirus was isolated from adult black bullhead (*Ameiurus melas*) from two different farms in Italy (Alborali et al., 1996). Morbidity and mortality were very high (80-90%), with clinical signs being unexpected spiral movements, swimming in a vertical position and death. Internal findings included haemorrhages on skin, spleen and liver. This catfish herpesvirus was shown to be different from IcHV-1, but appeared to be highly virulent for channel catfish fry and juveniles (Hedrick et al., 2003). Hence, the virus was later designated *Ictalurid herpesvirus 2* (Waltzek et al., 2009).

2.3 Carp herpesviruses

Pox disease of carp was described as early as 1563 by Conrad Gessner. Four hundred years later, herpesvirus-like particles were found to be associated with the pox-like lesions in carp (Schubert, 1966). The agent was eventually isolated in Japan, and designated *Cyprinid herpesvirus 1* (CyHV-1) (Sano et al., 1985a; Sano et al., 1985b). Infection trials showed that the virus was highly pathogenic for carp-fry, but not for older carp (Sano et al., 1990b; Sano et al., 1991). The majority of surviving carp-fry and a number of older carp developed papillomas several months after infection. Mortality and regression of the papillomas appeared to be temperature dependent (Sano et al., 1993).
The causative agent of herpesviral haematopoietic necrosis of goldfish was first identified in the early 1990s in Japan (Jung & Miyazaki, 1995), and later designated *Cyprinid herpesvirus 2* (CyHV-2). This virus may cause severe mortality especially among juvenile goldfish (Chang et al., 1999; Groff et al., 1998; Jeffery et al., 2007; Jung & Miyazaki, 1995), at water temperatures between 15 and 25 °C (Jeffery et al., 2007). Clinical signs include lethargy, anorexia and inappetence. Gross pathology includes pale gills, and swollen spleen and kidney (Jeffery et al., 2007). The disease has been reported in the USA (Goodwin et al., 2006; Goodwin et al., 2009; Groff et al., 1998), Taiwan (Chang et al., 1999), Australia (Stephens et al., 2004), UK (Jeffery et al., 2007), and Hungary (Doszpoly et al., 2011b). CyHV-2 seems to be widespread on commercial goldfish farms, with outbreaks occurring when fish are subjected to stress during permissive temperatures (Goodwin et al., 2009).
In the late 1990s, mass mortalities associated with gill and skin disease occurred in the koi and common carp (*Cyprinus carpio* spp.) industries worldwide (Haenen et al., 2004). Affected fish were lethargic, anorexic and showed increased respiratory movements (Bretzinger et al., 1999; Walster, 1999). The disease is characterized by epidermal lesions, extensive gill necrosis, and an enlarged anterior kidney showing moderate damage histologically. The course is acute or peracute in most cases, with high morbidity and mortality, depending on the water temperature (15-28 °C). EM analyses revealed the presence of herpesvirus-like particles in respiratory epithelial cells of gills of affected koi carp (Bretzinger et al., 1999), and River's postulates were fulfilled subsequently (Hedrick et al., 2000). The etiological agent koi herpesvirus was shown to differ from CyHV-1 (Gilad et al., 2002), and later designated *Cyprinid herpesvirus 3* (CyHV-3) (Waltzek et al., 2005). Common and koi carp are

among the most economically important aquaculture species worldwide, with CyHV-3 still being one of the most significant threats (Michel et al., 2010). CyHV-3 has therefore been the subject of advanced fundamental and applied research in the past decade.

2.4 Salmon herpesviruses

During the early 1970s a herpesvirus was isolated from a rainbow trout (*Oncorhynchus mykiss*) hatchery in the USA, which had increased post spawning mortalities (30-50%) for several years (Wolf, 1976). The virus could only be propagated in cell cultures of salmonid origin at low temperatures (10°C) (Wolf et al., 1978). General characteristics of a herpesvirus were demonstrated by EM. Rainbow trout fry could be infected with this virus, with mortality ranging from 50-100%, but related salmonid species could not (Wolf, 1976). Symptoms observed included inappetence, lethargy, dark pigmentation, pale gills, and sometimes haemorrhagic exophthalmia (Wolf & Smith, 1981). Visceral organs and the heart showed major pathological changes, with the liver and kidneys being prime targets for the virus. The disease failed to spread by cohabitation. The etiological agent was later designated *Salmonid herpesvirus 1* (SalHV-1).

In the same period a number of herpesviruses was isolated in Japan from different salmonid species, such as kokanee salmon (*Oncorhynchus nerka*) (Sano, 1976), masu salmon (*Oncorhynchus masou*) (Hayashi et al., 1986; Kimura et al., 1981b), yamame (*Oncorhynchus masou*) (Sano et al., 1983), coho salmon (*Oncorhynchus kisutch*) (Kumagai et al., 1994), and rainbow trout (Yoshimizu et al., 1995). The viruses appeared to be highly pathogenic particularly for young fry of different salmonid species (Kimura et al., 1983; Yoshimizu et al., 1995). The liver and kidney were the primary target organs, characterized by necrosis (Tanaka et al., 1984). Interestingly, surviving fish developed epithelial tumours around the mouth (Kimura et al., 1981a; Sano et al., 1983; Yoshimizu et al., 1987). Subsequent serological and DNA restriction endonuclease cleavage analysis demonstrated that all isolates could be considered as a single virus species, designated *Salmonid herpesvirus 2* (SalHV-2) (Hayashi et al., 1986; Hayashi et al., 1989; Hedrick et al., 1987; Yoshimizu et al., 1995).

A third salmonid herpesvirus caused high mortalities among hatchery-reared juvenile lake trout (*Salvelinus namaycush*) in the Great Lakes Region of the USA for several subsequent springs and falls (6-15°C) during the mid-1980s (Kurobe et al., 2009). Epidemics were characterized by the rapid onset of mortality, followed by a number of nonspecific clinical signs, including corkscrew swimming, lethargy, and periods of hyperexcitability (Bradley et al., 1989). External symptoms included haemorrhages in the eyes, fin and skin degeneration, and secondary fungus infections (Bradley et al., 1989; McAllister & Herman, 1989). Mortality could be as much as 100%, with fry being more susceptible than fingerlings. In the late 1980s herpesvirus-like particles were associated with the disease. Transmission experiments demonstrated that *Salmonid herpesvirus 3* (SalHV-3) was the etiologic agent of the epizootic epitheliotrophic disease restricted to lake trout. Propagation of the virus in cell culture is still impossible, which hampered detection until very recently (Kurobe et al., 2009).

A fourth salmonid herpesvirus has been described, but not yet characterized. In the late 1970s benign proliferative epidermal papillomatous lesions of cultured Atlantic salmon (*Salmo salar*) in Scandinavia and the UK were investigated (Bylund et al., 1980; Carlisle & Roberts, 1977). Papillomas developed in July and August, after which they sloughed, and in December nearly all were gone. The papillomas appeared as white plaques which raised several millimetres and were up to several centimetres in diameter. They were frequently multiple and found anywhere on the skin and fins posterior to the head. Morbidity and mortality were generally low. Virus-like particles were observed using EM in samples from papillomatous tissue (Carlisle, 1977), later characterized as a herpesvirus in Atlantic salmon from Russia (Shchelkunov et al., 1992). Attempts to isolate the observed virus in cell culture failed (Carlisle, 1977; Shchelkunov et al., 1992).

2.5 Sturgeon herpesviruses

In 1991 a herpesvirus was isolated from juvenile white sturgeon (*Acipenser transmontanus*) from a commercial farm in California, USA (Hedrick et al., 1991). The white sturgeon herpesvirus 1, later designated *Acipenserid herpesvirus 1* (AciHV-1), was associated with infections of the tegument and oropharyngeal mucosa, and mortality among the juvenile white sturgeons. Experimentally induced infections also resulted in mortality. AciHV-1 was later isolated from other farmed white sturgeons in California and Italy (Kelley et al., 2005; Kurobe et al., 2008).

Few years later another herpesvirus called white sturgeon herpesvirus 2, or *Acipenserid herpesvirus 2* (AciHV-2), was isolated from dermal lesions of subadult white sturgeon and ovarian fluids of a mature white sturgeon (Watson et al., 1995). Mortality among experimentally infected juvenile white sturgeons reached a cumulative total of 80%. AciHV-2 has since been isolated from wild white sturgeon in Idaho and Oregon (USA), from farmed shortnose sturgeon (*Acipenser brevirostrum*) from Canada, and from Siberian sturgeon (*Acipenser baeri*) in Russia (Doszpoly & Shchelkunov, 2010; Kelley et al., 2005; Kurobe et al., 2008; Shchelkunov et al., 2009).

2.6 Eel herpesvirus

Herpesvirus-like particles in wild European eels (*Anguilla anguilla*) were described for the first time in 1986 (Békési et al., 1986). A herpesvirus was later isolated from cultured European eels and Japanese eels (*A. japonica*) in Japan (Sano et al., 1990a). Serological, molecular, and sequence data indicated that Asian and European eel herpesvirus isolates can be considered as a single virus species (Chang et al., 2002; Lee et al., 1999; Rijsewijk et al., 2005; Sano et al., 1990a; Ueno et al., 1992; Ueno et al., 1996; Waltzek et al., 2009), designated *Anguillid herpesvirus 1* (AngHV-1). Clinical and pathological findings of the infection varied among and within outbreaks, and were predominantly apathy, haemorrhages and ulcerative lesions in skin and fins, haemorrhagic or pale and congested gills, a pale spleen, a pale and haemorrhagic liver, a distended gall bladder, and ascites (Chang et al., 2002; Davidse et al., 1999; Haenen et al., 2002; Lee et al., 1999; Sano et al., 1990a). AngHV-1 infection in cultured eels resulted in decreased growth rates and an increased mortality (Haenen et al., 2002). The virus is also frequently observed in wild European eels (Haenen et al., 2010; Jørgensen et al., 1994; van Ginneken et al., 2004).

2.7 Pilchard herpesvirus

In 1995, a massive epizootic occurred in adult Australasian pilchards (*Sardinops sagax neopilchardus*) in south Australia (O'Neill, 1995). In several months it spread thousands of kilometres bidirectionally along the Australian coastline, and then to New Zealand (Whittington et al., 1997). A similar event occurred a few years later in 1998/1999 (Murray et al., 2003). Affected pilchards showed progressive gill inflammation followed by epithelial hypertrophy and hyperplasia (Whittington et al., 1997). Consequent clinical symptoms included hypoxaemia and hypercapnea, resulting in an estimated mortality of at least 10%. Involvement of an infectious agent was suggested, and PCR analysis revealed the putative involvement of a herpesvirus (Tham & Moon, 1996), which was soon confirmed by EM (Hyatt et al., 1997). Diagnostic tools for detection of the pilchard herpesvirus have been developed (Crockford et al., 2005; Crockford et al., 2008), revealing that the virus is now endemic in Australian pilchard populations (Whittington et al., 2008). Although the pilchard herpesvirus has not yet been isolated in cell culture, hampering further studies, limited phylogenetic analysis showed its relation to other fish and frog herpesviruses (Doszpoly et al., 2011a).

2.8 Other fish herpesviruses

Several other herpesvirus-like particles have been observed and found to be associated with disease in other fish species. Many of these viruses have not been isolated yet, however, and limited sequence availability hampers official classification.

In the late 1970s a herpes-type viral infection of the epithelia of the skin and gills of turbot (*Scophthalmus maximus*) was found, presumably associated with heavy mortalities among farmed turbot (Buchanan & Madeley, 1978; Buchanan et al., 1978). Although the virus could not be isolated in cell culture, EM observations clearly demonstrated herpesvirus characteristics. The virus was tentatively named herpesvirus scophthalmi, later referred to as pleuronectid herpesvirus 1 (PlHV-1).

Few years later a herpesvirus was isolated from hyperplastic epidermal tissue from a walleye (*Stiozostedion vitreum vitreum*) taken in Saskatchewan, Canada (Kelly et al., 1983). The virus was isolated in a walleye ovarian cell line and identified as a herpesvirus based on size, morphology, and apparent pattern of replication. The virus was initially called herpesvirus vitreum, but later designated percid herpesvirus 1 (PeHV-1).

A year later the same research group observed typical herpesvirus particles in epidermal hyperplasia or blue spot disease of northern pike (*Esox lucius*) in several waters of central Canada (Yamamoto et al., 1984). The virus, tentatively designated esocid herpesvirus 1 (EsHV-1), could not be isolated in cell culture, however. EsHV-1 was later also observed in northern pike and muskellunge (*Esox masquinongy*) in the USA, with clinical signs present only for a short period when water temperatures were between 2 and 13 °C (Margenau et al., 1995), and in northern pike in Ireland (Graham et al., 2004).

In the early 1980s, in a quarantined population of golden ide (*Leuciscus idus*) imported from Germany to the USA, 5% of the fish developed carp pox-like lesions (McAllister et al., 1985). EM analysis showed herpesvirus-like particles associated with the lesions, but the virus could not be isolated in cell culture.

In 1985 herpesvirus-like particles were observed in so-called spawning papillomas on the skin and fins of smelt (*Osmerus eperlanus*) in Germany (Anders & Möller, 1985). Herpesvirus-like particles were also observed in similar epidermal tumours of rainbow smelt (*O. mordax*) during spawning-time in Canada and the USA (Herman et al., 1997; Morrison et al., 1996). Isolation and genomic analysis of the herpesvirus of smelt have failed so far (Jakob et al., 2010).

In the same year a viral dermatitis was observed in a small percentage of wild and captive smooth dogfish (*Mustelus canis*) (Leibovitz & Lebouitz, 1985). Most skin eruptions were found on the tail and fins, often exceeding 1 cm in diameter, and histologically characterized by epidermal cell degeneration. EM revealed the progressive development of cellular pathology associated with a specific epidermal viral infection, and viral particles showed the characteristics of a herpesvirus.

In the mid-1980s a new disease characterized by skin and fin opacity, and associated with high mortality occurred in larvae and juveniles of Japanese flounder (*Paralichthys olivaceus*) hatcheries in Japan (Iida et al., 1989; Miyazaki et al., 1989). Microscopically, epidermal cells at the surface were rounded, and histopathologically the epidermis appeared to be hyperplastic and necrotic (Iida et al., 1991; Miyazaki, 2005). Although the causative agent could not be isolated, herpesvirus-like particles were observed by EM. Infection trials showed that especially larvae <10 mm were susceptible, at water temperatures around 20 °C (Masumura et al., 1989).

After a stress-trigger, all three angelfish (*Pterophyllum altum*) in a fish tank showed loss of equilibrium and hung apathetic at the water surface (Mellergaard & Bloch, 1988). The fish had skin haemorrhages, pale gills and distended liver and spleen. Histopathological findings of the spleen were all suggestive of severe haemolytic anaemia. Herpesvirus-like particles were observed by EM in the nuclei of spleen macrophages and monocytes.

A wild redstriped rockfish (*Sebastes proriger*) demonstrated hepatic lesions, which were histologically suggestive of a herpesvirus-type infection (Kent & Myers, 2000). EM analysis of suboptimally preserved liver tissue revealed the presence of intranuclear particles, consistent in size and shape with herpesvirus capsids.

Recently, an outbreak of a novel disease characterized by a whirling syndrome and high mortality rates occurred in laboratory-reared tilapia larvae (*Oreochromis* spp.) (Shlapobersky et al., 2010). The disease was designated viral encephalitis of tilapia larvae. The morphological characteristics of virus particles found in the brains of diseased larvae as observed by EM were comparable to those of a herpesvirus.

2.9 Oyster herpesvirus

The first description of a herpesvirus-like virus in oysters originates from the United States (Farley et al., 1972). As for the fish and amphibian herpesviruses, it was only the virus morphology that identified this oyster virus as a herpesvirus. The principle susceptible species is the Japanese oyster (*Crassostrea gigas*), and the virus was designated *Ostreid herpesvirus 1* (OsHV-1). In Europe, where the virus was found for the first time in the early 1990s, OsHV-1 has been associated with high mortalities in oyster seedlings (Garcia et al., 2011). Herpesvirus-like particles - later confirmed to be OsHV-1 by molecular analyses - have also been observed in various other bivalve species, associated with mortalities (Arzul et al., 2001; Burge et al., 2011). Recently, an OsHV-1 variant, designated OsHV-1 μvar, was identified as the causative agent of high mortalities in juvenile oysters (Segarra et al., 2010).

2.10 Abalone herpesvirus

A second herpesvirus with an invertebrate host has been identified by EM in cultured abalone (*Haliotis diversicolor supertexta*) in Taiwan in early 2003 and in Australia in late 2005 (Chang et al., 2005; Tan et al., 2008). Abalones of all ages suffered from the disease, which was characterized by mantle recession and muscle stiffness, followed by high mortality within a few days. Histologically the nerve system appeared to be the primary target tissue, characterized by tissue necrosis with infiltration of haemocytes. The virus has been designated *Abalone herpesvirus 1* (AbHV-1).

3. Classification and taxonomy of the order *Herpesvirales*

Herpesviruses are large and complex DNA viruses with a distinctive virion morphology, which consists of four distinct structures: the core, capsid, tegument, and envelope (Davison et al., 2005a). The order *Herpesvirales* is subdivided into three families (Davison et al., 2009), which separated about 500 million years ago (McGeoch et al., 2006). The family *Herpesviridae* comprises the herpesviruses with mammalian, avian and reptilian hosts, and is further subdivided into the subfamilies *Alpha-*, *Beta-* and *Gammaherpesvirinae*, which fall into genera.

The family *Alloherpesviridae* comprises the piscine and amphibian herpesviruses (Waltzek et al., 2009). The criteria for the establishment of genera within the family *Alloherpesviridae* have not been defined yet, nor have rules been formulated for deciding whether species should belong to a particular genus. Currently, genera and their respective species are assigned largely based on available phylogenetic analyses, with phylogenetically closely related species assigned to the same genus. To date, four genera in the family *Alloherpesviridae* have been established: *Batrachovirus, Cyprinivirus, Ictalurivirus* and *Salmonivirus*, comprising a total of 11 different species (Table 1, Fig. 1). In the majority of the cases the classification follows the grouping of alloherpesviruses infecting the same host. At least another 14 herpesviruses infecting fish have been described, but not yet characterized sufficiently to allow classification.

The oyster herpesvirus OsHV-1 has been assigned to the genus *Ostreavirus* of the third herpesvirus family *Malacoherpesviridae*, which comprises the invertebrate herpesviruses (Davison et al., 2009; Davison et al., 2005b). The other invertebrate herpesvirus infecting abalone AbHV-1 has been shown to be related to OsHV-1 (Savin et al., 2010). Despite the similarities in capsid structure between the herpesviruses of mammals, birds and reptiles, fish and amphibians, and invertebrates, the three families are highly divergent. Only a single gene, encoding a DNA packaging enzyme complex distantly related to the ATPase subunit of bacteriophage T4 terminase, is convincingly conserved among all herpesviruses (Davison, 1992; 2002).

4. Conservation of herpesvirus capsid architecture & structural proteins

4.1 Capsid architecture of herpesviruses

Despite their diversity by genes, host range, and genome size, herpesvirus structure is conserved throughout the entire order *Herpesvirales*. Herpesvirus virions invariably consist of a large (diameter >100 nm) thick-walled icosahedral nucleocapsid (T=16), surrounded by a host-derived envelope with a diameter of about 200 nm, with an intervening proteinaceous layer called the tegument (Booy et al., 1996). This appearance is distinctively different from that of any other animal virus. Key to this morphological conservatism is the icosahedral nucleocapsid made up of hollow capsomers. The functionality of the genes involved in capsid assembly is largely conserved.

The capsid structures of alloherpesvirus IcHV-1 and malacoherpesvirus OsHV-1 have been studied by cryoelectron microscopy and three-dimensional image reconstruction (Booy et al., 1996; Davison et al., 2005b). Both viruses have capsids with diameters of approximately 116 nm, which is slightly smaller than the capsids of the human model herpesvirus, Herpes simplex virus type 1 (HSV-1, diameter 125 nm). The capsids of IcHV-1 and OsHV-1 are roughly hexagonal in outline and reconstruction revealed an icosahedral structure with a triangulation number of T=16. The icosahedral facets of IcHV-1 appeared to be flatter, and the shell is about 20% thinner (12.4 nm vs. 15 nm) than that of HSV-1, consistent with the smaller size of its major capsid protein. The hexons and pentons showed protrusions with an axial channel through each capsomer. The outer surface is composed of heterotrimeric complexes or triplexes at the sites of local threefold symmetry, and the inner surface has a relatively flat and featureless appearance. IcHV-1 and OsHV-1 capsids are therefore similar in overall appearance to those of all other herpesviruses studied to date.

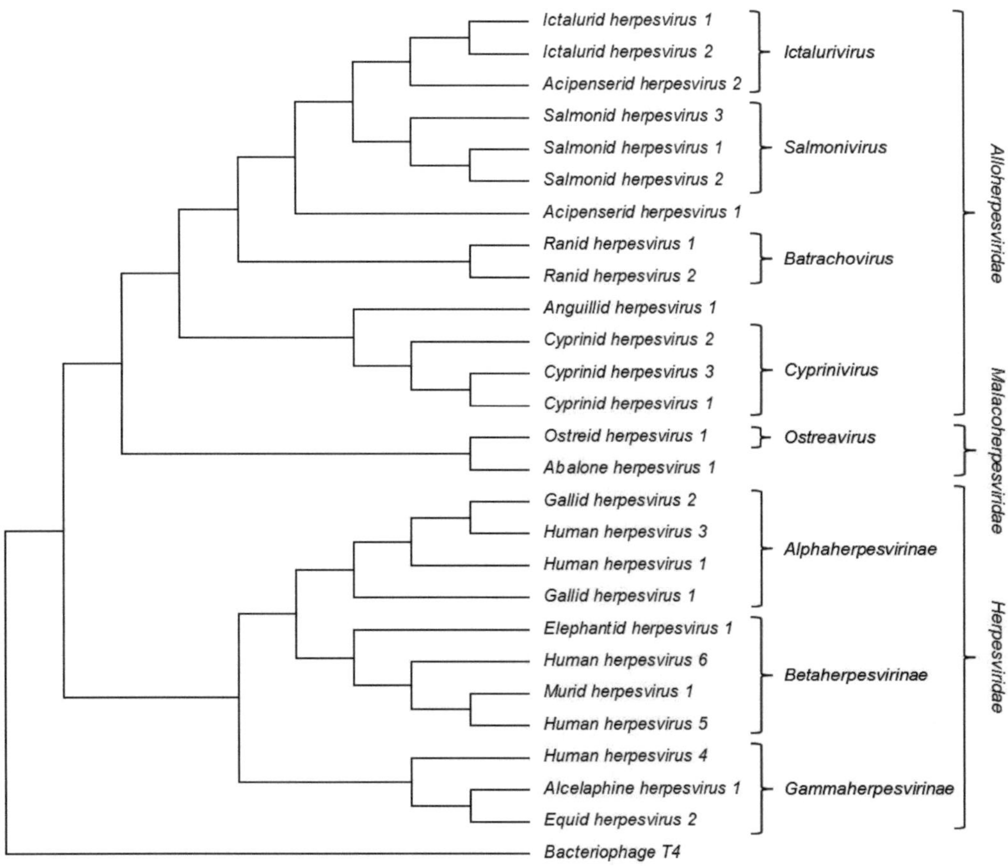

Fig. 1. Phylogenetic tree depicting the relationships (topology only) among viruses in the order *Herpesvirales*, based on partially deduced amino acid sequence of the terminase gene (107 residues, including gaps), analysed with the maximum likelihood method, using the JTT matrix (1,000 replicates), and rooted with bacteriophage T4

4.2 Structural proteins of *Alloherpesviridae*

Complete herpesvirus virions are made up of about 40 viral proteins. Recent mass spectrometry (MS) analyses showed that HSV-1 virions comprise at least 8 viral capsid proteins, 13 viral glycoproteins, 23 potential viral teguments, and 49 host proteins (Loret et al., 2008). When in 1995 the structural proteins of IcHV-1 were identified by MS (Davison & Davison, 1995), a total of 11 genes encoding 15 virion proteins was identified. Based on analyses of capsid, capsid-tegument, and envelope fractions, the proteins could be assigned to the different compartments of the virion.

More recent studies on the structural proteins of CyHV-3 and AngHV-1 used liquid chromatography tandem MS-based proteomic approaches. For CyHV-3 a total of 40 structural proteins was identified, which were classified based on homology and bioinformatic analyses as capsid (3), envelope (13), tegument (2) and unclassified (22) structural proteins (Michel et al., 2010). For AngHV-1, by analysing separately prepared fractions of capsid, tegument, and envelope, the identified proteins could also be functionally characterized. A total of 40 structural proteins was identified, of which 7 could be assigned to the capsid, 11 to the envelope, and 22 to the tegument (van Beurden et al., 2011).

The protein composition of fish herpesvirus capsids generally mirrors that of mammalian herpesvirus capsids. MS analyses of purified alloherpesvirus capsids demonstrated the presence of the major capsid protein, the capsid triplex protein 2, and, presumably, the capsid triplex protein 1 (Davison & Davison, 1995; van Beurden et al., 2011). The protease-and-scaffolding protein is only abundantly present in premature capsids, and later replaced by viral DNA during maturation. The small protein which forms the hexon tips in mammalian herpesviruses has not been found in alloherpesvirus capsids.

Conservation of tegument and envelope proteins among fish herpesviruses is rather limited (van Beurden et al., 2011). A large tegument protein was found to be partially conserved, and two envelope proteins might be conserved. The higher conservation of structural proteins between members of the family *Herpesviridae* resembles the greater evolutionary distance of the family *Alloherpesviridae*.

5. Genome organization and gene conservation

5.1 Genome properties

The single linear double stranded DNA genomes of herpesviruses vary greatly in size, ranging from 124 kbp for Simian varicella virus, to more than 250 kbp. This enormous variation is also present within the family *Alloherpesviridae*, in which IcHV-1 has the smallest genome of 134 kbp, and AngHV-1 and CyHV-3 represent the largest herpesvirus genomes known of 249 and 295 kbp, respectively (Table 2). G+C content varies from 32 to 75% within the family *Herpesviridae* (McGeoch et al., 2006), but seems to be more restricted among members of the family *Alloherpesviridae* (52.8 to 59.2%), and is rather low for OsHV-1 (38.7%).

5.2 Genome organization

Herpesvirus genomes characteristically contain one or two regions of unique sequence flanked by direct or inverted repeats (McGeoch et al., 2006). To date, six different classes of genome organization have been identified (Davison, 2007). The genome organization of six alloherpesviruses has been determined. The genomes of AngHV-1, CyHV-3, IcHV-1, RaHV-1 and RaHV-2 all consist of one long unique region (U) flanked by two short direct repeat regions (TR) at the termini (Fig. 2).This genome structure (A) is also represented among the *Betaherpesvirinae* (Davison, 2007). Interestingly, the terminal repeats of the ranid herpesviruses are considerably shorter (<1-kbp) than those of the fish herpesviruses (>10-kbp). Genome organization A does not seem to be a general feature of the *Alloherpesviridae*, since SalHV-1 is known to have a long unique region (U_L) linked to a short unique region (U_S) flanked by an inverted repeat (IR_S and TR_S) (Davison, 1998). This genome structure (D) is characteristic of *Alphaherpesvirinae* in the *Varicellovirus* genus (Davison, 2007).

Name	Genome length	Terminal repeat length	G+C content	Number of ORFs	ORF density per kpb	Refseq accession	Key reference
Anguillid herpesvirus 1	248,531 bp	10,634 bp	53.0%	136	0.57	NC_013668	(van Beurden et al., 2010)
Cyprinid herpesvirus 3	295,146 bp	22,469 bp	59.2%	156	0.57	NC_009127	(Aoki et al., 2007)
Ictalurid herpesvirus 1	134,226 bp	18,556 bp	56.2%	77	0.67	NC_001493	(Davison, 1992)
Ranid herpesvirus 1	220,859 bp	636 bp	54.6%	132	0.60	NC_008211	(Davison et al., 2006)
Ranid herpesvirus 2	231,801 bp	912 bp	52.8%	147	0.64	NC_008210	(Davison et al., 2006)
Ostreid herpesvirus 1	207,439 bp	7584 bp 9774 bp	38.7%	124	0.65	NC_005881	(Davison et al., 2005b)

Table 2. Genome characteristics of completely sequenced members of the families *Alloherpesviridae* and *Malacoherpesviridae*

Genome structure E is the most complex genome structure and characteristic of *Alphaherpesvirinae* in the *Simplexvirus* genus, and certain members of the genus *Cytomegalovirus* of the *Betaherpesvirinae* (Davison, 2007). The gross genome organization of OsHV-1 is a combination of class D and E genomes, consisting of two invertible unique regions (U_L & U_S), each flanked by inverted repeats (TR_L & IR_L and IR_S & TR_S), with an additional short unique sequence (X) between the inverted repeats (Davison et al., 2005b).

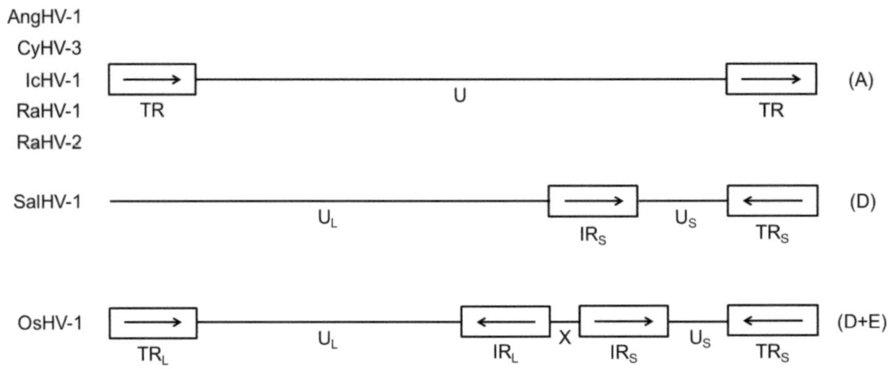

Fig. 2. Schematic representation of the genome organization of selected members of the families *Alloherpesviridae* and *Malacoherpesviridae*

5.3 Gene conservation

Herpesvirus genomes show a wide range in number of genes, ranging from about 70 (Varicella zoster virus) to more than 200 (Human cytomegalovirus) genes (Davison, 2007; McGeoch et al., 2006). Herpesvirus genes are divided into core genes and non-core genes.

The core genes are inherited from a common ancestor and fundamental to replication, being involved in capsid assembly and structure, DNA replication machinery, processing and packaging of DNA, egress of capsids from the nucleus, and control and modulation. The non-core genes represent accessory systems that developed more recently and fit a virus to a particular biological niche. These genes are involved in cellular tropisms, control of cellular processes, manipulation or evasion from the host immune system, and latency. Among the *Herpesviridae*, there is a subset of 43 core genes (McGeoch & Davison, 1999).

Only 13 genes are convincingly conserved among all members of the family *Alloherpesviridae* (Aoki et al., 2007). These genes encode proteins putatively involved in capsid morphogenesis, DNA replication and DNA packaging (Table 3). Five of the identified conserved genes encode proteins with unknown functions. With only 13 genes conserved among all family members, the family *Alloherpesviridae* appears to be considerably more divergent than the family *Herpesviridae*, reflecting the greater divergence of its host species.

Function	**AngHV-1**	**CyHV-3**	**IcHV-1**	**RaHV-1**	**RaHV-2**
ATPase subunit of terminase	ORF10	ORF33	ORF62	ORF42	ORF68
Primase	ORF21	ORF46	ORF63	ORF87	ORF121
Unknown	ORF22	ORF47	ORF64	ORF88	ORF122
Capsid triplex protein 2	ORF36	ORF72	ORF27	ORF95	ORF131
DNA helicase	ORF37	ORF71	ORF25	ORF93	ORF129
Unknown	ORF52	ORF80	ORF60	ORF84	ORF118
DNA polymerase	ORF55	ORF79	ORF57	ORF72	ORF110
Capsid protease and scaffolding protein	ORF57	ORF78	ORF28	ORF63	ORF88
Large envelope glycoprotein	ORF67	ORF99	ORF46	ORF46	ORF72
Unknown	ORF82	ORF61	ORF54	ORF75	ORF113
Unknown	ORF98	ORF107	ORF56	ORF73	ORF111
Unknown	ORF100	ORF90	ORF37	ORF52	ORF78
Major capsid protein	ORF104	ORF92	ORF39	ORF54	ORF80

Table 3. Conserved genes of the family *Alloherpesviridae*

The arrangement of homologous genes in AngHV-1 and CyHV-3 appears to be conserved in clusters (van Beurden et al., 2010). Several conserved gene blocks can be identified, either in the same or in inverse orientation. At the *Alloherpesviridae* family level, the 13 conserved genes seem to be conserved within the same clusters, which was previously shown also for IcHV-1 and SalHV-1 (Davison, 1998), and appears to apply for all completely sequenced *Alloherpesviridae* (Fig. 3). This resembles the seven blocks of core genes that are typically arranged throughout the family *Herpesviridae* (McGeoch et al., 2006).

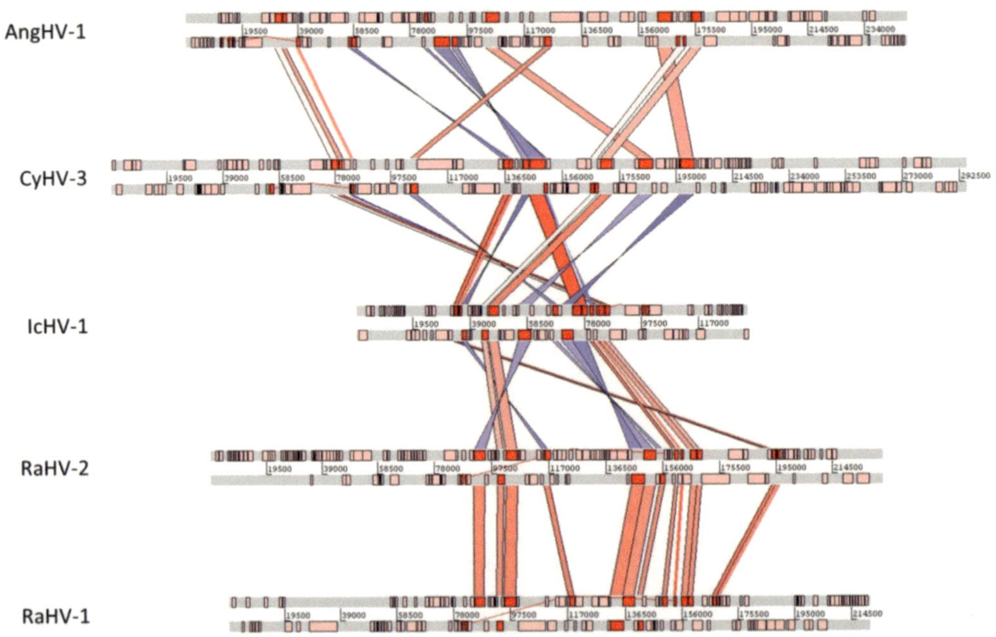

Fig. 3. Geneblock conservation throughout the family *Alloherpesviridae*: conserved genes are coloured red and connected through the genomes by coloured bars; red bars indicate similar and reading frame direction, blue bars indicate reversed reading frame direction; percentage sequence identity at amino acid level is indicated by bar colour intensity

6. Extended characterization of *Alloherpesviridae*

6.1 Gene expression

Gene expression of herpesviruses is regulated in a temporal fashion, with genes being classified on the basis of their expression kinetics as immediate early, early, and late genes (McGeoch et al., 2006). Temporal gene expression has been suggested for IcHV-1 based on polypeptide analyses of *in vitro* infection experiments (Dixon & Farber, 1980). Transcription studies of selected ORFs, especially of the terminal repeat region of IcHV-1, confirmed the temporal expression of these genes (Huang & Hanson, 1998; Silverstein et al., 1995; Silverstein et al., 1998; Stingley & Gray, 2000). Expression of certain ORFs of CyHV-3 at lower and higher temperatures *in vitro* has been studied using RT-PCR (Dishon et al., 2007). Initial experiments to determine the complete transcription profile of AngHV-1 by quantitative RT-PCR showed similar temporal expression kinetics as have been determined for members of the family *Herpesviridae* (van Beurden et al., unpublished results).

6.2 Latency

The ability to establish a latent infection is one of the hallmarks of herpesviruses. Latent infections are characterized by the absence of infectious virus particles and regular viral transcription and replication, but the presence of intact viral genomic DNA and transcription of latency associated transcripts. Accordingly, the presence of viral DNA (and not infectious virus) has been demonstrated in fish surviving infections with IcHV-1 and CyHV-3 (Eide et al., 2011a; Gray et al., 1999), whereas viral replication was absent in such fish (Eide et al., 2011b; Stingley et al., 2003). It has been shown *in vitro* that CyHV-3 is able to persist in cultured cells at a nonpermissive temperature, with viral propagation and viral gene transcription being turned off, and reactivated upon return to the permissive temperature (Dishon et al., 2007). Reactivation of fish herpesviruses *in vivo* has been demonstrated for AngHV-1 following dexamethasone treatment (van Nieuwstadt et al., 2001), and for CyHV-3 following temperature stress (Eide et al., 2011b; St-Hilaire et al., 2005).

6.3 Gene characterization

Identification and characterization of most alloherpesvirus ORFs is based on sequence homology and bioinformatics. Recent probabilistic mapping of IcHV-1 (Kunec et al., 2009), and complete transcriptome analysis of AngHV-1 (van Beurden et al., unpublished results), show, however, that there might still be a large discrepancy between the predicted and actual numbers of ORFs.

MS analysis of purified capsids resulted in the identification of the structural proteins of IcHV-1, CyHV-3 and AngHV-1 (Davison & Davison, 1995; Michel et al., 2010; van Beurden et al., 2011). Based on the localization of the structural proteins in the different virion compartments, several of these proteins could be functionally characterized. Two alloherpesvirus proteins have been characterized in more detail: IcHV-1 ORF50 has been shown to encode a secreted mucin-like glycoprotein (Vanderheijden et al., 1999), and CyHV-3 ORF81 has been identified as an envelope protein (Rosenkranz et al., 2008).

6.4 Virulence factors and vaccine development

In many herpesviruses the homologues of cellular enzymes are nonessential for virus replication *in vitro*, but relevant for virulence *in vivo*. Attenuated IcHV-1 and CyHV-3 strains with specific gene deletions have been developed and tested for virulence. Thymidine kinase-negative mutants of IcHV-1 resembled wild type IcHV-1 *in vitro*, but appeared to be much less pathogenic *in vivo* (Zhang & Hanson, 1995). Similarly, CyHV-3 recombinants possessing deletions within the viral ribonucleotide reductase, thymidine kinase and dUTPase genes were developed and tested for attenuation (Fuchs et al., 2011). The use of the attenuated strains as modern live vaccines in challenges with wild-type virus showed promising results.

Several other attempts of vaccine development have been undertaken for IcHV-1 and CyHV-3. For CyHV-3, immunization with wild type and attenuated virus has been tested in relation to different water temperatures (Ronen et al., 2003). For IcHV-1, experimental subunit and attenuated vaccines were developed and tested (Dixon, 1997). Also, DNA vaccination with several different ORFs has been tested for IcHV-1 (Nusbaum et al., 2002). Later, an overlapping and a full BAC have been developed for IcHV-1 (Kunec et al., 2008) and CyHV-3 (Costes et al., 2008), respectively. The latter was used to test attenuation after disruption of the thymidine kinase locus and deletion of ORF16. To date no satisfying vaccine has been developed nor registered for any of the fish herpesviruses.

7. Conclusions

In conclusion, herpesviruses of fish, amphibians and invertebrates form a potentially large group of important pathogens. Understanding the origins of the distantly related families

Alloherpesviridae and *Malacoherpesviridae* provides insights into the evolution of the family *Herpesviridae*. The association of many fish herpesviruses with severe diseases in important aquaculture species has stimulated fundamental and applied research. For a selected number of alloherpesviruses, complete genome sequences and structural analyses of the virus particles are now available and have revealed similarity to the basic composition of higher vertebrate herpesviruses. Extended characterization of gene expression, latency, the function of specific genes and virulence factors as well as vaccine development is currently ongoing. These studies will add to the control and prevention of fish herpesvirus associated diseases, and might serve as models for research on human and domestic animal herpesviruses.

8. Acknowledgements

We thank Alex Bossers (Central Veterinary Institute (CVI), part of Wageningen UR) for generating Fig. 3. We are grateful to Olga Haenen (CVI), Ben Peeters (CVI), Fred van Zijderveld (CVI), and Peter Rottier (Faculty of Veterinary Medicine, Utrecht University) for a critical reading of this book chapter.

9. References

Alborali, L., Bovo, G., Cappellaro, H. & Guadagini, P.F. (1996). Isolation of an herpesvirus in breeding catfish (*Ictalurus mela*). *Bull Eur Ass Fish Pathol*, Vol. 16, No. 4, pp. 134-137

Anders, K. & Möller, H. (1985). Spawning papillomatosis of smelt, *Osmerus eperlanus* L., from the Elbe estuary. *J Fish Dis*, Vol. 8, pp. 233-235

Anders, K. & Yoshimizu, M. (1994). Role of viruses in the induction of skin tumours and tumour-like proliferations of fish. *Dis Aquat Org*, Vol. 19, pp. 215-232

Aoki, T., Hirono, I., Kurokawa, K., Fukuda, H., Nahary, R., Eldar, A., Davison, A.J., Waltzek, T.B., Bercovier, H. & Hedrick, R.P. (2007). Genome sequences of three koi herpesvirus isolates representing the expanding distribution of an emerging disease threatening koi and common carp worldwide. *J Virol*, Vol. 81, No. 10, pp. 5058-5065

Arzul, I., Renault, T., Lipart, C. & Davison, A.J. (2001). Evidence for interspecies transmission of oyster herpesvirus in marine bivalves. *J Gen Virol*, Vol. 82, No. 4, pp. 865-870

Békési, L., Horváth, I., Kovács-Gayer, E. & Csaba, G. (1986). Demonstration of herpesvirus like particles in skin lesions of European eel (*Anguilla anguilla*). *J Appl Ichthyol*, Vol. 4, pp. 190-192

Booy, F.P., Trus, B.L., Davison, A.J. & Steven, A.C. (1996). The capsid architecture of channel catfish virus, an evolutionarily distant herpesvirus, is largely conserved in the absence of discernible sequence homology with herpes simplex virus. *Virology*, Vol. 215, No. 2, pp. 134-141

Bradley, T.M., Medina, D.J., Chang, P.W. & McClain, J. (1989). Epizootic epitheliotropic disease mof lake trout (*Salvelinus namaycush*): history and viral etiology. *Dis Aquat Org*, Vol. 7, pp. 195-201

Bretzinger, A., Fischer-Scherl, T., Oumouna, M., Hoffmann, R. & Truyen, U. (1999). Mass mortalities in Koi carp, *Cyprinus carpio*, associated with gill and skin disease. *Bull Eur Ass Fish Pathol*, Vol. 19, No. 5, pp. 182-185

Buchanan, J.S. & Madeley, C.R. (1978). Studies on *Herpesvirus scophthalmi* infection of turbot *Scophthalmus maximus* (L.) ultrastructural observations. *J Fish Dis*, Vol. 1, pp. 283-295

Buchanan, J.S., Richards, R.H., Sommerville, C. & Madeley, C.R. (1978). A herpes-type virus from turbot (*Scophthalmus maximus* L). *Vet Rec*, Vol. 102, No. 24, pp. 527-528

Burge, C.A., Strenge, R.E. & Friedman, C.S. (2011). Detection of the oyster herpesvirus in commercial bivalve in northern California, USA: conventional and quantitative PCR. *Dis Aquat Org*, Vol. 94, No. 2, pp. 106-116

Bylund, G., Valtonen, E.T. & Niemelä, E. (1980). Observations on erpidermal papillomata in wild and cultured Atlantic salmon *Salmo salar* L. in Finland. *J Fish Dis*, Vol. 3, pp. 525-528

Carlisle, J.C. (1977). An epidermal papilloma of the Atlantic samon II: Ultrastructure and etiology. *J Wildl Dis*, Vol. 13, No. 3, pp. 235-239

Carlisle, J.C. & Roberts, R.J. (1977). An epidermal papilloma of the Atlantic salmon I: Epizootiology, pathology and immunology. *J Wildl Dis*, Vol. 13, No. 3, pp. 230-234

Chang, P.H., Kuo, S.T., Lai, S.H., Yang, H.S., Ting, Y.Y., Hsu, C.L. & Chen, H.C. (2005). Herpes-like virus infection causing mortality of cultured abalone *Haliotis diversicolor supertexta* in Taiwan. *Dis Aquat Org*, Vol. 65, No. 1, pp. 23-27

Chang, P.H., Lee, S.H., Chiang, H.C. & Jong, M.H. (1999). Epizootic of herpes-like virus infection in Goldfish, *Carassius auratus* in Taiwan. *Fish Pathol*, Vol. 34, No. 4, pp. 209-210

Chang, P.H., Pan, Y.H., Wu, C.M., Kuo, S.T. & Chung, H.Y. (2002). Isolation and molecular characterization of herpesvirus from cultured European eels *Anguilla anguilla* in Taiwan. *Dis Aquat Org*, Vol. 50, No. 2, pp. 111-118

Costes, B., Fournier, G., Michel, B., Delforge, C., Raj, V.S., Dewals, B., Gillet, L., Drion, P., Body, A., Schynts, F., Lieffrig, F. & Vanderplasschen, A. (2008). Cloning of the koi herpesvirus genome as an infectious bacterial artificial chromosome demonstrates that disruption of the thymidine kinase locus induces partial attenuation in *Cyprinus carpio koi*. *J Virol*, Vol. 82, No. 10, pp. 4955-4964

Crockford, M., Jones, J.B., Crane, M.S. & Wilcox, G.E. (2005). Molecular detection of a virus, Pilchard herpesvirus, associated with epizootics in Australasian pilchards *Sardinops sagax neopilchardus*. *Dis Aquat Org*, Vol. 68, No. 1, pp. 1-5

Crockford, M., Jones, J.B., McColl, K. & Whittington, R.J. (2008). Comparison of three molecular methods for the detectioon of pilchard herpesvirus in archived parrafin-embedded tissue and frozen tissue. *Dis Aquat Org*, Vol. 82, pp. 37-44

Davidse, A., Haenen, O.L.M., Dijkstra, S.G., van Nieuwstadt, A.P., van der Vorst, T.J.K., Wagenaar, F. & Wellenberg, G.J. (1999). First isolation of herpesvirus of eel (Herpesvirus Anguillae) in diseased European eel (*Anguilla anguilla* L.) in Europe. *Bull Eur Ass Fish Pathol*, Vol. 19, No. 4, pp. 137-141

Davison, A.J. (1992). Channel catfish virus: a new type of herpesvirus. *Virology*, Vol. 186, No. 1, pp. 9-14

Davison, A.J. (1998). The genome of salmonid herpesvirus 1. *J Virol*, Vol. 72, No. 3, pp. 1974-1982

Davison, A.J. (2002). Evolution of the herpesviruses. *Vet Microbiol*, Vol. 86, No. 1-2, pp. 69-88

Davison, A.J. (2007). Comparative analysis of the genomes, In: *Human Herpesviruses: Biology, Therapy, and Immunoprophylaxis* A. Arvin, G. Campadelli-Fiume, E. Mocarski, P.S.

Moore, B. Roizman, R. Whitley & K. Yamanishi, Cambridge University Press, Cambridge

Davison, A.J., Cunningham, C., Sauerbier, W. & McKinnell, R.G. (2006). Genome sequences of two frog herpesviruses. *J Gen Virol*, Vol. 87, No. 12, pp. 3509-3514

Davison, A.J. & Davison, M.D. (1995). Identification of structural proteins of channel catfish virus by mass spectrometry. *Virology*, Vol. 206, No. 2, pp. 1035-1043

Davison, A.J., Eberle, R., Ehlers, B., Hayward, G.S., McGeoch, D.J., Minson, A.C., Pellett, P.E., Roizman, B., Studdert, M.J. & Thiry, E. (2009). The order Herpesvirales. *Arch Virol*, Vol. 154, No. 1, pp. 171-177

Davison, A.J., Eberle, R., Hayward, G.S., McGeoch, D.J., Minson, A.C., Pellet, P.E., Roizman, B., Studdert, M.J. & Thiry, E. (2005a). *Herpesviridae*, In: *Virus Taxonomy: VIIIth Report of the International Committee on Taxonomy of Viruses*, C.M. Fauquet, M.A. Mayo, J. Maniloff, U. Desselberger & L.A. Ball, pp. 193-212, Elsevier Academic Press, Amsterdam

Davison, A.J., Sauerbier, W., Dolan, A., Addison, C. & McKinnell, R.G. (1999). Genomic studies of the Lucke tumor herpesvirus (RaHV-1). *J Cancer Res Clin Oncol*, Vol. 125, No. 3-4, pp. 232-238

Davison, A.J., Trus, B.L., Cheng, N., Steven, A.C., Watson, M.S., Cunningham, C., Le Deuff, R.M. & Renault, T. (2005b). A novel class of herpesvirus with bivalve hosts. *J Gen Virol*, Vol. 86, No. 1, pp. 41-53

Dishon, A., Davidovich, M., Ilouze, M. & Kotler, M. (2007). Persistence of cyprinid herpesvirus 3 in infected cultured carp cells. *J Virol*, Vol. 81, No. 9, pp. 4828-4836

Dixon, P. (1997). Immunization with viral antigens: viral diseases of carp and catfish. *Dev Biol Stand*, Vol. 90, pp. 221-232

Dixon, R.A. & Farber, F.E. (1980). Channel catfish virus: physicochemical properties of the viral genome and identification of viral polypeptides. *Virology*, Vol. 103, No. 2, pp. 267-278

Doszpoly, A., Benkő, M., Bovo, G., LaPatra, S.E. & Harrach, B. (2011a). Comparative analysis of a conserved gene block from the genome of the members of the genus Ictalurivirus. *Intervirology*, pp. 1-8

Doszpoly, A., Benkő, M., Csaba, G., Dán, Á., Lang, M. & Harrach, B. (2011b). Introduction of the family Alloherpesviridae: The first molecular detection of herpesviruses of cyprinid fish in Hungary. *Magyar Allatorvosok Lapja*, Vol. 133, No. 3, pp. 174-181

Doszpoly, A., Kovacs, E.R., Bovo, G., LaPatra, S.E., Harrach, B. & Benko, M. (2008). Molecular confirmation of a new herpesvirus from catfish (*Ameiurus melas*) by testing the performance of a novel PCR method, designed to target the DNA polymerase gene of alloherpesviruses. *Arch Virol*, Vol. 153, No. 11, pp. 2123-2127

Doszpoly, A. & Shchelkunov, I.S. (2010). Partial genome analysis of Siberian sturgeon alloherpesvirus suggests its close relation to AciHV-2. *Acta Vet Hung*, Vol. 58, No. 2, pp. 269-274

Eide, K., Miller-Morgan, T., Heidel, J., Bildfell, R. & Jin, L. (2011a). Results of total DNA measurement in koi tissue by Koi Herpes Virus real-time PCR. *J Virol Methods*, Vol. 172, No. 1-2, pp. 81-84

Eide, K.E., Miller-Morgan, T., Heidel, J.R., Kent, M.L., Bildfell, R.J., Lapatra, S., Watson, G. & Jin, L. (2011b). Investigation of koi herpesvirus latency in koi. *J Virol*, Vol. 85, No. 10, pp. 4954-4962

Farley, C.A., Banfield, W.G., Kasnic, G.J. & Foster, W.S. (1972). Oyster herpes-type virus. *Science*, Vol. 178, pp. 759-760

Fawcett, D.W. (1956). Electron microscope observations on intracellular virus-like particles associated with the cells of the Lucke renal adenocarcinoma. *J Biophys Biochem Cytol*, Vol. 2, No. 6, pp. 725-741

Fijan, N., Petrinec, Z., Sulimanovic, D. & Zwillenberg, L.O. (1971). Isolation of the viral causative agent from the acute form of infectious dropsy of carp. *Veternarski arhiv*, Vol. 41, pp. 125-138

Fuchs, W., Fichtner, D., Bergmann, S.M. & Mettenleiter, T.C. (2011). Generation and characterization of koi herpesvirus recombinants lacking viral enzymes of nucleotide metabolism. *Arch Virol*, Vol. 156, No. 6, pp. 1059-1063

Garcia, C., Thebault, A., Degremont, L., Arzul, I., Miossec, L., Robert, M., Chollet, B., Francois, C., Joly, J.P., Ferrand, S., Kerdudou, N. & Renault, T. (2011). Ostreid herpesvirus 1 detection and relationship with *Crassostrea gigas* spat mortality in France between 1998 and 2006. *Vet Res*, Vol. 42: 73

Gilad, O., Yun, S., Andree, K.B., Adkison, M.A., Zlotkin, A., Bercovier, H., Eldar, A. & Hedrick, R.P. (2002). Initial characteristics of koi herpesvirus and development of a polymerase chain reaction assay to detect the virus in koi, *Cyprinus carpio koi. Dis Aquat Org*, Vol. 48, No. 2, pp. 101-108

Goodwin, A.E., Khoo, L., LaPatra, S.E., Bonar, A., Key, D.W., Garner, M., Lee, M.V. & Hanson, L. (2006). Goldfish Hematopoietic Necrosis Herpesvirus (Cyprinid Herpesvirus 2) in the USA: Molecular confirmation of isolates from diseased fish. *J Aquat Anim Health*, Vol. 18, pp. 11-18

Goodwin, A.E., Sadler, J., Merry, G.E. & Marecaux, E.N. (2009). Herpesviral haematopoietic necrosis virus (CyHV-2) infection: case studies from commercial goldfish farms. *J Fish Dis*, Vol. 32, No. 3, pp. 271-278

Graham, D.A., Curran, W.L., Geoghegan, F., McKiernan, F. & Foyle, K.L. (2004). First observation of herpes-like virus particles in northern pike, *Esox lucius* L., associated with bluespot-like disease in Ireland. *J Fish Dis*, Vol. 27, No. 9, pp. 543-549

Granoff, A. (1999). Amphibian herpesviruses (*Herpesviridae*), In: *Encyclopedia of Virology*, A. Granoff & R. Webster, pp. 51-53, Academic Press, London

Gravell, M. (1971). Viruses and renal carcinoma of Rana pipiens. X. Comparison of herpes-type viruses associated with Lucke tumor-bearing frogs. *Virology*, Vol. 43, No. 3, pp. 730-733

Gravell, M., Granoff, A. & Darlington, R.W. (1968). Viruses and renal carcinoma of *Rana pipiens*. VII. Propagation of a herpes-type frog virus. *Virology*, Vol. 36, No. 3, pp. 467-475

Gray, W.L., Williams, R.J., Jordan, R.L. & Griffin, B.R. (1999). Detection of channel catfish virus DNA in latently infected catfish. *J Gen Virol*, Vol. 80, No. 7, pp. 1817-1822

Groff, J.M., LaPatra, S.E., Munn, R.J. & Zinkl, J.G. (1998). A viral epizootic in cultured populations of juvenile goldfish due to a putative herpesvirus etiology. *J Vet Diagn Invest*, Vol. 10, No. 4, pp. 375-378

Haenen, O.L.M., Dijkstra, S.G., Tulden, P.W., Davidse, A., van Nieuwstadt, A.P., Wagenaar, F. & Wellenberg, G.J. (2002). Herpesvirus anguillae (HVA) isolations from disease outbreaks in cultured European eel, *Anguilla anguilla* in the Netherlands since 1996. *Bull Eur Ass Fish Pathol*, Vol. 22, No. 4, pp. 247-257

Haenen, O.L.M., Lehmann, J., Engelsma, M.Y., Stürenberg, F.-J., Roozenburg, I., Kerkhoff, S. & Klein Breteler, J. (2010). The health status of European silver eels, *Anguilla anguilla*, in the Dutch River Rhine Watershed and Lake IJsselmeer. *Aquaculture*, Vol. 309, No. 1-4, pp. 15-24

Haenen, O.L.M., Way, K., Bergmann, S.M. & Ariel, E. (2004). The emergence of Koi herpesvirus and its significance to European aquaculture. *Bull Eur Ass Fish Pathol*, Vol. 24, No. 6, pp. 293-307

Hayashi, Y., Kodoma, H., Ishigaki, K., Mikami, T., Izawa, H. & Sakai, D.K. (1986). Characteristics of a new herpesviral isolate from salmonid fish. *Jpn J Vet Sci*, Vol. 48, No. 5, pp. 915-924

Hayashi, Y., Kodoma, H., Mikami, T. & Izawa, H. (1989). Serological and genetica relationships of three herpesvirus strains from salmonid fish. *Arch Virol*, Vol. 104, pp. 163-168

Hedrick, R.P., Gilad, O., Yun, S., Spangenberg, J.V., Marty, G.D., Nordhausen, R.W., Kebus, M.J., Bercovier, H. & Eldar, A. (2000). A herpesvirus associated with mass mortality of juvenile and adult koi, a strain of common carp. *J Aquat Anim Health*, Vol. 12, No. 1, pp. 44-57

Hedrick, R.P., McDowell, T., Eaton, W.D., Kimura, T. & Sano, T. (1987). Serological relationships of five herpesviruses isolated from salmonid fishes. *J Appl Ichthyol*, Vol. 3, pp. 87-92

Hedrick, R.P., McDowell, T.S., Groff, J.M., Yun, S. & Wingfield, W.H. (1991). Isolation of an epitheliotropic herpesvirus from white sturgeon *Acipenser transmontanus*. *Dis Aquat Org*, Vol. 11, pp. 49-56

Hedrick, R.P., McDowelll, T.S., Gilad, O., Adkison, M. & Bovo, G. (2003). Systemic herpes-like virus in catfish *Ictalurus melas* (Italy) differs from Ictalurid herpesvirus 1 (North America). *Dis Aquat Org*, Vol. 55, No. 2, pp. 85-92

Herman, R.L., Burke, C.N. & Perry, S. (1997). Epidermal tumors of rainbow smelt with associated virus. *J Wildl Dis*, Vol. 33, No. 4, pp. 925-929

Huang, S. & Hanson, L.A. (1998). Temporal gene regulation of the channel catfish virus (Ictalurid herpesvirus 1). *J Virol*, Vol. 72, No. 3, pp. 1910-1917

Hyatt, A.D., Hine, P.M., Whittington, R.J., Kearns, C., Wise, T.G., Crane, M.S. & Williams, L.M. (1997). Epizootic mortality in the pilchard *Sardinops sagax neopilchardus* in Australia and New Zealand in 1995. II. Identification of a herpesvirus within the gill epithelium. *Dis Aquat Org*, Vol. 28, pp. 17-29

Iida, Y., Masumura, K., Nakai, T., Sorimachi, M. & Matsuda, H. (1989). A viral disease in larvae and juveniles of the Japanese flounder *Paralichthys olivaceus*. *J Aquat Anim Health*, Vol. 1, pp. 7-12

Iida, Y., Nakai, T., Sorimachi, M. & Masumura, K. (1991). Histopathology of a herpesvirus infection in larvae of Japanese flounder *Paralythys olivaceus*. *Dis Aquat Org*, Vol. 10, pp. 59-63

Jakob, N.J., Kehm, R. & Gelderblom, H.R. (2010). A novel fish herpesvirus of *Osmerus eperlanus*. *Virus genes*, Vol. 41, No. 1, pp. 81-85

Jeffery, K.R., Bateman, K., Bayley, A., Feist, S.W., Hulland, J., Longshaw, C., Stone, D., Woolford, G. & Way, K. (2007). Isolation of a cyprinid herpesvirus 2 from goldfish, Carassius auratus (L.), in the UK. *J Fish Dis*, Vol. 30, No. 11, pp. 649-656

Jørgensen, P., Castric, J., Hill, B., Ljungberg, O. & De Kinkelin, P. (1994). The occurrence of virus infections in elvers and eels (*Anguilla anguilla*) in Europe with particular reference to VHSV and IHNV. *Aquaculture*, Vol. 123, No. 1-2, pp. 11-19

Jung, S.J. & Miyazaki, T. (1995). Herpesviral haematopoietic necrosis of goldfish, *Carassius auratus* (L.). *J Fish Dis*, Vol. 18, pp. 211-220

Kelley, G.O., Waltzek, T.B., McDowell, T.S., Yun, S.C., LaPatra, S.E. & Hedrick, R.P. (2005). Genetic Relationships among Herpes-Like Viruses Isolated from Sturgeon. *J Aquat Anim Health*, Vol. 17, No. 4, pp. 297-303

Kelly, R.K., Nielsen, O., Mitchell, S.C. & Yamamoto, T. (1983). Characterization of Herpesvirus vitreum isolated from hyperplastic epidermal tissue of walleye, *Stizostedion vitreum vitreum* (Mitchill). *J Fish Dis*, Vol. 6, pp. 249-260

Kent, M.L. & Myers, M.S. (2000). Hepatic lesions in a redstriper rockfish (*Sebastes proriger*) suggestive of a herpesvirus infection. *Dis Aquat Org*, Vol. 41, pp. 237-239

Kimura, T., Yoshimizu, M. & Tanaka, M. (1981a). Studies on a new virus (OMV) from *Oncorhynchus masou* - II. Oncogenic nature. *Fish Pathol*, Vol. 15, No. 3/4, pp. 149-153

Kimura, T., Yoshimizu, M. & Tanaka, M. (1983). Scusceptibility of different fry stages of representative salmonid species to oncorhynchus masou virus (OMV). *Fish Pathol*, Vol. 17, No. 4, pp. 251-258

Kimura, T., Yoshimizu, M., Tanaka, M. & Sannohe, H. (1981b). Studies on a new virus (OMV) from *Oncorhynchus masou* - I. Characteristics and pathogenicity. *Fish Pathol*, Vol. 15, No. 3/4, pp. 143-147

Kucuktas, H. & Brady, Y.J. (1999). Molecular biology of channel catfish virus. *Aquaculture*, Vol. 172, No. 1-2, pp. 147-161

Kumagai, A., Takahashi, K. & Fukuda, H. (1994). Epizootics caused by salmonid herpesvirus type 2 infection in maricultured coho salmon. *Fish Pathol*, Vol. 29, No. 2, pp. 127-134

Kunec, D., Hanson, L.A., van Haren, S., Nieuwenhuizen, I.F. & Burgess, S.C. (2008). An overlapping bacterial artificial chromosome system that generates vectorless progeny for channel catfish herpesvirus. *J Virol*, Vol. 82, No. 8, pp. 3872-3881

Kunec, D., Nanduri, B. & Burgess, S.C. (2009). Experimental annotation of channel catfish virus by probabilistic proteogenomic mapping. *Proteomics*, Vol. 9, No. 10, pp. 2634-2647

Kurobe, T., Kelley, G.O., Waltzek, T.B. & Hedrick, R.P. (2008). Revised Phylogenetic Relationships among Herpesviruses Isolated from Sturgeons. *J Aquat Anim Health*, Vol. 20, No. 2, pp. 96-102

Kurobe, T., Marcquenski, S. & Hedrick, R.P. (2009). PCR assay for improved diagnostics of epitheliotropic disease virus (EEDV) in lake trout *Salvelinus namaycush*. *Dis Aquat Org*, Vol. 84, No. 1, pp. 17-24

Lee, N.-S., Kobayashi, J. & Miyazaki, T. (1999). Gill filament necrosis in farmed Japanese eels, *Anguilla japonica* (Temminck & Schlegel), infected with *Herpesvirus anguillae*. *J Fish Dis*, Vol. 22, No. 6, pp. 457-463

Leibovitz, L. & Lebouitz, S.S. (1985). A viral dermatitis of the smooth dogfish, *Mustelus canis* (Mitchill). *J Fish Dis*, Vol. 8, pp. 273-279

Loret, S., Guay, G. & Lippe, R. (2008). Comprehensive characterization of extracellular herpes simplex virus type 1 virions. *J Virol*, Vol. 82, No. 17, pp. 8605-8618

Lucké, B. (1934). A neoplastic disease of the kidney of the frog, *Rana pipiens*. *Am J Cancer*, Vol. 20, pp. 352-379

Lucké, B. (1938). Carcinoma in the Leopard Frog: Its Probable Causation by a Virus. *J Exp Med*, Vol. 68, No. 4, pp. 457-468

Lucké, B. & Schlumberger, H. (1949). Induction of metastasis of frog carcinoma by increase of environmental temperature. *J Exp Med*, Vol. 89, No. 3, pp. 269-278

Lunger, P.D. (1964). The Isolation and Morphology of the Luck'e Frog Kidney Tumor Virus. *Virology*, Vol. 24, pp. 138-145

Margenau, T.L., Marcquenski, S.V., Rasmussen, P.W. & MacConnell, E. (1995). Prevalence of Blue spot disease (Esocid herpesvirus-1) on northern pike and muskellunge in Wisconsin. *J Aquat Anim Health*, Vol. 7, pp. 29-33

Masumura, K., Iida, Y., Nakai, T. & Mekuchi, T. (1989). The effects of water temperature and fish age on a herpesvirus infection of Japanese flounder larvae, *Paralichthys olivaceus*. *Fish Pathol*, Vol. 24, No. 2, pp. 111-114

McAllister, P.E. & Herman, R.L. (1989). Epizootic mortality in hatchery-reared lake trout *Salvelinus namaycush* caused by a putative virus possibly of the herpesvirus group. *Dis Aquat Org*, Vol. 6, pp. 113-119

McAllister, P.E., Lidgerding, B.C., Herman, R.L., Hoyer, L.C. & Hankins, J. (1985). Viral diseases of fish: first report of carp pox in golden ide (*Leuciscus idus*) in North America. *J Wildl Dis*, Vol. 21, No. 3, pp. 199-204

McGeoch, D.J. & Davison, A. (1999). The molecular evolutionary history of the herpesviruses, In: *Origin and Evolution of Viruses*, E. Domingo, R. Webster & J. Holland, pp. 441-465, Academic Press, London

McGeoch, D.J., Rixon, F.J. & Davison, A.J. (2006). Topics in herpesvirus genomics and evolution. *Virus Res*, Vol. 117, No. 1, pp. 90-104

McKinnell, R.G. & Carlson, D.L. (1997). Lucke renal adenocarcinoma, an anuran neoplasm: studies at the interface of pathology, virology, and differentiation competence. *J Cell Physiol*, Vol. 173, No. 2, pp. 115-118

McKinnell, R.G. & Tarin, D. (1984). Temperature-dependent metastasis of the Lucke renal carcinoma and its significance for studies on mechanisms of metastasis. *Cancer Metastasis Rev*, Vol. 3, No. 4, pp. 373-386

Mellergaard, S. & Bloch, B. (1988). Herpesvirus-like particles in angelfish *Pterophyllum altum*. *Dis Aquat Org*, Vol. 5, pp. 151-155

Michel, B., Fournier, G., Lieffrig, F., Costes, B. & Vanderplasschen, A. (2010). Cyprinid herpesvirus 3. *Emerg Infect Dis*, Vol. 16, No. 12, pp. 1835-1843

Michel, B., Leroy, B., Stalin Raj, V., Lieffrig, F., Mast, J., Wattiez, R., Vanderplasschen, A. & Costes, B. (2010). The genome of cyprinid herpesvirus 3 encodes 40 proteins incorporated in mature virions. *J Gen Virol*, Vol. 91, No. 2, pp. 452-462

Miyazaki, K., Fujiwara, K., Kobara, J., Matsumoto, N., Abe, M. & Nagano, T. (1989). Histopathology associated with two viral diseases of larval and juvenile fishes: epidermal necrosis of the Japanese flounder *Paralichthys olivaceus* and epithelial necrosis of black sea bream *Acanthopagrus schlegeli*. *J Aquat Anim Health*, Vol. 1, No. 2, pp. 85-93

Miyazaki, T. (2005). Ultrastructural features of herpesvirus-infected cells in epidermal lesions in larvae of the Japanese flounder *Paralichthys olivaceus*. *Dis Aquat Org*, Vol. 66, No. 2, pp. 159-162

Mizell, M., Toplin, I. & Isaacs, J.J. (1969). Tumor induction in developing frog kidneys by a zonal centrifuge purified fraction of the frog herpes-type virus. *Science*, Vol. 165, No. 898, pp. 1134-1137

Morrison, C.M., Leggiardro, C.T. & Martell, D.J. (1996). Visualization of viruses in tumors of rainbow smelt *Osmerus mordax*. *Dis Aquat Org*, Vol. 26, pp. 19-23

Murray, A.G., O'Callaghan, M. & Jones, B. (2003). A model of spatially eviolving herpesvirus epidemics causing mass mortality in australian pilchard *Sardinops sagax*. *Dis Aquat Org*, Vol. 54, pp. 1-14

Naegele, R.F., Granoff, A. & Darlington, R.W. (1974). The presence of the Lucke herpesvirus genome in induced tadpole tumors and its oncogenicity: Koch-Henle postulates fulfilled. *Proc Natl Acad Sci U S A*, Vol. 71, No. 3, pp. 830-834

Nusbaum, K.E., Smith, B.F., DeInnocentes, P. & Bird, R.C. (2002). Protective immunity induced by DNA vaccination of channel catfish with early and late transcripts of the channel catfish herpesvirus (IHV-1). *Vet Immunol Immunopathol*, Vol. 84, No. 3-4, pp. 151-168

O'Neill, G. (1995). Ocean anomaly triggers record fish kill. *Science*, Vol. 268, No. 5216, p. 1431

Rafferty, K.A., Jr. (1965). The cultivation of inclusion-associated viruses from Lucke tumor frogs. *Ann N Y Acad Sci*, Vol. 126, No. 1, pp. 3-21

Rijsewijk, F., Pritz-Verschuren, S., Kerkhoff, S., Botter, A., Willemsen, M., van Nieuwstadt, T. & Haenen, O. (2005). Development of a polymerase chain reaction for the detection of Anguillid herpesvirus DNA in eels based on the herpesvirus DNA polymerase gene. *J Virol Methods*, Vol. 124, No. 1-2, pp. 87-94

Ronen, A., Perelberg, A., Abramowitz, J., Hutoran, M., Tinman, S., Bejerano, I., Steinitz, M. & Kotler, M. (2003). Efficient vaccine against the virus causing a lethal disease in cultured *Cyprinus carpio*. *Vaccine*, Vol. 21, No. 32, pp. 4677-4684

Rosenkranz, D., Klupp, B.G., Teifke, J.P., Granzow, H., Fichtner, D., Mettenleiter, T.C. & Fuchs, W. (2008). Identification of envelope protein pORF81 of koi herpesvirus. *J Gen Virol*, Vol. 89, No. 4, pp. 896-900

Sano, M., Fukuda, H. & Sano, T. (1990a). Isolation and characterization of a new herpesvirus from eel, In: *Pathology in Marine Sciences*, F.O. Perkins & T.C. Cheng, pp. 15-31, Academic Press, San Diego

Sano, N., Moriwake, M. & Sano, T. (1993). *Herpesvirus cyprini*: thermal effects on pathogenicity and oncogenicity. *Fish Pathol*, Vol. 28, No. 4, pp. 171-175

Sano, T. (1976). Viral diseases of cultured fishes in Japan. *Fish Pathol*, Vol. 10, pp. 221-226

Sano, T., Fukuda, H. & Furukawa, M. (1985a). Herpesvirus cyprini: biological and oncogenic properties. *Fish Pathol*, Vol. 20, No. 4, pp. 381-388

Sano, T., Fukuda, H., Furukawa, M., Hosoya, H. & Moriya, Y. (1985b). A herpesvirus isolated from carp papilloma in Japan, In: *Fish and Shellfish Pathology*, A.E. Ellis, pp. 307-311, Academic Press, London

Sano, T., Fukuda, H., Okamoto, N. & Kaneko, F. (1983). Yamame tumor virus: lethality and oncogenicity. *Bull Jpn Soc Sci Fish*, Vol. 49, No. 8, pp. 1159-1163

Sano, T., Morita, N., shima, N. & Akimoto, M. (1990b). A preliminary report on pathogenicity and oncogenicity of cyprinid herpesvirus. *Bull Eur Ass Fish Pathol*, Vol. 10, No. 1, pp. 11-13

Sano, T., Morita, N., Shima, N. & Akimoto, M. (1991). *Herpesvirus cyprini*: lethality and oncogenicity. *J Fish Dis*, Vol. 14, pp. 533-543

Savin, K.W., Cocks, B.G., Wong, F., Sawbridge, T., Cogan, N., Savage, D. & Warner, S. (2010). A neurotropic herpesvirus infecting the gastropod, abalone, shares ancestry with oyster herpesvirus and a herpesvirus associated with the amphioxus genome. *Virol J*, Vol. 7: 308

Schubert, G.H. (1966). The infective agent in carp pox. *Bull Off Int Epiz*, Vol. 65, No. 7-8, pp. 1011-1022

Segarra, A., Pepin, J.F., Arzul, I., Morga, B., Faury, N. & Renault, T. (2010). Detection and description of a particular Ostreid herpesvirus 1 genotype associated with massive mortality outbreaks of Pacific oysters, *Crassostrea gigas*, in France in 2008. *Virus Res*, Vol. 153, No. 1, pp. 92-99

Shchelkunov, I.S., Karaseva, T.A. & Kadoshnikov, Y.U.P. (1992). Atlantic salmon papillomatosis: visualization of herpesvirus-like paticles in skin growths of affected fish. *Bull Eur Ass Fish Pathol*, Vol. 12, No. 1, pp. 28-31

Shchelkunov, I.S., Shchelkunova, T.I., Shchelkunov, A.I., Kolbassova, Y.P., Didenko, L.V. & Bykovsky, A.P. (2009). First detection of a viral agent causing disease in farmed sturgeon in Russia. *Dis Aquat Org*, Vol. 86, No. 3, pp. 193-203

Shlapobersky, M., Sinyakov, M.S., Katzenellenbogen, M., Sarid, R., Don, J. & Avtalion, R.R. (2010). Viral encephalitis of tilapia larvae: Primary characterization of a novel herpes-like virus. *Virology*, Vol. 399, No. 2, pp. 239-247

Silverstein, P.S., Bird, R.C., van Santen, V.L. & Nusbaum, K.E. (1995). Immediate-early transcription from the channel catfish virus genome: characterization of two immediate-early transcripts. *J Virol*, Vol. 69, No. 5, pp. 3161-3166

Silverstein, P.S., van Santen, V.L., Nusbaum, K.E. & Bird, R.C. (1998). Expression kinetics and mapping of the thymidine kinase transcript and an immediate-early transcript from channel catfish virus. *J Virol*, Vol. 72, No. 5, pp. 3900-3906

St-Hilaire, S., Beevers, N., Way, K., Le Deuff, R.M., Martin, P. & Joiner, C. (2005). Reactivation of koi herpesvirus infections in common carp *Cyprinus carpio*. *Dis Aquat Org*, Vol. 67, No. 1-2, pp. 15-23

Stephens, F.J., Raidal, S.R. & Jones, B. (2004). Haematopoietic necrosis in a goldfish (*Carassius auratus*) associated with an agent morphologically similar to herpesvirus. *Aust Vet J*, Vol. 82, No. 3, pp. 167-169

Stingley, R.L. & Gray, W.L. (2000). Transcriptional regulation of the channel catfish virus genome direct repeat region. *J Gen Virol*, Vol. 81, No. 8, pp. 2005-2010

Stingley, R.L., Griffin, B.R. & Gray, W.L. (2003). Channel catfish virus gene expression in experimentally infected channel catfish, *Ictalurus punctatus* (Rafinesque). *J Fish Dis*, Vol. 26, No. 8, pp. 487-493

Tan, J., Lancaster, M., Hyatt, A., van Driel, R., Wong, F. & Warner, S. (2008). Purification of a herpes-like virus from abalone (*Haliotis* spp.) with ganglioneuritis and detection by transmission electron microscopy. *J Virol Methods*, Vol. 149, No. 2, pp. 338-341

Tanaka, M., Yoshimizu, M. & Kimura, T. (1984). *Oncorhynchus masou* virus: Pathological changes in masu salmon (*Onchorhynchus masou*), chum salmon (*O. keta*), coho salmon (*O. kisutch*) fry infected with OMV by immersion method. *Bull Jpn Soc Sci Fish*, Vol. 50, No. 3, pp. 431-437

Tham, K.M. & Moon, C.D. (1996). Polymerase chain reaction amplification of the thymidine kinase and protein kinase-related genes of channel catfish virus and a putative pilchard herpesvirus. *J Virol Methods*, Vol. 61, No. 1-2, pp. 65-72

Ueno, Y., Kitao, T., Chen, S.-N., Aoki, T. & Kou, G.-H. (1992). Characterization of A Herpes-like Virus Isolated from Cultured Japanese Eels in Taiwan. *Fish Pathol*, Vol. 27, No. 1, pp. 7-17

Ueno, Y., Shi, J.-W., Yoshida, T., Kitao, T., Sakai, M., Chen, S.-N. & Kou, G.H. (1996). Biological and serological comparisons of eel herpesvirus in Formosa (EHVF) and Herpesvirus anguillae (HVA). *J Appl Ichthyol*, Vol. 12, No. 1, pp. 49-51

van Beurden, S.J., Bossers, A., Voorbergen-Laarman, M.H., Haenen, O.L.M., Peters, S., Abma-Henkens, M.H., Peeters, B.P., Rottier, P.J. & Engelsma, M.Y. (2010). Complete genome sequence and taxonomic position of anguillid herpesvirus 1. *J Gen Virol*, Vol. 91, No. 4, pp. 880-887

van Beurden, S.J., Leroy, B., Wattiez, R., Haenen, O.L.M., Boeren, S., Vervoort, J.J.M., Peeters, B.P.H., Rottier, P.J.M., Engelsma, M.Y. & Vanderplasschen, A.F. (2011). Identification and localization of the structural proteins of anguillid herpesvirus 1. *Vet Res*, Vol. 42: 105

van Ginneken, V., Haenen, O., Coldenhoff, K., Willemze, R., Antonissen, E., van Tulden, P., Dijkstra, S., Wagenaar, F. & van den Thillart, G. (2004). Presence of eel viruses in eel species from various geographic regions. *Bull Eur Ass Fish Pathol*, Vol. 24, No. 5, pp. 268-272

van Nieuwstadt, A.P., Dijkstra, S.G. & Haenen, O.L. (2001). Persistence of herpesvirus of eel Herpesvirus anguillae in farmed European eel *Anguilla anguilla*. *Dis Aquat Org*, Vol. 45, No. 2, pp. 103-107

Vanderheijden, N., Hanson, L.A., Thiry, E. & Martial, J.A. (1999). Channel catfish virus gene 50 encodes a secreted, mucin-like glycoprotein. *Virology*, Vol. 257, No. 1, pp. 220-227

Walster, C.I. (1999). Clinical observations of severe mortalities in Koi carp, *Cyprinus carpio*, with gill disease. *Fish Vet Journal*, Vol. 3, pp. 54-58

Waltzek, T.B., Kelley, G.O., Alfaro, M.E., Kurobe, T., Davison, A.J. & Hedrick, R.P. (2009). Phylogenetic relationships in the family *Alloherpesviridae*. *Dis Aquat Org*, Vol. 84, pp. 179-194

Waltzek, T.B., Kelley, G.O., Stone, D.M., Way, K., Hanson, L., Fukuda, H., Hirono, I., Aoki, T., Davison, A.J. & Hedrick, R.P. (2005). Koi herpesvirus represents a third cyprinid herpesvirus (CyHV-3) in the family Herpesviridae. *J Gen Virol*, Vol. 86, No. 6, pp. 1659-1667

Watson, L.R., Yun, S.C., Groff, J.M. & Hedrick, R.P. (1995). Characteristics and pathogenicity of a novel herpesvirus isolated from adult and subadult white sturgeon *Acipenser transmontanus*. *Dis Aquat Org*, Vol. 22, pp. 199-210

Whittington, R.J., Crockford, M., Jordan, D. & Jones, B. (2008). Herpesvirus that caused epizootic mortality in 1995 and 1998 in pilchard, *Sardinops sagax neopilchardus* (Steindachner), in Australia is now endemic. *J Fish Dis*, Vol. 31, No. 2, pp. 97-105

Whittington, R.J., Jones, J.B., Hine, P.M. & Hyatt, A.D. (1997). Epizootic mortality in the pilchard *Sardinops sagax neopilchardus* in Australia and New Zealand in 1995. I. Pathology and epizootiology. *Dis Aquat Org*, Vol. 28, pp. 1-16

Wolf, K. (1976). Fish viral diseases in North America, 1971-75, and recent research of the Eastern fish disease laboratory, U.S.A. *Fish Pathol*, Vol. 10, No. 2, pp. 135-154

Wolf, K. (1988). Channel catfish virus disease, In: *Fish viruses and fish viral diseases*, K. Wolf, pp. 21-42, Cornell University Press, Ithaca, New York

Wolf, K. & Darlington, R.W. (1971). Channel catfish virus: a new herpesvirus of ictalurid fish. *J Virol*, Vol. 8, No. 4, pp. 525-533

Wolf, K., Darlington, R.W., Taylor, W.G., Quimby, M.C. & Nagabayashi, T. (1978). Herpesvirus salmonis: Characterization of a New Pathogen of Rainbow Trout. *J Virol*, Vol. 27, No. 3, pp. 659-666

Wolf, K. & Smith, C.E. (1981). *Herpesvirus salmonis*: pathological changes in parenterally-infected rainbow trout, *Salmo gairdneri* Richardson, fry. *J Fish Dis*, Vol. 4, pp. 445-457

Yamamoto, T., Kelly, R.K. & Nielsen, O. (1984). Epidermal hyperplasias of northern pike (*Esox lucius*) associated with herpesvirus and C-type particles. *Arch Virol*, Vol. 79, No. 3-4, pp. 255-272

Yoshimizu, M., Fukuda, H., Sano, T. & Kimura, T. (1995). Salmonid herpesvirus 2. Epizootiology and serological relationship. *Vet Res*, Vol. 26, No. 5-6, pp. 486-492

Yoshimizu, M., Tanaka, M. & Kimura, H. (1987). *Oncorhynchus masou* virus (OMV): Incidence of tumor development among experimentally infected representative salmonid species. *Fish Pathol*, Vol. 22, No. 1, pp. 7-10

Zhang, H.G. & Hanson, L.A. (1995). Deletion of thymidine kinase gene attenuates channel catfish herpesvirus while maintaining infectivity. *Virology*, Vol. 209, No. 2, pp. 658-663

Part 4

Current Treatments and Future Treatment Targets

11

Nucleoside and Nucleotide Analogues for the Treatment of Herpesvirus Infections: Current Stage and New Prospects in the Field of Acyclic Nucleoside Phosphonates

Marcela Krečmerová
Institute of Organic Chemistry and Biochemistry Academy of Sciences of the Czech Republic,
Czech Republic

1. Introduction

Viral infections have accompanied humankind from time immemorial. Herpesvirus infections, especially those caused by HSV-1 and HSV-2, are among the most common viral infections at all. The control and treatment of the virus has changed through history, starting with cauterization with hot iron, recommended in ancient Rome, through the most diverse herbal treatments and naturopathic remedies including miracle diets. Fundamental change in the approach to the whole issue occurred in the second half of the twentieth century with discoveries in the field of nucleic acid chemistry. Explanation of nucleic acid structure initiated not only enormous interest and the subsequent boom of molecular biology and genetics but also the formation of a new field of organic chemistry – chemistry of nucleic acid components: nucleosides, nucleotides and oligonucleotides.

2. Chemically modified nucleosides: First generation of antimetabolites of nucleic acids

It was shown that chemically modified nucleosides or nucleobases can work as antimetabolites in the process of nucleic acid metabolism. The word "antimetabolite" means, generally, a chemically modified molecule of a natural metabolite able to influence some enzyme reactions. Antimetabolites can influence processes in cells (neoplasia) as well as processes in cell parasites, e.g. viruses, parasites, and fungi. The first generation of antimetabolites is distinguished by a maximum structural resemblance to natural metabolites. Many nucleoside or nucleobase analogues from this group were found to be effective cytostatics: cytosine arabinoside (Cytarabine, Ara-C), an antileukemic agent used for the treatment of acute myeloid leukemia and non-Hodgkin's lymphoma, 6-mercaptopurine (Purinethol®, 6-MP) used for the acute lymphoblastic leukemia, 5-fluorouracil (Efudex® , 5-FU), a thymidylate synthase inhibitor used for the treatment of colon, rectal, stomach, skin, breast and pancreatic cancer, and finally, antileukemic agents 5-azacytidine (Vidaza®) and 2´-deoxy-5-azacytidine (decitabine, Dacogene®), so far the most successful agents approved for therapy of myelodysplastic syndrom. Discoveries of these great molecules came in the sixtieth decade of the last century, a period of the beginning of great development of nucleoside chemistry. This chemistry was substantially supported by the pharmaceutical industry with the intent to finally find an effective medicine against the terror of mankind known as cancer. In these times, viral infections were not in the forefront.

3. Acyclic analogues of nucleosides: The second generation of antimetabolites

The situation had changed by the end of the 1960s and at the beginning of the 1970s. The turning point was a large "epidemy" of genital herpes (HSV-2) in the USA, especially widespread due to the promiscuous lifestyle of the time. This sexually transmitted disease became a common problem for the whole society, and a fast solution got priority. The great success came with the synthesis and clinical development of acyclovir (Zovirax) by Burroughs-Wellcome. So far this drug is one of the most frequently used drugs against HSV-1 and HSV-2 infections. Among others, development of acyclovir resulted in the first Nobel Prize targeted to the pharmaceutical industry: in 1988 the Nobel Prize winners for medicine were Gertrude B. Elion and Georg Hitchings from the above mentioned company.
Acyclovir, 9-(2-hydroxyethoxymethyl)guanine, similar to the many other antiherpetic agents (penciclovir, ganciclovir and their prodrug forms), belongs to the group of acyclic nucleoside analogues, compounds having the sugar furanose ring substituted with a polyhydroxylic carbon chain (Fig. 1). These compounds represent the so-called second generation of antimetabolites where the structural resemblance to a natural metabolite is only present in some basic aspects and the necessary steric arrangement can be formed by its subsequent contact with a target metabolic enzyme.

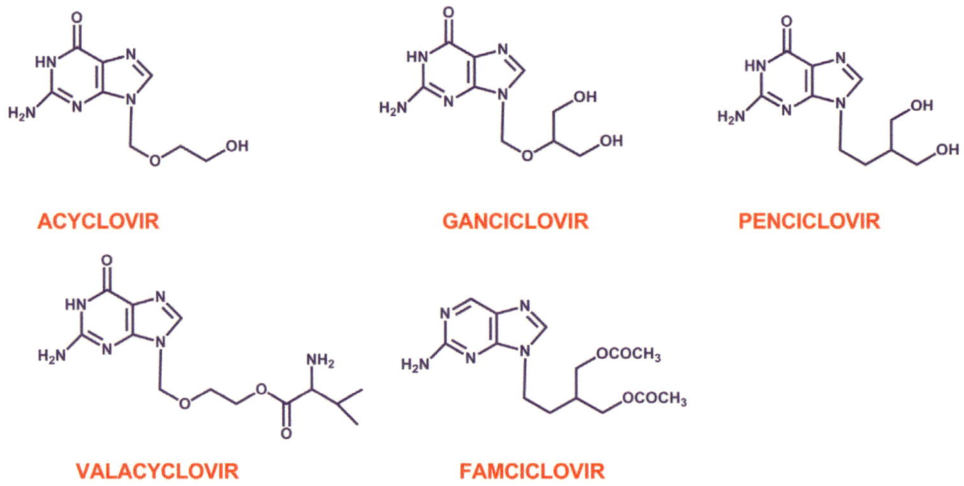

Fig. 1. Structures of the most commonly-used antiherpetic drugs from the family of acyclic nucleoside analogues

Fundamental developments in this field were also made in Prague at the Institute of Organic Chemistry and Biochemistry in the laboratory of Antonin Holy. His synthetic effort and close collaboration with the Belgian virologist Erik De Clercq resulted in many new acyclic nucleoside analogues whose activity against herpes viruses was confirmed. The most potent agents were found to be N^9-alkyl derivatives of adenine with hydroxyl group(s) on the alkyl chain (*RS*)-3-(adenin-9-yl)-2-hydroxypropanoic acid (AHPA, especially in the form of alkyl esters), D-eritadenine and the broad-spectrum antiviral agent (*S*)-(2,3-dihydroxypropyl)adenine (DHPA) (De Clercq et al. 1978, De Clercq & Holý 1985, Holý et al. 1982). Antiviral potency of these adenosine analogues concerns their inhibition of SAM-dependent methylation reactions via inhibition of S-adenosylhomocysteine (SAH) hydrolase. SAH is the product of S-adenosylmethionine (SAM) mediated transmethylation reactions and it is itself a feedback inhibitor of these reactions. If SAH hydrolase is inhibited, SAH accumulates and thereby all biological processes that require intensive methylations are suppressed. One such situation is the maturation of viral mRNA, i.e., 5'-cap formation and subsequent blocking virus replication. The most effective inhibitor of SAH hydrolase, DHPA became an approved drug for the topical treatment of herpes labialis (HSV-1) in the former Czechoslovakia, marketed under the name Duvira® gel (Fig. 2).

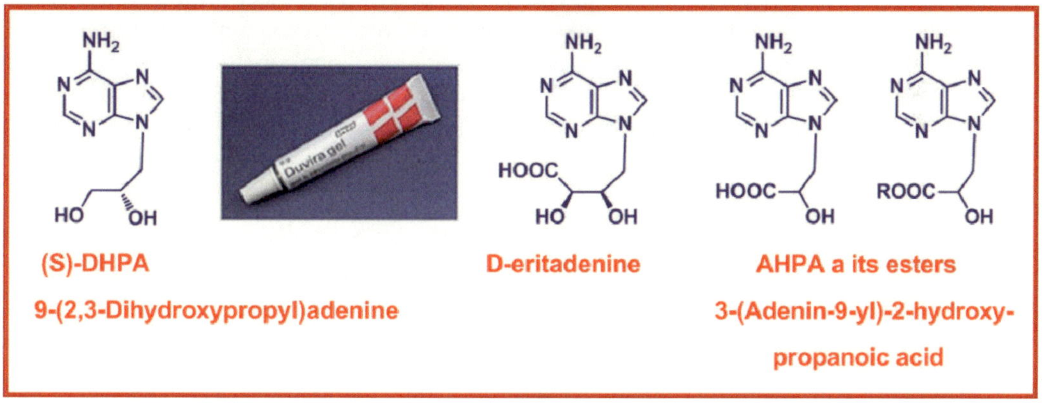

Fig. 2. Aliphatic analogues of adenosine as inhibitors of SAH hydrolase: DHPA ("Duvira gel"), D-eritadenine and AHPA esters

4. Acyclic nucleoside phosphonates

The necessary condition for any antimetabolite to be of use in enzyme reactions is its phosphorylation. Unfortunately, the direct medical application of phosphates of the antimetabolites has no advantage due to their instability. To overcome this problem, in the mid-1980s, our Prague team lead by Antonin Holy came up with the revolutionary idea of preparation of phosphonomethyl derivatives: compounds stabilized by the introduction of a methylene bridge between a phosphonic acid residue and the rest of the molecule. During the short time, acyclic nucleoside phosphonates (ANPs) were revealed as compounds with an extraordinary broad spectrum of biological activities: antiviral, cytostatic, antiparasitic or immunomodulatory. Some of them are commercially available pharmaceuticals effective against serious viral infections (cidofovir, adefovir and tenofovir) (Holý, 2003; De Clercq & Holý, 2005). Several comprehensive reviews on ANPs as antiviral agents have been published recently (Holý & De Clercq, 2010; De Clercq, 2011).

The mentioned compounds represent three different types of ANPs: HPMP derivatives, i.e. (*S*)-[3-hydroxy-2-(phosphonomethoxy)propyl] derivatives (e.g. HPMPC, cidofovir), PME derivatives, i.e. 2-(phosphonomethoxy)ethyl derivatives (e.g. PMEA, adefovir) and PMP derivatives, i.e. (*R*)-2-(phosphonomethoxy)propyl derivatives (e.g. PMPA, tenofovir).

4.1 (*S*)-[3-Hydroxy-2-(phosphonomethoxy)propyl] derivatives (HPMP derivatives) – Synthesis and activity of HPMPA and its aza/deaza analogues

HPMP derivatives are active against DNA viruses; the activity is bound always to *S* enantiomers. The first described ANP was 9-(*S*)-[3-hydroxy-2-(phosphonomethoxy)propyl]adenine (HPMPA), a compound derived from above mentioned DHPA by the introduction of a phosphonomethyl group (De Clercq et al., 1986; Holý & Rosenberg, 1987).

Synthesis of (*S*)-HPMP derivatives mostly utilizes basically catalyzed nucleophilic opening of the oxirane ring in (2*S*)-2-[(trityloxy]methyl]oxirane or (*R*)-glycidol butyrate with an appropriate nucleobase, e.g. *N*[4]-benzoylcytosine, *N*[6]-benzoyladenine or 2,6-bis(benzoylamino)purine (Webb et al., 1988; Brodfuehrer et al., 1994). This reaction proceeds regioselectively to *N*[9] position of the purine or *N*[1] position of the pyrimidine base. The intermediary formed 2,3-dihydroxypropyl derivatives are subsequently etherified with dialkyl (diethyl or diisopropyl) ester of tosyloxymethanephosphonate in the presence of sodium hydride. After removal of benzoyl groups and trityl, phosphonic ester groups are deprotected by the treatment with bromotrimethylsilane followed by hydrolysis (Holý, 1993)(Fig. 3).

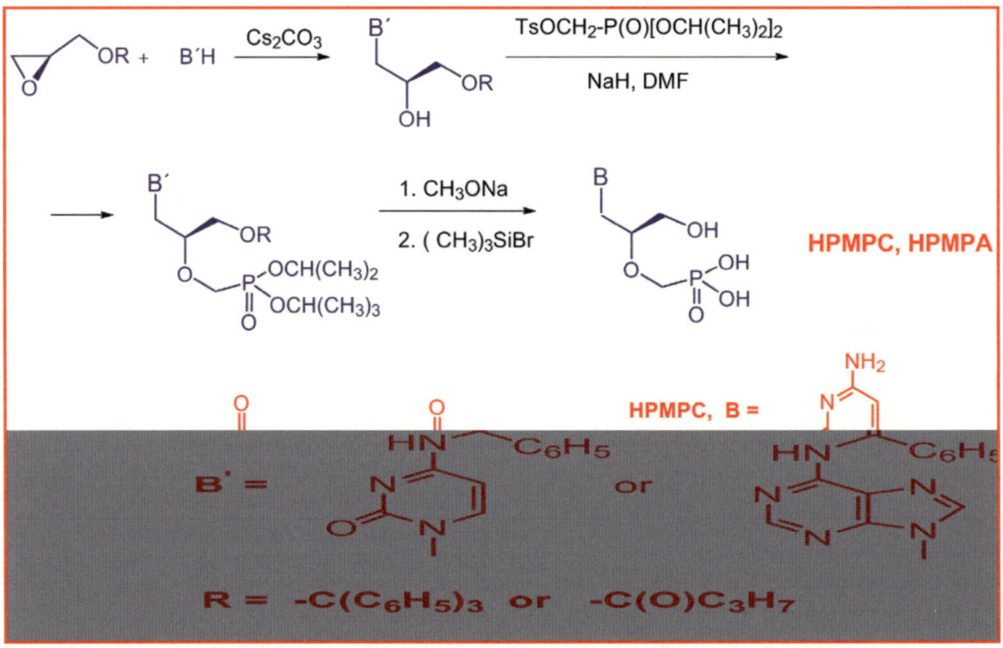

Fig. 3. Synthetic scheme for the preparation of (*S*)-[3-hydroxy-2-(phosphonomethoxy)propyl] derivatives of adenine and cytosine (HPMPC and HPMPA) from appropriate oxiranes

Preparation of diisopropyl tosyloxymethanephosphonate consists of the treatment of diisopropyl phosphite with paraformaldehyde and triethyl amine followed by tosylation

(Holý, 1993). Another possibility for the introduction of a phosphonomethyl ether group based on use of diisopropyl bromomethylphosphonate (Göbel et al., 1992) is also recommended (Holý, 2005; Oh & Hong, 2008). Most recently, a novel, very efficient and environmentally friendly synthesis of diisopropyl bromomethylphosphonate (and other dialkylhaloalkylphosphonates in general), has been developed in our Institute using a microwave-assisted Michaelis–Arbuzov reaction of dihaloalkanes. Diisopropyl bromomethylphosphonate thus can be prepared by reaction of dibromomethane with triisopropyl phosphite (Jansa et al., 2011). Syntheses of both agents are depicted in Fig. 4.

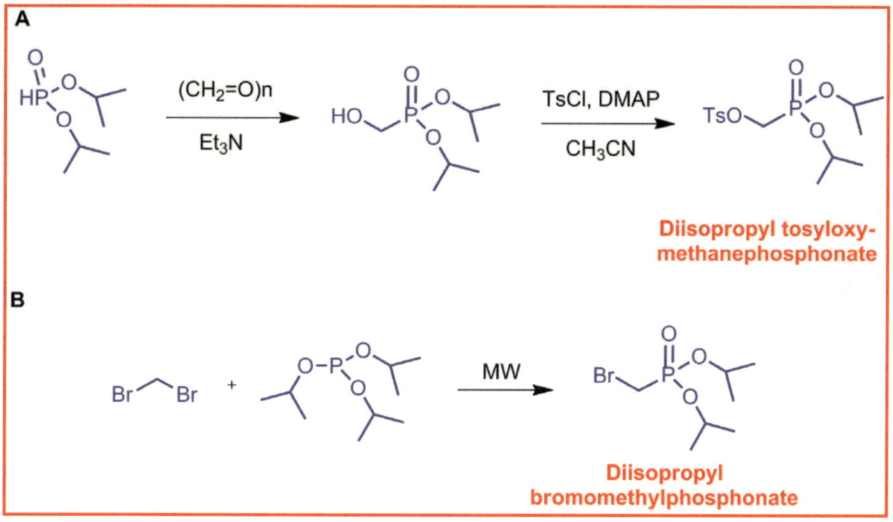

Fig. 4. Syntheses of reagents for an introduction of a phosphonomethyl residue to the molecule of acyclic nucleoside analogues: synthesis of the "Holy´s tosylate", diisopropyl tosyloxymethanephosphonate and the microwave assisted approach to diisopropyl bromomethylphosphonate by Jansa

(S)-HPMPA is a compound with a broad spectrum of anti DNA-virus activities, so far not clinically developed. It efficiently inhibits herpesviruses (Andrei et al., 1992) including clinical isolates of varicella zoster virus (Andrei et al., 1995), HHV-6 (Reymen et al., 1995) and HHV-8 (Neyts & De Clercq, 1997). HHV-6 is one of the recently discovered members of the betaherpesviridae family. It is involved in pathogenesis of several diseases including the childhood disease exanthema subitum (roseola) (Yamanishi et al. 1988) and lymphoproliferative disorders, and it probably takes part in the progression of chronic fatigue syndrome (Komaroff, 2006). HHV-6 has also been proposed to be a cofactor in the progression of AIDS; high levels of HHV-6 have been found in many AIDS patients. The comparative study of effectiveness of diverse kinds of ANP towards HHV-6 revealed, besides HPMPA, also several other active (S)-HPMP derivatives: (S)-HPMPC, (S)-cHPMPC, (S)-3-deaza-HPMPA, (S)-3-deaza-cHPMPA, (S)-HPMPG, (S)-cHPMPG and (R)-HPMPG, their EC_{50} values ranging from 1 to 11 /μM and their selectivity index ranging from 6 to 30 (Reymen et al., 1995).

A special attention is now paid to the investigation of HPMPA prodrugs to improve the pharmacokinetic profile of this ANP, especially the development of alkoxyalkyl esters (Beadle et al., 2006). It is based on etherification of the appropriate hydroxy derivate with

alkoxyalkyl tosyloxymethanephosphonate, a phosphonomethyl residue containing an agent having the lipophilic group already preattached. This compound can be prepared in three steps from diethyl tosyloxymethanephosphonate: deprotection of ethyl ester groups with bromotrimethylsilane, transformation to chloridate by the action of oxalyl chloride, and reaction with alkoxyalkanols under basic conditions. The starting material for syntheses of HPMPA esters is (*S*)-9-(3-trityloxy-2-hydroxypropyl)-N^6-trityladenine, an intermediate in preparation of HPMPA according to Webb's method (Webb, 1989).
The whole process is outlined in Figure 5.

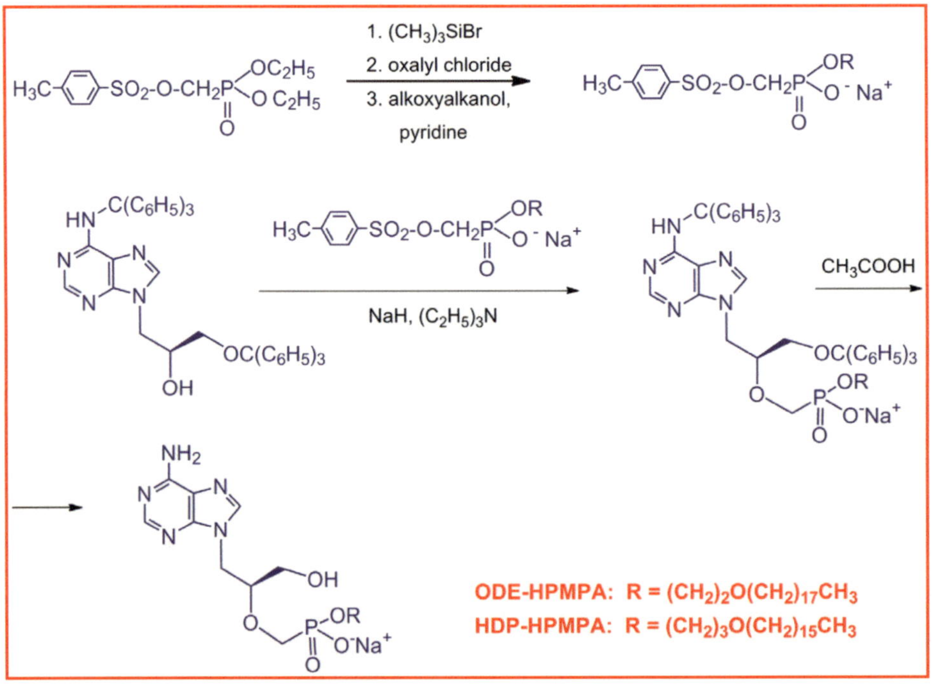

Fig. 5. Synthesis of alkoxyalkyl ester prodrugs of HPMPA.

Excellent anti-DNA virus effects were also found at other HPMP derivatives, e.g. 2,6-diaminopurine counterpart of HPMPA, (*S*)-HPMPDAP. Recently, a detailed investigation of this compound and its ester prodrugs has been performed (Krečmerová et al., 2010a). This research, originally targeted to antipoxvirus agents, also selected, among others, several candidates with excellent antiherpetic effects. Remarkable broad-spectrum antiherpetic effects were found at some base modified ANPs (aza/deaza analogs). Anti-DNA-viral activity was found especially at (S)-8-aza-HPMPA and (*S*)-3-deaza-HPMPA.
Syntheses of deazapurines, i.e. purines lacking one nitrogen atom in position 1, 3 or 7 and their nucleosides and ANPs, were developed by Holý and Dvořáková (Dvořáková et al., 1993; Dvořáková & Holý, 1993). Activity of (*S*)-3-deazaHPMPA against herpesviruses is comparable to that of the parent compound (*S*)-HPMPA, especially in case of VZV and CMV (Dvořáková et al., 1990). (*S*)-3-deaza-HPMPA, and its cyclic form, (*S*)-3-deaza-cHPMPA are also highly active against HHV-6 infections (Naesens and De Clercq, 2006). Evaluation of a series of diverse ANPs for activity against HHV-6 in HSB-2 cells showed 3-

deaza-HPMPA as a compound with the highest selectivity index (Reymen et al., 1995). In spite of all the progress in this topic, there is so far no approved drug for the treatment of HHV-6 infections (De Bolle et al., 2005). Moreover there is also another difficulty: no animal model for HHV-6 testing. These facts substantiate further intensive exploration of ANPs, especially 3-deaza-HPMPA and HPMPA, as potential drug candidates for the treatment of HHV-6 infections.

The synthesis of acyclic nucleotide analogues derived from 8-azapurine was first reported in 1996 (Holý et al., 1996). In the HPMP series, only (S)-HPMP-8-azaadenine exhibits remarkable inhibitory potency to all DNA viruses tested. The best data were found for HSV-1, TK⁻ HSV, HSV-2, VZV, TK⁻ VZV and vaccinia virus. In particular, exquisitely inhibitory effects were found for VZV with MIC 0.2-2 µg/mL. In general, the antiviral potency of HPMP-8-azaA is mostly comparable to (*S*)-HPMPA. Its 2,6-diaminopurine counterpart, (*S*)-HPMP-8-aza-DAP is approximately two orders of magnitude less potent of an inhibitor of these viruses than HPMP-8-azaA. Other structural types of 8-azapurine ANPs (PMP and (*S*)-FPMP derivatives) are not markedly inhibitory to any of the DNA viruses tested. In a series of PME derivatives, only PME-8-azaguanine was inhibitory to HSV-1, the thymidine kinase (TK⁻) deficient HSV-1 strains, HSV-2, CMV, both TK⁺ and TK⁻ VZV strains and vaccinia virus (Holý et al., 1996). Structures of the most important anti-DNA viral HPMP derivatives are depicted in Fig. 6.

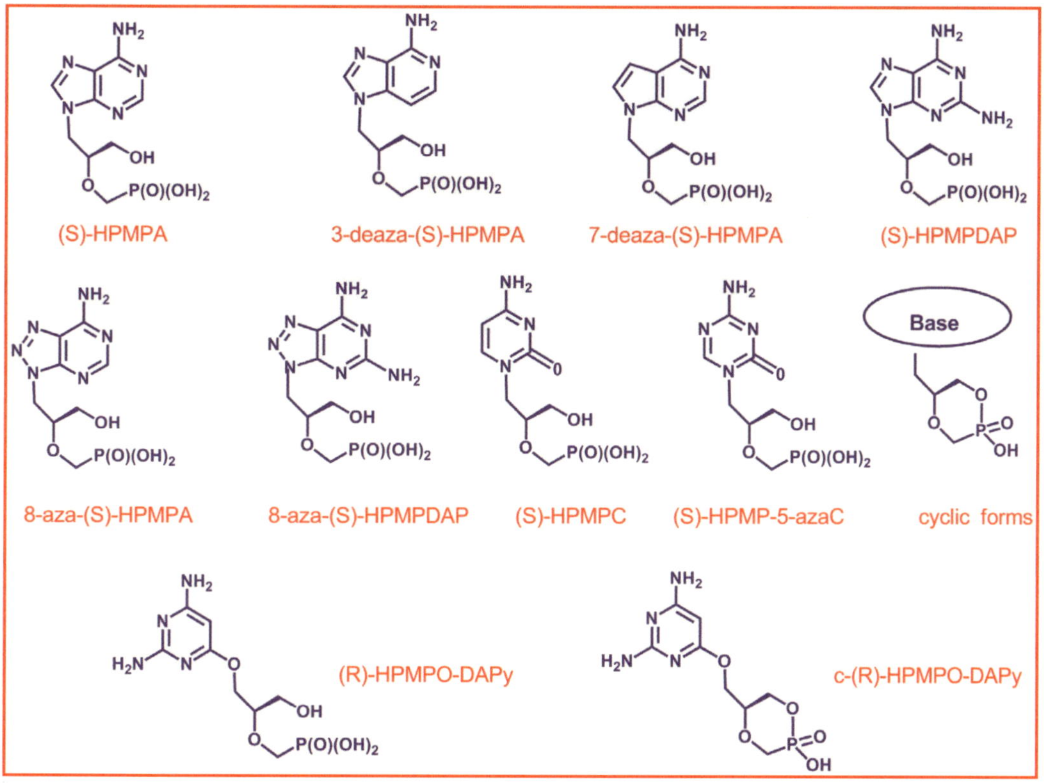

Fig. 6. HPMP derivatives: acyclic nucleoside phosphonates with a broad spectrum of activities against herpes- and other DNA virus infections

4.2 Cidofovir (HPMPC)

Cidofovir, 1-(*S*)-[3-hydroxy-2-(phosphonomethoxy)propyl]cytosine, is a broad spectrum anti DNA virus agent whose spectrum of activities covers all types of human herpesviruses [HSV-1, HSV-2, varicella-zoster virus (VZV), Epstein–Barr virus, CMV, HHV-6, HHV-7 and HHV-8 – and also thymidine kinase-deficient (TK–) HSV and VZV, and protein kinase-deficient (PK–) CMV variants], and polyoma-, papilloma-, adeno- and poxviruses. The large scale of cidofovir activities has already been a topic of many reviews, e.g. (Hitchcock et al., 1996; Naesens & De Clercq, 1997; De Clercq, 1998; Naesens et al., 1997).

Cidofovir was the first acyclic nucleoside phosphonate utilized in clinical practice: in 1996 this drug was approved by the FDA for the treatment of cytomegalovirus retinitis in AIDS patients. The drug is marketed by Gilead Sciences, Inc. under the commercial name Vistide™ and it is applied to patients in the form of intravenous injections (Fig. 7). CMV retinitis is a systemic infection commonly seen in patients suffering from AIDS. It is most easily characterized by the cloudiness which can appear in the patient's retina. If untreated, the virus will attack retina cells and develop into lesions. These lesions can eventually lead to vision impairment or permanent blindness. Cidofovir suppresses CMV replication by the selective inhibition of viral DNA polymerase and therefore prevention of viral replication and transcription (Wachsman et al., 1996; Lalezari et al., 1997). A serious side-effect of cidofovir (and all other ANPs) is its dose-dependent nephrotoxicity. To surmount this problem, cidofovir must be administered in conjunction with probenecid (Bagnis et al., 1999; Lacy et al., 1998).

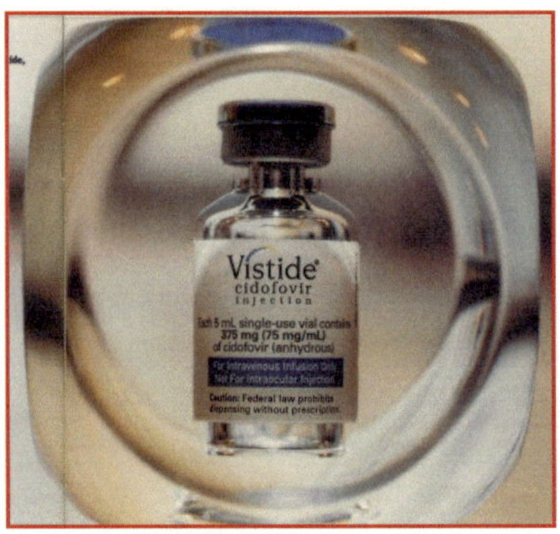

Fig. 7. Vistide™ - cidofovir injections. The first approved acyclic nucleoside phosphonate in clinical practice

At the present time, cidofovir is also important (off label) particularly for the treatment of severe cases of (malignizing) papillomatoses (anogenital, laryngeal)(Calista, 2000; Bielamovicz et al., 2002), progressive multifocal leukoencephalopathy caused by JC virus (Gasnault et al., 2001), adenovirus infections (Legrand et al., 2001) and some rather obscure severe infections caused by poxviruses (vaccinia, orf, molluscum contagiosum) (Bray &Wright, 2003). The attractiveness of cidofovir is dramatically enhanced by its supreme activity against smallpox virus and related monkey pox virus; both of these highly infectious viruses can be easily cultivated and purposely used in a bioterrorist attack. For this purpose, the cidofovir prodrug, hexadecyloxypropyl ester CMX001, is currently clinically investigated (Chimerix, Inc., California). Moreover, CMX001 is also being developed to treat cytomegalovirus (CMV) and BK virus - potentially deadly diseases for immunocompromised patients (www.chimerix-inc.com).

4.3 5-Azacytosine analogue of cidofovir (HPMP-5-azaC): Higher potency with a lower toxicity

Great success in our search for antiviral compounds came with the discovery of ANPs bearing a triazine ring, especially 5-azacytosine as a base component (Krečmerová et al., 2007a). The 5-azacytosine analogue of cidofovir, i.e. 1-(*S*)-[3-hydroxy-2-(phosphonomethoxy)propyl]-5-azacytosine (HPMP-5-azaC), shows antiviral activities similar - or in some cases higher - compared to cidofovir, better selectivity, and lower toxicity.

Synthesis of (*S*)-HPMP-5-azaC can be performed in two different manners. The first approach is based on nucleophilic opening of an oxirane ring in (2*S*)-2-[(trityloxy]methyl]oxirane with 5-azacytosine under basic conditions, e.g. in a presence of sodium hydroxide. The reaction gives regiospecifically the only N-1 substituted product, 1-[(2*S*)-2-hydroxy-3-(triphenylmethoxy)propyl]-5-azacytosine), in excellent yield. Its further treatment with diisopropyl tosyloxymethylphosphonate in the presence of excess sodium hydride in *N,N*-dimethylformamide gave fully protected phosphonate ester, which was subsequently treated with bromotrimethylsilane followed by hydrolysis. This process leads simultaneously to a removal of trityl group and phosphonate protecting diisopropyl ester groups under formation of the final HPMP-5-azaC (Fig. 8).

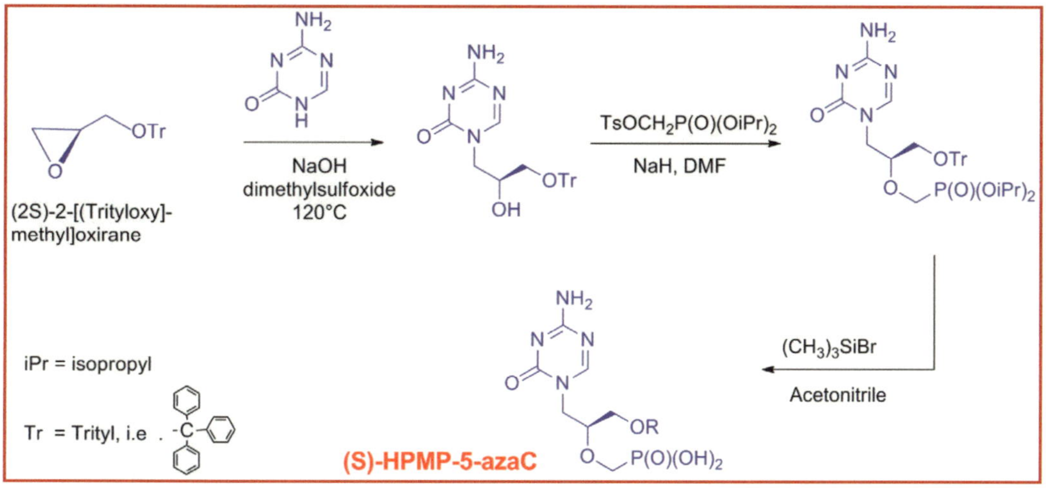

Fig. 8. Synthesis of (*S*)-HPMP-5-azaC from (2S)-2-[(trityloxy)methyl]oxirane. The stepwise approach

The second approach is based on alkylation of 5-azacytosine with an appropriate chiral synthon, i.e. the whole aliphatic part activated with a suitable leaving group, usually tosyl or halogen (Fig. 9). Preparation of "(*S*)-HPMP synthon", i.e. diisopropyl ester of (1*S*)-[2-hydroxy-1-tosyloxymethyl)ethoxy]methylphosphonate followed the protocol originally developed for its racemic form (Hocek et al., 1996). Also in this case, (2*S*)-2-[(trityloxy]methyl]oxirane was selected as a starting material. The oxirane ring was first opened by nucleophilic reaction with sodium benzylate to give (2*S*)-1-benzyloxy-3-

trityloxypropan-2-ol. The next steps are introduction of a phosphonomethyl residue using diisopropyl bromomethanephosphonate, removal of the trityl group with acetic acid, tosylation, and the final deprotection of benzyl group by catalytic hydrogenation. Removal of benzyl group just in this step, i.e. still in a stage of the synthon is necessary. Its removal in some of the following steps would not be possible due to a sensitivity of 5-azacytosine towards catalytic hydrogenation leading to 5,6-dihydro-5-azacytosine derivatives. Diisopropyl (1*S*)-[2-hydroxy-1-tosyloxymethyl)ethoxy]methylphosphonate (HPMP-synthon) was used for the final condensation with a sodium salt of 5-azacytosine. This condensation proceeds exclusively to form the desired N-1 isomer, i.e. diisopropyl ester of HPMP-5-azaC, accompanied by N-3 and O-isomers in a small amount only. This reaction was revealed as an advantageous approach to HPMP-5-azaC, especially for its larger-scale syntheses (Krečmerová et al., 2010b). The final deprotection of ester groups was performed by the standard procedure with bromotrimethylsilane, followed by hydrolysis.

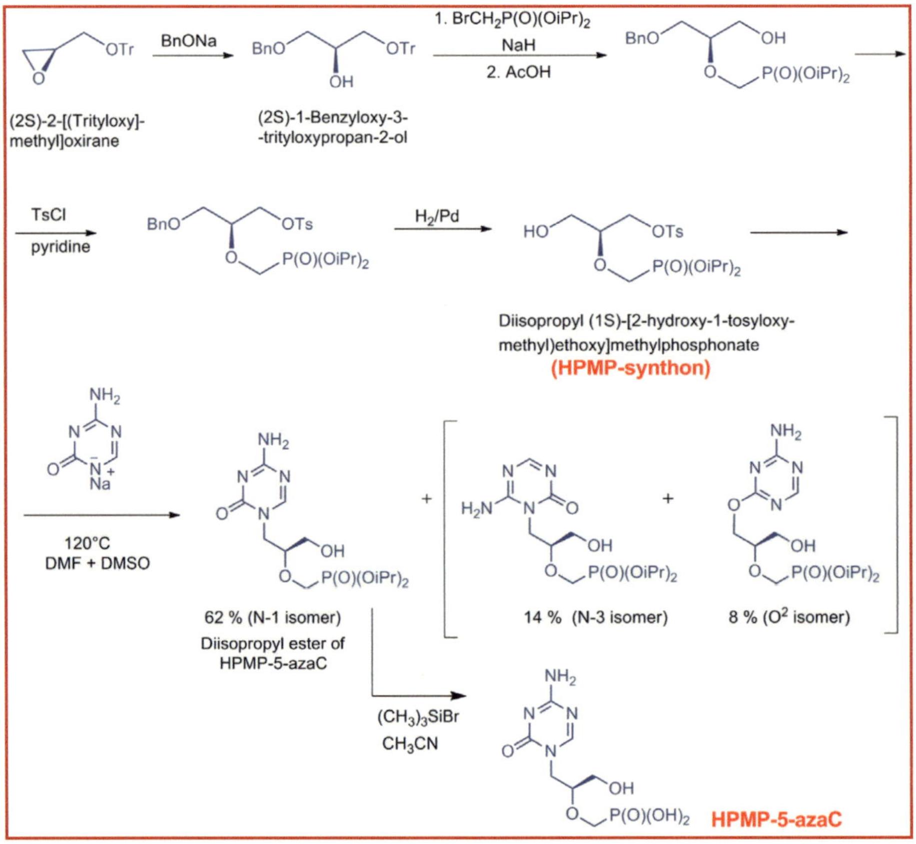

Fig. 9. Synthesis of (*S*)-HPMP-5-azaC by the synthon approach

HPMP-5-azaC showed potent and selective activity against several DNA viruses, including different herpesviruses (HSV-1, HSV-2, VZV, HCMV and HHV-6), adenovirus (Ad2) and poxvirus (vaccinia virus) with 50% effective concentration (EC_{50}) values of 0.71μg/mL for Ad2, 2.56 μg/mL for vaccinia virus and 0.02-0.6 μg/mL for herpesviruses. The antiviral activity of HPMP-5-azaC was comparable to cidofovir against HSV-1, HSV-2 and vaccinia virus, or 2 to 7 times more active against VZV, HCMV, HHV-6 and Ad2. HPMP-5-azaC proved to be 2 times less cytotoxic for HEL cells than (*S*)-HPMPC but 2-fold more toxic for human T-lymphoblast HSB-2 cells. For all these DNA viruses, HPMP-5-azaC showed a 2- to 16-times higher antiviral selectivity index (ratio of CC_{50} to EC_{50}) than (*S*)-HPMPC (cidofovir) (Krečmerová et al., 2007a).

In contrast to cidofovir, HPMP-5-azaC has more complicated metabolic profile, and, similar to other N-1 substituted 5-azacytosine derivatives (riboside, 2′-deoxyriboside, arabinoside), it decomposes in alkaline conditions (Dračínský et al., 2008). The first step is a reversible ring opening of the sym-triazine to the N-formylguanidine derivative which can close back to the cyclic structure. This hydrolytic reaction is slow and reaches equilibrium within several days. However, the reversible ring-opening hydrolysis is accompanied by irreversible deformylation reaction of the intermediary formyl derivative that gives rise to antivirally inactive 2-{[(2*S*)-3-hydroxy-2-(phosphonomethoxy)propyl]carbamoylguanidine. Among these decomposition products (Fig. 10), the N-formylguanidine derivative, which can close back to the cyclic structure, showed activity with equivalent EC_{50} values to those obtained for the original compound HPMP-5-azaC (VZVand HCMV) or at 3- to 25-fold higher EC_{50}'s for HSV-1, HSV-2, HHV-6, Ad2 and vaccinia virus. In contrast, the final decomposition product, the carbamoylguanidine derivative, is antivirally inactive (Krečmerová et al., 2007a).

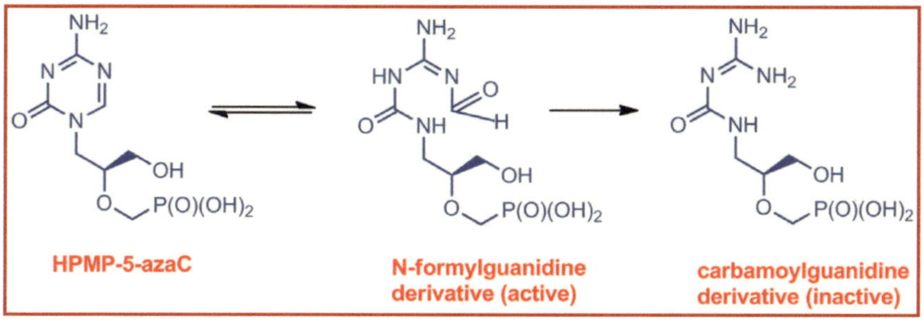

Fig. 10. The course of decomposition of (*S*)-HPMP-5-azaC in alkaline conditions

Investigation of the intracellular metabolism of HPMP-5-azaC revealed its phosphorylation to mono- and diphosphate (60 fold higher then cidofovir) and deaminated uracil product (HPMP-5-azaU) as a minor component (6%). HPMP-5-azaC also showed about 45-fold higher incorporation into cellular DNA than cidofovir. In general, HPMP-5-azaC has a favorable metabolic profile that is characterized by low sensitivity to catabolic deamination and high efficiency for phosphorylation and DNA incorporation (Naesens et al., 2008).

Discovery of the unique antiviral activity of HPMP-5-azaC resulted in the necessity to also prepare some kinds of prodrugs: the cyclic form of 1-(*S*)-[3-hydroxy-2-(phosphonomethoxy)propyl]-5-azacytosine (cHPMP-5-azaC) and its esters. Transformation of HPMP-5-azaC to its cyclic form was realized by the action of dicyclohexylcarbodiimidide (DCC) and *N,N*,-dicyclohexyl-4-morpholinocarboxamidine. To assess the role of ester structure in antiviral activity, four diverse ester types were synthesized: alkyl (octadecyl), alkenyl (erucyl, i.e. (*Z*)-docos-13-enyl), pivaloyloxymethyl (POM) and alkoxyalkyl (2-(hexadecyloxy)ethyl, HDE). The most successful esterification method was the reaction of tetrabutylammonium salt of cHPMP-5-azaC with alkyl bromides or with chloromethyl pivalate, respectively (Fig. 11) (Krečmerová et al., 2007b).

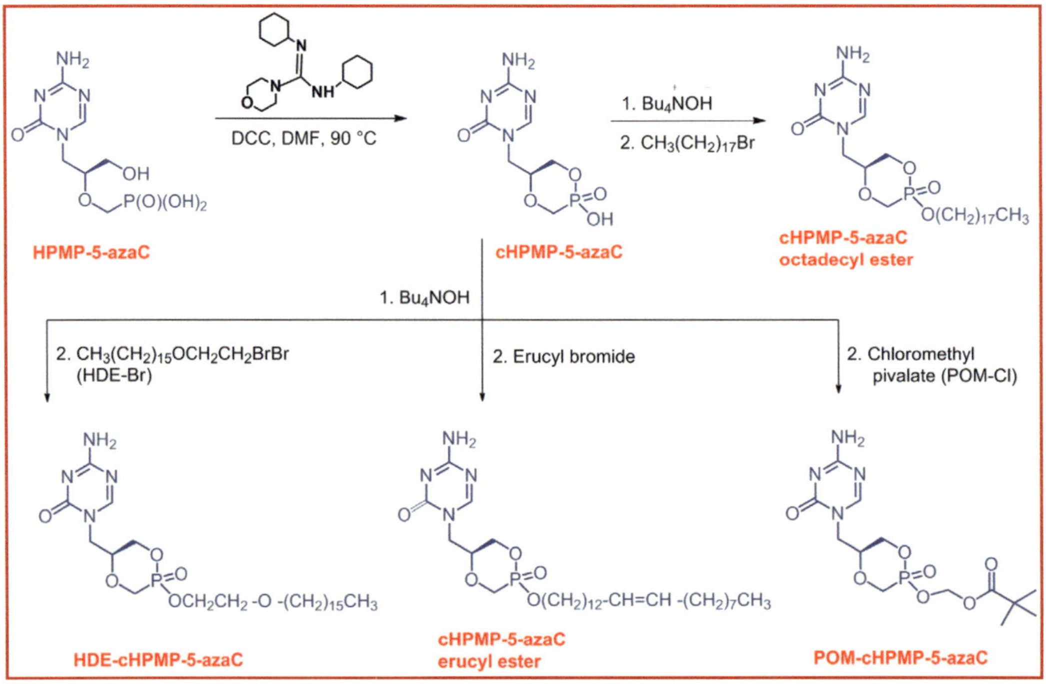

Fig. 11. Synthesis of ester prodrugs derived from the cyclic (*S*)-HPMP-5-azaC

cHPMP-5-azaC was able to inhibit the replication of poxviruses (vaccinia virus), and different herpesviruses, including herpes simplex virus type 1 (HSV-1) and type 2 (HSV-2), thymidine kinase-deficient HSV-1 [acyclovir resistant (ACV^r)], varicella-zoster virus (VZV), human cytomegalovirus (HCMV) and human herpesvirus 6 (HHV-6) with EC_{50} values in the range of 0.06 to 3.1 µg/ml. cHPMP-5-azaC did not affect cell morphology or cell growth (measured on HEL cells). This resulted in selectivity indices (ratio of CC_{50} to EC_{50}) varying from >47 (vaccinia virus) to >1500 (HCMV). The potency of the new triazine analogues HPMP-5-azaC and cHPMP-5-azaC was comparable to that of HPMPC and cHPMPC; however, HPMP-5-azaC and cHPMP-5-azaC proved to be approximately 2 times less cytostatic for HEL cells than HPMPC and cHPMPC, resulting in a superior selectivity.

When the different ester prodrugs, i.e. octadecyl, (erucyl), alkoxyalkyl (HDE) and pivaloyloxymethyl (POM), were evaluated, the HDE emerged as the most active one, with EC_{50} values in the range of 0.003 to 0.008 µg/mL for HSV, ≤0.0008 to ≤.0014 µg/mL for VZV, ≤0.00014 to ≤0.00038 µg/mL (HCMV), 0.008 to 0.037 µg/mL for HHV-6 and 0.037 µg/mL for vaccinia virus. This resulted in 58- (vaccinia virus), 100- (mean for HSV strains), 123- (mean for VZV strains) to 250-fold (mean for HCMV strain) increase in antiviral activity when compared to cHPMP-5-azaC. Not only an improvement in the antiviral activity, but also an increase in selectivity, was observed for HDE-cHPMP-5-azaC. Thus, selectivity indices for HDE-cHPMP-5-azaC were found 43 (HHV-6A), 70 (HHV-6B), 173 (vaccinia virus), 1160 (HSV), ≥5800 (VZV) and ≥24600 (HCMV), as compared to 74 (HHV-6A), 11 (HHV-6B), >47 (vaccinia virus), >180 (HSV), >740 (VZV) and >1540 (HCMV) for the free cHPMP-5-azaC.

Although a marked increase in antiviral potency was noted for the octadecyl ester compared to free cHPMP-5-azaC against HCMV (EC_{50} = 0.0014-0.0037 µg/mL), only a slight increase in activity against VZV or a decrease in potency against HSV was observed. Despite the fact

that the octadecyl ester did not affect cell growth up to a concentration of 100 μg/mL, it produced an alteration of cell morphology at a concentration ≥20 μg/mL.
The esterification of cHPMP-5-azaC to the erucyl prodrug resulted in a loss of activity against vaccinia virus and no improvement or slight decrease in activity against HSV and VZV. The pivaloyloxymethyl ester has a good potency against HCMV (EC_{50} <0.032 μg/mL), but generally, its EC_{50} values are equivalent to those of the free cHPMP-5-azaC.
Progress in the investigation of HPMP-5-azaC and its derivatives is currently still under way. The compound finished its preclinical stage of investigation; its eventual clinical development can be supported by the very promising results in *in vivo* models of poxvirus and herpesvirus infections, as well as by our recent progress on the development of new types of ester prodrugs. These results can substantially improve oral bioavailability of the compound and pharmacological properties in general. HPMP-5-azaC also has a potent activity and selectivity against polyomaviruses: murine polyoma virus, primate simian virus 40 strains and BK virus in human primary renal cells. These findings highlight HPMP-5-azaC and its derivatives as potential drug candidates against polyomavirus associated nephropathies in kidney transplant patients, a diagnosis so far with no FDA approved treatment (Topalis et al., 2011).

4.4 (*S*)-HPMPDAP and its prodrugs – Synthesis of ester prodrugs in HPMP series

In our recent collaborative project with the Rega Institute in Belgium, we have performed a very detailed study of the antiviral efficacy of (S)-HPMPDAP against various DNA viruses, including poxviruses [i.e. vaccinia virus (VACV)] and herpesviruses [i.e. herpes simplex virus type 1 (HSV-1)] and type 2 (HSV-2), thymidine kinase-deficient HSV-1 (acyclovir-resistant, ACV^r), varicella-zoster virus (VZV), human cytomegalovirus (HCMV), and human herpesvirus 6 (HHV-6)]. In the case of HSV-1, HSV-1 ACV^r, HSV-2, and VZV, EC_{50} values for (S)-HPMPDAP and its cyclic form and (*S*)-HPMPC were similar. In contrast, (*S*)-HPMPC was more inhibitory towards HCMV than (*S*)-HPMPDAP or its cyclic form (Krečmerová et al., 2010a).
(S)-HPMPDAP, similar to other acyclic nucleoside phosphonates, represents a compound with a low bioavailability caused by the high polarity of a phosphonic group; its utilization in a prodrug form is thus highly desirable (Fig. 12).
ANPs lacking a free hydroxyl group in a side chain (PME and PMP derivatives) are mostly developed in a form of neutral bis(esters) or bis(amidates). In contrast to them, no prodrugs are commercially available in the case of HPMP derivatives, compounds having a free hydroxyl group in a side chain. Synthesis of their diesters is problematic due to a formation of corresponding cyclic phosphonates. So far, the most promising prodrugs seem to be alkoxyalkyl monoesters (Kern et al., 2002). One representative of this group, hexadecyloxypropyl ester of cidofovir (CMX001) is currently developed as antipox virus agent in clinical Phase II (www.chimerix-inc.com).
The alkoxyalkyl ester prodrugs of (*S*)-HPMPDAP, i.e. hexadecyloxypropyl, octadecyloxyethyl and hexadecyloxyethyl derivatives, emerged as the most potent and selective compounds against VACV with EC_{50} values consistently in the range of 0.00074-0.0012 μM. Although the alkoxyalkyl ester prodrugs proved more toxic than the parent compound (*S*)-HPMPDAP, either for HEL cell morphology or HEL cell growth, they were more selective than (*S*)-HPMPDAP, with selectivity indices [ratio = CC_{50} / EC_{50}] higher than 10,000 compared to >625 for (*S*)-HPMPDAP. The alkoxyalkyl ester prodrugs of the cyclic form of (*S*)-HPMPDAP (both *cis* and *trans* isomers) inhibited VACV replication with EC_{50}

values that were 10-fold (ODE ester, *trans*), 48-fold (HDP ester), 100-fold (ODE ester *cis*) and 100- to 200-fold (HDE, *cis* and *trans*) lower than that of cyclic(*S*)-HPMPDAP. The EC_{50} values obtained for the alkoxyalkyl ester prodrugs of cyclic(*S*)-HPMPDAP were about 3- to 70-fold higher against vaccinia virus than the corresponding monoester prodrugs of (*S*)-HPMPDAP, and they had selectivity indices of 1,200 to 8,000.

The alkoxyalkyl ester prodrugs of (*S*)-HPMPDAP and its cyclic form also proved remarkably potent and selective against HSV-1, HSV-2, HSV-1 ACV^r, VZV, and HCMV, with EC_{50} values in the range of 0.007-0.0008 μM. Lower activities of the alkoxyalkyl ester prodrugs of cyclic(*S*)-HPMPDAP than of the corresponding alkoxyalkyl ester prodrugs of (S)-HPMPDAP were also observed against HSV and VZV. The alkoxyalkyl ester prodrugs also showed potent activity against HCMV, with EC_{50} values at least 225-fold lower than those for the corresponding parent compound. The alkoxyalkyl ester prodrugs proved rather toxic against the lymphoblast HSB-2 cells; and the only compounds, the HDP derivatives of (*S*)-HPMPDAP and cyclic(*S*)-HPMPDAP, respectively, showed selective activity against HHV-6 at non-toxic concentrations.

Although the POM esters (both monoester and *cis* and *trans* isomers of the cyclic form), 2,2,2-(trifluoro)ethyl esters, the butylsalicylyl derivatives, and prodrugs based on peptidomimetics proved less active than the alkoxyalkyl ester prodrugs, they appeared to be less cytotoxic and cytostatic. The POM derivate of cyclic(*S*)-HPMPDAP, either the diastereoisomeric mixture or the *trans* isomer, was able to inhibit VACV replication with EC_{50} values similar to those observed with the parent compounds, while 2,2,2-(trifluoro)ethyl esters, the butylsalicylyl derivatives, and peptidomimetic esters showed EC_{50} values 4- to 16-fold higher than the parent compounds. The POM, 2,2,2-(trifluoro)ethyl, butylsalicylyl derivatives, and prodrugs based on peptidomimetics also proved active against HSV, VZV, and HCMV, with EC_{50}'s similar or 10-fold higher than those of the parent drugs. Both types of POM esters (cyclic and monoester) also displayed potent and selective activity against HHV-6. The EC_{50} values and the selectivity indices for these compounds against HHV-6 were equivalent to those observed for (*S*)-HPMPDAP.

As mentioned above, despite the great experience in development of phosphonate and phosphate prodrugs, preparation of prodrugs in HPMP series remained long problematic (Hecker & Erion, 2008). In our recent work on HPMPDAP prodrugs, we managed to work out conditions for the selective transformation of a free HPMP derivative to the corresponding POM monoester in one reaction step. Reaction can be achieved by the action of chloromethyl pivalate in DMF in the presence of *N,N*,-dicyclohexyl-4-morpholinecarboxamidine; the reaction conditions were optimized so that no cyclization or formation of decomposition products occurred (Krečmerová et al., 2010a). This procedure was also found generally useful for preparation of other POM HPMP monoesters (e.g. HPMPC, HPMP-5-azaC, HPMPA). Preparation of cyclic HPMP POM esters can be performed by the action of chloromethyl pivalate and a tetrabutyl ammonium salt of an appropriate cyclic phosphonate (Fig. 13).

Besides procedures based on alkylation of tetrabutylammonium salt of the cyclic phosphonate, we focused on development of new approaches based on activation of a phosphonic acid residue with hexafluorophosphate coupling agents - PyBOP, PyBroP or HATU. Such reagents are currently used as coupling agents, especially in peptide chemistry (Han & Kim, 2004). This approach proved successful, e.g. in preparation of 2,2,2-(trifluoro)ethyl esters, so far known only in PME series (Sekyia et al., 2002; Kamiya et al.,

2002). Also in this case, the desired 2,2,2-(trifluoroethyl) monoester could be prepared from a free phosphonic acid (HPMPDAP) in one reaction step without any protection (Fig. 14).

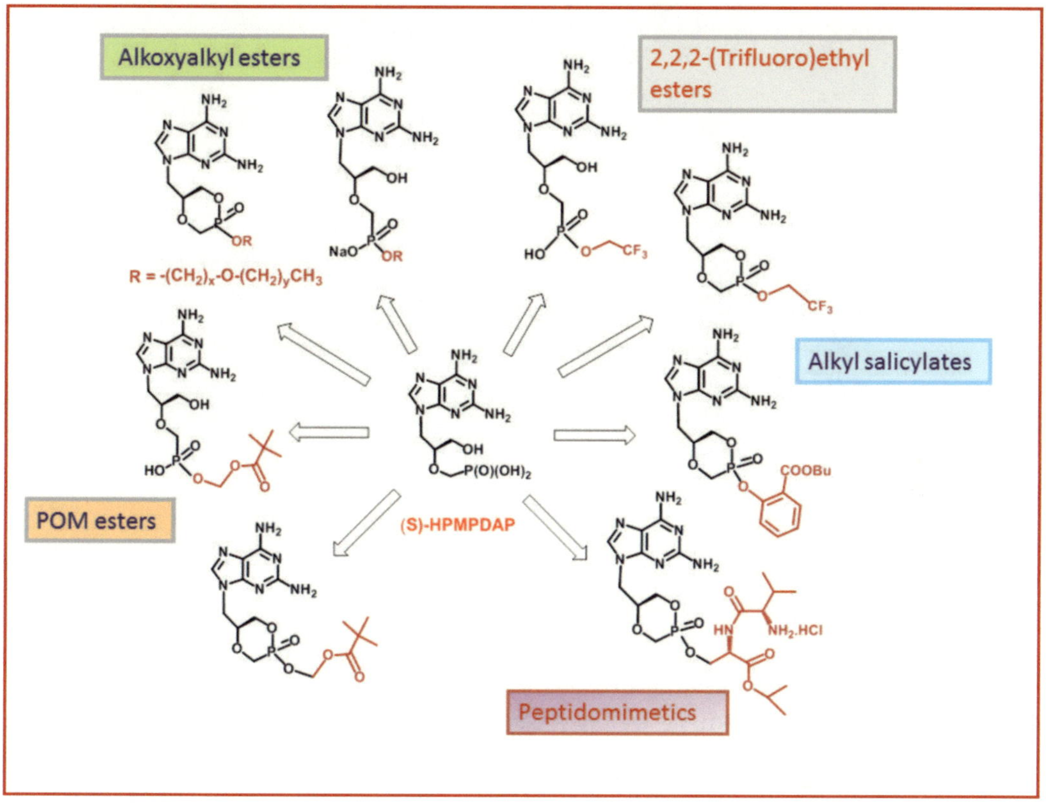

Fig. 12. Structurally diverse types of (*S*)-HPMPDAP prodrugs prepared for investigation of their anti-poxvirus and anti-herpesvirus activities

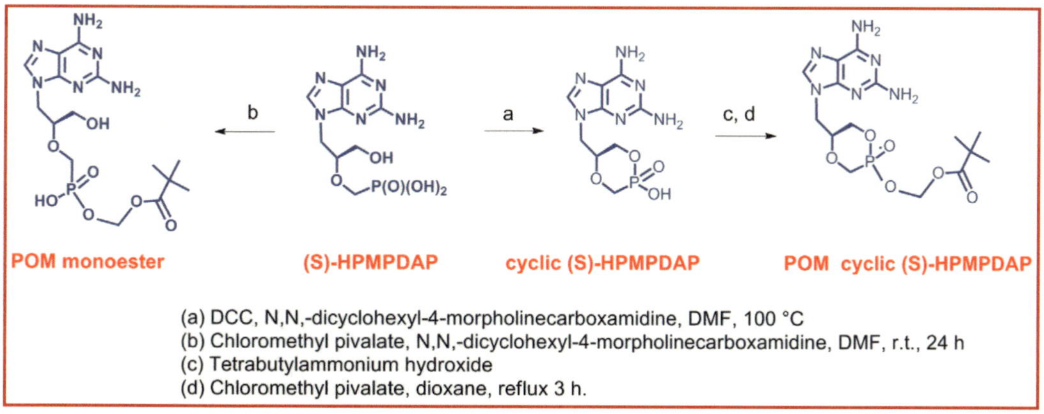

Fig. 13. Synthesis of POM esters of (*S*)-HPMPDAP. The reactions were successfully applied also for HPMPC, HPMP-5-azaC and HPMPA.

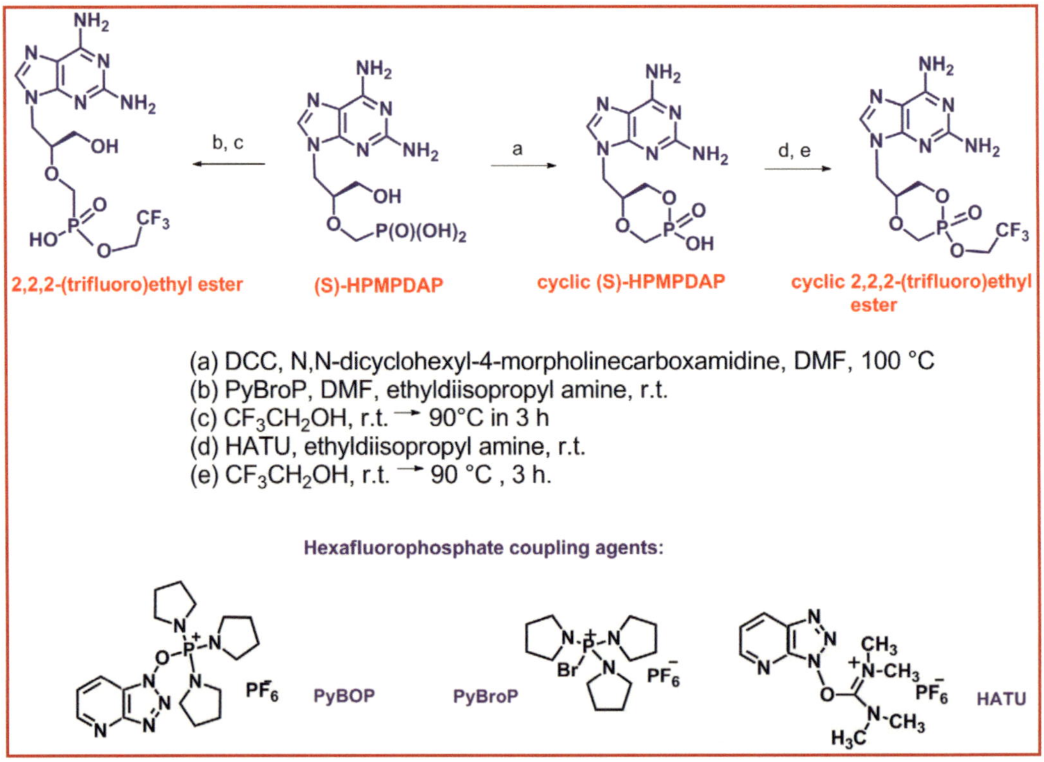

Fig. 14. Structures of some hexafluorophosphate coupling agents and their utilization in synthesis of 2,2,2-(trifluoro)ethyl ester prodrugs of (S)-HPMPDAP

Also, synthesis of other types of HPMP prodrugs can be simplified using the above-mentioned coupling agents, e.g. synthesis of salicylyl esters or peptidomimetic prodrugs ((Krečmerová et al., 2010a; Peterson et al., 2011).

4.5 PME derivatives, open-ring analogues and other structures

In a (phosphonomethoxy)ethyl (PME) series, special attention should be paid to the adenine derivative 9-(2-phosphonomethoxyethyl)adenine (PMEA), 2,6-diaminopurine derivative (PMEDAP) and its N6-substituted analogues. The activity of PME-derivatives against DNA viruses is generally lower compared to their counterparts in the HPMP-series (Holý, 2003). The most active compound is 9-(2-phosphonomethoxyethyl)-2,6-diaminopurine (PMEDAP). PME-derivatives of adenine and 2,6-diaminopurine reveal remarkable activity against HHV-6 *in vitro* (Reymen et al., 1995; Manichanh et al., 2000). PMEDAP is also highly effective against HCMV; it inhibits the expression of HCMV late antigens.

N6-substitutution on the 6-amino group of PMEDAP by one or two alkyl, aryl or cycloalkyl group lead to the compounds with pronounced activities against herpesviruses, especially cytomegalovirus, VZV and EBV (Snoeck et al., 1997; Meerbach et al., 1998). Despite its excellent antiviral parameters, PMEDAP has never been systematically investigated as an antiviral agent. Its main clinical potential lies in its cytostatic effects.

During the past decade, we have also systematically investigated a novel group of base modified ANP, the "open-ring" analogues (Fig. 15). They are characterized by an aliphatic chain (PME-, PMP and/or HPMP-group) linked to the position 6 of 2,4-diaminopyrimidine (DAPy) *via* the oxygen atom. These compounds can be thought of as mimics of the appropriate 2,6-diaminopurine derivatives with an open imidazole ring. Their antiviral activity is essentially identical to that of the parent compounds, including their enantiomeric specificity (De Clercq et al., 2005). The 6-[2-(phosphonomethoxy)ethoxy]-2,4-diaminopyrimidine (PMEO-DAPy) and its 5-substituted derivatives offer antiviral potential similar to adefovir, mostly against retroviruses and HBV. (R)-HPMPO-DAPy has antiviral potential similar to cidofovir (herpes-, adeno, pox-, polyoma and papilllomaviruses) (De Clercq, 2011).

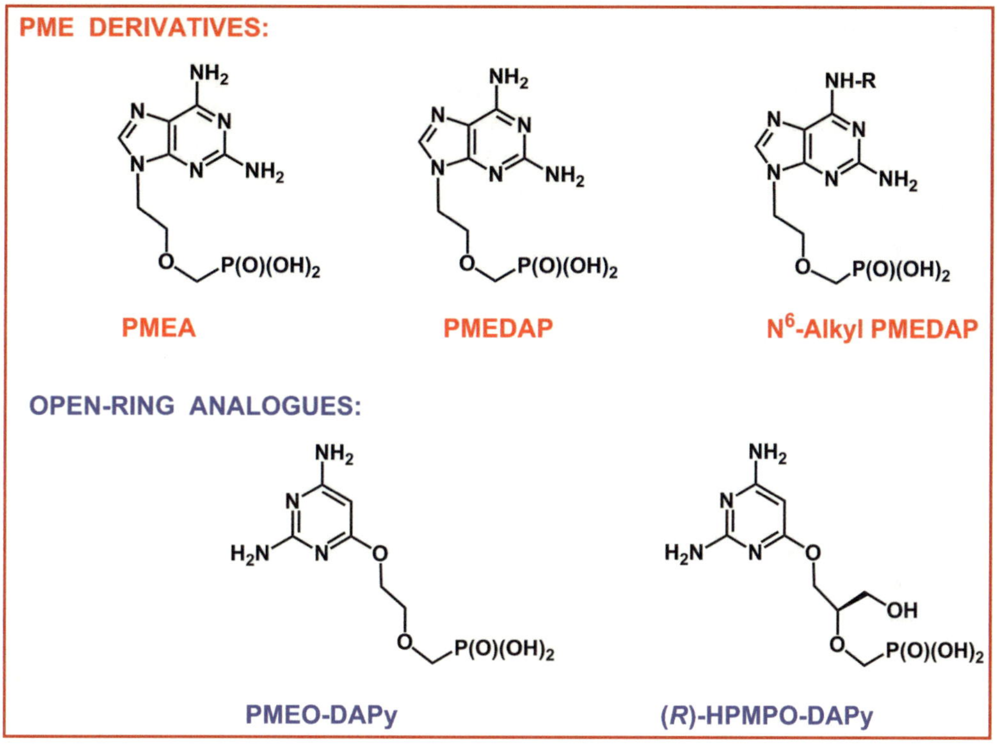

Fig. 15. Structures of selected (phosphonomethoxy)ethyl (PME) derivatives and "open-ring" analogues

5. Animal herpesviruses

The last chapter should be devoted to a special part of virology - animal viruses (Giguère et al., 2006). Their study is important from a veterinary viewpoint in general but many of them can cause diseases which are economically devastating. There is a wide variety of different herpesviruses with different biological characteristics. In animals the most important herpesviruses belong to the Alphaherpesviridae.

Pseudorabies virus causing Aujeszky's disease in pigs is now extensively studied as a model for basic processes during lytic herpesvirus infection and for unravelling molecular mechanisms of herpesvirus neurotropism. The disease is caused by porcine herpesvirus 1, also called pseudorabies virus (PRV) or suid herpesvirus-1 (SHV-1). PRV is considered to be the most economically important viral disease of swine in areas where hog cholera has been eradicated ("Hog cholera" is an alternative name of classical swine fewer (CSF), an infectious disease caused by a pestivirus CSFV from the family *Flaviviridae*) (Fenner et al., 1993). Pseudorabies is endemic in most parts of the world. Pigs are the only natural host for the Aujeszky's virus. Clinical signs in pigs vary depending on the age of the pigs involved. In neonatal pigs, the incubation period is 2-4 days, and signs of central nervous system disease (shivering, inco-ordination and hind leg weakness) are seen. In weaned pigs, respiratory disease is the predominant problem. Sneezing, coughing and laboured breathing is accompanied by fever and weight loss. Mortality rates tend to decrease as the age of the affected pigs rises. Clinical signs can be present for 6-10 days. In uncomplicated cases, the animals often recover. (Lee & Wilson, 1979). Other domestic and wild mammals, such as cattle, sheep, goats, cats, dogs and raccoons (Thawley & Wright, 1982), are also susceptible to this virus. For these hosts, the disease is usually fatal and no effective treatment is available. The main symptoms in dogs include intense itching, jaw and pharyngeal paralysis, howling, and death. In cats, the disease is so rapidly fatal that there are usually no symptoms. Death usually occurs within 48 hours. Vaccines are available only for swine.

Bovine herpesvirus 1 causes several diseases in cattle: infectious bovine rhinotracheitis (IBR), infectious pustular vulvovaginitis (IPV), balanoposthitis, conjunctivitis, abortion, encephalomyelitis, and mastitis. The respiratory form is most common. The viral infection itself is not life-threatening but predisposes to secondary bacterial pneumonia, which may result in death. (Jones & Chowdhury, 2007, 2010). Immunization with modified live or inactivated virus vaccine generally provides adequate protection against clinical disease.

The avian herpesvirus 1 (also called Gallid herpesvirus 1, GaHV-1) is phylogenetically different from both abovementioned viruses and serves to underline similarity and diversity within the Alphaherpesviridae. The virus is a causative agent of laryngotracheitis in poultry. (Hidalgo, 2003). A vaccine is available but it does not prevent latent infections.

Herpesvirus infections are one of the main reasons of animal abortions (Chénier et al., 2004; Smith, 1997). Abortion or neonatal diseases may follow infection with not only alpha-herpesviruses but also beta and gamma-herpesviruses. The alpha-herpesvirus, equine herpesvirus-1 (EHV-1), causes single or epizootic abortions or neonatal deaths in horses, and the closely related virus EHV-4 causes sporadic equine abortions. In cattle, the alpha-herpesviruses, bovine herpesvirus-1 (infectious bovine rhinotracheitis virus) and bovine herpesvirus-5 (bovine encephalitis virus), and a gamma-herpesvirus, bovine herpesvirus-4, have all been implicated as causes of abortion. In pigs, suid herpesvirus-1 (SHV-1: pseudorabies virus), an alpha-herpesvirus, and SHV-2 (porcine cytomegalovirus), a beta-herpesvirus, each cause abortion or neonatal piglet losses. Caprine herpesvirus-1, canine herpesvirus and feline herpesvirus-1, all alpha-herpesviruses, cause abortions or neonatal deaths in goats, dogs and cats, respectively.

5.1 Investigation of antiviral activity of acyclic nucleoside phosphonates against animal herpesviruses

Many years of lasting research on acyclic nucleoside phosphonates (ANPs) as exceptional drugs and/or drug candidates against human viral infections gave an impetus for their study as antivirals in veterinary medicine. The well- researched candidate is cidofovir, active against equine herpes virus type 1, bovine herpesvirus type 1, feline herpesvirus type 1 and caprine herpesvirus type 1. Remarkable effects against animal herpesviruses were also observed at HPMPA and finally at PMEDAP, 9-(phosphonomethoxypropyl)-2,6-diaminopurine, a compound mostly investigated for its cytostatic effects.

Recently, several extensive studies have been paid to the treatment of caprine herpesvirus 1 (CpHV-1) infections by cidofovir.

Caprine herpesvirus 1 (CpHV-1) is responsible for recidivous genital disease in adult goats, characterized by confluent vesicles evolving to ulcers and crusts on the vulvar rima and vaginal mucosa (Tempesta et al., 1999). Several biological similarities exist between CpHV-1 and the human genital herpesvirus type 2, such as the preferential tropism for the genital tract, the vesicular ulcerative nature of the topical lesions, and the tendency to become latent in the sacral ganglia (Lafferty et al., 1987; Tempesta et al., 1999). This makes the genital CpHV-1 infection of goats a reliable animal model for comparative studies. In described experiments, goats were infected experimentally by the vaginal route with CpHV-1 and then treated topically at different time intervalas after infection. The administration of 1% cidofovir cream onto vaginal mucosa was able to prevent the onset of genital lesions and to decrease significantly the titers of the virus shed by the infected animals, notably in the groups treated shortly after infection (24 and 48 h). The efficacy of cidofovir against caprine herpesvirus infection was higher when the treatment was started shortly after infection than when lesions were already present and advanced (Tempesta et al., 2007, 2008). Concerning other drugs effective against CpHV-1, the attention of researchers has been focused in recent years also on the study of acyclovir and ganciclovir.

In horses, two herpesvirus infections mostly occur: equine herpesviruses 1 (EHV-1) and 4 (EHV-4) (Patel & Heldens, 2005). Although both viruses may cause febrile rhinopneumonitis, EHV-1 is the main cause of abortions, paresis and neonatal foal deaths. The lesion central to these three conditions is necrotising vasculitis and thrombosis resulting from lytic infection of endothelial cells lining blood capillaries. The initiation of infection in these lesions is likely to be by reactivated EHV-1 from latently infected leukocytes. However, host factors responsible for reactivation remain poorly understood. Although vaccines are available, they are not fully protective and outbreaks of disease may occur in vaccinated herds. Therefore, there is an urgent need for effective antiviral treatment.

It was found that ganciclovir is the most potent compound and therefore a valuable candidate for the treatment.

Ganciclovir displays the best overall activity against EHV-1infection in vitro, without affecting cell viability. However, due to the high cost price, there is no direct clinical application possible. Therefore, acyclovir seems to be a more valuable candidate for antiviral therapy against EHV-1. As acyclovir has been patented since 1997 and generic alternatives are available, it seems attractive to use this drug for the treatment of horses during an outbreak (Wilkins et al., 2005). However, the bioavailability of orally administered acyclovir is a serious restriction (Bentz al., 2006). Bioavailability of only 2.8%, resulting in low plasma concentrations, is inadequate to expect any clinically relevant antiviral efficacy. The oral prodrug of acyclovir, valacyclovir seems to be more effective due to its higher bioavailability (Ormrod & Goa, 2000). Recently, a large study comparing the effect of several antiviral drugs - acyclovir, ganciclovir, cidofovir, adefovir, 9-(2-phosphonylmethoxyethyl)-2,6-diaminopurine (PMEDAP) and foscarnet against three abortigenic (94P247, 97P70 and 99P96) and three neuropathogenic isolates (97P82, 99P136 and 03P37) of EHV-1 was performed (Garré, B. et al., 2007). Ganciclovir was most potent in reducing plaque number, followed by PMEDAP and acyclovir. Adefovir and cidofovir were less effective and foscarnet was the least effective compound. There were no differences detected for acyclovir, ganciclovir, adefovir and PMEDAP between the abortigenic and neuropathogenic isolates. Although cidofovir is not highly efficient in reducing plaque number, it is able to significantly reduce plaque size at very low concentrations. Cidofovir was 40-fold more effective in reducing plaque size than in reducing plaque number (Garré, B. et al., 2007).

A similar comparative study was also performed for feline herpesvirus. Feline herpesvirus 1 (FHV-1) is a common cause of respiratory and ocular disease in cats. Especially in young kittens that have not yet reached the age of vaccination, but have already lost maternal immunity, severe disease may occur. In the study, the efficacy of six antiviral drugs - acyclovir, ganciclovir, cidofovir, foscarnet, adefovir and 9-(2-phosphonylmethoxyethyl)-2, 6-diaminopurine (PMEDAP), against FHV-1 was compared in Crandell-Rees feline kidney (CRFK) cells using reduction in plaque number and plaque size as parameters. The capacity to reduce the number of plaques was most pronounced for ganciclovir, PMEDAP and cidofovir. All antiviral drugs were able to significantly reduce plaque size when compared with the untreated control. As observed for the reduction in plaque number, ganciclovir, PMEDAP and cidofovir were most potent in reducing plaque size. Adefovir and foscarnet were intermediately potent. The most remarkable effect was observed for cidofovir and ganciclovir. None of the products were toxic for CRFK cells at antiviral concentrations (van der Meulen, K. et al., 2006).

6. Conclusion

For a long time, viral infections remained a major medical problem worldwide due to a lack of therapy, prevention, or vaccination strategy, and also due to the rapid development of resistance. Four decades of intensive research in the field of nucleic acid component chemistry brought the fundamental changes in the treatment of most viral infections. Discovery of acyclic nucleoside phosphonates and their systematic investigation resulted in marketed drugs effective so far against fatal infections (AIDS, HBV, CMV infections in immunocompromised patients, etc.). The fundamental research in the field resulted in many excellent active structures so far waiting for clinical investigation, e.g. "open-ring" analogues, HPMP-5-azaC, HPMPDAP, and many other structures described in the text. Investigation of these compounds still remains a significant challenge for the pharmaceutical industry.

7. Acknowledgment

This work was performed as a part of the research project of the IOCB AVOZ40550506. Financial support of the Centre for New Antivirals and Antineoplastics 1M0508 by the Ministry of Education, Youth and Sports of the Czech Republic is greatly acknowledged.

8. References

Andrei, G.; Snoeck, R.; Goubau, P., Desmyter, J. & De Clercq, E. Comparative activity of various compounds against clinical strains of herpes simplex virus. *European Journal of Clinical Microbiology & Infectious Diseases.* Vol. 11, No. 2, (February, 1992), pp. 143 - 151, ISSN 0934-9723

Andrei, G.; Snoeck, R.; Reymen, D.; Liesnard, C.; Goubau, P.; Desmyter, J. & De Clercq, E. Comparative activity of selected antiviral compounds against clinical isolates of varicella-zoster virus. *European Journal of Clinical Microbiology & Infectious Diseases*. Vol. 14, No. 4, (April 1995), pp. 318 - 329, ISSN 0934-9723

Bagnis, C.; Izzdine, H. & Deray, G. Renal tolerance of cidofovir. *Therapie*. Vol. 54, No. 6, (November - December 1999), pp. 689 - 691, ISSN 0040-5957

Beadle, J.R.; Wan, W.B.; Ciesla, S.L.; Keith, K.A.; Hartline, C.; Kern, E.R. & Hostetler, K.Y. Synthesis and Antiviral Evaluation of 9-(*S*)-(3-Hydroxy-2-phosphonomethoxypropyl)adenine against Cytomegalovirus and Orthopoxviruses. *Journal of Medicinal Chemistry*. Vol. 49, No. 6, (March 2006), pp. 2010-2015, ISSN 0022- 2623

Bentz, B.G.; Maxwell, L.K.; Erkert, R.S.; Royer, C.M.; Davis, M.S.; MacAllister, C.G. & Clarke, C.R. Pharmacokinetics of acyclovir after single intravenous and oral administration to adult horses. *Journal of Veterinary Internal Medicine*. Vol. 20, No. 3, (May-June 2006), pp. 589–594, ISSN 0891-6640

Bielamowicz, S.; Villagomez, V.; Stager, S. V. & Wilson, W. R. Intralesional cidofovir therapy for laryngeal papilloma in an adult cohort. *Laryngoscope*. Vol. 112, No. 4, (April 2002), pp. 696-699, ISSN 0023-852X

Bray, M. & Wright, M. E. Progressive vaccinia. *Clinical Infecious Diseases*. Vol. 36, No. 6, (March 2003), pp. 766-774, ISSN 1058-4838

Brodfuehrer, P.R., Howell, H.G., Sapino, C. & Vemishetti, P. A practical synthesis of (S)-HPMPC. *Tetrahedron Letters*. Vol. 35, No. 20, (May 1994), pp. 3243-3246, ISSN 0040-4039

Calista, D. Topical cidofovir for severe cutaneous human papillomavirus and molluscum contagiosum infections in patients with HIV/AIDS. A pilot study. *Journal of the European Academy of Dermatology and Venereology*. Vol. 14, No. 6, (November 2000), pp. 484-488, ISSN 0926-9959

Chénier, S.; Montpetit, C. & Hélie, P. Caprine herpesvirus-1 abortion storm in a goat herd in Quebec. *Canadian Veterinary Journal – Revue Veterinaire Canadienne*. Vol. 45, No. 3 (March 2004), pp. 241-243, ISSN 0008-5286

De Bolle, L.; Naesens, L. and De Clercq, E. Update on human herpesvirus 6 biology, clinical features, and therapy. *Clinical Microbiology Reviews*. Vol. 18, No. 1, (January 2005), pp. 217–245, ISSN 0893-8512

De Clercq E. Towards an effective chemotherapy of virus infections: Therapeutic potential of cidofovir [(S)-1-[3- hydroxy-2-(phosphonomethoxy)propyl]cytosine, HPMPC] for the treatment of DNA virus infections. *Collection of Czechoslovak Chemical Communications*. Vol. 63, No. 4, (April 1998), pp. 480-506, ISSN 0010- 0765

De Clercq, E. Acyclic nucleoside phosphonates: An unfinished story. *Collection of Czechoslovak Chemical Communications*. Vol. 76, No. 7, (July 2011), pp. 829-842, ISSN 0010-0765

De Clercq, E.; Andrei, G.; Balzarini, J.; Leyssen, P.; Naesens, L.; Neyts, J. ; Pannecouque, C.; Snoeck, R.; Ying, C.; Hocková, D. & Holý, A. Antiviral potential of a new generation of acyclic nucleoside phosphonates, the 6-[2-(phosphonomethoxy)alkoxy]-2,4-diaminopyrimidines. *Nucleosides Nucleotides Nucleic Acids. Special Issue* . Vol. 24, No. 5-7, (2005), pp. 331-341, ISSN 1525-7770

De Clercq, E.; Descamps, J.; De Somer, P. & Holý, A. (S)-9-(2,3-Dihydroxypropyl)adenine: An Aliphatic Nucleoside Analog with Broad-Spectrum Antiviral Activity. Science. Vol. 200, No. 4341, (May 1978), pp. 563-565, ISSN 0036-8075

De Clercq, E. & Holý, A. Alkyl Esters of 3-Adenin-9-yl-2-hydroxypropanoic Acid: A New Class of Broad-spectrum Antiviral Agents. *Journal of Medicinal Chemistry.* Vol. 28, No. 3, (March 1985), pp. 282-287, ISSN 0022-2623

De Clercq, E.; Holy, A. Acyclic nucleoside phosphonates: a key class of antiviral drugs. *Nature Reviews Drug Discovery.* Vol. 4, No. 11, (November 2005) pp. 928-940, ISSN 1474-1776

De Clercq, E.; Holý, A.; Rosenberg, I.; Sakuma, T.; Balzarini, J. & Maudgal, P.C. A novel selective broad-spectrum anti-DNA virus agent. *Nature.* Vol. 323, No. 6087, (October, 1986), pp. 464-467, ISSN 0028-0836

Dračínský, M.; Krečmerová, M. & Holý, A. Study of chemical stability of antivirally active 5-azacytosine acyclic nucleoside phosphonates using NMR spectroscopy. *Bioorganic & Medicinal Chemistry.* Vol. 16, No. 14, (July 2008), pp. 6778-6782, ISSN 0968-0896

Dvořáková, H. & Holý, A. Synthesis and biological effects of N-(2-phosphonomethoxyethyl) derivatives of deazapurine bases. *Collection of Czechoslovak Chemical Communications.* Vol. 58, No. 6, (June 1993), pp. 1419-1429, ISSN 0010-0765

Dvořáková, H.; Holý, A. & Alexander, P. Synthesis and biological effects of 9-(3-hydroxy-2-phosphonomethoxypropyl) derivatives of deazapurine bases. *Collection of Czechoslovak Chemical Communications.* Vol. 58, No. 6, (June 1993), pp. 1403-1418, ISSN 0010-0765

Dvořáková, H.; Holý, A.; Snoeck, R.; Balzarini, J. & De Clercq, E. Acyclic nucleoside and nucleotide analogues derived from 1-deaza and 3-deazaadenine. *Collection of Czechoslovak Chemical Communications.* Vol. 55, Special issue No. 1, (1990), pp. 113-116, ISSN 0010-0765

Fenner, F.J. ; Gibbs, E.P.J. ; Murphy, F.A. ; Rott, R. ; Studdert, M.J. & White, D.O. *Veterinary Virology (2nd ed.).* Academic Press, Inc. ISBN 0-12-253056-X

Garré, B.; van der Meulen, K.; Nugent, J.; Neyts, J.; Croubels, S.; De Backer, P. & Nauwynck, H. In vitro susceptibility of six isolates of equine herpesvirus 1 to acyclovir, ganciclovir, cidofovir, adefovir, PMEDAP and foscarnet. *Veterinary Microbiology.* Vol. 122, No. 1-2, (May 2007), pp. 43–51, ISSN 0378-1135

Gasnault, J.; Kousignian, P.; Kahraman, M.; Rahoiljaon, J.; Matheron, S.; Delfraissy, J. F. & Taoufik Y. Cidofovir in AIDS-associated progressive multifocal leukoencephalopathy: A monocenter observational study with clinical and JC virus load monitoring. *Journal of Neurovirology.* Vol. 7, No. 4, (August 2001), pp. 375-381, ISSN 1355-0284

Giguère, S.; Prescott, J:F. & Baggot, J.D., Editors. *Antimicrobial therapy in veterinary medicine, Fourth Edition.* Wiley- Blackwell 2006, ISBN 978-0-8138-0656-3

Göbel, R.; Richter, F. & Weichmann, H. Synthesis and reactivity of methylene bridged diphosphoryl compounds. *Phosphorus, Sulfur and Silicon.* Vol. 73, No. 1-4, (1992), pp. 67-80, ISSN 0308-664X

Han, S.-Y. & Kim, Y.-A. Recent development of peptide coupling reagents in organic synthesis. *Tetrahedron,* Vol. 60, No. 11, (March 2004), pp. 2447-2467, ISSN 0040-4020

Hecker, S.J. & Erion, M.D. Prodrugs of Phosphates and Phosphonates. *Journal of Medicinal Chemistry.* Vol. 51, No. 8, (April 2008), pp. 2328-2345, ISSN 0022-2623

Hidalgo, H. Infectious Laryngotracheitis: A Review. *Brazilian Journal of Poultry Science.* Vol. 5, No. 3, (September - December 2003), pp. 157-168, ISSN 1516-635X

Hitchcock, M.J.M.; Jaffe, H.S.; Martin, J.C. & Stagg, R.J. Cidofovir, a new agent with potent anti-herpesvirus activity. *Antiviral Chemistry & Chemotherapy.* Vol. 7, No. 3, (May 1996), pp. 115 - 127, ISSN 0956-3202

Hocek, M.; Masojídková, M.; Holý, A.; Andrei, G.; Snoeck, R.; Balzarini, J. & de Clercq, E. Synthesis and antiviral activity of acyclic nucleotide analogues derived from (6-aminomethyl)purines and purine-6- carboxamidines. *Collection of Czechoslovak Chemical Communications.* Vol. 61, No. 10, (October 1996), pp. 1525-1537, ISSN 0010-0765

Holý, A. Syntheses of enantiomeric N-(3-hydroxy-2-phosphonomethoxypropyl) derivatives of purine and pyrimidine bases. *Collection of Czechoslovak Chemical Communications.* Vol. 58, No. 3, (March 1993), pp. 649-674, ISSN 0010-0765

Holý, A. Phosphonomethoxyalkyl analogs of nucleotides. *Current Pharmaceutical Design.* Vol. 9, No. 31, (2003), pp. 2567-2692, ISSN 1381-6128

Holý, A. Synthesis of acyclic nucleoside phosphonates. In: "Current Protocols in Nucleic Acid Chemistry", Unit 14.2. John Wiley & Sons, Inc., Published Online October 1, 2005, DOI: 10.1002/0471142700.nc1402s22

Holý, A. & De Clercq, E. (2010). In: "Anti-DNA virus Agents". *Burger´s Medicinal Chemistry, Drug Discovery, and Development, Seventh Edition,* D.J. Abraham & D.P. Rotella (Ed.), pp. 221-258, John Wiley & Sons, Inc., (September 2010), ISBN 978-0-470-27815-4.

Holý, A. & Rosenberg, I. Stereospecific syntheses of 9-(S)-(3-hydroxy-2-phosphonylmethoxypropyl)adenine (HPMPA). *Nucleic Acids Symp Ser.* Vol. 18, (1987), pp. 33 - 36

Holý, A.; Votruba, I. & De Clercq, E. Studies on S-adenosyl-L-homocysteine hydrolase. 5. Synthesis and antiviral activity of stereoisomeric eritadenines. *Collection of Czechoslovak Chemical Communications.* Vol. 47, No.5, (May 1982), pp. 1392-1407, ISSN 0010-0765

Holý, A.; Dvořáková, H.; Jindřich, J.; Masojídková, M.; Buděšínský, M.; Balzarini, J.; Andrei, G. & De Clercq, E. Acyclic nucleotide analogs derived from 8-azapurines: synthesis and antiviral activity. *Journal of Medicinal Chemistry.* Vol. 39, No. 20, (September 1996), pp. 4073-4088, ISSN 0022-2623

Jansa, P.; Holý, A.; Dračínský, M.; Baszczyňski, O.; Česnek, M. & Janeba, Z. Efficient and "green" microwave- assisted synthesis of haloalkylphosphonates *via* the Michaelis–Arbuzov reaction. *Green Chemistry.* Vol. 13, No. 4, (2011), pp. 882-888, ISSN 1463-9262

Jones, C.; & Chowdhury, S. A review of the biology of bovine herpesvirus type 1 (BHV-1), its role as a cofactor in the bovine respiratory disease complex and development of improved vaccines. *Animal Health Research Reviews.* Vol. 8, No. 2, (December 2007), pp. 187-205, ISSN 1466-2523

Jones, C.; & Chowdhury, S. Bovine herpesvirus type 1(BHV-1) is an important cofactor in the bovine respiratory disease complex. *Veterinary Clinics of North America: Food Animal Practice.* Vol. 26, No. 2, (July 2010), pp. 303-321, ISSN 0749-0720

Kamiya, N., Kubota, A., Iwase, Y., Sekiya, K., Ubasawa, M. & Yuasa, S. Antiviral activities of MCC-478, a novel and specific inhibitor of hepatitis B virus. *Antimicrobial Agents and Chemotherapy.* Vol. 46, No. 9, (September 2002, pp. 2872-2877, ISSN 0066-4804

Kern, E. R.; Hartline, C.; Harden, E.; Keith, K.; Rodriguez, N.; Beadle, J. R. & Hostetler, K. Y. Enhanced inhibition of orthopox virus replication in vitro by alkoxyalkyl esters of cidofovir and cyclic cidofovir. *Antimicrobial Agents and Chemotherapy*. Vol. 46, No. 4, (April 2002), pp. 991-995, ISSN 0066- 4804

Komaroff, A.L. Is human herpesvirus-6 a trigger for chronic fatigue syndrome? *Journal of Clinical Virology*. Vol. 37, Suppl. 1, (December 2006), pp. S39-S46, ISSN 1386-6532

Krečmerová, M.; Holý, A.; Pískala, A.; Masojídková, M.; Andrei, G.; Naesens, L.; Neyts, J.; Balzarini, J.; De Clercq, E. & Snoeck, R. Antiviral activity of triazine analogues of 1-(*S*)-[3-hydroxy-2- (phosphonomethoxy)propyl]cytosine (cidofovir) and related compounds. *Journal of Medicinal Chemistry*. Vol. 50, No. 5, (March 2007a), pp. 1069-1077, ISSN 0022-2623

Krečmerová, M.; Holý, A.; Pohl, R.; Masojidková, M.; Andrei, G.; Naesens, L.; Neyts, J.; Balzarini, J.; De Clercq, E. & Snoeck, R. Ester prodrugs of cyclic 1-(S)-[3-hydroxy-2-(phosphonomethoxy)propyl]-5- azacytosine: Synthesis and antiviral activity. *Journal of Medicinal Chemistry*. Vol. 50, No. 23,(November 2007b), pp. 5765-5772, ISSN 0022-2623

Krečmerová, M.; Holý, A.; Andrei, G.; Pomeisl, K.; Tichý, T.; Břehová, P.; Masojídková, M.; Dračínský, M.; Pohl, R.; Laflamme, G.; Naesens, L.; Hui, H.; Cihlar, T.; Neyts, J.; De Clercq, E.; Balzarini J. & Snoeck, R. Synthesis of ester prodrugs of 9-(S)-[3-hydroxy-2-(phosphonomethoxy)propyl]-2,6-diaminopurine (HPMPDAP) as anti-poxvirus agents. *Journal of Medicinal Chemistry*. Vol. 53, No. 19, (October 2010a), pp. 6825-6837, ISSN 0022-2623

Krečmerová, M.; Masojídková, M. & Holý, A. Acyclic nucleoside phosphonates with 5-azacytosine base moiety substituted in C-6 position. *Bioorganic & Medicinal Chemistry*. Vol. 18, No. 1, (January 2010b), pp. 387-395, ISSN 0968-0896

Lacy, S.A.; Hitchcock, M.J.M.; Lee, W.A.; Tellier, P. & Cundy, K.C. Effect of oral probenecid coadministration on the chronic toxicity and pharmacokinetics of intravenous cidofovir in cynomolgus monkeys. *Toxicological Sciences*. Vol. 44, No. 2, (August 1998), pp. 97 - 106, ISSN 1096-6080

Lafferty, W.E.; Coombs, R.W.; Benedetti, J.; Critchlow, C. & Corey, L. Recurrences after oral and genital herpes simplex virus infection. Influence of site of infection and viral type. *New England Journal of Medicine*. Vol. 316, No. 23, (June 1987), pp. 1444-1449, ISSN 0028-4793

Lalezari, J.; Schacker, T.; Feinberg, J.; Gathe, J.; Lee, S.; Cheung, T.; Kramer, F.; Kessler, H.; Corey, L.; Drew, W.L.; Boggs, J.; McGuire, B.; Jaffe, H.S. & Safrin, S. A randomized, double-blind, placebo-controlled trial of cidofovir gel for the treatment of acyclovir-unresponsive mucocutaneous herpes simplex virus infection in patients with AIDS. *Journal of Infectious Diseases*. Vol. 176, No. 4, (October 1997), pp. 892 - 898, ISSN 0022-1899

Lee, J.Y.S. & Wilson, M.R. A Review of Pseudorabies (Aujesky´s Disease) in Pigs. *Canadian Veterinary Journal* Vol. 20, No. 3, (March 1979), pp. 65–69, ISSN 0008-528

Legrand, F.; Berrebi, D.; Houhou, N.; Freymuth, F.; Faye, A.; Duval, M.; Mougenot, J. F.; Peuchmaur, M. & Vilmer, E. Early diagnosis of adenovirus infection and treatment with cidofovir after bone marrow transplantation in children. *Bone Marrow Transplantation*. Vol. 27, No. 6, (March 2001), pp. 621-626, ISSN 0268-3369

Manichanh, C.; Grenot, P.; Gautheret-Dejean, A.; Debré, P.; Huraux, J.M.; & Agut, H. Susceptibility of human herpesvirus 6 to antiviral compounds by flow cytometry analysis. *Cytometry*. Vol. 40, No. 2, (June 2000), pp. 135 – 140, ISSN 0196-4763

Meerbach, A.; Holy, A.; Wutzler, P.; De Clercq, E. & Neyts, J. Inhibitory effects of novel nucleoside and nucleotide analogues on Epstein-Barr virus replication. *Antiviral Chemistry & Chemotherapy*. Vol. 9, No. 3, (May 1998), pp. 275 – 282, ISSN 0956-3202

Van der Meulen, K.; Garré, B.; Croubels, S. & Nauwynck, H. In vitro comparison of antiviral drugs against feline herpesvirus 1. *BMC Veterinary Research*. Vol. 2, (April 2006), article No.13, ISSN 1746-6148

Naesens, L.; Andrei, G.; Votruba, I.; Krečmerová, M.; Holý, A.; Neyts, J.; DeClercq, E. & Snoeck R. Intracellular metabolism of the new antiviral compound, 1-(S)-[3-hydroxy-2-(phosphonomethoxy)propyl]-5- azacytosine. *Biochemical Pharmacololgy*. Vol. 76, No. 8, (October 2008), pp. 997-1005, ISSN 0006-2952

Naesens, L. & De Clercq, E. Therapeutic potential of HPMPC (cidofovir), PMEA (adefovir) and related acyclic Nucleoside phosphonate analogues as broad- spectrum antiviral agents. *Nucleosides & Nucleotides*. Vol. 16, No. 7-9 (1997), pp. 983 - 992, ISSN 0732-8311

Naesens, L. & De Clercq, E. Antiviral activity of diverse classes of broad-acting agents and natural compounds in HHV-6-infected lymphoblasts. *Journal of. Clinical Virology*. Vol. 37, Suppl. 1, Meeting Abstract: 56, (December 2006)), pp. S69–S75, ISSN 1386-6532.

Naesens, L.; Snoeck, R.; Andrei, G; Balzarini, J.; Neyts, J. & De Clercq, E. HPMPC (cidofovir), PMEA (adefovir) and related acyclic nucleoside phosphonate analogues: A review of their pharmacology and clinical potential in the treatment of viral infections. *Antiviral Chemistry & Chemotherapy*. Vol. 8, No. 1, (January 1997), pp. 1–23, ISSN ISSN 0956-3202

Neyts, J. & De Clercq, E. Antiviral drug susceptibility of human herpesvirus 8. *Antimicrobial Agents and Chemotherapy*. Vol. 41, No. 12, (December 1997), pp. 2754 -2756, ISSN 0066-4804

Oh, C.H. & Hong, J.H. Design, synthesis and anti-HIV activity of homologous PMEA derivatives. *Nucleosides Nucleotides & Nucleic Acids*. Vol. 27, No. 2, (2008), pp. 186-195, ISSN 1525-7770

Ormrod, D. & Goa, K. Valaciclovir – A review of its use in the management of herpes zoster. *Drugs*. 59, No. 6, (June 2000), pp. 1317-1340, ISSN 0012-6667

Patel, J.R. & Heldens, J. Equine herpesviruses 1 (EHV-1) and 4 (EHV-4) - epidemiology, disease and immunoprophylaxis: A brief review. *Veterinary Journal*. Vol. 170, No. 1, (July 2005), pp. 14-23, ISSN 1090-0233

Peterson, L.W.; Kim, J.S.; Kijek, P.; Mitchell, S.; Hilfinger, J.; Breitenbach, J.; Borysko, K.; Drach, J.C.; Kashemirov, B.A. & McKenna, C.E. Synthesis, transport and antiviral activity of Ala-Ser and Val-Ser prodrugs of cidofovir. *Bioorganic & Medicinal Chemistry Letters*. Vol. 21, No. 13, (July 2011), pp. 4045- 4049, ISSN 0960-894X

Reymen, D.; Naesens, L.; Balzarini, J.; Holý, A.; Dvořáková, H. & De Clercq E. Antiviral activity of selected acyclic nucleoside analogues against human herpesvirus 6. *Antiviral Research*. Vol. 28, No. 4, (December 1995), pp. 343 – 357, ISSN 0166-3542

Sekiya, K., Takashima, H., Ueda, N., Kamiya, N., Yuassa, S., Fujimura, Y. & Ubasawa, M. 2-Amino-6-arylthio- 9-[2-(phosphonomethoxy)ethyl]purine bis(2,2,2-trifluoroethyl)

esters as novel HBV-specefic antiviral reagents. *Journal of Medicinal Chemistry*. Vol. 45, No. 14, (July 2002), pp. 3138–3142, ISSN 0022-2623

Smith, K.C. Herpesviral abortion in domestic animals. Veterinary Journal. Vol. 153, No. 3, (May 1997), pp 253- 268, ISSN 1090-0233

Snoeck, R.; Andrei, G.; Holy, A. & De Clercq, E. Activity of N^6-substituted adenine and 2,6-diaminopurine acyclic nucleoside phosphonates against human cytomegalovirus (CMV) and other herpesviruses. Abstract Book 1997. 6th International Cytomegalovirus Workshop, Orange Beach, Alabama, USA. March 5-9, 1997

Tempesta, M.; Pratelli, A.; Corrente, M. & Buonavoglia, C. A preliminary study on the pathogenicity of a strain of caprine herpesvirus 1. *Comparative Immunology, Microbiology and Infectious Diseases.* Vol. 22, No. 2, (April 1999), pp. 137–143, ISSN 0147-9571

Tempesta, M.; Pratelli, A.; Greco, G.; Martella, V.. & Buonavoglia, C. Detection of caprine herpesvirus 1 in sacral ganglia of latently infected goats by PCR. *Journal of Clinical Microbiology.* Vol. 37, No. 5, (May 1999), pp. 1598-1599, ISSN 0095-113

Tempesta, M.; Camero, M.; Bellacio, A.L.; Thiry, J.; Crescenzo, G.; Neyts, J.; Thiry, E. & Buonavoglia, C. Cidofovir is effective against caprine herpesvirus 1 infection in goats. *Antiviral Research.* Vol. 74, No. 2, (May 2007), pp. 138-141, ISSN 0166-3542

Tempesta, M.; Crescenzo, G.; Camero, M.; Bellacicco, A.L.; Tarsitano, E.; Decaro, N.; Neyts, J.; Martella, V. & Buonavoglia, C. Assessing the Efficacy of Cidofovir against Herpesvirus-Induced Genital Lesions in Goats Using Different Therapeutic Regimens. *Antimicrobial Agents and Chemotherapy.* Vol. 52, No. 11, (November 2008), pp. 4064-4068, ISSN 0066-4804

Thawley, D.G. & Wright, J.C. Pseudorabies virus infection in raccoons: A review. *Journal of Wildlife Diseases.* Vol. 18, No. 1, (January 1982), pp. 113-116, ISSN 0090-3558

Topalis, D.; Lebeau, I.; Krečmerová, M.; Andrei, G. & Snoeck, R. Activity of different classes of acyclic nucleoside phosphonates against BK virus in primary human renal cells. *Antimicrobial Agents and Chemotherapy.* Vol. 55, No. 5, (May 2011), pp. 1961-1967, ISSN 0066-4804

Wachsman, M.; Petty, B.G.; Cundy, K.C.; Jaffe, H.S.; Fisher, P.E.; Pastelak, A. & Lietman, P.S. Pharmacokinetics, safety and bioavailability of HPMPC (cidofovir) in human immunodeficiency virus-infected subjects. *Antiviral Research.* Vol. 29, No. 2-3, (March 1996), pp. 153 – 161, ISSN 0166- 3542

Webb, R.R. The bis-trityl route to (*S*)-HPMPA. *Nucleosides & Nucleotides.* Vol. 8, No. 4, (1989), pp. 619-624, ISSN 0732-8311

Webb, R.R., Wos, J.A., Bronson, J.J. & Martin, J.C. Synthesis of (S)-N-(3-hydroxy-2-phosphonylmethoxy)- propylcytosine, (S)-HPMPC. *Tetrahedron Letters.* Vol. 29, No. 43, (1988), pp. 5475-5478, ISSN 0040-4039

Wilkins, P.A.; Papich, M. & Sweeney, R. Pharmacokinetics of acyclovir in adult horses. *Journal of Veterinary Emergency and Critical Care.* Vol. 15, No. 3 (September, 2005), pp. 174-178, ISSN 1479-3261

Yamanishi, K.; Okuno, T.; Shiraki, K.; Takahashi, M.; Kondo, T.; Asano, Y. & Kurata, T. Identification of human herpesvirus-6 as a causal agent for exanthema subitum. *Lancet.* Vol. 1, No. 8594, (May 1988), pp. 1065- 1067, ISSN 0140-6736

12

Evidence-Based Treatment of Postherpetic Neuralgia

Rafael Galvez[1] and Maria Redondo[2]

[1]Pain Unit, Anesthesiology Department, Virgen de las Nieves Hospital, Granada,
[2]General Practitioner, Specialist in Family and Community Medicine, Badajoz,
Spain

1. Introduction

Postherpetic neuralgia (PHN) is the most common and feared complication of herpes zoster (HZ); it is mainly reported among the elderly and is described as painful and refractory. It is a complication rather than a continuation of acute HZ, and is defined as persistent pain in HZ-involved areas that continues for > 3 months after disappearance of the vesicles (Rowbotham & Fields, 1989). It is considered one of the most important neuropathic pains for the reasons set out in table 1.

1. There is an elevated incidence of PHN among the elderly. PHN occurs in 10.20% of all HZ patients but in >50% of elderly HZ patients.
2. Neurosensory lesions frequently have a pain component (Rowbotham &Petersen 2001) - Sensitive: dysesthesia, paresthesia, allodynia… - Motor: paresis, paralysis…
3. There is a high associated comorbidity in previously healthy individuals: loss of nocturnal sleep, loss of appetite, marked functional limitation, and major emotional component, which all impair the long-term quality of life of patients (Jensen et al, 2007)
4. The pain is highly intense and often disproportionate to the initial injury.
5. It is characterized by a high chronicity, although only around 50% of patients developing PHN are moderately symptomatic at 1 year after onset.
6. Diverse pathophysiological mechanisms are involved in the different spontaneous and evoked symptoms in PHN, resulting in: - A very heterogeneous symptomatology that varies between one patient and another. - Symptoms that change over time - Highly complex and difficult treatment, with the need to test and combine different therapies to obtain a satisfactory outcome. - Only partial pain relief
7. These patients consume large amounts of healthcare resources, making PHN an important institutional and public health problem (Gauthier et al, 2009).
8. PHN and diabetic neuropathy (DPN) are the models preferentially selected and required by the FDA and EMA in controlled trials for any drug or technique seeking approval against peripheral neuropathic pain.

Table 1. Clinical relevance of postherpetic neuralgia (Watson & Evans, 1986; Robotham& Fields, 1989; Helgason et al, 2000; Dubinsky et al, 2004; Scholz & Woolf 2007).

Mixed inflammatory and neuropathic pain is experienced in acute HZ, whereas neuropathic pain is highly predominant in PHN and the symptoms persist over time (Rowbotham et al, 2001). The clinical symptoms presented by these patients are very heterogeneous, and some are spontaneous while others are evoked. Spontaneous symptoms frequently include a constant deep and burning pain and an intermittent intense and lancing pain throughout the painful area, leaving it hypersensitive and painful for some minutes. Other disagreeable symptoms are pruritus and painless, but nevertheless disabling, sensations of coldness or numbness (Anne et al, 2005; Treede et al, 2008).

SPONTANEOUS PAIN (due to spontaneous firing of axons or dorsal horn neurons): - Burning, constant pain - Cramping and dysesthesia - Lancing and paroxysmal pain
EVOKED PAIN (due to damage in peripheral and central sensory neurons): - Hyperalgesia (mechanical and thermal) - Allodynia (mechanical and thermal)
OTHER CLASSIC SYMPTOMS: - Positive: hyperhidrosis, pruritus, tic - Negative: hypoesthesia, paresis, paralysis

Table 2. Classic PHN symptomatology

The characteristics of PHN often lead to two well-known situations:

a. Desperation of the affected patients and their relatives.
b. Frustration of the professionals treating it.

As a result, patients complaining of PHN are often referred by primary care centers and emergency departments to the Pain Unit or Neurology and Dermatology specialists in an attempt to seek a definitive solution that cannot, unfortunately, be completely achieved.

Treatments are either partially or totally ineffective for many people with PHN. The development of PHN may be prevented by the antiviral agents used to treat the rash. Once PHN is established, various well-known selection drugs and techniques may alleviate the pain (Dubinsky et al, 2004). The recent appearance of specific evidence-based analgesic guidelines and algorithms for neuropathic pain, including PHN, offers an excellent opportunity to improve pain management in these patients.

2. Background and objectives

Despite the social and public health importance of PHN, there is a wide variability in its routine clinical management by different healthcare professionals. The objective of this chapter was to review and update the different treatments available for PHN in light of the analgesic drugs and techniques that have appeared in this field (especially pharmacological therapy), from the time of its detection and diagnosis in primary care to its treatment in the Pain Unit if not controlled. We also describe current approaches to PHN in the most recent clinical guidelines, according to the available evidence, and offer a practical view of analgesia for the different professionals involved in PHN. No attempt is made to review the available evidence, given the existence of excellent guidelines published in different specialist journals.

3. Analgesic strategy

As with other neuropathic pains, the approach to PHN is complex but always in the pursuit of clear and, when possible, viable objectives (see Table 3), usually shared by the specialist and primary healthcare professional (Dubinsky et al, 2004; Galvez, 2009; Dworking et al, 2010). The majority of PHN patients are initially and sometimes exclusively attended at the level of primary care, which is the entry gate into the health system in many countries and therefore plays a key role in the prevention of PHN. In the case of children, it is the pediatrician who has the possibility to educate parents to vaccinate their children against chickenpox and thereby reduce its incidence, explaining that when this infection reactivates, e.g., in an immunodepressed state, it can produce re-infection by HZ virus, which is the virus that produces chickenpox in children, emphasizing that the severest complication of this re-infection is HZ and subsequently PHN. Since 2008, HZ vaccines have been recommended that can be administered to over-70-year-olds, the age group most susceptible to complications (Anne & Mounsey, 2005; Redondo et al, 2007).

1. To relieve the pain by drugs/techniques with reduced adverse effects that are acceptable to the patient.
2. To recover nocturnal sleep.
3. To reduce symptoms related to hypersensitivity and allodynia by at least 3 points on the 11-point Likert scale.
4. To improve the ability of the patient to deal with the pain.
5. To stabilize the patient's emotional state.

Table 3. Analgesic objectives in PHN

The analgesic strategy is based on the application of the drugs with the strongest scientific evidence on their effectiveness in PHN, but with reduced and tolerable adverse effects. Table 4 contains a summary of this global strategy.

1. Immediate initiation of treatment (PHN worsens with passage of time)
2. Communication of correct information and realistic expectations to the patient
3. Analgesia using drugs with the best evidence on their usefulness in PHN
4. Evidence-based pharmacological therapy as the main approach
5. Active rehabilitation program
6. Educational resources for patients with neuropathic pain
7. Some invasive techniques in certain cases

Table 4. Key points of PHN treatment strategy (Turk &Stieg, 1987; Dubinsky et al, 2004; Argoff et al, 2004; Baron et al, 2010)

Antidepressants (tricyclic antidepressants, …)
Antiepileptics (gabapentinoids, carbamazepine…)
Tramadol and opioids (morphine, oxycodone, methadone...)
Other drugs acting on modifications generated in the synapses of injured neurons (N-methyl-D-aspartate receptor antagonists, etc.)
Topical agents (5% lidocaine patch, capsaicin cream or patch...)
Other drugs (baclofen, mexiletine, clonidine…)
Some techniques: nerve blocks, transcutaneous electrical nerve stimulation, spinal cord stimulation, intrathecal infusion …

Table 5. Main drugs used in PHN

However, despite the ever-expanding therapeutic arsenal of drugs and techniques against PHN (table 5), there is little scientific evidence on the majority of analgesic treatments and they are rarely compared in head-to-head trials (Dubinsky et al, 2004). In fact, analgesic responses are frequently highly disparate, even among patients in similar situations of PHN and treated with identical analgesic regimens, explaining the need to individualize PHN therapy (Papagallo & Haldey, 2003)

Classically, the symptoms and signs of pain in PHN have been treated globally, regardless of the specific clinical symptoms. However, a new approach has been developed over the past decade, which proposes the selective analgesic treatment of the different spontaneous or evoked symptoms that arise (Jensen & Baron 2003; Hanson, 2003). A recent article described six clinical subtypes of neuropathic pain according to the predominant symptoms, each with a different profile and obtained from a sample of 2100 patients with diabetic neuropathy (DPN) or PHN (Arning & Baron, 2009; Baron et al, 2009; Wasner & Baron, 2009; Baron et al, 2010). Treatment may vary as a function of the clinical subtype of neuropathic pain and the symptoms detected. However, considerable research remains to be done before protocols can be established for the treatment of distinct subtypes and symptoms in daily clinical practice.

4. Analgesic pharmacology

Analgesic pharmacotherapy is considered the basis of PHN treatment, and there has been a major strategic change with the proposal of a series of specific drugs for this type of pain. It is recognized by the scientific community that the classic Analgesic Ladder of the WHO, based on the use of analgesics as a function of pain intensity, does not adequately address PHN pain or other types of peripheral neuropathic pain which do not respond satisfactorily to therapy with classic analgesics (non-steroidal anti-inflammatory drugs [NSAIDs] and opioids). There is a need to evaluate other drugs considered as basic analgesic pillars in PHN, including antiepileptics, certain antidepressants, and one or other opioid that has evidenced analgesic effectiveness in this type of neuropathic pain (McCleane, 2004; Dubinsky, 2004; Backonja et al, 2006; Jensen et al, 2009; Martinez-Salio et al, 2009). It has been proposed that the analgesic management ladder (figure 1) for peripheral neuropathic pain (e.g., PHN) would include the reference analgesic drugs cited above, unlike those established in the classic WHO ladder (Galvez et al, 2006; Galvez et al, 2007).

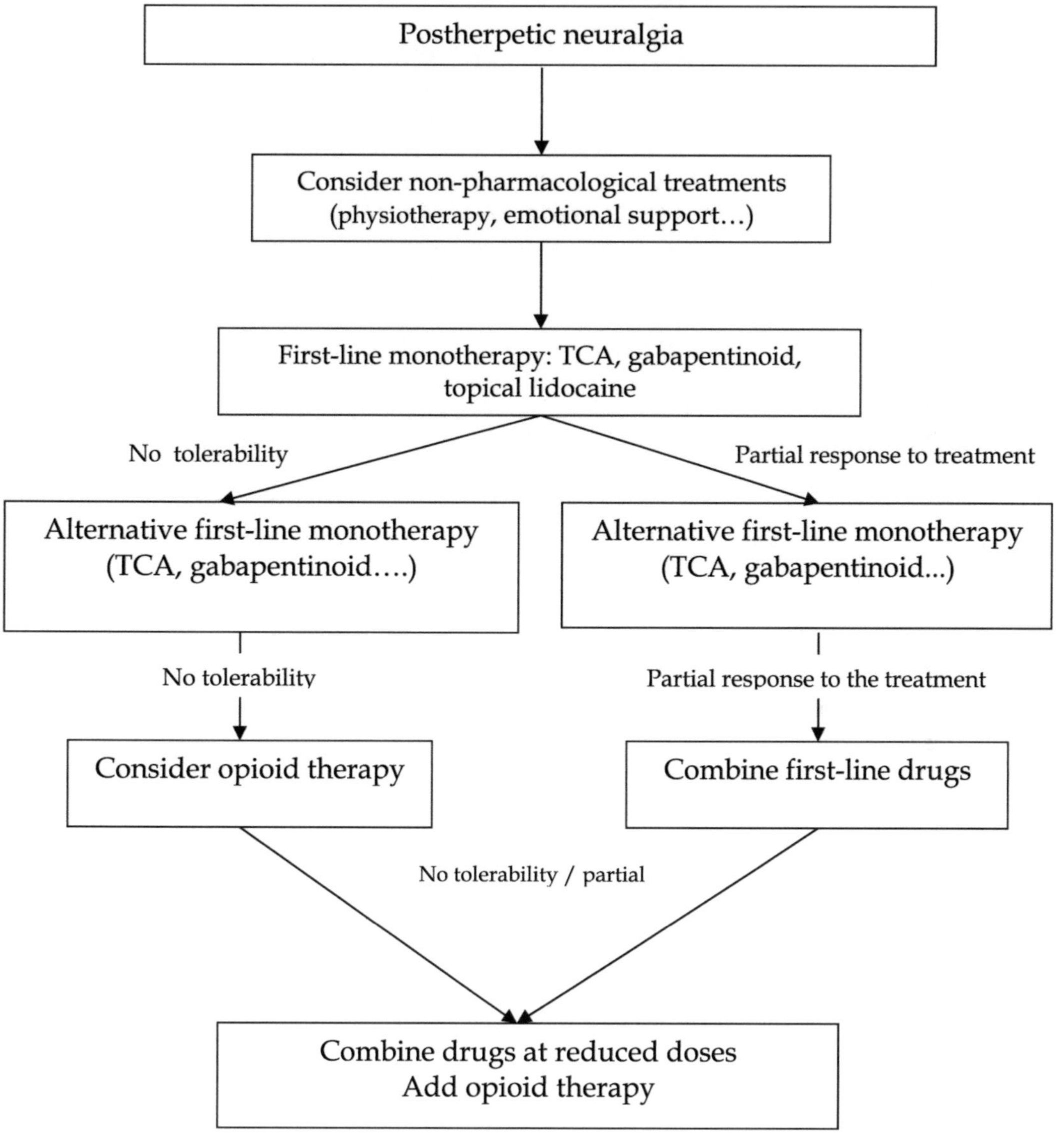

Fig. 1. Proposed Algorithm for PHN

The first step of the new ladder for neuropathic pain calls for certain antiepileptic drugs (AEDs), such as gabapentinoids (gabapentin or pregabalin), and some antidepressants, such as tricyclic antidepressants (TCAs) or serotonin and norepinephrine reuptake inhibitors (SNRIs), e.g., venlafaxine and duloxetine. Some topical treatments, such as lidocaine or capsaicin patches, can be considered. Opioids like oxycodone or tramadol have demonstrated effectiveness in neuropathic pain but are on the second or third step of the ladder due to their adverse effects. If the pain is not alleviated, the second step is the combination of first-step drugs with tramadol. On the third step, the first-step drugs are maintained and combined with potent opiates (morphine, oxycodone, methadone, fentanyl transdermal, or buprenorphine transdermal) (Gilron et al, 2005). Nerve blocks or transcutaneous electrical nerve stimulation (TENS) can be useful at any point. If these drugs and techniques fail, patients must be referred to more specialized departments, e.g., the Pain Unit or Neurosurgery, for more invasive techniques such as Dorsal Root Entry Zone (DREZ), Spinal Cord Stimulation (SCS), or spinal infusions.

1st STEP	2nd STEP	3red STEP
TCAs, SNRIs GABAPENTINOID TOPICAL AGENTS Lidocaine or capsaicin patches	COMBINATION OF 1st STEP DRUGS + TRAMADOL	COMBINATION OF 1st STEP DRUGS + POTENT OPIOID

Fig. 2. Neuropathic Pain Analgesic Ladder

5. Antidepressants

For more than 30 years, antidepressants have played an important role in the treatment of chronic pain. The most widely known and used drugs have been TCAs (amitriptyline, imipramine, chlorimipramine, and desipramine) (Mc Quay et al, 1996). TCAs have a proven analgesic effect in neuropathic pain that is independent of their effect on the state of mind, with reports that the analgesic effect appears before the antidepressant effect and that a lower dose is required for analgesia than for the treatment of depression (Mc Quay et al, 1996; Saarto & Wifen 2005). TCAs have different action mechanisms with primarily analgesic effects. The main mechanism is the modulation of neurotransmitters by inhibiting the reuptake of serotonin (5HT) and noradrenaline (NA) at presynaptic level, increasing their bioavailability. NA and 5HT are involved in modulating pathways mediated by endorphins at both central nervous system (CNS) and spinal cord level. There is also evidence that they antagonize N-methyl-D-aspartate (NMDA) receptors and block muscarinic, cholinergic, histamine H1, and alpha-adrenergic receptors, which may participate in the modulation of the nociceptive response. TCAs also act on sodium channels in neuronal tissue, thereby stabilizing peripheral nerves and modulating the hyperexcitability of neurons at CNS level.

As already noted, PHN is a major cause of chronic pain among the elderly, in whom TCAs have also been traditionally used. Meta-analysis of TCA trials for this indication found that they are able to significantly relieve pain in PHN (Watson et al, 1982; Mc Quay et al, 1996; Saarto & Wifen 2005; Sindrup et al, 2005). Amitriptyline has proven effective as an analgesic

and is the most widely used drug with the best outcomes. In a recent controlled trial, nortriptyline showed practically the same efficacy as opioids in PHN (Raja et al, 2002).
The adverse effects of TCAs are largely related to their anticholinergic action: dryness of the mouth, constipation, urinary retention, and tachycardia. The blocking of alpha-1 adrenergic receptors can produce orthostatic hypotension, and the blocking of histamine receptors is associated with sedation and weight gain. All of these adverse effects can be minimized by slow titrations. The adverse effect that causes greatest concern is the alteration of cardiac conduction (through inhibition of noradrenalin reuptake). The response is dose-dependent, and it is recommended to start treatment at low doses (10 mg in over 65-year-olds and 25 mg in others) before bedtime and to titrate the dose very slowly according to the clinical response, without exceeding 75 mg/day. TCAs have a lower NNT (number needed to treat) value in comparison to other analgesic drugs in neuropathic pain and are attributed with the best evidence in clinical guidelines. Amitriptyline has an NNT of 2.2 for PHN, but its adverse effects, lack of recommendation in the elderly, and the small sample size of studies have relegated it behind antiepileptics for certain PHN cases (Saarto & Wifen 2005; Dworking et al, 2007). Nortriptyline, maprotiline, and desipramine have also proven effective, but less so than amitriptyline.
The SNRIs duloxetine and venlafaxine are efficacious in painful polyneuropathy but have not been studied in PHN. Selective serotonin reuptake inhibitors (SSRIs) have shown little effectiveness in neuropathic pain and practically none in PHN (McQuay et al, 1996; Saarto & Wifen 2005).

5.1 Conclusions

TCAs have shown lower NNT values in comparison to other drugs against PHN. Amitriptyline has demonstrated the strongest evidence on effectiveness. Other non-tricyclic antidepressants have shown no evidence of efficacy in PHN.

6. Anticonvulsant drugs (AEDs)

AEDs or anticonvulsants have been used in pain management since the 1960s and represent a very important therapeutic option in chronic neuropathic pain, especially when this is lancing or burning. Since the initial use of carbamazepine, a new generation of antiepileptic drugs have been incorporated into clinical practice (>40 controlled trials) with characteristics that distinguish them from the classical drugs, including greater tolerability, fewer pharmacological interactions, and novel action mechanisms (Robotham et al, 1998; Rice et al 2001; Dworking et al, 2003; Sabatowsky et al, 2004; Van Seventer et al, 2006). A Cochrane meta-analysis (Wifen et al, 2005) yielded significant evidence to support the efficacy of AEDs in the treatment of PHN, especially calcium channel $\alpha 2$-δ ligands (gabapentin and pregabalin) (Wifen et al, 2005; Gilron et al, 2011). The results evidenced their effectiveness, highlighting the use of pregabalin and later gabapentin in PHN treatment. There have only been small observational studies on carbamazepine in PHN, with no controlled trials.
AEDs took their place as analgesics in neuropathic pain, which is accompanied by hyperexcitability and lancing pains suggestive of a somatosensory lesion. Although the action mechanism differs among AEDs and is not fully understood, it is known that they can alter pathophysiological mechanisms implicated in the genesis and/or maintenance of neuropathic pain, primarily by stabilizing the neuronal membrane and reducing the number of repetitive discharges in nerves lesioned by different mechanisms (Tremont-Lukats et al, 2000).

Structurally, gabapentin is analogous to gamma-aminobutyric acid (GABA) but does not interact with its receptors. Its action mechanism has not been fully elucidated but appears to be related to specific alpha-2-delta subunits of calcium channels. Pregabalin, which appeared after gabapentin, is a GABA analog but does not bind to the receptor or develop GABAergic activity, and its action mechanism, although not completely understood, is also based on its capacity to bind to the alpha-2-delta protein subunit of voltage-dependent calcium channels. In PHN, effective doses range between 1200 and 2400 mg/day for gabapentin but between only 220 and 600 mg/day for pregabalin. Their adverse effects are observed in more than 30% of patients and are related to the CNS, notably somnolence, vertigo and the loss of concentration, which are closely linked to the speed of dose titration and sensitivity of the patient. As a result, around 15-30% of patients cannot tolerate these drugs and abandon treatment (Dworking et al, 2007; Jensen et al, 2009).

6.1 Conclusions

There is good-quality evidence that gabapentinoids are the most effective antiepileptic drugs in PHN. Pregabalin is somewhat more effective than gabapentin. A slow titration is necessary to reduce adverse effects.

7. Opioids

Since the editorial by Dubner in *Pain* at the beginning of the 1990s (Dubner, 1991), evidence has begun to emerge on the use of opioids to treat neuropathic pain. The first systematic Cochrane review appeared in 1999 (Dellemin et al, 1999), followed by a meta-analysis in 2006 that included 23 clinical trials and clearly evidenced the efficacy of opioids in neuropathic pain (Eisenberg et al, 2006).

Opioid analgesics are agonists of presynaptic and postsynaptic opioid receptors. Their efficacy has been reported in several randomized controlled trials in different peripheral neuropathic pain disorders. Their effectiveness is probably lower for certain symptoms, such as thermal hyperalgesia and allodynia, due to the involvement of fibers with no opioid receptors. The same may be true for static mechanical allodynia and hyperalgesia (Dickenson AH et al, 2005; Trescot AM et al, 2008; Besson M et al, 2008).

In more recent reviews, morphine, oxycodone, and methadone have demonstrated a similar effectiveness to that of TCAs in PHN, but opioids are relegated to the second analgesic line due to their possible adverse effects (Watson et al, 1998; Przewlocki et al, 2005). The most recent studies have been on oxycodone in PHN and DPN, showing an acceptable effectiveness. Combined gabapentin and morphine was very useful in neuropathic cancer pain (Keskinbora et al, 2007).

Tramadol exerts a weak opiate effect on mu receptors in comparison to opioids and a weak monoaminergic effect in comparison to TCAs and AEDs. However, the adverse effect profile of tramadol is more acceptable than that of TCAs and AEDs, and tolerance and dependence complications are uncommon. Tramadol has demonstrated effectiveness but in studies offering low-quality evidence (Boureau et al, 2003). Its administration starts with an oral dose of 12.5-25 mg every 6 or 8 hours, with rescue doses of the same amount remaining available until the pain is controlled and then passing to sustained formulations up to a maximum recommended dose of 400 mg/day (Hollingshead et al,2006; Eisemberg et al, 2006).

7.1 Conclusions

These drugs have an effect on neuropathic pain but are not considered first-line drugs due to issues around dependence, cognitive impairment, tolerance, and possible hormonal problems.

8. Topical drugs

The ease and effectiveness of topical applications have led to the increasing introduction of topical drugs with local analgesic effects. However, despite the thinness of skin, only drugs with certain characteristics are able to pass through it, limiting the use of this administration route. Topical drugs can be in cream, ointment, lotion, spray, or patch form. Topical analgesics provide pain relief with minimal risk of systemic toxicity or drug-drug interactions, because they are formulated to produce a local effect while avoiding high plasma concentrations and adverse systemic events. Among patients with PHN, especially those with peripheral symptoms, various topical agents have proven effective and represent a viable treatment option. Topical treatment also offers a therapeutic approach to patients in whom systemic treatment is contraindicated.

9. Lidocaine

The analgesic effectiveness of topical local anesthetics has long been known, based on the direct binding of the local anesthesia with anomalous sodium channels of skin nerve endings (which participate in the maintenance of both spontaneous and evoked neuropathic pain), blocking them and thereby stabilizing the neuronal membrane and the production of ectopic discharges (Robotham, 1995). The first drug to be used was EMLA cream, a mixture of lidocaine and prilocaine, which had already shown some effectiveness in some PHN patients (Wheeler JG 1991; Stow, 1989). Subsequently, after a report on the usefulness of 5% lidocaine-medicated plaster (LMP) in PHN (Robotham, 1996; Galer et al, 1999) as a new topical treatment and its FDA approval for PHN pain in 1999, multiple studies evaluated this therapy. In 2007, the Cochrane Library produced a review (Khalick, 2007) of three articles on lidocaine treatment of PHN, although two of these were on lidocaine gel and only one used 5% LMP. The authors of the review concluded that there was inadequate evidence to recommend 5% LMP as a first-line analgesic against PHN.

A new exhaustive review of articles on 5% LMP (up to May 2010) was recently published, comparing its effects in PHN with those of other therapies or placebo (Wolff, 2011). Out of 2417 references, it included 32 articles reporting on 20 studies on 5% LMP. Patches (10 x 14 cm) containing 700 mg lidocaine each were daily placed for a maximum of 12 hours and then removed, generally using 3 or sometimes 4 patches simultaneously to cover the painful area. The 5% LMP patch showed effectiveness *versus* placebo, especially for allodynia, one of the most important and disagreeable symptoms in PHN. Pain relief was achieved, and there were no cases of anesthesia or loss of cutaneous sensitivity Comparison between 5% LMP and pregabalin showed them to have the same efficacy for pain relief, while 5% LMP had a greater positive effect on almost all quality of life dimensions (in the SF-36 survey), with much lower adverse effects, and received a higher overall rating by patients. In the meta-analysis, only gabapentin and 5% LMP produced a reduction in baseline pain (on VAS scale) in comparison to placebo, and this reduction was larger with 5% LMP. Pain relief was greater with gabapentin or 5% LMP than with capsaicin or pregabalin. Topical lidocaine in

patients with various localized peripheral neuropathic pain syndromes had a good NNT, leading to the recommendation of lidocaine plaster for PHN patients (Woolf 2011).
All articles reported the good tolerability and low (< 3%) systemic absorption of lidocaine (Davies, 2004), with the consequent scarcity of adverse systemic reactions. Patients receiving pregabalin reported dizziness, somnolence, and tiredness whereas the only effect in those treated with 5% LMP was local irritation and mild erythema (in 6-28% of cases). The dropout from treatment was also more frequent among pregabalin-treated patients. The review by Woolf noted various major limitations in studies, primarily the small sample sizes in most reports and the short treatment duration, which was usually 4 weeks. A further limitation was the scarcity of studies directly comparing 5% LMP with other drugs, so that comparisons had to be indirect (Liedgens et al, 2008). There was only one head-to-head study, comparing 5% LMP and pregabalin (Baron 2009; Rehm 2010). Comparative economic analysis of six-month courses of 5% LMP, gabapentin, and pregabalin found 5% LMP to be the most cost-effective treatment (Dakin et al, 2007); moreover, these authors concluded that the good tolerability and efficacy of 5% LMP places it as first-line topical analgesic treatment in PHN. In this sense, another economic study has ended favourable toward 5% LMP (Ritchie et al, 2010).

9.1 Conclusions

Lidocaine has demonstrated high analgesic effectiveness in PNH, especially in the form of 5% patches, and is indicated as first-line drug for the treatment of localized pain.

10. Capsaicin

Capsaicin is an alkaloid substance of natural origin and is the main chemical compound (70%) in capsaicinoids, which include more than 90 varieties of chili. Capsaicin is a selective agonist of transient receptor potential vanilloid type 1 (TRPV1), preferentially bound to small-diameter amyelinic nociceptive nerve fibers such as C fibers, capable of synthesizing and releasing primarily substance P and other excitatory neurotransmitters (Green 1988; Bjerring 1989). The topical application of capsaicin initially activates C-fiber nociceptors by depolarization of the neuronal membrane and alteration of calcium and sodium ions, producing an initial erythematous sensation and skin reddening. However, if this contact with capsaicin is maintained, it leads to a transient and reversible desensitization and degradation of TRPV1-expressing cutaneous nerve endings, without altering other sensations (Nolano 1999; Szolcsany 2004).
The cream started to be applied at low capsaicin concentrations (0.025% and 0.075%) several times a day, obtaining pain relief, although; h moderate and short-lived, as well as producing local discomfort, occasionally refractory, which sometimes led to the suspension of the treatment (Berstein et al, 1989; Peikert et al, 1991; Watson et al, 1993). A high-concentration (8%) capsaicin dermal patch (179 mg capsaicin; 280 cm^2) was recently introduced, which is applied for 60 minutes in the peripheral pain area after its treatment with topical local anesthesia to avoid the initial burning pain. The relief obtained persists for around 12 weeks. One week after exposure to the 8% capsaicin patch there was also an 80% reduction in the density of the majority of epidermal nerve fibers (ENFs) in treated areas compared to untreated areas of healthy volunteers. It has been demonstrated that reinnervation practically returns to normality at 224 weeks after patch application (Kennedy 2010). These data support its topical utilization for different symptoms related to peripheral neuropathic pain.

In 2009, a Cochrane review was conducted of randomized, double blind placebo-controlled studies of at least six weeks duration in which topical capsaicin was used to treat neuropathic pain (Derry et al, 2009). Six studies (389 participants in total) compared the regular application of low-dose (0.075%) capsaicin cream with placebo cream, reporting a very good NNT for any pain relief. Two initial studies (709 participants in total) compared a single application of 8% capsaicin patch with placebo patch, finding a good NNT for < 30% pain relief over 12 weeks. The authors concluded that capsaicin may provide a degree of pain relief to some patients with painful neuropathic conditions, either through the repeated application of a low-dose (0.075%) cream or the single application of a high-dose (8%) patch. Earlier studies with repeated applications of low-dose capsaicin have not convincingly demonstrated good efficacy, while the single application of an 8% capsaicin patch has emerged as a new strategy.

Jones et al in 2011 reviewed the evidence on the 8% capsaicin patch in PHN pain, finding that its topical application decreased pain linked to TPRV1 receptors and transiently reduced the number of nociceptive nerve endings at the application site. Their review was based on two pivotal studies in which the 8% patch was compared with 0.04% capsaicin. The primary endpoint of both trials was the reduction in numerical pain rating scale (NPRS) score. The 8% capsaicin patch reduced the pain from baseline to weeks 2-8 (by 29.6% and 32%), a significantly greater reduction ($P \leq 0.01$) than found in 0.04% capsaicin-treated controls to weeks 2-8 (19.9% and 24.4%). At the end of week 12, the reduction in pain was more pronounced ($P \leq 0.03$) in the 8% capsaicin group (by 29.9% and 32.3%) than in the controls (by 20.4% and 25%). Around 40% of all treated patients were responders, considered an acceptable proportion in controlled trials of other analgesics in neuropathic pain. Applications of 8% patch can be repeated a maximum of once every 3 months, as needed. In conclusion, the author concluded that one 8% capsaicin patch every 3 months offers acceptable efficacy in comparison to other PHN treatments requiring daily doses.

With regard to safety, the systemic absorption is low, and drug interactions are not expected, with virtually no systemic repercussions. All remains of capsaicin metabolites have practically disappeared at 6 hours after removing the capsaicin patch (Babbar et al, 2010; Irving et al, 2010). The only adverse effect is a mild increase in blood pressure in some patients during application of the 8% patch. There have also been reports of eye and airway irritation due to aerosolization of capsaicin during patch removal or inhalation of the dried cream (Rains et al, 1995). The most common adverse drug reactions with capsaicin are at the application site, with burning reported by 60% of patients using 0.075% capsaicin cream (Dubinsky 2004) and mild or moderate erythema (63%) and burning pain (42%) described by 63% and 42% of patients, respectively, at the 8% capsaicin patch site. It is often necessary to administer analgesics or local cold during the first 24-72 hours after patch application.

Withdrawals due to adverse events were nearly all due to skin reactions. In two single-dose studies, 37 patients (15%) withdrew out of 242 patients receiving 0.075% capsaicin cream, whereas only three patients (0.7%) had to cease treatment out of 430 patients receiving 8% capsaicin patches. Withdrawals were more frequent with repeated low-dose capsaicin applications than with a single high-dose patch application (Derry et al, 2009).

A 48-week study was conducted to test the long-term efficacy and tolerability of the 8% capsaicin patch (Backjonja et al, 2010), finding virtually no changes in analgesic efficacy over the passage of time and no increase in treatment dropout or topical adverse effects.

Another recent study indirectly compared the cost-effectiveness of 8% capsaicin patch with that of other PNH treatments (Angstrom et al, 2011), evaluating the analgesic improvement, adverse effects, and cost per quality-adjusted life-year (QALY) of the treatments. It reported that the 8% capsaicin patch and topical lidocaine patch were significantly more effective in comparison to oral agents used to treat PHN. The cost-effectiveness and cost per QALY of the 8% capsaicin patch were similar to those of the lidocaine patch and superior to those of the oral products.

10.1 Conclusions

The 8% capsaicin patch is effective to reduce PHN pain, and its usefulness is supported by stronger evidence in comparison to other topical agents. Studies have demonstrated some benefit from the use of 0.075% capsaicin cream in PHN.

11. Other topical drugs

Other trials of topical drugs in PHN have not yielded noteworthy results. A crossover trial of single doses of indomethacin, aspirin, and diclofenac in solutions with diethyl-ether against placebo (Beneditti, 1996) found that solutions prepared with aspirin and indomethacin were effective in PHN, but not those with diclofenac. However, the data were inadequate for conclusions to be reached.

A double-blind multiple-dose cross-over study comparing 3% benzydamine cream with placebo in PHN treatment (Mc Quay et al, 1990) found no significant differences, which the authors attributed to the short treatment periods studied.

12. Other modalities for PHN

Interventional treatment is indicated when the pharmacological treatment is not effective or cannot be tolerated by the patient. It can also be considered in patients who need continued high-dose treatment to control the pain and may prefer an invasive or surgical approach.

In a randomized, controlled, single-blind study, four weekly injections of 60 mg of preservative-free methylprednisolone were administered intrathecally or into the epidural space in PHN patients. There was a substantial benefit for the intrathecal group at 1 and 24 weeks after completion of the treatment, with a good NNT, but no improvement was observed in the epidural group. In a double-blind, randomized, controlled clinical trial, 277 patients with PHN were randomized for the intrathecal administration of 60 mg of preservative-free methylprednisolone in 3 ml of 3% lidocaine, or 3 mL of 3% lidocaine alone, or no lumbar puncture. In the methylprednisolone group, 90% of the patients reported good to excellent pain relief at the end of the treatment, which continued during 2 years of follow-up. No adverse events were reported during the 2-year follow-up period (Kikuchi et al, 1999; Kotani et al, 2000).

The aim of neuromodulation treatments of pain is to use minimally invasive and reversible techniques that can be modified as a function of changes in patient symptoms. Implantable systems with opioids or ziconotide are used in patients with refractory pain (Cruccu et al, 2007; Deer et al, 2007), but there is scant evidence on their use in PHN patients.

Electricity has been used to relieve pain for thousands of years. TENS, defined by the American Physical Therapy Association as the application of electrical stimulation to the skin for pain control, is non-invasive, inexpensive, safe, and easy to use. TENS has multiple indications and has demonstrated some efficacy in PHN (Nonahan &Kumbang 2008; Cruccu et al, 2007). However, the scientific evidence on its use in PHN is limited and does not allow definitive recommendations to be made (McQuay H, et al, 1998). For its part, the usefulness of spinal cord stimulation has not been supported by a randomized controlled trial (Benzon et al, 2009)

13. Clinical guidelines for PHN treatment

Over the past decade, numerous European and American guidelines on neuropathic pain have emerged. Most of them are specific to peripheral neuropathic pain (e.g., PHN) but their preparation has been difficult because almost all of the studies only offer comparisons with placebo and were conducted in small samples of patients for short time periods, despite the chronicity of the disease (Feder et al, 99). There is also a shortage of data on long-term outcomes and on the usefulness of combining different drugs. Methodological limitations include the retrospective calculation of data from studies with different experimental designs and results. Taking this into account, most of the proposals for the treatment of neuropathic pain are based on cost-effectiveness estimations using indirect indicators such as the NNT (number needed to treat to obtain 50% pain relief in one patient) and NNH (number of patients needed for harm, i.e., for withdrawal of one patient from the study due to adverse effects), positively rating treatments with a low NNT and high NNH. Table 6 provides a global summary of the analgesic evidence.

a. Finnerup established an algorithm for peripheral neuropathic pain (including PHN) in 2005 (Finnerup et al, 2005) and published a revised version in 2007 (Finnerup et al, 2007), based on the available evidence and with many limitations. However, it served as a guide for analgesic treatment in neuropathic pain. They reviewed 105 randomized clinical trials against placebo that were considered to offer high-quality evidence, gathered by a search of Medline, EMBASE and the Cochrane Database, taking the NNT and NNH as reference. Studies of oncologic neuropathic pain and those with a sample of < 10 patients were excluded.
b. Recommendations:
- Based on the results of these studies, the authors recommend that localized pain in PHN be treated by the topical administration of the 5% lidocaine patch. When the pain is more widespread, they recommend initiating monotherapy with TCAs or gabapentinoids (oral gabapentin oral or pregabalin) as first-line analgesics.
- Second-line drugs are the new SNRIs, such as venlafaxine and especially duloxetine, although the studies have been in peripheral neuropathic pain.
- Opioids, including tramadol, can be considered as third-line options because they have an effect on neuropathic pain, but they are associated with dependency, tolerance, cognitive impairment, and even long-term hormonal disorders.

c. In 2006 (Attal et al, 2006), a group of experts in neuropathic pain from the EFNS published guidelines on the pharmacological management of neuropathic pain according to the quality of evidence in studies available in Medline or the Cochrane Database. They only analyzed controlled trials (from 1966 to 2006) considered class I or II trials according to the EFNS classification, using the NNT value as reference. They mainly took account of the drugs' analgesic efficacy to reduce the signs and symptoms of neuropathic pain and of their adverse effects, but they also considered the repercussions on the quality of life and state of mind of the patient.

d. Recommendations in PHN:
- First-line analgesics: TCAs, pregabalin, and gabapentin, with grade A evidence.
- Second-line: SNRIs (e.g., duloxetine and venlafaxine), although their effectiveness and lesser adverse effects in comparison to TCAs mean that the new SNRI antidepressants are often prioritized.
- Lower-quality evidence is available for opioids (tramadol and oxycodone) and lamotrigine.
- When the pain relief is inadequate, they proposed using combinations of first-line drugs that do not interact and have complementary action mechanisms, despite the scant scientific evidence on this approach, and as a last resort, combinations with opioids.

e. In 2007 (Moulin et al, 2007), the Canadian Pain Society published evidence-based guidelines on the clinical management of neuropathic pain, directed at Canadian healthcare professionals. The main treatment lines and a concise management algorithm were included. They only considered well-designed controlled clinical trials against a placebo or effective substance with a minimum of 10 patients, gathered from Medline and the Cochrane Database. Recommendations were based on four criteria: analgesic efficacy with at least grade 1B evidence, tolerability, ease of management, and cost-effectiveness.

f. Recommendations for PHN:
- First-line analgesics: TCAs (amitriptyline and imipramine) or antiepileptics (gabapentin and pregabalin). If the drug fails or cannot be tolerated, it is recommended to try another from the same group.
- Second-line: SNRIs (e.g., venlafaxine and duloxetine) due to the weaker evidence and their higher cost. Lidocaine patches.
- Third-line: opioids such as tramadol and oxycodone for moderate or intense pain.
- Fourth-line: cannabinoids, methadone, SSRIs and other AEDs.
- Non-pharmacological procedures, such as physiotherapy, moderate exercise and psychological support are recommended alongside the different drugs.

g. A group of neuropathic pain experts from the IASP (Dworking et al, 2007) provided an evidence-based update on recommendations for neuropathic pain management. They reviewed articles (from 1966 to 2007) in Medline and the Cochrane Database on controlled clinical trials (grade 1b evidence or higher) as well as relevant book chapters and other publications. They highlighted the lack of head-to-head studies of the drugs, making it difficult to clearly establish their relative efficacy or safety. The main criteria applied for establishing recommendations were: degree of efficacy of the drug in neuropathic pain, its safety and tolerability, drug-drug interactions, ease of management, impact on patient quality of life, improvement in comorbidities associated with neuropathic pain (sleep, anxiety, etc.), costs associated with the therapy, the potential risk of abuse and addiction, and the risk of overdose.

Recommendations:
- First-line: TCAs, SNRIs (duloxetine and venlafaxine), calcium channel alpha2delta ligands (pregabalin and gabapentin), and topical lidocaine.
- Second-line: opioids (morphine, oxycodone, methadone) and tramadol, based on trials with grade A evidence, the clinical experience of the experts, and guidelines on the management of opioids in non-oncologic pain, although it can be considered as first-line treatment in certain circumstances (more intense pain or during titration of other drugs).

- Third-line: capsaicin, mexiletine, or NMDA receptor antagonists, based on controlled trials with grade B evidence alongside the clinical experience of the experts, although these drugs can be used as first-line treatment in certain specific situations.
- For non-responding patients, they recommended trying combinations among first-line drugs with different action methods or even with a third-line drug, although there is scant evidence on these strategies.

h. In 2009 (Attal et al,2009), the group of experts in neuropathic pain of the EFNS again published an update, using Medline and the Cochrane Database and classifying trials according to the etiology. All class I and II randomized controlled trials were considered.

Recommendations

- First-line: TCAs (amitriptyline or imipramine 25-150mg/day), pregabalin (150-600 mg/day), and gabapentin (1200-3600 mg/day), supported by the strongest evidence. As topical analgesics, 5% lidocaine patch (maximum of 3 patches at a time, with special indication in the elderly) and 8% capsaicin patch.
- Second- or third-line: 0.075% capsaicin cream and valproate, with weaker supporting evidence. Opioids such as morphine, oxycodone, or methadone and tramadol (200-400 mg/day), with good evidence in PHN but in 2nd or 3rd line due to their adverse effects.
- When first-line treatments fail, combinations are recommended, despite the little evidence available. The association of morphine with gabapentin has shown some effectiveness in PHN.

DRUG	N N T
1. TCAs (tricyclic antidepressants)	2.8 (2.2-3.8) Amitriptyline (better evidence)
2. SNRIs	N D
3. Gabapentin	3.8 (3.1-5.1),
4. Pregabalin	3.7 (3.2-4.4),
5. Opioids	2.6 (1.9-4.1) Oxycodone (better evidence)
6. Tramadol	4.8 (2.6-27)
7. NMDA antagonists	N E
8. 5% Lidocaine patch	UK
9. 8% Capsaicin patch	UK
10. Capsaicin cream	3.2 (2.2-5.9)

ND: No data available; NE: No efficacy in PHN; UK: Unknown

Table 6. NNT of pharmacological therapies in PHN (Dubinsky et al, 2004; Argoff et al, 2004; Finnerup et al, 2007; Attal et al, 2010; Baron et al, 2010)

14. Conclusions (Hemperstal 2005; Baron, 2010; Dubinsky et al, 2004; O´Connor et al, 2009)

1. A multidisciplinary approach is needed, using pharmacological and non-pharmacological treatments.
2. The optimum individual pharmacological regimen in PHN should balance analgesia with harm in terms of side-effects, comorbidities, and drug interactions.
3. Drugs providing the greatest pain relief with fewest side-effects should be identified.
4. Drugs with strongest evidence as first-line analgesics should be used. TCAs (amitriptyline, imipramine), calcium channel α2-δ ligands (gabapentin, pregabalin), topical 5% lidocaine patch, and topical 8% capsaicin patch have shown consistent efficacy in randomized controlled clinical trials and meta-analyses in PHN (Table 6). Figure 1.
5. Some opioid analgesics and tramadol may be indicated if there is no response to other drugs. Despite the evidence on their efficacy, they are relegated to the second-line due to the possible adverse effects. They can only be considered as first-line treatment in certain circumstances (severe pain or poor tolerability of first-line drugs).
6. Topical agents may be first-line in PHN patients who are elderly or with the presence of multiple diseases, despite weak evidence.
7. There is no evidence-based treatment of PHN with NSAIDs.
8. In clinical practice, a combination of two or more drugs is often needed to achieve satisfactory pain relief, although there have been few trials to support this clinical observation. Regular assessment is mandatory.

15. References

[1] Anne L, Mounsey MD, Leah G, Matthew MD, David C, Slawson MD (2005). Herpes Zoster and Postherpetic Neuralgia: Prevention and Management. *Am Fam Physician*.1075:1080-82 ISSN 1745-509X. PMID:16190505 [PubMed - indexed for MEDLINE]

[2] Argoff, CE, Katz, N, Backonja M. (2004) Postherpetic Neuralgia. J *Pain Symptom Manag* 28:396–411. ISSN 1531-3433.

[3] Armstrong, E.; Malone, D.; McCarberg, B.; Panarites, Ch.; Pham, S.; Armstrong, E.P.; Malone, D.C.; Panarites, C.J.; Pham, S.V.(2011). Cost-effectiveness analysis of a new 8% capsaicin patch compared to existing therapies for postherpetic neuralgia. *Current Medical Research and Opinion* 27(5): 939-950.ISSN 0300-7995

[4] Arning K, Baron R. (2009) Evaluation of symptom heterogeneity in neuropathic pain using assessments of sensory functions. *Neurotherapeutics* 6: 738–48. ISSN:1933-7213, OCLC: 71782307

[5] Attal N, Cruccu G, Haanpää M, Hansson P, Jensen TJ, Nurmikko T et al. (2006) EFNS guidelines on pharmacological treatment of neuropathic pain. *Eur J Neu* Nov; 13 (11): 1153-69._ISSN: 1136-9450. DEPÓSITO LEGAL: M-4580-1996

[6] Attal N, Cruccu G, Baron R, Haanpa¨a M, Hansson P, Jensen TJ, and Nurmikko T. (2010)EFNS guidelines on the pharmacological treatment of neuropathic pain: 2009

revision. *European Journal of Neurology* Online Library. DOI: 10.1111/j.1468-1331.2010.02999.

[7] Babbar S, Marier JF, Mouksassi MS, et al. (2009) Pharmacokinetic analysis of capsaicin after topical administration of a highconcentration capsaicin patch to patients with peripheral neuropathic pain. *Ther Drug Monit.* 31:502–510. DOI: 10.1097/FTD.0b013e3181a8b200 PMID: 19494795

[8] Backonja M.M, Irving G, Argoff C. (2006) Rational multidrug therapy in the treatment of neuropathic pain. *Curr Pain Head Reports* 10: 34-8. REVIEW PMID: 16499828 [PubMed - indexed for MEDLINE]

[9] Backonja M.M.; Malan TP; Vanhove, GF.; Tobias, J. (2010) NGX-4010, a High-Concentration Capsaicin Patch, for the Treatment of Postherpetic Neuralgia: a randomized, doble-blind, controlled study with an opel label extension. *Pain Medicine* 11(4):600-608. PMID:20113411 [PubMed - indexed for MEDLINE]

[10] Baron R, Tolle TR, Gockel U, Brosz M, Freynhagen R. (2009). A cross-sectional cohort survey in 2100 patients with painful diabetic neuropathy and postherpetic neuralgia: differences in demographic data and sensory symptoms. Pain 146: 34–40. PMID: 19592166 [PubMed - indexed for MEDLINE]

[11] Baron R, Mayoral V, Leijon G, Binder A, Steigerwald I, Serpell M. (2009) Efficacy and safety of 5% lidocaine (lignocaine) medicated plaster in comparison with pregabalin in patients with postherpetic neuralgia and diabetic polyneuropathy.Interim analysis from an open-label, two-stageadaptive, randomized, controlled trial. Clin *Drug Investig* 29:231–41. www.ncbi.nlm.nih.gov/pubmed/19301937 doi: 10.2165/00044011-200929040-00002

[12] Baron R, Binden A, Wasner G. (2010) Neuropathic pain: diagnosis, pathophysiological mechanisms and treatment. *Lancet Neurol* 9:807-19. Print ISSN: 1060-0280; Online ISSN: 1542-6270…

[13] Benzon HT, Chekka K, Darnule A, Chung B, Wille O, Malik K. (2009) Evidence-based case report: the prevention and management of postherpetic neuralgia with emphasis on interventional procedures. *Reg Anesth Pain Med.* Sep-Oct; 34(5):514-21. Review PubMed PMID: 19920429

[14] Bernstein JE, Korman NJ, Bickers DR, Dahl MV, Millikan LE. (1989) Topical capsaicin treatment of chronic postherpetic neuralgia. *J Am Acad Dermatol.* Aug; 21(2 Pt 1):265-70. PMID: 2768576. [PubMed - indexed for MEDLINE]

[15] Besson M, Piguet V, Dayer P, Desmeules J. (2008) New Approaches to the Pharmacotherapy of Neuropathic Pain. *Expert Rev Clin Pharmacol.* 1(5):683-693DOI 10.1586/17512433.1.5.683

[16] Bjerring P, Arendt-Nielsen L (1989) Use of a new argon laser technique to evaluate changes in sensory and pain thresholds in human skin following topical capsaicin treatment. *Skin Pharmacol* 2:162-167. (DOI:10.1159/000210813)

[17] Boureau F, Legallicier P, Kabir-Ahmadi M. (2003) Tramadol in postherpetic neuralgia: a randomized, double-blind, placebo-controlled trial. *Pain* 104:323–31. PII: S0304-3959(03)00020-4 doi:10.1016/S0304-3959(03)00020-4 PMID:12855342 [PubMed - indexed for MEDLINE]

[18] Cruccu G, Aziz TZ, Garcia-Larrea L, Hansson P, Jensen TS, Lefaucheur JP et al. (2007) EFNS guidelines on neurostimulation therapy for neuropathic pain. *Eur J Neurol.* Sep;14(9):952-70. In :http://www.guideline.gov/summary/summary.aspx7doc_id =11372&nbr=5909#1146.

[19] Dakin H, Nuijten M, Liedgens H, Nautrup BP. (2007) Cost-effectiveness of a lidocaine 5% medicated plaster relative to gabapentin for postherpetic neuralgia in the United Kingdom. *Clin Ther* 29:1491–507. PMID: 17825701[PubMed - indexed for MEDLINE]

[20] Davies PS, Galer BS. (2004) Review of lidocaine patch 5% studies in the treatment of postherpetic neuralgia. *Drugs* 64:937–47. Print ISSN: 0003-2999; Online ISSN: 1526-7598 .

[21] De Benedittis G, Lorenzetti A. (1996) Topical aspirin/diethyl ether mixture versus indomethacin and diclofenac/diethyl ether mixtures for acute herpetic neuralgia and postherpetic neuralgia: a double blind crossover placebo-controlled study. *Pain* 65:45-52. PMID:8826489[PubMed - indexed for MEDLINE]

[22] Deer T, Krames ES, Hassenbusch SJ, Burton A, Caraway D, Dupen S et al. (2007) Polyanalgesic Consensus Conference 2007: Recommendations for the Management of Pain by Intrathecal (Intraspinal) Drug Delivery: Report of an Interdisciplinary Expert Panel. *Neuromodulation* 10(4): 300-28. DOI: 10.1111/j.1525-1403.2007.00128.x

[23] Dellemijn P. (1999) Are opioids effective in relieving neuropathic pain? *Pain* 80: 453-62. ISSN: 0304-3959

[24] Derry S, Lloyd R, Moore RA, McQuay HJ. (2009) Topical capsaicin for chronic neuropathic pain in adults. *Cochrane Database of Systematic Reviews* 2009, Issue 4. Art. No.: CD007393. DOI: 10.1002/14651858.CD007393.pub2.

[25] Dickenson AH, Suzuki R. (2005) Opioids in neuropathic pain: clues from animals studies. *Eur J Pain* 9: 113-6. ISSN: 1090-3801

[26] Dubinsky RM, Kabbani H, El-Chami Z, Boutwell C, Ali H; Quality (2004) Standards Subcommittee of the American Academy of Neurology. Practice parameter: treatment of postherpetic neuralgia: an evidence-based report of the Quality Standards Subcommittee of the American Academy of Neurology. *Neurology*. Sep 28; 63(6):959-65. Print ISSN: 0028-3878; Online ISSN: 1526-632X ...

[27] Dubner R. (1991) A call for more science, not more rethoric, regarding opioids and neuropathic pain. *Pain* 47; 1-2._ISSN 0304-3959 CODEN PAINDB

[28] Dworkin RH, Corbin AE, Young JP, Jr., et al. (2003) Pregabalin for the treatment of postherpetic neuralgia: a randomized, placebo-controlled trial. *Neurology* 60:1274–1283. Print ISSN: 0028-3878. Online ISSN: 1526-632X

[29] Dworkin RH, Backonja M, Rowbotham MC, Allen RR, Argoff CR, Bennett GJ et al. (2003)Advances in neuropathic pain. *Arch Neurol* 60: 1524-34. PMID:14623723 [PubMed - indexed for MEDLINE]

[30] Dworkin RH, O´Connor AB, Backonja M, Farrar JT, Finnerup NB, Jensen TS et al. (2007) Pharmacologic management of neuropathic pain: evidence-based recommendations. *Pain* Dec 5; 132(3): 237-51. [ISSN] 1872-6623

[31] Dworkin RH, O'Connor AB, Audette J, et al. (2010) Recommendations for the pharmacological management of neuropathic pain: an overview and literature update. *Mayo Clin Proc* 85: S3–14. [ISSN] 1942-5546

[32] Eisenberg E, McNicol ED, Carr DB. (2006) Efficacy of mu-opioid agonists in the treatment of evoked neuropathic pain: review of randomized controlled trials. *Eur J Pain* 10: 667-76. [ISSN] 1090-3801

[33] Feder G, Eccles M, Grol R, Griffiths C, Grimshaw J. (1999) Clinical guidelines. Using clinical guidelines. *Br J Med* 318: 728-30._[PMID: 10074024]

[34] Finnerup NB et al. (2005) Algorithm for neuropathic pain treatment: an evidence based proposal. *Pain* 118(3): 289-305. PubMed: 16213659Available from www.ncbi.nlm.nih.gov

[35] Finnerup NB, Otto M, Jensen TS, Sindrup SH. (2007) An evidence-based algorithm for the treatment of neuropathic pain. *Med Gen Med* May 15; 9(2): 36. doi:10.1016/j.pain.2005.08.013

[36] Galer BS, Rowbotham MC, Perander J, Friedman E. (1999) Topical lidocaine patch relieves postherpetic neuralgia more effectively than a vehicle topical patch: results of an enriched enrollment study. *Pain* 80: 533–538. doi:10.1016/S0304-3959(98)00244-9

[37] Gálvez R, Ruiz S, Romero J. (2006) Propuesta de nueva Escalera Analgésica para el dolor neuropático. *Rev Soc Esp Dolor* 6: 377-80.

[38] Gálvez R, Ruiz S, Romero J. (2007) A neuropathic pain ladder. Neuropathic Pain: II International congress of NeuPSIG. Poster.*Abstract Book*. Berlin.

[39] Gálvez Mateos R. Manual práctico de Dolor Neuropático. (2009) ISBN: 978-84-8086-456-5. Ed. Elsevier. Madrid.

[40] Gauthier A, Breuer J, Carrington D, Martin M, Remy V. (2009) Epidemiology and cost of herpes zoster and post-herpetic neuralgia in the United Kingdom. *Epidemiol Infect* 137:38–47. PMID:18466661[PubMed - indexed for MEDLINE] doi:10.1017/S0950268808000678

[41] Gilron I, Bailey JM, Tu D, Holden RR, Weaver DF, Houlden RL. (2005) Morphine, gabapentin, or their combination for neuropathic pain. *N Engl J Med* 352: 1324–1334. PMID:15800228 [PubMed - indexed for MEDLINE]

[42] Gilron I, Wajsbrot D, Therrien F, Lemay J. (2011) Pregabalin for peripheral neuropathic pain: a multicenter, enriched enrollment randomized withdrawal placebo-controlled trial. *Clin J Pain*. Mar-Apr; 27(3):185-93.PubMed PMID: 21178603.

[43] Green BG, Flammer LJ. (1988) Capsaicin as a cutaneous stimulus: Sensitivity and sensory qualities on hairy skin. *Chem Senses* 13:367-384. Monell chemical senses center advancing discovery in taste and smell .Monell Publications 1969-2009 doi: 10.1093/chemse/13.3.367

[44] Hanson P. (2003) Dificulties in stratifying neuropathic pain by mechanisms. *Eur J Pain* 7:353-357. PMID:12821406 [PubMed - indexed for MEDLINE]

[45] Helgason S, Petursson G, Gudmundsson S, Sigurdson JA. (2000) Prevalence of postherpetic neuralgia after a first episode of herpes zoster: prospective study with long term follow-up. *BMJ* 321:794–796.PMCID: PMC27491

[46] Hempenstall K, Nurmikko TJ, Johnson RW, A'Hern RP, Rice ASC. (2005) Analgesic therapy in postherpetic neuralgia: a quantitative systematic review. *PLoS Med* 2:628–44. PMID: 16013891[PubMed - indexed for MEDLINE)

[47] Hollingshead J, Dühmke RM, Cornblath DR. (2006) Tramadol for neuropathic pain. *Cochrane Database Syst Rev* 3: CD003726.

[48] Irving, G.; Backonja, M.M.; Vanhove, GF.; Lu, SP; Tobias, J. A (2010) Multicenter, Randomized, Double-Blind, Controlled Study of NGX-4010, a High-Concentration Capsaicin Patch, for the Treatment of Postherpetic Neuralgia. *Pain Medicine* 12(1): 99-109. PMID: 20937130 Owner: NLM Status: MEDLINE

[49] Jensen TS, Baron R. (2003) Translation of symptoms and signs into mechanisms in neuropathic pain. *Pain* 102:1-8. PII: S0304-3959(03)00006-X doi:10.1016/s0304-3959(03)00006-x

[50] Jensen MP, Chodroff MJ, Dworkin RH. The impact of neuropathic pain on health-related quality of life: review and implications. Neurology 2007 apr 10; 68(15): 1178-82. PMID:17420400 [PubMed - indexed for MEDLINE]

[51] Jensen TS, Madsen CS, Finnerup NB. (2009) Pharmacology and treatment of neuropathic pains. *Curr Opin Neurol* 22: 467–74. ISSN 1096-1186

[52] Jones VM, Moore KA, Peterson DM. (2011) Capsaicin 8% Topical Patch (Qutenza)- A Review of the Evidence. *J of Pain and Palliative Care Pharmacotherapy* 25(1): 32-41. PMID:21426216 [PubMed - indexed for MEDLINE]

[53] Kennedy WR, Vanhove GF, Lu SP, et al. (2010) A randomized, controlled, open-label study of the long-term effects of NGX-4010, a high-concentration capsaicin patch, on epidermal nerve fiber density and sensory function in healthy volunteers. *J Pain*. 11:579–587. PMID: 20400377 [PubMed - indexed for MEDLINE].PII: S1526-5900(09)00816-5. doi:10.1016/j.jpain.2009.09.019

[54] Keskinbora K, Pekel AF, Aydinli I. (2007) Gabapentin and an opioid combination versus opioid alone for the management of neuropathic cancer pain: a randomized open trial. *J Pain Symptom Manage*. 34:183-9. PMID: 17604592. [PubMed - indexed for MEDLINE] PII: S0885-3924(07)00321-1 doi:10.1016/ j.jpainsymman. 2006. 11.013

[55] Khaliq W, Alam S, Puri NK. (2007) Topical lidocaine for the treatment of postherpetic neuralgia. *Cochrane Database Syst Rev*. Reviews Issue 2 John Wiley & Sons, Ltd Chichester, UK. DOI: 10 1002/14651858 CD004846 pub2.

[56] Kikuchi A, Kotani N, Sato T, Takamura K, Sakai I, Matsuki A. (1999) Comparative therapeutic evaluation of intrathecal versus epidural methylprednisolone for long-term analgesia in patients with intractable postherpetic neuralgia. *Reg Anesth Pain Med* 24:287–293. Online ISSN 1471-6771

[57] Kotani N, Kushikata T, Hashimoto H, et al. (2000) Intrathecal methylprednisolone for intractable postherpetic neuralgia. *N Engl J Med* 343:1514–1519. ISSN: 0028 4793. CODEN: NEJMA. DOI: 10.1056/NEJM200011233432102 PubMed ID: 11087880

[58] Liedgens H, Hertel N, Gabriel A et al. (2008) Cost-effectiveness analysis of a lidocaine 5% medicated plaster compared with gabapentin and pregabalin for treating postherpetic neuralgia: a german perspective. *Clin Drug Investig* 2008;28:583–601.PMID:18666805[PubMed - indexed for MEDLINE]

[59] Martínez-Salio A, Gómez De la Cámara A, Ribera Canudas MV, Montero Homs J, Blanco Tarrío E, Collado Cruz A, Ferrero Méndez A, Molet Teixidó J, Oteo-Alvaro A, Gálvez Mateos R, Zamorano Bayarri E, Peña Arrebola A, Pardo Fernández J. (2009) *Med Clin.* Oct 31; 133 (16):629-36. PMID:19640552[PubMed - indexed for MEDLINE]

[60] McCleane G. (2004) Pharmacological strategies in relieving neuropathic pain. *Expert Opin Pharmacother*, 5, 6:1299-1312. (doi:10.1517/14656566.5.6.1299)

[61] McQuay H.J., D. Carroll, A. Moxon, C.J. Glynn and R.A. Moore. (1990) Benzydamine cream for the treatment of post-herpetic neuralgia: minimum duration of treatment periods in a cross-over trial. *Pain* 40, 2: 130-135. doi:10.1016/0304-3959(90)90063-J PMID:2308759 [PubMed - indexed for MEDLINE]

[62] McQuay HJ, Tramer M, Nye Ba, Carrol D, Wiffen PJ, Moore RA. (1996) A systematic review of antidepressants in neuropatic pain. *Pain* 68: 217-227. PMID:9121808[PubMed - indexed for MEDLINE]

[63] McQuay H, Moore A. (1998) Transcutaneous electrical nerve stimulation (TENS) in chronic pain. En McQuay H, Moore A eds. An evidence-based resource for pain relief. Oxford: Editorial Oxford University Press 207-211. Print ISSN: 0031-9023; Online ISSN: 1538-6724.

[64] Moulin DE, Clark AJ, Gilron I, Ware MA, Watson CP, Sessle BJ et al. (2007) Pharmacological management of chronic neuropathic pain - consensus statement and guidelines from the Canadian Pain Society. *Pain Res Manag*. Spring;12 (1):13-21. [ISSN] 1203-6765

[65] Nolano M, Simone DA, Wendelschafer-Crabb G, Johnson T, Hazen E, Kennedy WR. (1999) Topical capsaicin in humans: Parallel loss of epidermal nerve fibers and pain sensation. *Pain* 81:135-145. doi:10.1016/S0304-3959(99)00007-X

[66] Nonaham KE, Kumbang J. (2008) Transcutaneous electrical nerve stimulation (TENS) for chronic pain. Cochrane Database Syst Rev. Jul 16; (3): CD003222.

[67] O'Connor AB, Dworkin RH. Treatment of neuropathic pain: an overview of recent guidelines. *Am J Med* 2009; 122: S22–32. [ISSN] 1555-7162

[68] Pappagallo M, Haldey EJ. (2003) Pharmacological management of postherpetic neuralgia. *CNS Drugs* 17(11):771-80. PMID: 12921490 [PubMed - indexed for MEDLINE]

[69] Peikert A, Hentrich M, Ochs G. (1991) Topical 0.025% capsaicin in chronic post-herpetic neuralgia: Efficacy, predictors of response and long-term course. *J Neurol* 238:452–6. DOI: 10.1007/BF00314653

[70] Przewlocki R, Przewlocka B. (2005) Opioids in neuropathic pain. *Current Pharmaceuthical Desing* 11: 3013-25. PMID: 16178760 [PubMed - indexed for MEDLINE]

[71] Rains C, Bryson HM. (1995) Topical Capsaicin. A review of its pharmacological properties and therapeutic potential in postherpetic neuralgia, diabetic neuropathy and osteoarthritis. *Drugs Aging* 7(4):317–28.PMID:8535059 [PubMed - indexed for MEDLINE]

[72] Raja SN, Haythornthwaite JA, Pappagallo M, Clark MR, Travison TG, Sabeen S et al. (2002) Opioids versus antidepressants in postherpetic neuralgia: a randomized,

placebo-controlled trial. *Neurology* 59: 1015–21. PMID:12370455[PubMed - indexed for MEDLINE]

[73] Redondo Fernández, J. Costillo Rodríguez y M. Jiménez Rodríguez. (2007) Abordaje de la neuralgia postherpética en Atención Primaria: situación actual del tratamiento farmacológico. *Semergen*. 33(2):80-5. ISSN: 1138-3593. Depósito Legal: M-22691-1977.

[74] Rehm S, Binder A, Baron R. (2010) Post-herpetic neuralgia: 5% lidocaine medicated plaster, pregabalin, or a combination of both? A randomized, open, clinical effectiveness study. *Curr Med Res Opin* 26:1607–19 doi:10.1185/03007995.2010.483675.

[75] Rice ACS, Maton S. (2001) Gabapentin in postherpetic neuralgia: a randomised, double blind, placebo controlled study. *Pain* 94:215–224. PMID: 11690735 [PubMed - indexed for MEDLINE]

[76] Ritchie M, Liedgens H, Nuijten M. (2010) Cost effectiveness of lidocaine 5% medicated plaster compared with pregabalin for the treatment of postherpetic neuralgia in the UK: Markov model analysis. Clin Drug Investig 30:71–87.doi: 10.2165/11533310-000000000-00000. PMID:[PubMed - indexed for MEDLINE]

[77] Rowbotham MC, Fields HL. (1989) Postherpetic neuralgia: the relation of pain compliant, sensory disturbance and skin temperature. *Pain* 39:129-144. PMID: 2594392 [PubMed - indexed for MEDLINE]

[78] Rowbotham MC, Davies PS, Fields HL. (1995) Topical lidocaine gel relieves postherpetic neuralgia. *Ann Neurol* Feb; 37 (2):246-53. PMID:7847866 [PubMed - indexed for MEDLINE]

[79] Rowbotham MC, Davies PS, Verkempinck C, et al. (1996) Lidocaine patch: Double-blind controlled study of new treatment method for post-herpetic neuralgia. *Pain* 65:39-44. PMID: 8826488 [PubMed - indexed for MEDLINE]

[80] Rowbotham MC, Harden N, Stacey B, Bernstein P, Magnus-Miller L. (1998) Gabapentin for the treatment postherpetic neuralgia: a randomized controlled trial. *JAMA* 280:1837–42. doi: 10.1001/jama.280.21.1837

[81] Rowbotham MC, Petersen KL. (2001) Zoster-associated pain and neural dysfunction. *Pain* 93:1–5.PMID:11406332 [PubMed - indexed for MEDLINE]

[82] Saarto T, Wiffen PJ. (2005)Antidepressants for neurophatic pain. The *Cochrane Database of Systematic Reviews*, Issue 3. Art. No.: CD005454. DOI:10.1002/ 14651858. CD005454.

[83] Sabatowski R, Galvez R, Cherry DA, Jacquot F, Vincent E, Maisonobe P et al 1008-045 Study Group. (2004) Pregabalin reduces pain and improved sleep and mood disturbances in patients with postherpetic neuralgia: results of a randomised, placebo-controlled clinical trial. *Pain* 109:26–35, ISSN: 0025-7753.

[84] Scholz J, Woolf CJ. (2007) The neuropathic pain triad: neurons, immune cells and glia. *Nat Neurosci* 10: 1361–68.PMID:17965656 [PubMed - indexed for MEDLINE]

[85] Sindrup SH, Otto M, Finnerup NB, Jensen TS. (2005)Antidepressants in the treatment of neuropathic pain. *Basic Clin Pharmacol Toxicol*. Jun; 96(6):399-409. DOI: 10.1111 /j.1742-7843.2005. pto_96696601.x

[86] Stow PJ, Glynn CJ, Minor B. (1989) EMLA cream in the treatment of post-herpetic neuralgia: efficacy and pharmacokinetic profile. *Pain* Dec; 39 (3): 301-5. PMID: 2616182 [PubMed - indexed for MEDLINE]

[87] Szolcsanyi J (2004) Forty years in capsaicin research for sensory pharmacology and physiology. *Neuropeptides* 38:377-384.PMID:15567473[PubMed - indexed for MEDLINE]

[88] Treede RD, Jensen TS, Campbell JN, Cruccu G, Dostrovsky JO, Griffin JW et al. (2008) Neuropathic pain: redefinition and a grading system for clinical and research purposes. *Neurology.* Apr 29; 70(18):1630-5. PMID: 18003941 [PubMed - indexed for MEDLINE]

[89] Tremont-Lukats I, Megeff C, Backonja M. (2000) Anticonvulsivants for neurophatic pain syndromes. *Drugs* 60:5:1029-52. [ISSN] 0012-6667.

[90] Trescot AM, Helm S, Hansen H, Benyamin R, Glaser SE, Adlaka R, P atel S, Manchikanti L. Opioids in the management of chronic non-cancer pain: an update of American Society of the Interventional Pain Physicians' (ASIPP) Guidelines. *Pain Physician.* 2008 Mar;11 (2 Suppl):S5-S62. ISSN 1533-3159 | www.painphysicianjournal.com | Index Medicus/MEDLINE/PubMed | Listed in Excerpta Medica/EMBASE |

[91] Turk D, Stieg RL. (1987) Chronic pain: the necessity of interdisciplinary communication. *Clin J Pain* 3: 163-7, ISSN 1068-9583.

[92] Van Seventer R., Feister H.A., Young Jr, Stoker M., Versavel M., & Rigaudy L. (2006) Efficacy and tolerability of twice-daily pregabalin for treating pain and related sleep interference in postherpetic neuralgia: a 13-week, randomized trial. *Current Medical Research and Opinion* 22: 375-84. (doi: 10.1185/ 030079906X80404)

[93] Wasner G, Baron R. (2009) Pain: clinical pain assessment: from bedside to better treatment. Nat Rev Neurol 5: 359-61. PMID: 19578341[PubMed - indexed for MEDLINE]

[94] Watson CP, Evans RJ, Reed K, Merskey H, Goldsmith L, Warsh J. (1982) Amitriptyline versus placebo in postherpetic neuralgia. *Neurology* 32: 671–673.PMID:19578341[PubMed - indexed for MEDLINE]

[95] Watson PN, Evans RJ.(1986) Postherpetic neuralgia. A review. *Arch Neurol* 43:836–840.PMID:2873807[PubMed - indexed for MEDLINE]

[96] Watson DC, Tyler KL, Bickers DR, Millikan LE, Smith S, Coleman E. (1993) A randomized vehicle-controlled trial of topical capsaicin in the treatment of postherpetic neuralgia. *Clin Ther.* May-Jun; 15(3):510-26. PMID:8364943 [PubMed - indexed for MEDLINE]

[97] Watson CPN, Babul N. (1998) Eficacy of oxycodone in neuropathic pain: a randomized trial in postherpetic neuralgia. Neurology 50:1837–41.PMID:9633737 [PubMed - indexed for MEDLINE

[98] Wheeler JG. (1991) EMLA cream and herpetic neuralgia [letter]. *Med J Aust Jun* 3; 154 (11): 781. PMID: 1875823 [PubMed - indexed for MEDLINE]

[99] Wiffen P, Collins S, McQuay H, Carrol D, Jadad A, Moore A. (2005) Anticonvulsants drugs for acute and chronic pain *Crochrane Database Syst Re.*

http://www.update -software.com.CD001133. PMID: 16034857 [PubMed - indexed for MEDLINE]

[100] Wolff RF, Bala MM, Westwood M, Kessels AG, Kleijnen J. (2011) 5% lidocaine-medicated plaster vs other relevant interventions and placebo for post-herpetic neuralgia (PHN): a systematic review. *Acta Neurol Scand* 123: 295–309. DOI: 10.1111/j.1600-0404.2010.01433.x

13

Antiviral Activity of Lactoferrin and Ovotransferrin Derived Peptides Towards Herpesviridae

Francesco Giansanti[1], Loris Leboffe[2] and Giovanni Antonini[2]
[1]*Department of Basic and Applied Biology, University of L'Aquila, L'Aquila*
[2]*Department of Biology, Roma TRE University, Roma, Italy,*

1. Introduction

1.1 Marek's disease virus (MDV)

Marek's disease virus (MDV) belongs to the alphaherpesvirus family, like Herpes simplex viruses 1 and 2 (HSV-1 and HSV-2) and varicella zoster virus (VZV). Marek's Disease Virus (MDV) is the etiologic agent of Marek's Disease (MD), a highly contagious malignant lymphoma of chickens. (Morimura, *et al.* 1998).

Marek's Disease (MD) was first described by József Marek in 1907 as fowl paralysis caused by mononuclear infiltration into the sciatic nerve plexi (Marek, 1907). Marek's Disease (MD) is a lymphoproliferative and neuropatic disease of domestic chickens and, less commonly, turkeys and quails (Payne & Venugopal, 2000).

Generally, four different clinical forms of the disease are recognized in flocks infected with MDV: A) Classical or neuronal form; B) Acute form; C) Transient paralysis and D) Acute mortality syndrome.

1.2 MDV life cycle

The infection occurs by inhalation of infected dust (Beasley, *et al.* 1970) in the poultry house environment contaminated with the viruses shed from the feather follicle epithelium of infected birds. According to the current model of MDV pathogenesis, it is thought that the virus is transported by macrophages from the lungs to the lymphoid tissues of the spleen, thymus and the *bursa* of *Fabricius*, where virus targets the lymphocyte subsets, the major cells of the host immune system (Fig. 1). These cells could transport MDV to the lymphoid tissues via the lymph or blood, where it can be detected as early as 18 h post-infection (Adldinger & Calnek, 1973)

Calnek and coworkers (Calnek, 1985; Calnek, 1986; Schat, 1987) developed a model for the pathogenesis of MD in the early 1980s which remains valid (Fig. 2). MDV is first detected in the spleen 3 days post-exposure after exposure by inhalation. The virus causes an early cytolytic infection in B cells, which are presumed to be the primary target for viral replication (Schat *et al.*, 1980; Calnek *et al.*, 1982; Shek *et al.*, 1983). Resting T cells are refractory to infection; successively, T cells become activated and susceptible to MDV infection (Calnek *et al*,. 1984 a, b).

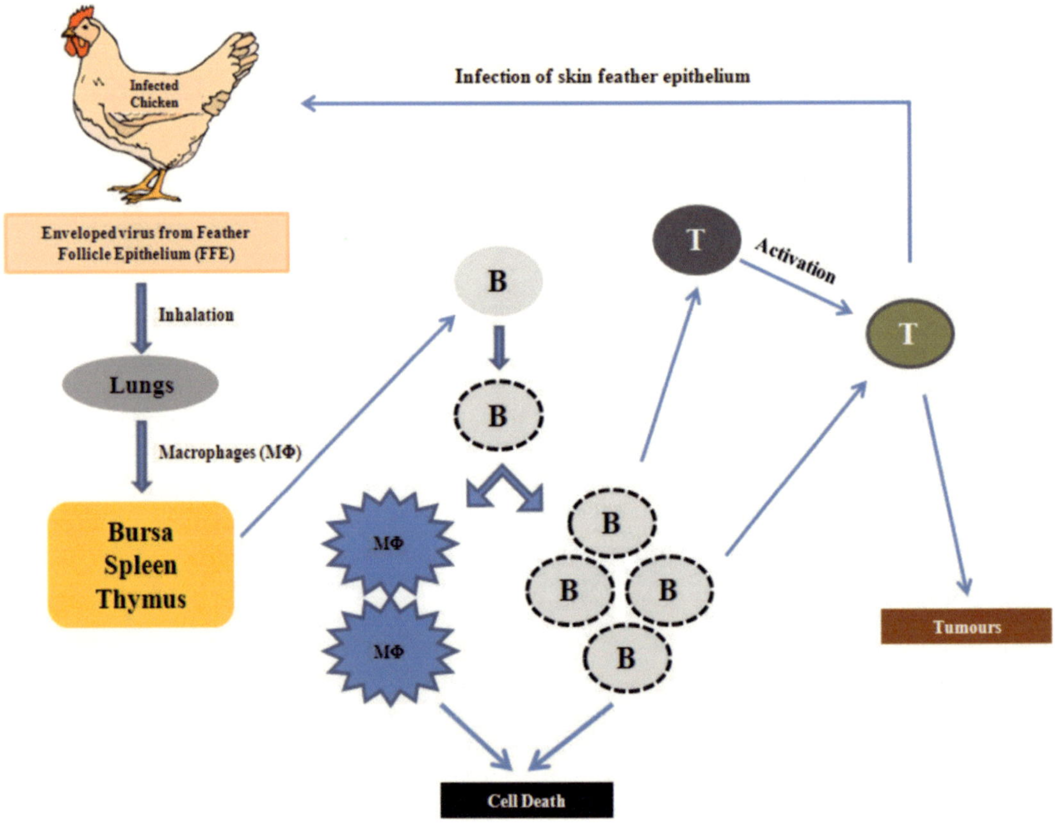

Fig. 1. Pathogenesis of MD. Feather follicle epithelium (FFE); B-cells (B); T-cells (T); macrophages (M) (Modified from: Nair, 2005).

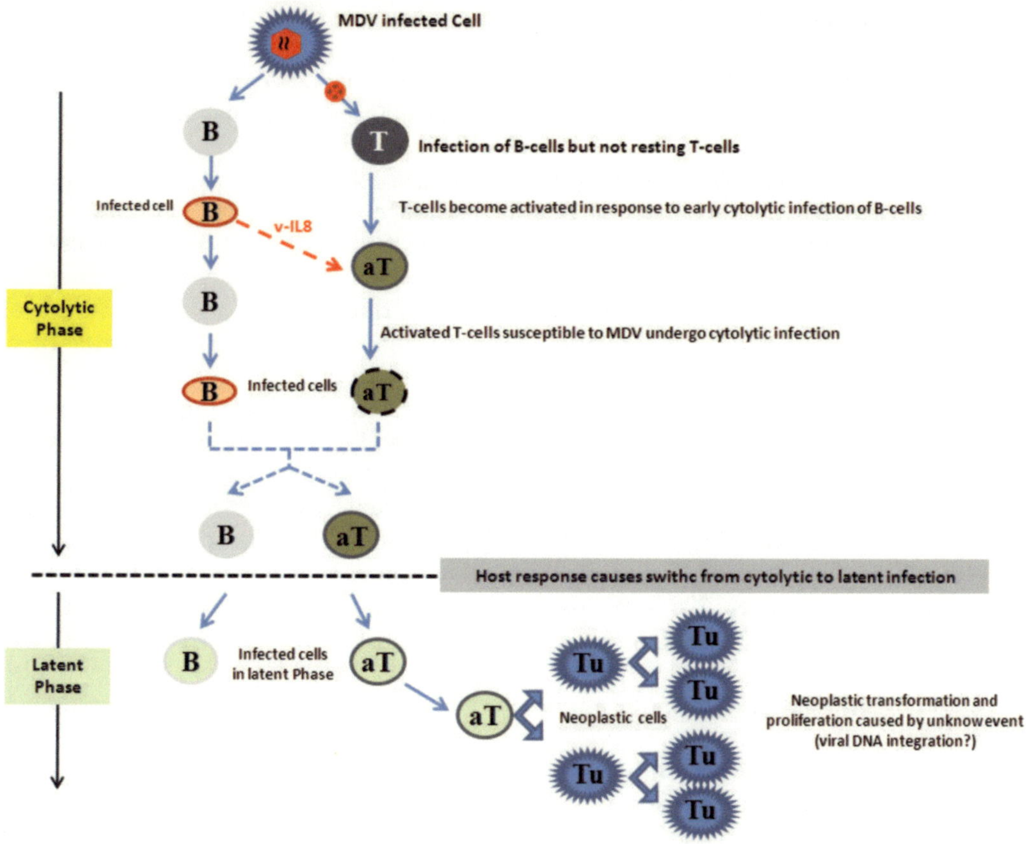

Fig. 2. Sequential events in lymphocyte infections with MDV (Modified from: Calnek, 1985)

It was hypothesized (Schat & Xing, 2000; Schat, 2001) that, during the lytic infection, the MDV transfer from B to T cells may be facilitated by the production of vIL-8. This is a CXC chemokine and it was described as a homologue of IL-8 (vIL-8) (Parcells *et al.*, 2001); vIL-8 is the first reported CXC chemokine encoded by an alphaherpesvirus (Liu *et al.*, 1999). The majority of these T cells are $CD4^{+}TCR\alpha\beta_1^{+}$, but a small percentage of infected cells are $CD8^{+}TCR\alpha\beta_2^{+}$ (Sugano *et al.*, 1987; Martins-Green, 2001). Moreover, MDV-driven tumors are dominated by a highly restricted number of $CD4^{+}$ clones. Further, the responding $CD8^{+}$ T cell infiltrate is oligoclonal, indicating recognition of a limited number of MDV antigens (Mwangi *et al.*, 2011).

These early cytolytic events result in atrophic changes in the *bursa* of *Fabricius* and thymus, leading to severe debilitation of the immune system and marked immunosuppression. One week post-infection, when virus levels peak, MDV switches from early cytolytic to latent infection, probably due to cell-mediated immune responses (Buscaglia *et al.*, 1988; Schat & Xing, 2000). During latency, clinical signs of the infection diminish, productive viral antigen cannot be detected in the *bursa*, thymus and spleen, and within 2 weeks the lymphocyte populations in the bursal follicles and thymic cortex return to normal.

1.3 Defence mechanisms against MDV infection

1.3.1 Nonspecific immune responses

Against MDV infections, the organisms establish both nonspecific and specific immune responses. The cells involved in these responses are NK cells and macrophages. It has been hypothesized that avian NK cells are able to recognize target cells as mammalian NK cells do (Kaufman, 1996; Kaufman & Salomonsen, 1997; Kaufman & Venugopal, 1998). Macrophages play an important role in resistance to MDV infection both *in vitro* and *in vivo*; their depletion leads to a lower immunity versus MD and reduces protective efficacy of vaccination (Gupta *et al.*, 1989). They are thought to be critical during the early stages after MDV infection, but are also important during the later stages of pathogenesis (Calnek, 2001); they limit MDV replication or have a detrimental role (Lee. *et al.*, 1978 a,b).

Macrophages are involved in virus phagocytosis, but no replication, or antigenic changes at the cell surface have been observed (Haffer & Sevoian, 1979; Haffer *et al.*, 1979). MDV antigen expression was not evident after co-culturing of either bone marrow-derived macrophages or macrophage cell lines with MDV-infected lymphocytes, suggesting the requirement for *in vivo* conditions. These data indicate that macrophages could be a primary target for cytolytic infection *in vivo*, in addition to facilitating transportation of the virus, as proposed by Calnek (Calnek, 2001). Macrophages from MDV-infected chickens are also able to inhibit the DNA synthesis of MD lymphoblastoid cell lines (Lee *et al.*, 1978 b) and suppress the mitogen response of T lymphocytes (Lee *et al.*, 1978 a,b); these effects have also been found in macrophages isolated from uninfected chickens (Sharma, 1980; Von Bulow & Klasen, 1983).

Macrophages are also able to produce large quantities of Nitric Oxide (NO) (Hussain & Qureshi, 1997); depletion of these cells causes the suppression of NO production and so the increase of viral load in the blood, tumour incidence and tumour load (Rivas *et al.*, 2003). Moreover, in addition the high levels of IL-1β, IL-6, IL-12, iNOS, and type 1 and 2 IFNs, the relative expression levels of IL-4, IL-10, and IL-13 were significantly upregulated in the infected chickens during the lytic phase of infection compared to uninfected controls. This observation suggests that an immune response with a Th-2 characteristic is induced by a very virulent plus MDV strain during the lytic phase of infection, and there is no significant MDV-specific immune response in the latent phase of infection (Heidari *et al.*, 2008)

1.3.2 Specific immune responses

Specific immune responses are antigen-dependent and require lymphocyte activation to produce specific antibodies and antigen-specific $CD4^+$ and $CD8^+$ T cells. Cell-mediated immune responses (CMI) and virus neutralizing antibodies are important in herpesvirus infections in general (Mester & Rouse, 1991) and have been described after natural infection with oncogenic MDV and after inoculation with vaccine strains. It was suggested that CTL (Cytotoxic T Limphocytes) responses are also important for the elimination of MDV-infected cells (Ross, 1977; Kodama *et al.*, 1979). Although immune defences against infected cells are predominantly mediated by CTL, humoral immune responses also play an important role in herpesvirus infections (Medveczky *et al.*, 1998). Antibodies to the virus envelope neutralise viral infectivity, kill lytically infected cells by antibody-dependent cell cytotoxicity (ADCC), and protect against reinfections with EBV (Chubb & Churchill, 1969).

1.3.3 Induction of apoptosis

Apoptosis of virus-infected cells can be beneficial to the host if cells are eliminated before virus assembly. It is therefore not surprising that certain viruses code for proteins inhibiting apoptosis during the early phase of replication but facilitate the process during the later stages of replication. Apoptosis occurs during MDV infection in $CD4^+CD8^+$ thymus tissues in the first week after infection (Morimura *et al.,* 1996), during the second week in $CD4^+$ T cells in peripheral blood (Morimura *et al.,* 1995) and spleen cells from chickens 7 days post infection with the JM-16 strain of MDV (Schat & Xing, 2000). However, it is likely that the Meq protein is responsible for the prevention of apoptosis. This protein is expressed in most, if not all, MD tumour cell lines and overexpression of *meq* in the rodent cell line Rat-2 caused transformation of these cells. The transformed cells became highly resistant to the induction of apoptosis (Liu *et al.,* 1998). It is of interest to note that *meq* is transcribed during the lytic infection without an apparent effect on apoptosis. However, the regulation of *meq* transcription is very complex and alternate splicing has been described (Peng & Shirazi, 1996). Recently was described that the Meq oncoprotein interacts directly with p53 and inhibits p53-mediated transcriptional activity and apoptosis, providing a valuable insight into the molecular basis for the function of *meq* in MDV oncogenesis (Deng *et al.,* 2010)
Moreover, expression of pp38 in tumour cells may be correlated with the induction of apoptosis (Schat & Xing, 2000). This hypothesis is interesting in view of the finding that pp38 expression in MD tumour cell lines is generally low and is apparently inversely related to the expression of *meq* and a small RNA antisense to ICP4 (Ross *et al.,* 1997). Expression of pp38 in tumour cell lines can be upregulated by transfection with ICP4 (Pratt *et al.,* 1994). There are very recent data that involve microRNAs (highly conserved among different field strains of MDV1), and they are expressed in lytic and latent infections and in MDV1-derived tumors. This evidence suggests that these small molecules are very important to the virus, and that they play some roles in immune evasion, anti-apoptosis, or proliferation (Burnside & Morgan, 2011). All these data suggest that the fate of tumour cells depends on an intricate balance between the expression and phosphorylation of Meq (Liu *et al.,* 1999), pp38, ICP4 and the small antisense RNA to ICP4 (Gimeno & Cortes, 2010).

1.3.4 MD vaccination

It is thought that the economic impact of MD on the global poultry industry accounts for at least US $1 bn yearly (Nair, 2005). The first MDV vaccine was obtained with an oncogenic strain repeatedly passaged *in vitro;* it was able to prevent MD tumors in chickens challenged with oncogenic MDV (Churchill & Chubb, 1969) but not to prevent the infection with field viruses. The first attenuated vaccine was used in the UK in 1970 but was quickly replaced by an HVT vaccine (Turkey Herpes Virus) (Witter *et al.,* 1970). Introduction of HVT as a live vaccine resulted in significant reduction of MD incidence and was extensively used because of its efficacy and economical production in tissue culture (Okazaki *et al.,* 1970; Purchase & Okazaki, 1971). However, within 10 years, new outbreaks of clinical MD occurred in vaccinated flocks (Eidson *et al.,* 1978; Witter *et al.,* 1980) and vvMDV isolated from these birds had a greater pathogenic effect than field viruses present before vaccine introduction (Witter, 1983). It was probably due to imperfect vaccination practices and, in some countries, wrong hygienic conditions that led to reservoirs of viruses in poultry houses (Bourne, 1996). In response to the increasing number of MD outbreaks in vaccinated flocks, in the 1980s, new vaccines based on the non-oncogenic serotype-2 MDV were introduced in bivalent combination with HVT (Calnek *et al.*, 1983; Witter *et al.*, 1984). The use of polyvalent vaccine provided a better protection against MDV challenge (Witter, 1992). This strategy was initially effective, but in the 1990s new and more virulent MDV pathotypes (vv + MDV) were isolated from flocks vaccinated with bivalent vaccines. In Europe, the problems have been less severe and in the Netherlands a very effective MDV vaccine, based on a weakly oncogenic serotype-1 MDV (CVI988), has been available (Rispens *et al.*,1972; Geerligs *et al.*, 1999; Witter, 2001, Baigent *et al.*, 2006; Schat & Baranowski, 2007). All these vaccination strategies are unfortunately due to the rapid variability of virus; vaccines are poorly effective in preventing infection in time (Gimeno, 2008).

1.3.5 Mechanisms of Herpesviruses infection

Attachment of HSV to cells occurs upon binding of gC to GAGs that decorate heparan sulphate or chondroitin sulphate (Spear *et al.*, 1992). This step enhances HSV infectivity, but is not an absolute requirement, as cells defective in heparin sulphate and chondroitin sulphate exhibit a 100-fold reduced susceptibility to infection, yet can be infected (Gruenheid *et al.*, 1993). A large variety of viruses use heparan sulphate proteoglycans as receptors; their broad expression argues that they cannot be responsible for any specific viral tropism. Herpes simplex virus type 1 (HSV-1) infects a wide range of cells and causes disease in a variety of different tissues.

Electron microscopy studies suggested that this virus enters host cells by means of either endocytosis or fusion between the membranes of the virus and the cell (Hodnichak *et al.*, 1984). The envelope of the HSV-1 virion contains at least ten different viral glycoproteins, several of which project as distinct spikes from the membrane surface and are likely to interact sequentially or simultaneously with different binding sites on the cell surface (Fuller & Lee, 1992; Herold *et al.*, 1994). The initial attachment of virions to cells is shown to be mediated independently by interactions of either glycoprotein C (gC) or glycoprotein B (gB) with heparan sulphate moieties of cell surface proteoglycans (Campadelli-Fiume *et al.*, 1990; Spear *et al.*, 1992; Shieh *et al.*, 1992; Gruenheid *et al.*, 1993; Herold *et al.*, 1994; Trybala *et al.*, 1994).

Heparin, an anionic related glycosaminoglycan, has been demonstrated to block HSV-1 adsorption to cells (WuDunn & Spear, 1989). There is also evidence that glycoprotein D (gD) may interact with its own cell receptor (Johnson *et al.*, 1990), and oligomers of glycoprotein H (gH) and glycoprotein L (gL) are also known to be required for HSV-1 penetration (Fuller & Lee, 1992; Forrester *et al.*, 1992; Roop *et al.*, 1993). Moreover, it has been suggested that the low-density lipoprotein receptor present in coated pits may interact with domains in gB, gC or gD allowing the virions to penetrate by an endocytosis process (Becker *et al.*, 1994).

Heparan sulphate, the primary cell surface receptor for HSV-1, is a ubiquitous and multifunctional constituent of most mammalian cell plasma membranes and of extracellular matrices, and has been also identified as a binding site for human and bovine lactoferrin (Ji & Mahley, 1994; Mann *et al.*, 1994; Wu *et al.*, 1995). The evidence that heparan sulphate proteoglycans and the low density lipoprotein receptor-related protein are capable of binding to lactoferrin, and acting as receptors for initial cell-HSV-1 interactions, suggested the idea that lactoferrin could interfere with early events of viral infection.

In previous studies the efficacy of Lactoferrin and Ovotransferrin to prevent the *in vitro* infection of chicken cell lines with MDV was demonstrated (Giansanti *et al.*, 2002, 2005). The efficacy of Lactoferrin and its derivative peptides against a variety of viruses as rotavirus and HSV was also demonstrated (Gruenheid *et al.*, 1993; Siciliano *et al.*, 1999; Spear *et al.*, 2000; Superti *et al.*, 2001)

2. Lactoferrin

Lactoferrin (Lf) is a non-haem iron-binding protein that is part of the transferrin protein family, along with serum transferrin (sTf), ovotransferrin (Otrf), melanotransferrin and the inhibitor of carbonic anhydrase. Lf is produced by mucosal epithelial cells in various mammalian species, including humans, cows, goats, horses, dogs, and several rodents (González-Chávez *et al.*, 2009). This glycoprotein has protective functions and it is found in mucosal secretions, including tears, saliva, vaginal fluids, semen (van der Strate *et al.*, 2001), nasal and bronchial secretions, bile, gastrointestinal fluids, urine (Öztas & Özgünes, 2005) and, most highly, in milk and colostrum (up to 7 g/L) (Rodriguez *et al.*, 2005) making it the second most abundant protein in milk after caseins (Connely, 2001). It can also be found in bodily fluids such as blood plasma and amniotic fluid, and in considerable amounts in secondary neutrophil granules (15 $\mu g/10^6$ neutrophils) (Bennett & Kokocinski, 1987; González-Chávez *et al.*, 2009), where it plays a significant physiological role. Lf possesses a great iron-binding affinity with the ability to retain the metal over a wide pH range (Aisen & Leibman, 1972) including extremely acidic pH. It also exhibits a great resistance to proteolysis. In addition to these differences, Lf net positive charge and its distribution in various tissues make it a multifunctional protein (Valenti & Antonini 2005; Baker & Baker, 2009).

2.1 Lactoferrin structure

Lf is an 80 kDa glycosylated protein of ca. 700 aminoacids (711 aa for hLf and 689 aa bLf) with high homology among species. It is a simple polypeptide chain folded into two symmetrical lobes (N and C lobes) which are highly homologous with one another (33–41% homology) (Anderson *et al.*, 1987, 1989; Baker, 1994; Moore *et al.*, 1997; Sharma *et al.*, 1998; Baker & Baker, 2009). These two lobes are connected by a hinge region containing parts of an α-helix between residues 333 and 343 in human Lf (hLF), which provides additional flexibility to the molecule. The polypeptide chain includes amino acids 1–332 for the N lobe and 344–703 for the C lobe, and is made up of α-helix and β-pleated sheet structures that create two domains for each lobe (domains I and II) (Moore *et al.*, 1997). Each lobe can be further divided into two subdomains (N1 and N2 in the N-lobe and C1 and C2 in the C-lobe) that form a cleft inside of which the iron is bound. The subdomain N1 contains residues 1-90 and 251-333, while N2 contains the residues 91-250) (Baker *et al.*, 1998; Moore *et al.*, 1997; Baker & Baker, 2009). Each lobe can bind a metal atom in synergy with the carbonate ion ($CO_3{}^{2-}$). Lf notably binds Fe^{2+} and Fe^{3+} ions, but also Cu^{2+}, Zn^{2+} and Mn^{2+} ions (Aisen & Harris, 1989; Baker *et al.*, 1994, 2005; Baker & Baker, 2009).

2.2 Antinfective activities of Lf

Lf is involved in several physiological functions, including: regulation of iron absorption in the bowel; immune response; and antioxidant, anticarcinogenic and anti-inflammatory properties. Protection against microbial infection is the most widely studied function to date (Sanchez *et al.*, 1992; Brock, 1995; Lonnerdal & Iyer; 1995; Vorland, 1999; Brock, 2002; Valenti & Antonini, 2005; Baker & Baker, 2009; Leboffe *et al.*, 2009). The antimicrobial activity of LF is mostly due to two different mechanisms: the first one is iron sequestration in sites of infection, which deprives the microorganism of this metal, thus creating a bacteriostatic effect. The other mechanism is the direct interaction of LF with the infectious agents. Positively charged amino acids of LF can interact with anionic molecules on some bacterial, viral, fungal and parasite surfaces, causing cell lysis (Bullen, 1981; Braun & Braun, 2002; Valenti & Antonini, 2005). Considering the physiological capabilities of Lf in host defence, in addition to current pharmaceutical and nutritional needs, Lf is considered to be a nutraceutical, and for several decades investigators have searched for the most convenient way to produce it (González-Chávez *et al.*, 2009).

Molecular mechanims of Lf antiparasitic activity are more complex. Antiparasitic activities of Lf often appear to involve interference with iron acquisition by some parasites, e.g. *Pneumocystis carinii*, while Lf appears to act as a specific iron donor in other parasites such as *Trichomonas foetus;* in the latter case, Lf could be expected to enhance infection. Preincubation of *Toxoplasma gondii* and *Eimeria stiedai* sporozoites with an Lf-derived peptide, lactoferricin, reduces their infectivity in animal models. Lf antiparasitic activity is also sometimes mediated by interaction with host cells. Thus, iron-saturated Lf enhances intramacrophage killing of *T. cruzi* amastigotes and decreases intra-erythrocytic growth of *Plasmodium falciparum*. Lf is able to inhibit the invasion of cultured cells by *Plasmodium* spp. sporozoites through specific binding to HS. In the case of *Plasmodium berghei*, Lf reduces invasion by inhibiting the binding of the plasmodial CS protein, with or without HS, suggesting the possibility that Lf can also bind to the same site on LDL receptor-related protein (LRP) as the CS protein (see Leboffe *et al.*, 2009).

The antiviral activity of hLf was firstly demonstrated in mice infected with the polycythemia-inducing strain of the Friend virus complex (FVC-P) (Lu *et al.*, 1987). Since 1995, potent antiviral activity of hLf and bLf has been demonstrated against both enveloped and naked viruses, like *Cytomegalovirus* (CMV) (Harmsen *et al.*, 1995; Andersen *et al.*, 2001), *Herpes simplex virus* (HSV) (Marchetti *et al.*, 1996, 1998; Siciliano *et al.*, 1999; Valenti & Antonini, 2005), *Human immunodeficiency virus* (HIV) (Swart *et al.*, 1996; Puddu *et al.*, 1998), as well as *Human hepatitis C* (HCV) and *human hepatitis B* (HBV) viruses (Ikeda *et al.*, 1998; Hara *et al.*, 2002).

3. Ovotransferrin

Ovotransferrin is the iron-binding glycoprotein belonging to the family of transferrin iron-binding glycoproteins, found in avian egg white and in avian serum. Contrary to the mammalian genome, the avian genome contains only one transferrin gene which is expressed both in liver and oviduct, being present in most bodily fluids, including serum and egg albumen where its concentration reaches values as high as 12 g/L (Stevens, 1991). The expression of this avian transferrin gene is modulated by iron level in liver and by steroid hormones in oviduct. The liver and oviduct products are known as avian serum transferrin and ovotransferrin, respectively (Dierich *et al.*, 1987). Avian serum transferrin is devoted to iron transport and delivery, while ovotransferrin displays protective functions, similarly to mammalian lactoferrin.

3.1 Ovotransferrin structure

Strong similarities could be observed between mammalian serum transferrin, lactoferrin and ovotransferrin; despite few differences in aminoacids sequences, the overall 3D structure is strictly conserved. The polypeptide chain is folded into two lobes, each containing a single iron-binding site. The two lobes have very similar structures, as expected from the sequence identity of 37.4% with mammalian lactoferrin (Jeltsch & Chambon, 1982; Williams *et al.*, 1982). The polypeptide chain includes amino acids 1-329 for the N lobe and 330-686 for the C lobe (Thakurta *et al.*, 2003). Interestingly, the two half molecules of ovotransferrin corresponding to the N-terminal and C-terminal lobes, obtained by a limited proteolysis procedure, have the ability to re-associate non-covalently in solution (Oe *et al.*, 1988). Most of the secondary structural elements are comparable between the two lobes. The main differences between the two lobes are in the loop regions, as expected by sequence insertions and deletions in the primary structure. Each lobe is comprised of two distinct, similar-sized α/β sub-domains (N-terminal lobe with N1 and N2 subdomains; C-terminal lobe with C1 and C2 subdomains). The two sub-domains are linked by two antiparallel β-strands that allow them to adopt either open or closed conformations. Iron (III) ions bound to Otrf are hexacoordinated, and the two iron-binding sites are located in the inter-sub-domain cleft of each lobe (Kurokawa *et al.*, 1995; Kurokawa *et al.*, 1999; Mizutani *et al.*, 1999, 2000; Lindley *et al.*, 1993; Kuser *et al.*, 2002; Thakurta *et al.*, 2003) being very similar each other and to those reported for human lactoferrin and for human serum transferrin (Anderson *et al.*, 1989).

3.2 Antinfective activities of ovotransferrin

Ovotransferrin antibacterial activity partially depends on its ability to bind and sequester iron, essential for bacterial growth (Alderton *et al.*, 1946, Bullen *et al*,. 1978). This activity is bacteriostatic, and the effect can be reversed by addition of exogenous iron ions. Other studies suggested that the antibacterial activity of Otrf is not simply due to the removal of iron from the medium, but probably involves further, more complex mechanisms (Ibrahim *et al.*, 2000). Ovotransferrin, as well as serum transferrin and lactoferrin, were also shown to permeate the *E. coli* outer membrane and to access the inner membrane, where they caused permeation of ions in a selective manner (Aguilera *et al.*, 2003). The importance of the presence of cationic sequences on the surface of Otrf in exploiting the antibacterial activity has been clearly pointed out by Ibrahim (Ibrahim *et al.*, 1998) using a peptide called OTAP-92 obtained by limited proteolysis, consisting of 92 amino acid residues located within the 109–200 sequence at the lip of the N2 domain of the N lobe

In relation to the antifungal activity of Otrf, a direct interaction of iron-loaded protein with Candida cells has been reported (Valenti *et al.*, 1985), like bovine and human lactoferrin (Leboffe *et al.*, 2009). The inhibiting activity of Otrf was tested against one hundred strains of Candida spp; the anti-mycotic effect was not coupled to iron sequestration, but rather related to Otrf binding on the Candida cell surface (Valenti *et al.*, 1985; Valenti *et al.*, 1986; Superti *et al.*, 2007 a, b).

Ovotransferrin's antibacterial activity was established many years ago while the antiviral activity of Otrf was demonstrated only recently towards the Marek's disease virus (MDV), an avian herpesvirus (Giansanti *et al.*, 2002). In addition, it was found that following infection with MDV on Chichen Embryo Fibroblasts (CEF), a variety of host genes were transcribed, including ovotransferrin (Morgan *et al.*, 2001). Moreover, *in vitro* viral infection of chicken embryo fibroblasts caused a slight increase of ovotransferrin release, whereas viral re-infection of lymphoblastoid cells *in vitro* caused a remarkable ovotransferrin release in a virus concentration-dependent manner (Giansanti *et al.*, 2007). Finally, the production of nitric oxide (NO), a molecule naturally exerting an antiviral activity, was observed in MDCC-MSB1 (Chicken hematopoietic lymphoblastic cell line) following reinfection and/or Otrf and lactoferrin (Lf) or following treatment with the cytokines IL-8 and IFN-γ), thus suggesting a possible role as a complementary or alternative strategy against MDV infection spread (Giardi *et al.,* 2009).

4. Antiviral activity of intact lactoferrin

The antiviral effect of lactoferrin was first believed to be linked to its iron-binding property, similarly to other iron-chelating substances known as inhibitors of herpesvirus ribonucleotide reductases (Spector *et al.*, 1989, 1991). In contrast, lactoferrin effect towards HSV-1 infection does not appear related to iron-withholding since no significant differences in the HSV-1 inhibition were found between lactoferrins in apo- and iron-saturated form. The infection inhibition occurs during the very early phases of the viral multiplication cycle, since the highest inhibitory effect took place when lactoferrin was added during the attachment step. In fact, the binding of [^{35}S]methionine-labelled HSV-1 virions to Vero cells was strongly inhibited when bLf was added. bLf interacts with both Vero cell surfaces and HSV-1 particles, suggesting that the hindrance of cellular receptors and/or of viral attachment proteins may be involved in its antiviral mechanism (Marchetti *et al.*, 1996). The antiviral effect of lactoferrin correlates well with its affinity for the virus receptor binding sites. In fact, polyanionic glycosaminoglycan chains of heparan sulphate and apo-lipoprotein-E receptor have been shown to interact with highly cationic lactoferrin (Pierce *et al.*, 1991).
Consequently, it can be assumed that the capability of lactoferrin to inhibit HSV-1 infection at the level of viral attachment may rely to a large extent on its competitive interaction with cell receptors for HSV-1 which can hinder the binding of the virus attachment proteins. bLf is a better inhibitor than hLf, with a selectivity index being over 10-fold higher. This effect of bLf on HSV-1 infection probably involves more than a simple mechanism of interference at the level of cell receptors. A direct interaction of bovine lactoferrin with virus particles has been demonstrated by the findings that virus binds efficiently to bLf immobilized on a solid-phase surface, as revealed by an ELISA method, and causes the rapid agglutination of bLf coated latex beads. It can be put forward that the lower activity of hLf against HSV-1 (or the absence of antiviral activity anti HSV-1 of the hen's Ovotransferrin), as compared with that of bLf, is linked to differences in the molecular structure. Bovine lactoferrin is 69% identical to human lactoferrin (49% to Ovotransferrin), but, in spite of this high degree of similarity, their comparison shows that the glycan chains of the molecules and the number of disulphide bridges vary (Metz-Boutigue *et al.*, 1984; Pierce *et al.*, 1991). These variations are likely to contribute to the differences in the functional domains responsible for the binding properties of the lactoferrins to host cells and viral particles (Marchetti *et al.*, 1996).

4.1 Antiviral activity of lactoferrin peptides

Antimicrobial peptides are produced by a wide variety of organisms as their first line of defense, the so-called innate immune strategy (Hancock, 2001). Hundreds of such peptides have been isolated (Hancock & Chapple, 1999), suggesting their importance in the innate immune system (Hancock & Diamond, 2000). Antimicrobial peptides are typically relatively short (12 to 100 amino acids), positively charged, amphiphilic and have been isolated from single-celled microorganisms, amphibians, birds, fish plants and mammals, including man

(Wang & Wang, 2004; Ganz, 2005). Several antimicrobial peptides have been shown to also inhibit viral infection. The spectrum of viruses that are affected primarily comprises the enveloped RNA and DNA viruses. In most cases it has been concluded that antiviral activity is exerted at a very early stage in the viral multiplication cycle, either by direct action of the peptides on the virus itself (Aboudy *et al.*, 1994; Robinson *et al.*, 1998) or at the virus-cell interface (Belaid *et al.*, 2002). It has also been demonstrated that antimicrobial peptides regulate multiple cellular genes (Scott *et al.*, 2002), findings which support peptide stimulation of the cellular immune response (Andersen *et al.*, 2004). A reasonable hypothesis is that the products of a subset of these peptide-upregulated genes are able to suppress endotoxic responses that lead to production of pro-inflammatory cytokines while upregulating other genes assisting in resolving infections (Bowdish *et al.*, 2005 a, b; Bowdish & Hancock, 2005; Jenssen, 2005).

bLf derived peptide lactoferricin B (bovine lactoferrin fragment bLf17–41), generated from pepsin digestion of such protein, besides activities reported against bacteria, fungi, protozoa, and tumors (Bellamy *et al.*, 1992; Yoo *et al.*, 1998; Omata *et al.*, 2001), exerts a small, although significant, antiviral activity towards herpes simplex virus (Andersen *et al.*, 2004), human cytomegalovirus (Andersen *et al.*, 2001), and adenovirus (Di Biase *et al.*, 2003). In solution, lactoferricin B adopts a twisted beta-sheet structure that becomes markedly amphipathic with the hydrophobic groups lining up on one face of the peptide, while the opposite face contains most of the basic residues (Vogel *et al.*, 2002; Zhou *et al.*,2004) possibly interacting with glycosaminoglycan viral receptors. The N-terminus of lactoferrin binds to surface glycosaminoglycans (Mann *et al.*, 1994; Wu *et al.*, 1995), which are initial binding sites for HASV-1 virus (WuDunn & Spear, 1989; Roderiquez *et al.*, 1995) and a direct lactoferrin interaction with viral particles has been hypothetized (Marchetti *et al.*, 1996; Swart et al., 1996; Yi *et al.*, 1997). In an attempt to identify other lactoferrin amino acid sequences contributing to the antiviral activity, the antiviral activity of a library of peptide fragments, derived from the tryptic digestion of bLf, was analysed towards HSV1, a susceptible enveloped virus. The pool of fragments deriving from tryptic digestion of bLf showed antiviral activity toward HSV-1, suggesting that the inhibition of viral infection could not be exclusively linked to native, undigested bLf (Siciliano *et al.*, 1999).

Moreover, the protective effect towards HSV-1 infection possessed by low and high molecular weight peptides, deriving from tryptic digestion of bLf, was analyzed. Among high molecular weight peptides, the fraction with amino acid sequence 1–280, belonging to the N-lobe, was ten-fold more effective towards HSV-1 infection than the fraction representing the whole C-lobe. On the other hand, the fraction 1-280 was still six-fold less active than native bLf, which exerted the maximal antiviral activity. The different antiviral activity of the C-lobe and N-lobe toward HSV-1 cannot be explained on the basis of their different glycosylation sites (three glycosylation sites present in C-lobe while only one in N-lobe) since their removal from undigested bLf did not affect anti HSV-1 activity (Sicilano *et al.*, 1999). The absence of antiviral activity of the large fraction with amino acid sequence 86–258, which corresponds to the N2 domain, has been correlated to the lack of amino acid sequences 1–85 and/or 259–280, present in the effective fraction 1–280 which contains the N2 domain together with part of the N1 domain. Furthermore, it was observed that, among the low molecular weight fragments, only the association of two small peptides (ADRDQYELL (bLf222–230) and EDLIWK (bLf264–269) was effective. Considering their molecular mass, these peptides showed a much lower antiviral activity than that displayed by undigested bLf and by the fraction 1-280. Interestingly, these small peptides did not display any antiviral activity when they were separately tested.

It is important to note that effective fraction 1–280 contains both amino acid sequences of the two small co-purified peptides (amino acid sequences 222– 230 and 264–269), while ineffective fraction 86–258 does not contain the amino acid sequence 264–269 (Siciliano *et al.,* 1999). In the three-dimensional structure of iron-saturated bLf, these two small peptides are exposed to the solvent at the bLf surface and are located at opposite sites of the N-lobe (belonging to N2 and N1 domains respectively) (Moore *et al.,* 1997). The markedly reduced antiviral activity displayed by the two associated peptides (amino acid sequences 222–230 and 264–269) could therefore be correlated with the lack of the correct folding when they are separated from the protein.
All together, these results suggest that in bovine lactoferrin, both amino acid sequences and their conformations are involved in protection form HSV-1 infection (Siciliano *et al.,* 1999). Therefore it was concluded that the cluster of positive charges present in bLf has to be considered to be crucial for anti-herpesvirus activity. Interestigly, it should be noted that the anti HSV-1 active fragments belonging to the N-lobe of bLf do not have anti-rotavirus activity, while other peptides, belonging to the C-lobe, possess anti-rotavirus activity. The antiviral activity of lactoferrin towards viruses belonging to different families appears, therefore to be due to specific, although different, mechanisms, depending on the inhibited virus (Superti *et al.,* 2001)

5. Antiviral activity of intact ovotransferrin

Contrary to the antiviral activity of lactoferrin, the antiviral activity of ovotransferrin was not demonstrated until a model of chicken embryo fibroblasts infected with Marek's Disease Virus (MDV) was used (Giansanti *et al.,* 2002).
MDV belongs to the Herpesviridae family, and is currently grouped within the Alphaherpersvirinae subfamily, together with the herpesvirus of turkey (HVT) (Calnek, 2001). It possesses a 166–184 kb, double-stranded DNA genome. Like many herpesviruses (Izumiya *et al.,* 2001), MDV is highly cell-associated. MDV infection of susceptible cells is generally cytocidal, but latency can also be established. The virus-induced pathological changes, known as the cytopathic effect (CPE), take place in both the cytoplasm and the nucleus when the lytic cycle is ongoing. MDV has been shown to induce the synthesis of ovotransferrin in infected chicken embryo fibroblasts (Morgan *et al.,* 2001). In chicken embryo fibroblast primary cultures, Otrf is effective in inhibiting infection by the herpesvirus of Marek disease. In this experimental avian herpes virus system, Otrf was more active than bLf or hLf. As already shown in human HSV model (Marchetti *et al.,* 1996), iron saturation of the proteins did not influence the inhibiting activity of the iron-binding proteins, even though it could be expected that conditions increasing iron availability may facilitate virus infection since this metal ion is essential for nucleic acids and protein synthesis. These similarities suggested that Otrf inhibits MDV replication in a way similar to that utilized by hLf and bLf in inhibiting HSV-1 replication.

5.1 Antiviral activity of ovotransferrin peptides

Like lactoferrin, Otrf displays antiviral activity, though only when tested in homologous cell systems using primary cultures of chicken embryo fibroblasts infected with Marek's disease virus. Lactoferricin B (bovine lactoferrin fragment bLf17–41) and two peptides, derived from the tryptic digestion of bLf, fragments ADRDQYELL (bLf222–230) and EDLIWK (bLf264–269), have been found to display antiviral activity towards herpes simplex virus (Siciliano *et al.,* 1999), although, the antiviral activity of lactoferricin B and of these two other peptides was much lower than that of the intact protein, and this was tentatively attributed to the lack of correct folding of such fragments when they are separated from the protein. Therefore, fragments in hOtrf having sequence and/or structural homologies with the fragments with antiviral activity found in bLf were identified and tested for their antiviral activity with the aim of evaluating their possible involvement in the antiviral activity of the intact ovotransferrin. No fragment was identified in hOtrf having sequence homology with bLf fragment lactoferricin B (bLf17–41). On the contrary, two fragments having sequence homology with bLf fragments ADRDQYELL (bLf222–230) and EDLIWK (bLf264–269) were identified in hOtrf. The first one was the fragment DQKDEYELL (hOtrf219-227), while the second one was the fragment KDLLFK. Interestingly, the latter fragment KDLLFK is repeated twice in hOtrf, both in N-lobe (hOtrf269-361) and in C-lobe (hOtrf633–638). Moreover, hOtrf fragments DQKDEYELL and KDLLFK are located at the surface of the protein. As concerning structural homologies in the intact proteins, the hOtrf fragment KDLLFK possesses into the intact hOtrf a conformation similar to that possessed by the fragment EDLIWK in intact bLf (see figure 3). Similarly, the fragment LQMDDFELL (hOtrf561–569) displays the greatest structural homology in intact hOtrf with the fragments ADRDQYELL into intact bLf (see figure 3).

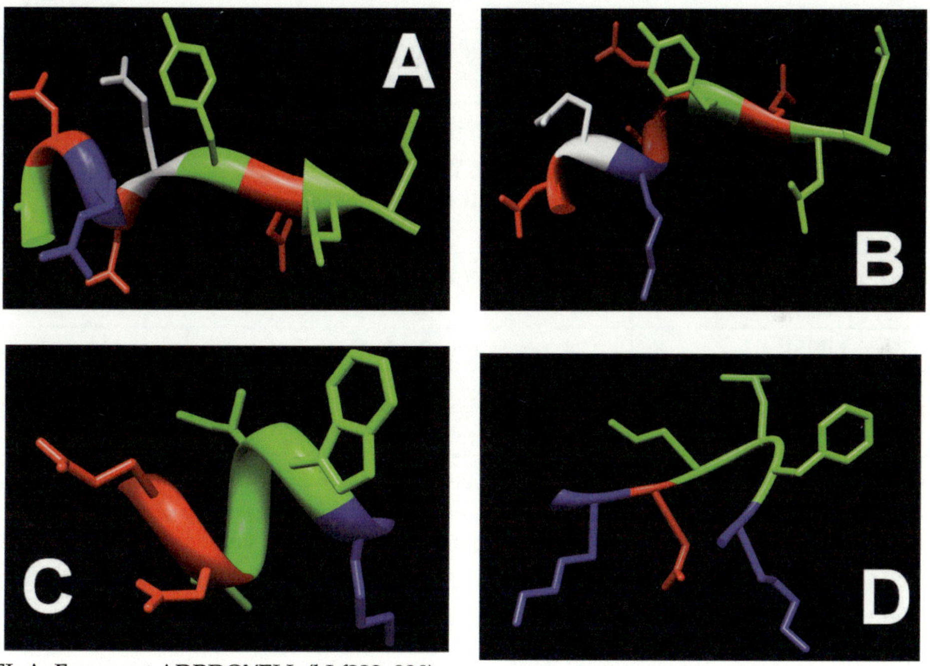

PANEL A: Fragment ADRDQYELL (bLf222–230),
PANEL B: Fragment DQKDEYELL (hOtrf219-227)
PANEL C: Fragment EDLIWK (bLf264–269)
PANEL D: Fragment KDLLFK (hOtrf269-361 and hOtrf633-638).
The fragments are shown with the conformation they have in the intact proteins: bovine lactoferrin (bLf) and hen's ovotransferrin (hOTrf). The ribbons indicate the presence of alpha-elices. In Panel A, the arrow indicates a.a. sequence direction. The colors indicate aminoacid properties: Green: hydrophobic; Blue: negatively charged; Red: positively charged; White: polar.
Molecular graphics images were produced using the UCSF chimera package (Pettersen *et al.*, 2004)

Fig. 3. Lactoferrin and ovotransferrin fragments with anti-herpesvirus activity

However, NMR spectroscopy indicated that, as expected, all these peptides do not have a favourite conformation in solution, as they are too short to have any secondary structure. All the fragments were then chemically synthesized and the corresponding peptides were tested on CEF/ MDV system for their cytotoxic and antiviral activities, hOtrf and bLf being used as positive control proteins. The peptide LNNSRA, with no sequence or structural homologies, was used as negative control. The maximal antiviral activities were shown by the positive control intact proteins (hOtrf and bLf) and no antiviral activity was shown by the negative control peptide LNNSRA. The peptides LQMDDFELL (hOtrf561-569) and KDCIIK (hOtrf378-383), which have little or no sequence homologies with the corresponding bLf fragment despite structural homologies in the intact proteins, showed little or no antiviral activity. On the contrary, the peptides in hOtrf having greatest sequence homology, DQKDEYELL (hOtrf219-227) and KDLLFK (hOtrf269-361 and hOtrf633-638), with the bLf peptides with antiviral activity ADRDQYELL (bLf222-230) and EDLIWK (bLf264-269) showed significant antiviral activity towards MDV.

PEPTIDES	**Characteristic**	**Selectivity index (SI)**
ADRDQYELL ($bLf_{222-230}$)	Control Blf fragment with antiviral activity	≥ 50
DQKDEYELL ($Otrf_{219-227}$)	hOtrf fragment with sequence homology with $bLf_{222-230}$	≥ 125 *
EDLIWK ($bLf_{264-269}$)	Control Blf fragment with antiviral activity	≥ 20
KDLLFK ($Otrf_{269-361}$) and ($Otrf_{633-638}$)	hOtrf fragment with sequence homology with $bLf_{264-269}$	≥ 40 *
LNNSRA	negative control	1
Hen Ovotransferrin	positive control	≥ 1600
Bovine lactoferrin	positive control	≥ 1000

Selectivity index (SI) is expressed as the ratio between the effective dose required to inhibit fluorescence by 50% and the effective dose required for 50 % cytotoxicity. Statistically significant differences ($P < 0.05$) of the hOtrf fragment selectivity index as compared with that of the corresponding bLf fragment.

Table 1. Bovine lactoferrin and hen ovotransferrin fragments: Characteristics and Selectivity Index (SI) towards Marek Disease Virus (modified from Giansanti *et al.*, 2002).

The antiviral activities of these two hOtrf peptides were about the double of those shown by the corresponding bLf derived peptides with sequence homologies. It is worth noting that these two hOtrf fragments possess significant antiviral activity such as the corresponding homologous fragments in bLf, suggesting that these fragments could indeed have a role in the exploitation of antiviral activity towards herpes viruses of those proteins when they are in native conformation. However, the presence of hydrophobic and positively charged residues is possibly a condition needed but not sufficient for the antiviral activity of bLf and hOtrf derived peptides, since the conformations they assume in the intact proteins may also be required (Giansanti *et al.*, 2005)

6. Conclusions

The results reported here suggest that clusters of positive charges present in the N-lobe of both bovine lactoferrin and hen's ovotransferrin are the most responsible for the anti-herpesvirus activity. The antiviral activity of these proteins is exerted at a very early stage in the viral multiplication cycle, possibly by interference at the virus-cell interface by binding to cell surface glycosaminoglycans. Few protein short peptides display anti-herpesviridae activity, although hundreds-fold less than the intact proteins, indicating that, for the exploitation of the maximal antiviral activity, the correct folding of aminoacids containing these clusters of positive charges is also required.

7. Acknowledgements

Prof Dario Botti, Dr. Maria T. Massucci and Dr. Maria F. Giardi, Department of Basic and Applied Biology, University of L'Aquila, are gratefully acknowledged for valuable discussions.

8. References

Aboudy, Y., Mendelson, E., Shalit, I., Bessalle, R. & Fridkin, M. (1994) Activity of two synthetic amphiphilic peptides and magainin-2 against herpes simplex virus types 1 and 2. *Int. J. Pept. Protein Res.* 43: 573–582

Adldinger, H., & Calnek, B.W., (1973) Pathogenesis of Marek's disease: early distribution of virus and viral antigens in infected chickens. *J. National Cancer Inst.* 50:1287–1298.

Aguilera, O., Quiros, L. M. & Fierro, J.F. (2003) Transferrins selectively cause ion efflux through bacterial and artificial membranes, *FEBS Letters,* 548:5-10.

Aisen, P. & Harris, D.C. (1989). Physical biochemistry of the transferrins. In: *Iron carriers and iron proteins.* Vol. 5, pp. 241–351, Edited by: T. Loehr. VCH Publishers, New York.

Aisen, P. & Leibman, A. (1972) Lactoferrin and transferrin: a comparative study. *Biochim Biophys Acta;* 257:314–23.

Alderton, G., Ward, W. H. & Fevold, H. L. (1946) Identification of the bacteria-inhibiting iron-binding protein of egg white as conalbumin, *Arch Biochem.* 11:9-13.

Andersen, H. J., Jenssen, H., Sandvik, K. & Gutteberg, T. J. (2004) The anti-HSV activity of lactoferrin and lactoferricin is dependent on the presence of heparan sulfate at the cell surface. *J. Med. Virol.* 74: 262–271

Andersen, J.H., Osbakk, S.A., Vorland, L.H., Traavik, T. & Gutteberg, T.J. (2001). Lactoferrin and cyclic lactoferricin inhibit the entry of human cytomegalovirus into human fibroblasts. *Antiviral Res.* 51:141–149.

Anderson, B.F., Baker, H.M., Dodson, E.J., Norris, G.E., Rumball, S.V., Waters, J.M. & Baker, E.N. (1987). Structure of human lactoferrin at 3.2-Å resolution. *Proc. Natl. Acad. Sci. USA* 84:1769–1773.

Anderson, B.F., Baker, H.M., Norris, G.E., Rice, D.W. & Baker, E.N. (1989) Structure of human lactoferrin: crystallographic structure analysis and refinement at 2.8 Å resolution, *J. Mol. Biol.* 209:711–734.

Baigent, S.J., Smith, L.P., Nair, V.K., Currie, R.J. (2006) Vaccinal control of Marek's disease: current challenges, and future strategies to maximize protection. Vet Immunol Immunopathol. 112(1-2):78-86.

Baker, E.N. & Baker H.M. (2009) A structural framework for understanding the multifunctional character of lactoferrin. *Biochimie*. 91(1):3-10.

Baker, E.N. (1994). Structure and reactivity of transferrins. *Adv. Inorg. Chem.* 41: 389–463.

Baker, E.N., Anderson, B.F., Baker, H.M., MacGillivray, R.T., Moore, S.A., Peterson, N.A., Shewry, S.C., & Tweedie, J.W. (1998). Three-dimensional structure of lactoferrin. Implications for function, including comparisons with transferrin. *Adv. Exp. Med. Biol.* 443: 1–14.

Beasley, J. N., Patterson, L. T. & McWade, D. H. (1970) Transmission of Marek's disease by poultry house dust and chicken dander. *Am. J. Vet. Res.* 31:339–344.

Becker, Y., Tabor, E., Asher, Y., Grifman, M., Kleinman, Y. & Yayon, A. (1994) Entry of herpes simplex virus type 1 into cells Early steps in virus pathogenicity. In: *Pathogenicity of human herpes viruses due to specific pathogenicity genes* Becker, Y. & Darai. G. (Eds), pp. 3-20. Springer Verlag, Berlin.

Belaid, A., Aouni, M., Khelifa, R., Trabelsi, A., Jemmali, M. & Hani, K. (2002) In vitro antiviral activity of dermaseptins against herpes simplex virus type 1. *J. Med. Virol.* 66:229–234

Bellamy, W., Takase, M., Wakabayashi, H., Kawase, K. & Tomita, M. (1992) Antibacterial spectrum of lactoferricin B, a potent bactericidal peptide derived from the N-terminal region of bovine lactoferrin. *J. Appl. Bacteriol.* 73:472–479.

Bennett, R.M. & Kokocinski, T. (1987) Lactoferrin content of peripheral blood cells. *Br J Haematol*; 39:509–21

Bowdish, D. M. & Hancock, R. E. W. (2005) Anti-endotoxin properties of cationic host defence peptides and proteins. *J. Endotox. Res.* 11: 230–236

Bowdish, D. M., Davidson, D. J. & Hancock, R. E. W. (2005) A re-evaluation of the role of host defence peptides in mammalian immunity. *Curr. Protein Pept. Sci.* 1: 35–51

Bowdish, D. M., Davidson, D. J., Lau, Y. E., Lee, K., Scott, M. G. & Hancock, R. E. W. (2005) Impact of cationic host defence peptides on anti-infective immunity. *J. Leukocyte Biol.* 77: 451–459

Braun, V. & Braun M. (2002). Active transport of iron and siderophore antibiotics. *Curr. Opin. Microbiol.*, 5:194–201.

Brock, J.H. (2002) The physiology of lactoferrin. *Biochem Cell Biol.*80(1):1-6.

Bullen, J. J. (1981). The significance of iron in infection. *Rev. Infect. Dis.* 3:1127–1138.

Bullen, J.J.¸ Rogers, H.J. & Griffiths, E. (1978) Role of iron in bacterial infection, *Curr Top Microbiol Immunol.* 80:1-35.

Burnside, J. & Morgan, R. (2011) Emerging roles of chicken and viral microRNAs in avian disease. *BMC Proceedings* 5(4):S2

Buscaglia, C., Calnek B. W. & Schat, K. A. (1988) Effect of immunocompetence on the establishment and maintenance of latency with Marek's disease herpesvirus. *J. Gen. Virol.* 69:1067–1077.

Calnek, B. W. (1985). Pathogenesis of Marek's disease. In: Calnek BW, Spencer JL, editors. pp (374–90) Proc. Int. Symp. Marek's Disease. Kennett Square, USA: American Association of Avian Pathologists.

Calnek, B. W. (1986) Marek's disease - a model for herpesvirus oncology. *CRC Crit. Rev. Microbiol.* 12:293–320.

Calnek, B. W. (2001) Pathogenesis of Marek's disease virus infection. In: *Current Topics in Microbiology and Immunology,* Hirai, K. (Ed.),. Pp (25-55), Springer, Berlin.

Calnek, B. W., Schat, A. K., Peckham, M. C. & Fabricant, J. (1983) Field trials with a bivalent vaccine (HVT and SB-1) against Marek's disease. *Avian Dis.* 27:844–849.

Calnek, B., W., Schat, A. K., Heller, E. D. & Buscaglia, C. (1984a) In vitro infection of T lymphoblasts with Marek's disease virus. In: An International Symposium on Marek's Disease, Cornell University, Ithaca. pp (173–187).

Calnek, B. W., Schat, A. K., Ross, L. N. J. & Chen, C. H. (1984b) Further characterization of Marek's disease virus-infected lymphocytes. II. In vitro infection. *Int. J. Cancer* 33:399–406.

Calnek, B. W., Schat, K. A., Shek, W. R. & Chen, C. L. H. (1982) In vitro infection of lymphocytes with Marek's disease virus. *J. National Cancer Inst.* 69:709–713.

Calnek, B.W. (2001) Pathogenesis of Pathogenesis of Marek's virus infection. *Curr. Top. Microbiol. Immunol.* 255:25–55.

Campadelli-Fiume, G., Stirpe, D., Boscaro, A., Avitabile, E., Foá-Tomasi, L., Barker, D. & Roizman, B. (1990) Glycoprotein C-dependent attachment of herpes simplex virus to susceptible cells leading to productive infection. *Virology.* 178(1):213-22.

Chubb, R. C. & Churchill, A. E. (1969) Effect of maternal antibody on Marek's disease. *Vet. Rec.* 85:303–305.

Churchill, A. E. & Chubb, R. C. (1969) The attenuation, with loss of oncogenicity, of the herpes-type virus of Marek's disease (strain HPRS-16) on passage in cell culture. *J. Gen. Virol.* 4:557–564.

Connely, O.M. (2001) Antiinflammatory activities of lactoferrin. *J Am Coll Nutr;* 20(5):389S–95S.

Deng, X., Li, X., Shen, Y., Qiu, Y., Shi, Z., Shao, D., Jin, Y., Chen, H., Ding, C., Li, L., Chen, P. & Ma Z. (2010) The Meq oncoprotein of Marek's disease virus interacts with p53 and inhibits its transcriptional and apoptotic activities. *Virology Journal* 7:348

Di Biase, A.M., Pietrantoni, A., Tinari, A. , Siciliano, R. , Valenti, P., Antonini, G., Seganti, L. & Superti, F. (2003) Effect of bovine lactoferricin on enteropathogenic Yersinia adhesion and invasion in HEp-2 cells. *J. Med. Virol.* 69:495–502.

Dierich, A., Gaub, M.P., LePennec, J.P., Astinotti, D. & Chambon, P. (1987) Cell-specificity of the chicken ovalbumin and conalbumin promoters. *EMBO J.* 6(8):2305-12

Eidson, C. S., Page, R. K. & Kleven, S. H. (1978) Effectiveness of cell-free or cell-associated turkey herpesvirus vaccine against Marek's disease in chickens as influenced by maternal antibody, vaccine dose, and time of exposure to Marek's disease virus. *Avian Dis.* 22:583–597.

Forrester, A., Farrell, H., Wilkinson, G., Kaye, J., Davis-Poynter, N. & Minson, T. (1992) Construction and properties of a mutant of herpes simplex virus type 1 with glycoprotein H coding sequences deleted. *J Virol.* 66(1):341-8.

Fuller, A.O. & Lee, W.C. (1992) Herpes simplex virus type 1 entry through a cascade of virus-cell interactions requires different roles of gD and gH in penetration. *J Virol.* 66(8):5002-12.

Ganz, T. (2005) Defensins and other antimicrobial peptides: a historical perspective and an update. *Comb. Chem. High Throughput Screen.* 3: 209–217

Geerligs, H. J., Weststrate, M. W., Pertile, T. L., Rodenberg, J., Kumar, M. & Chu, S. (1999) Efficacy of a combination vaccine containing MDV CVI 988 strain and HVT against challenge with very virulent MDV. *Acta Virol.* 43:198–200.

Giansanti, F., Giardi, M. F., Massucci, M. T., Botti, D. & Antonini, G. (2007) Ovotransferrin expression and release by chicken cell lines infected with Marek's disease virus, *Biochem Cell Biol.,* 85(1):150-155.

Giansanti, F., Massucci, M. T., Giardi, M. F., Nozza, F., Pulsinelli, E., Nicolini, C., Botti, D., & Antonini, G. (2005) Antiviral activity of ovotransferrin derived peptides. *Biochemical and Biophysical Research Communications* 331:69–73.

Giansanti, F., Rossi, P., Massucci, M. T., Botti, D., Antonini, G., Valenti, P. & Seganti, L. (2002) Antiviral activity of ovotransferrin discloses an evolutionary strategy for the defensive activities of lactoferrin. *Biochem. Cell. Biol.* 80:125-130.

Giardi, M. F.¸ La Torre, C., Giansanti, F. & Botti, D. (2009) Effects of transferrins and cytokines on nitric oxide production by an avian lymphoblastoid cell line infected with Marek's disease virus, *Antiviral Research,* 81:248–252.

Gimeno, I.M. & Cortes, A.L..(2010) Evaluation of factors influencing replication of serotype 1 Marek's disease vaccines in the chicken lung. *Avian Pathol.* 39(2):71-9).

Gimeno, I.M. (2008) Marek's disease vaccines: a solution for today but a worry for tomorrow? *Vaccine.*18;26 Suppl 3:C31-41.

González-Chávez, S.A., Arévalo-Gallegos, S. & Rascón-Cruz. Q. (2009) Lactoferrin: structure, function and applications. *Int J Antimicrob Agents.* 33(4):301.

Gruenheid, S., Gatzke, L., Meadows, H. & Tufaro F. (1993) Herpes simplex virus infection and propagation in a mouse cell mutant lacking heparan sulfate proteoglycans. *J. Virol.* 67:93–100

Gupta, M. K., Chauhan, H. V. S., Jha, G. J. & Singh, K. K. (1989) The role of the reticuloendothelial system in the immunopathology of Marek's disease. *Vet. Microbiol.* 20:223–234.

Haffer, K. & Sevoian, M. (1979) In vitro studies on the role of the macrophages of resistant and susceptible chickens with Marek's disease. *Poult. Sci.* 58:295–297.

Haffer, K., Sevoian, M. & Wilder, M. (1979) The role of the macrophage in Marek's disease: in vitro and in vivo studies. *Int. J. Cancer* 23:648–656.

Hancock, R. E. W. & Chapple, D. S. (1999) Peptide antibiotics. *Antimicrob. Agents Chemother.* 43: 1317–1323

Hancock, R. E. W. & Diamond, G. (2000) The role of cationic antimicrobial peptides in innate host defences. *Trends Microbiol.* 8: 402–410

Hancock, R. E. W. (2001) Cationic peptides: effectors in innate immunity and novel antimicrobials. *Lancet Infect. Dis.* 1: 156–164

Hara, K., Ikeda, M., Saito, S., Matsumoto, S., Numata, K., Kato, N. (2002). Lactoferrin inhibits hepatitis B virus infection in cultured human hepatocytes. *Res. Hepatol.* 24:228–236.

Harmsen, M.C., Swart, P.J., de Béthune M.P., Pawels, R., De Clercq, E., The, T.H. & Meijer, D.K.F. (1995). Antiviral effects of plasma and milk proteins: lactoferrin shows a potent activity against both human immunodeficiency virus and human cytomegalovirus replication *in vitro. J. Infect. Dis.* 172: 280–388.

Heidari, M., Zhang, H.M. & Sharif, S., (2008) Marek's disease virus induces Th-2 activity during cytolytic infection. *Viral Immunol.* 21(2):203-14.

Herold, B.C., Visalli, R.J., Susmarski, N., Brandt, C.R., Spear, P.G. (1994) Glycoprotein C-independent binding of herpes simplex virus to cells requires cell surface heparan sulphate and glycoprotein B. *J Gen Virol.* 75 (Pt 6):1211-22.

Hodnichak, C.M., Turley-Shoger, E., Mohanty, J.G. & Rosenthal, K.S. (1984) Visualization of herpes simplex virus type 1 attachment to target cells using Staphylococcus aureus as a morphologic tag. *J Virol Methods.* 8(3):191-8.

Hussain, I. & Qureshi, M. A. (1997) Nitric oxide synthase activity and mRNA expression in chicken macrophages. *Poult. Sci.* 76:1524–1530.

Ibrahim, H. R. , Sugimoto, Y. & Aoki, T. (2000) Ovotransferrin antimicrobial peptide (OTAP-92) kills bacteria through a membrane damage mechanism. *Biochimica et Biophysica Acta,* 1523:196-205.

Ibrahim, H. R., Iwamori, E., Sugimoto, Y. & Aoki, T. (1998) Identification of a distinct antibacterial domain within the N-lobe of Ovotransferrin. *Biochimica et Biophysica Acta,* 1401:289–303.

Ikeda, M., Nozaki, A., Sugiyama, K., Tanaka, T., Naganuma, A., Tanaka, K., Sekihara, H., Shimotohno, K., Saito, M. & Kato,V. (2000) Characterization of antiviral activity of lactoferrin against hepatitis C virus infection in human cultured cells. *Virus Res.* 66:51-63.

Ikeda, M., Sugiyama, K., Tanaka, T., Tanaka, K., Sekihara, H., Shimotohno, K. & Kato, N.(1998). Lactoferrin markedly inhibits hepatitis C virus infection in cultured human hepatocytes. *Biochem. Biophys. Res. Commun.*245:549–553.

Izumiya, Y., Jang, H. K., Ono, M. & Mikami, T. (2001) A complete genomic DNA sequence of Marek's disease virus type 2, strain HPRS24. *Curr. Top. Microb. Immunol.* 255: 191–221.

Jeltsch, J. M., Chambon, P. (1982) The complete nucleotide sequence of the chicken ovotransferrin mRNA. *Eur J Biochem.* 122(2):291-295.

Jenssen, H. (2005) Anti herpes simplex virus activity of lactoferrin/lactoferricin - an example of antiviral activity of antimicrobial protein/ Peptide. *Cell. Mol. Life Sci.* 62:3002–3013.

Ji, Z.S. & Mahley, R.W. (1994) Lactoferrin binding to heparan sulfate proteoglycans and the LDL receptor-related protein. Further evidence supporting the importance of direct binding of remnant lipoproteins to HSPG. *Arterioscler Thromb.* 14(12):2025-31.

Johnson, D.C., Burke, R.L. & Gregory, T. (1990) Soluble forms of herpes simplex virus glycoprotein D bind to a limited number of cell surface receptors and inhibit virus entry into cells. *J Virol.* 64(6):2569-76.

Kaufman, J. & Salomonsen, J. (1997) The minimal essential MHC revisited: both peptide-binding and cell surface expression level of MHC molecules are polymorphisms selected by pathogens in chickens. *Hereditas* 127:67–73.

Kaufman, J. & Venugopal, K. (1998) The importance of MHC for Rous sarcoma virus and Marek's disease virus—some Paynefull considerations. *Avian Pathol.* 27:82–87.

Kaufman, J. (1996). Structure and function of the major histocompatibility complex of chickens. In: *Poultry Immunology,* Davison F., Payne L. N., Morris T. R. (Eds.). pp (27-82), Carfax Publishing Company, Aberdeen, UK.,

Kodama, H., Mikami, T., Inoue, M. & Izawa, H. (1979) Inhibitory effects of macrophages against Marek's disease virus plaque formation in chicken kidney cell cultures. *J. Nat. Cancer Inst.* 63:1267–1271.

Kurokawa, H., Dewan, J.C., Mikami, B., Sacchettini, J.C. & Hirose, M.(1999) Crystal structure of hen apo-ovo transferrin: both lobes adopt an open conformation upon loss of iron, *J. Biol. Chem.* 274 (40):28445–28452.

Kurokawa, H., Mikami, B. & Hirose, M. (1995) Crystal structure of diferric hen ovotransferrin at 2.4 Å resolution, *J. Mol. Biol.* 254:196–207.

Kuser, P., Hall, D.R., Haw, M.L., Neu, M., Evans R.W. & Lindley, P.F. The mechanism of iron uptake by transferrins: the X-ray structures of the 18 kDa NII domain fragment of duck ovotransferrin and its nitrilotriacetate complex, *Acta Cryst. D* 58 (2002) 777–783.

Leboffe, L., Giansanti, F. & Antonini, G. (2009) Antifungal and Antiparasitic Activities of Lactoferrin, *Anti-Infective Agents in Medicinal Chemistry,* 14:114-127.

Lee, L. F., Sharma, J. M., Nazerian, K. & Witter, R. L. (1978a) Suppression and enhancement of mitogen response in chickens infected with Marek's disease virus and the herpesvirus of turkeys. *Infect. Immun.* 21:474–479.

Lee, L. F., Sharma, J. M., Nazerian, K. & Witter, R. L. (1978b) Suppression of mitogen-induced proliferation of normal spleen cells by macrophages from chickens inoculated with Marek's disease virus. *J. Immunol.* 120:1554–1559.

Lindley, P.F., Bajaj, M., Evans, R.W., Garatt, R.C., Hasnain, S.S., Jhoti, H., Kuser, P., Neu, M., Patel, K., Sarra, R., Strange, P. & Walton, A. (1993) The mechanism of iron uptake by transferrins: the structure of an 18 kDa NII-domain fragment from duck ovotransferrin at 2.3 Å resolution, *Acta Cryst. D* 49:292–304.

Liu, J. L., Lin, S. F., Xia, L., Brunovskis, P., Li, D., (1999) Davidson I. et al. MEQ and v-IL8: cellular genes in disguise? *Acta Virol.* 43: 94–101.

Liu, J. L., Ye, Y., Lee, L. F. & Kung, H. J. (1998) Transforming potential of the herpesvirus oncoprotein MEQ: morphological transformation, serum-independent growth, and inhibition of apoptosis. *J. Virol.* 72:388–395.

Lönnerdal, B. & Iyer, S. (1995) Lactoferrin: molecular structure and biological function. *Annu Rev Nutr.* 15:93-110.

Lu, L., Hangoc, G., Oliff, A., Chen, L.T., Shen, R.N. & Broxmeyer, H.E. (1987) Protective influence of lactoferrin on mice infected with the polycythemia-inducing strain of Friend viruscomplex. *Cancer Res.* ;47(15):4184-8.

Mann, D.M., Romm, E. & Migliorini, M. (1994) Delineation of the glycosaminoglycan-binding site in the human inflammatory response protein lactoferrin, *J. Biol. Chem.* 269:23661-23667.

Marchetti, M., Longhi, C., Conte, M. P., Pisani, S., Valenti, P. and Seganti, L. (1996) Lactoferrin inhibits herpes simplex virus type 1 adsorption to Vero cells. *Antiviral Research* . 29, 221-231

Marchetti, M., Longhi, C., Conte, M.P., Pisani, S., Valenti, P. & Seganti, L. (1996). Lactoferrin inhibits herpes simplex virus type 1 adsorption to Vero cells. *Ativiral Res.* 29:221–231.

Marchetti, M., Pisani, S., Antonini, G., Valenti, P., Seganti, L. & Orsi, N. (1998) Metal complexes of bovine lactoferrin inhibit in vitro replication of herpes simplex virus type 1 and 2. *BioMetals* 11:89-94.

Marek, J. (1907) Multiple Nervenentzündung (Polyneuritis) bei Hühnern. *Deutsche Tierärztliche Wochenschrift* 15:417–421.

Martins-Green, M. (2001) The chicken Chemotactic and Angiogenic Factor (cCAF), a CXC chemokine. *The Int J of Biochem & Cell Biol* 33:427–432.

Medveczky, P. G., Friedman, H. & Bendinelli, M. (1998). *Herpesviruses and Immunity*. Plenum Press, New York and London.

Mester, J. C. & Rouse, B. T. (1991) The mouse model and understanding immunity to herpes simplex virus. *Rev. Inf. Dis.* 13:935–945.

Metz-Boutigue, M.H., Jolles, J., Mazurier, J., Schoentgen, F., Legrand, D., Spik, G., Montreuil, J. & Jolles, P. (1984) Human lactotransferrin: amino acid sequence and structural comparisons with other transferrins. *Eur. J. Biochem.* 145, 659-676

Mizutani, K., Yamashita, H., Kurokawa, H., Mikami, B. & Mikami, B. (1999) Alternative structural state of transferrin. The crystallographic analysis of iron-loaded but domain-opened ovotransferrin N-lobe, *J. Biol. Chem.* 274:10190–10194.

Mizutani, K., Yamashita, H., Mikami, B. & Hirose, M. (2000) Crystal structure at 1.9 Å resolution of the apoovotransferrin N-lobe bound by sulfate anions: Implications for the domain opening and iron release mechanism, *Biochemistry.* 39:3258–3265.

Moore, S.A,, Anderson, B.F., Groom, C.R., Haridas, M., & Baker, EN. (1997) Three-dimensional structure of diferric bovine lactoferrin at 2.8 Å resolution. *J Mol Biol.* 274(2):222-36.

Morgan, R.W., Sofer, L., Anderson, A.S., Bernberg, E.L., Cui, J. & Burnside, J. (2001) Induction of host gene expression following infection of chicken embryo fibroblasts with oncogenic Mareks disease virus. *J. Virol.* 75:533–539.

Morimura, T., Hattori, M., Ohashi, K., Sugimoto, C. & Onuma, M. (1995) Immunomodulation of peripheral T cells in chickens infected with Marek's disease virus: involvement in immunosuppression. *J. Gen. Virol.* 76:2979–2985.

Morimura, T., Ohashi, K., Kon, Y., Hattori, M., Sugimoto, C. & Onuma, M. (1996) Apoptosis and CD8-down-regulation in the thymus of chickens infected with Marek's disease virus. *Arch. Virol.* 141:2243–2249.

Morimura, T., Ohashi, K., Sugimoto, C. & Onuma, M. Pathogenesis of Marek's (1998) Disease and possibile mechanisms of immunity induced by MD vaccine. *J. Vet. Med. Sci.* 60:1-8.

Mwangi, W.N., Smith, L.P., Baigent, S.J., Beal, R.K., Nair, V. & Smith, A.L.(2011) Clonal Structure of Rapid-Onset MDV-Driven CD4+ Lymphomas and Responding CD8+ T Cells. *PLoS Pathog.* 7(5):e1001337. Epub 2011 May 5).

Nair, V. (2005) Evolution of Marek's disease – A paradigm for incessant race between the pathogen and the host. *Vet. J.* 170:175–183.

Nazerian, K., Solomon, J. J., Witter, R. L. & Burmester, B. R. (1968) Studies on the etiology of Marek's disease. II. Finding of a herpesvirus in cell culture. *Proc. Soc. Exp. Biol. Med.* 127:177-182.

Oe, H., Doi, E. & Hirose, M. (1988) Amino-terminal and carboxyl-terminal half-molecules of ovotransferrin: preparation by a novel procedure and their interactions, *J Biochem.* 103(6): 1066-1072.

Okazaki, W., Purchase, H. G. & Burmester, B. R. (1970) Protection against Marek's disease by vaccination with a herpesvirus of turkeys. *Avian Dis.* 14:413–429.

Omata, Y., Satake, M., Maeda, R., Saito, A., Shimazaki, K., Yamauchi, K. , Uzuka, Y., Tanabe, S., Sarashina, T. & Mikami, T. (2001) Reduction of the infectivity of Toxoplasma gondii and Eimeria stiedai sporozoites by treatment with bovine lactoferricin, *J. Vet. Med. Sci.* 63:187–190.

Öztas¸ Yes¸ im ER, Özgünes¸ N. (2005) Lactoferrin: a multifunctional protein. *Adv Mol Med*;1:149–54.

Pappenheimer, A. M., Dunn, L. C. & Cone, V. (1926) A study of fowl paralysis (neuro-lymphomatosis gallinarum). *Storrs Agric. Exp. Stat. Bull.* 143:186–190.

Parcells, M. S., Lin, S-F, Dienglewicz, R. L., Majerciak, V., Robinson, D. R., Chen, H-C (2001) Marek's disease virus (MDV) encodes an interleukin-8 homolog (vIL-8): characterization of the vIL-8 protein and a vIL-8 deletion mutant MDV. *J. Virol.* 75: 5159–5173.

Payne, L. N. & Venugopal, K. (2000) Neoplastic Diseases: Marek's Disease, avian leukosis and reticuloendoteliosis. *Rev. Sci. Tech. Off. Int. Efiz.* 19:544-564.

Peng, Q. & Shirazi, Y. (1996) Characterization of the protein product encoded by a splicing variant of the Marek's disease virus Eco-Q gene (Meq). *Virology* 226:77–82.

Pettersen, E.F., Goddard, T.D., Huang, C.C., Couch, G.S., Greenblatt, D.M., Meng, E.C., Ferrin, T.E., UCSF Chimera: a visualization system for exploratory research and analysis, *J. Comput. Chem.* 25 (13): 1605–1612.

Pierce, A., Colavizza, D., Benaissa, M., Maes, P., Tartar, A., Montreuil, J. & Spik, G. (1991) Molecular cloning and sequence analysis of bovine lactotransferrin. *Eur. J. Biochem.* 196, 177-184.

Pratt, W. D., Cantello, J., Morgan, R. W. & Schat, K. A. (1994) Enhanced expression of the Marek's disease virus specific phosphoprotein after stable transfection of MSB-1 cells with the Marek's disease homologue of ICP4. *Virology* 201:132–136.

Puddu, P., Borghi, P., Gessani, S., Valenti, P., Belardelli, F. & Seganti, L. (1998) Antiviral effect of bovine lactoferrin saturated with metal ions on early steps of human immunodeficiency virus type 1 infection. *Int. J. Biochem. Cell Biol.* 30:1055-1062.

Purchase, H. G. & Okazaki, W. (1971) Effect of vaccination with herpesvirus of turkeys (HVT) on horizontal spread of Marek's disease herpesvirus. *Avian Dis.* 15:391–397.

Qureshi, M. A., Heggen, C. L. & Hussain, I. (2000) Avian macrophage: effector functions in health and disease. *Dev. Comp. Immunol.* 24:103–119.

Rispens, B. H., Vloten, Van, H. J., Mastenbroek, H., Maas, H. J. L. & Schat, K. A. (1972) Control of Marek's disease in the Netherlands. I. Isolation of an avirulent Marek's disease virus (strain CVI988) and its use in laboratory vaccination trials. *Avian Dis.* 16:108–125.

Rivas, C., Djeraba, A., Musset, E., van Rooijen, N., Baaten, B. & Quere, P. (2003) Intravenous treatment with liposome-encapsulated dichloromethylene bisphosphonate (Cl2MBP) suppresses nitric oxide production and reduces genetic resistance to Marek's disease. *Avian Pathol.* 32:139–149.

Robinson, W. E., Jr, McDougall, B., Tran, D. & Selsted, M. E. (1998) Anti-HIV-1 activity of indolicidin, an antimicrobial peptide from neutrophils. *J. Leukoc. Biol.* 63: 94–100

Roderiquez, G., Oravecz, T., Yanagishita, M., Bou-Habib, D.C., Mostowski, H. & Nocross, M.A. (1995). Mediation of human immunodeficiency virus type 1 binding by interaction of cell surface heparan sulfate proteoglycans with the V3 region of envelope gp120-gp41. *J. Virol.* 357:393-399.

Rodriguez, D.A., Vazquez, L. & Ramos, G. (2005) Antimicrobial mechanisms and potential clinical application of lactoferrin. *Rev Latinoam Microbiol* 47:102–11.

Roop, C., Hutchinson, L. & Johnson, D.C. (1993) A mutant herpes simplex virus type 1 unable to express glycoprotein L cannot enter cells, and its particles lack glycoprotein H. *J Virol.* 67(4):2285-97

Ross, L. J. N. (1977) Antiviral T cell-mediated immunity in Marek's disease. *Nature* 268:644–646.

Ross, N., O'Sullivan, G., Rothwell, C., Smith, G., Burgess, S. C., Rennie, M., Lee, L. F. and Davison, T. F. (1997) Marek's disease virus *Eco*R1-Q gene (*meq*) and a small RNA antisense to ICP4 are abundantly expressed in CD4+ cells carrying a novel lymphoid marker, AV37, in Marek's disease lymphomas. *J. Gen. Virol.* 78:2191–2198.

Sánchez, L., Calvo, M., Brock, J.H. (1992) Biological role of lactoferrin. *Arch Dis Child.* 67(5):657-61.

Schat, K. A & Xing, Z. (2000) Specific and non-specific immune responses to Marek's disease virus. *Dev. Comp. Immunol.* 24: 201-221.

Schat, K. A. (1987) Marek's disease - a model for protection against herpesvirus-induced tumors. *Cancer Surveys.* 6:1–37.

Schat, K. A. (2001). Specific and nonspecific immune responses to Marek's disease virus. In: *Current Progress on Marek's Disease Research.* Schat KA, Morgan RW, Parcells MS and Spencer JL (eds.). pp (123-126). American Association of Avian Pathologists, Kennett Square, PA.

Schat, K. A., Calnek, B. W. & Fabricant, J. (1980) Influence of the bursa of Fabricius on the pathogenesis of Marek's disease. *Infect. Immun.* 31:199–207.

Schat, K.A. & Baranowski, E. (2007) Animal vaccination and the evolution of viral pathogens. *Rev. sci. tech. Off. int. Epiz.,* 26 (2), 327-338.

Scott, M. G., Davidson, D. J., Gold, M. R., Bowdish, D. M. & Hancock, R. E. W. (2002) The human antimicrobial peptide LL-37 is a multifunctional modulator of innate immune responses. *J. Immunol.* 169: 3883–3891

Sharma, A.K., Paramasivam, M., Srinivasan, A., Yadav, M.P. & Singh, T.P. (1998). Three-dimensional structure of mare diferric lactoferrin at 2.6 Å resolution. *J. Mol. Biol.* 289: 303–317.

Sharma, J. M. (1980) In vitro suppression of T-cell mitogenic response and tumor cell proliferation by spleen macrophages from normal chickens. *Infect. Immun.* 28:914–922.

Shek, W., Calnek, B. W., Schat, K. & Chen, C. (1983) Characterization of Marek's disease virus-infected lymphocytes: discrimination between cytolytically and latently infected cells. *J. National Cancer Inst.* 70:485–491.

Shieh, M.T., WuDunn, D., Montgomery, R.I., Esko, J.D. & Spear, P.G. (1992) Cell surface receptors for herpes simplex virus are heparan sulfate proteoglycans. *J Cell Biol.* 116(5):1273-81.

Siciliano, R., Rega, B., Marchetti, M., Seganti, S., Antonini, G & Valenti, P. (1999) Bovine Lactoferrin Peptidic Fragments Involved in Inhibition of Herpes Simplex Virus. Type 1 Infection *Biochemical and Biophysical Research Communications* 264, 19–23.

Spear, P. G., Eisenberg, R. J. & Cohen, G. H. (2000) Three classes of cell surface receptors for alphaherpesvirus entry. *Virology*.275:1–8.

Spear, P.G. & Longnecker, R. (2003) Herpesvirus Entry: an Update. *J. Virol.* 77:10179–10185.

Spear, P.G., Shieh, M.T., Herold, B.C., WuDunn, D. & Koshy, T.I. (1992) Heparan sulfate glycosaminoglycans as primary cell surface receptors for herpes simplex virus. *Adv Exp Med Biol.* 313:341-53.

Spector, T., Harrington, J.A. & Porter, D.J.T. (1991) Herpes and human ribonucleotide reductases: inhibition by 2-acetylpyridine 5-[(2-chloroanilino)thiocarbonyl] thiocarbonohydrazone (348U87). *Biochem. Pharmacol.* 42, 91-96

Spector, T., Harrington, J.A., Morrison, R.W. Jr, Lambe, C.U., Nelson, D.J., Averett, D.R., Biron, K. & Furman, P.A. (1989) 2-Acetylpyridine 5-[(dimethylamino)thiocarbonyl] thiocarbono-hydrazone (1110U81), a potent inactivator of ribonucleotide reductase of herpes simplex and varicellazoster viruses and a potentiator of a acyclovir. *Proc. Natl. Acad. Sci. USA* 86, 1051 - 1055.

Stevens, L. (1991) Egg white proteins. *Comp Biochem Physiol B.*100(1):1-9.

Stout, R. D. (1993) Macrophage activation by T cells: cognate and non-cognate signals. *Curr. Opin. Immunol.* 5:398–403.

Sugano, S., Stoeckle, M. Y. & Hanafusa, H. (1987) Transformation by Rous sarcoma virus induces a novel gene with homology to a mitogenic platelet protein. *Cell* 49: 321–328.

Superti, F. Ammendolia, M.G., Berlutti, F. & Valenti, P. (2007 a). Ovotransferrin, In: *Bioactive Egg Compounds*, Huopalahti, R., Lopez-Fandino, R., Antonand, M., Schade, R. Eds, pp (43–48), Springer-Verlag, Berlin, Germany,

Superti, F., Ammendolia, M. G., Berlutti, F., Valenti, P. (2007 b) Ovotransferrin in *Bioactiv Egg Compounds, Part I, Subpart Ib,* 43-50.

Superti, F., Ammendolia, M.G., Valenti, P. & Seganti, L. (1997) Antirotaviral activity of milk proteins: lactoferrin prevents rotavirus infection in the enterocyte-like cell line HT-29, *Med. Microbiol. Immunol.* 186:83-91.

Superti, F., Siciliano, R., Rega, B., Giansanti, F., Valenti, P. & Antonini, G. (2001) Involvement of bovine lactoferrin metal saturation, sialic acid and protein fragments in the inhibition of rotavirus infection. *Biochimica et Biophysica Acta* 1528:107-115.

Swart, P.J., Kuipers, M.E., Smit, C., Pauwels, R., deBéthune M.P., de Clercq, E., Meijer, D.K.& Huisman J.G. (1996) Antiviral effects of milk proteins: acylation results in polyanionic compounds with potent activity against human immunodeficiency virus types 1 and 2 in vitro. *AIDS Res Hum Retroviruses.* 12(9):769-75.

Thakurta, P. G., Choudhury, D., Dasgupta, R. & Dattagupta, J. K. (2003) Structure of diferric hen serum transferrin at 2.8 Å resolution, *Acta Crystallogr., Sect.D*, 59:1773-1781.

Trybala, E., Bergström, T., Svennerholm, B., Jeansson, S., Glorioso, J.C. & Olofsson, S. (1994) Localization of a functional site on herpes simplex virus type 1 glycoprotein C involved in binding to cell surface heparan sulphate. *J Gen Virol.* 75 (Pt 4):743-52.

Valenti, P., Visca, P., Antonini G. & Orsi, N. (1985) Antifungal activity of ovotransferrin toward genus. Candida, *Mycopathologia,* 89:169–175.

Valenti, P., Visca, P., Antonini, G. & Orsi, N. (1986) Interaction between lactoferrin and ovotransferrin and Candida cells, *FEMS Microbiol Lett,* 33:271–275.

Valenti, P. & Antonini, G. (2005) Lactoferrin: an important host defence against microbial and viral attack. *Cell Mol Life Sci.* 62(22):2576-87.

van der Strate BWA, Belijaars L, Molema G, Harmsen MC, Meijer DK. (2001) Antiviral activities of lactoferrin. *Antiviral Res;* 52:225–39.

Vogel, H.J., Schibli, D.J., Jing, W. , Lohmeier-Vogel, E.M., Epand, R.F. & Epand, R.M. (2002) Towards a structure–function analysis of bovine lactoferricin and related tryptophan- and arginine-containing peptides. *Biochem. Cell Biol.* 80:49–63.

Von Bulow, V. & Klasen, A. (1983) Effects of avian viruses on cultured chicken bone-marrow-derived macrophages. *Avian Pathol.* 12:179–198.

Vorland, L.H. (1999) Lactoferrin: a multifunctional glycoprotein. *APMIS.*107(11):971-81.

Wang, Z. & Wang G. (2004) APD: the Antimicrobial Peptide Database. *Nucleic Acids Res.* 32: D590–D592

Williams, J., Elleman, T.C., Kingston, I.B., Wilkins, A.G. & Kuhn, K.A. (1982) The primary structure of hen ovotransferrin, *Eur. J. Biochem.* 122(2):297-303.

Witter, R. L. (1983) Characteristics of Marek's disease viruses isolated from vaccinated commercial chicken flocks: association of viral pathotype with lymphoma frequency. *Avian Dis.* 27:113–132.

Witter, R. L. (1992) Influence of serotype and virus strain on synergism between Marek's disease vaccine viruses. *Avian Pathol.* 21:601–614.

Witter, R. L., Calnek, B. W., Buscaglia, C., Gimeno I. M. & Schat K. A. (2005) Classification of Marek's disease viruses according to pathotype: philosophy and methodology. *Avian Pathology* 34(2), 75-90

Witter, R. L., Nazerian, K., Purchase, H. G. & Burgoyne, G. H. (1970) Isolation from turkeys of a cell-associated herpesvirus antigenically related to Marek's disease virus. *Am. J. Vet. Res.* 31:525–538.

Witter, R. L., Sharma, J. M., Lee, L. F., Opitz, H. M. & Henry, C. W. (1984) Field trials to test the efficacy of polyvalent Marek's disease vaccines in broilers. *Avian Dis.* 28:44–60.

Witter, R.L. (2001). Marek's disease vaccines - past, present and future (Chicken vs virus - a battle of the centuries). In *Current progress on Marek's disease research* , Schat, K.A., Morgan, R.W., Parcells, M.S. & Spencer, J.L. eds. pp (1-9). American Association of Avian Pathologists, Kennett Square, Pennsylvania.

Wu, H.F., Monroe, D.M. & Church, F.C. (1995) Characterization of the glycosaminoglycan-binding region of lactoferrin, *Arch. Biochem. Biophys.* 317:85-92.

WuDunn, D. & Spear, P.G. (1989) Initial interaction of herpes simplex virus with cells is binding to heparan sulfate, *J. Virol.* 69:2233-2239.

Yi, M., Kaneko, S., Yu, D.Y. & Murakami, S. (1997) Hepatitis C virus envelope proteins bind lactoferrin. *J. Virol.* 71:5997-6002.

Yolken, R.H., Willoughby, R.E., Wee, S.B., Misku, R. & Vonderfecht, S. (1987) Sialic acid glycoproteins inhibit in vitro and in vivo replication of rotaviruses. *J. Clin. Invest.* 79:148-154.

Yoo, Y.C., Watanabe, S., Watanabe, R., Hata, K., Shimazaki, K. & Azuma, I. (1998) Bovine lactoferrin and lactoferricin inhibit tumour metastasis in mice. *Adv. Exp. Med. Biol.* 443:285–291.

Zhou, N., Tieleman, D.P. & Vogel, H.J. (2004) Molecular dynamics simulations of bovine lactoferricin: turning a helix into a sheet. *Biometals* 17:217–223.